Handbook of Reproductive Biology

Handbook of
Reproductive Biology

Edited by Francisco Armstrong

hayle
medical

New York

Hayle Medical,
750 Third Avenue, 9th Floor,
New York, NY 10017, USA

Visit us on the World Wide Web at:
www.haylemedical.com

ISBN: 978-1-63241-864-7

Cataloging-in-Publication Data

Handbook of reproductive biology / edited by Francisco Armstrong.
p. cm.
Includes bibliographical references and index.
ISBN 978-1-63241-864-7
1. Reproduction. 2. Biology. 3. Human reproduction. 4. Reproductive technology. I. Armstrong, Francisco.
QH471 .H36 2020
571.8--dc23

Table of Contents

Preface

Human reproduction is a form of sexual reproduction, which results in human fertilization, due to sexual intercourse between a man and a woman. Human reproduction begins with copulation, followed by a period of 9-month gestation that lasts until childbirth. During gestation, the fetus grows and develops. While in the uterus, the baby undergoes a zygote stage, embryonic stage and a period characterized by development of all major organs. This can be achieved with the aid of reproductive technology, such as artificial insemination. The field of reproductive technology encompasses all uses of technology in human reproduction such as contraception, assisted reproductive technology and others. Assisted reproductive technology refers to the use of reproductive technology to treat infertility or low fertility. It is effective in individuals suffering from ovulatory disorders. Reproductive analysis enables family planning and monitoring of follicular dynamics, ovarian reserve and semen analysis. Germinal choice technology, artificial wombs, reprogenetics and in vitro parthenogenesis are the reproductive techniques that are undergoing development. An important research direction in reproductive biology is the exploration of same sex procreation. This book contains some path-breaking studies in the field of reproductive biology. It will also provide interesting topics for research, which interested readers can take up. It aims to equip students and experts with the advanced topics and upcoming concepts in this area.

This book is the end result of constructive efforts and intensive research done by experts in this field. The aim of this book is to enlighten the readers with recent information in this area of research. The information provided in this profound book would serve as a valuable reference to students and researchers in this field.

At the end, I would like to thank all the authors for devoting their precious time and providing their valuable contribution to this book. I would also like to express my gratitude to my fellow colleagues who encouraged me throughout the process.

Editor

Effectiveness of Omega-3 fatty acid for polycystic ovary syndrome

Kailin Yang[1†], Liuting Zeng[1†], Tingting Bao[2] and Jinwen Ge[1*]

Abstract

Objective: To assess the effectiveness and safety of omega-3 fatty acid for patients with PCOS.

Methods: In this meta-analysis, data from randomized controlled trials were obtained to assess the effects of omega-3 fatty acid versus placebo or western medicine in women with PCOS. The study's registration number is CRD42017065859. The primary outcomes included the change of homeostatic model assessment (HOMA) of insulin resistance, total cholesterol (TC), triglyceride (TG) and adiponectin.

Result: Nine trials involving 591 patients were included. Comparing with the control group, omega-3 fatty acid may improve HOMA index (WMD -0.80; 95% CI -0.89, − 0.71; P<0. 00001), decrease TC and TG level [TC: (WMD -9.43; 95% CI -11.90, − 6.95; P<0. 00001); TG: (WMD -29.21; 95% CI -48.08, − 10.34; $P = 0.002$)], and increase adiponectin level (WMD 1.34; 95% CI 0.51, 2.17; $P = 0.002$).

Conclusion: Based on current evidence, omega-3 fatty acid may be recommended for the treatment of PCOS with insulin resistance as well as high TC (especially LDL-C) and TG.

Keywords: Omega-3 fatty acid, Polycystic ovary syndrome, Systematic review, Meta-analysis

Background

Polycystic ovary syndrome (PCOS) is a common reproductive endocrine disease estimated to affect 6–10% of women of reproductive age [1, 2], which is associated with a variety of factors, including menstrual irregularity, insulin resistance, diabetes, and obesity [3]. The pathogenesis of PCOS is not yet clear, but genetics and lifestyle factors contribute significantly to the development of the PCOS [4]. The prevalence of metabolic syndrome (Reproductive disorders, infertility, metabolic disorders) in PCOS patients is higher than that in the general population [5]. The negative effects of these PCOS-related symptoms impaired the quality of women's life and led them to undeniable pressure.

The recommended treatments for PCOS women, especially for PCOS patients with obesity, are lifestyle and nutrition interventions and weight loss [6, 7]. The current study shows that metabolic disorders in patients with PCOS may be improved by the intervention of dietary factors such as anti-inflammatory foods [8]. Among dietary factors, omega-3 fatty acids play an important role in immune regulation, insulin sensitivity, cellular differentiation, and ovulation [8, 9]. This dietary supplement may be used for improving excessive oxidative stress-caused folliculogenesis disorder and hyperinsulinemia in women with PCOS [10–12]. Omega-3 fatty acids supplementation also has a beneficial effect on some cardiometabolic risk factors in women with PCOS [13], which is achieved through reducing the synthesis of prostaglandins by competitive inhibition of cyclooxygenase 2 (COX-2) [9] and increasing the activity of antioxidant enzymes [14, 15].

* Correspondence: 40831556@qq.com
†Equal contributors
[1]Hunan University of Chinese Medicine, Changsha 410208, Hunan Province, China
Full list of author information is available at the end of the article

Table 1 Inclusion criteria

P (Participants)	Women with a diagnosis of polycystic ovary syndrome
I (Intervention)	Omega-3 fatty acid with no limits on the type, dose, frequency and so on
C (Comparisons)	Blanks, placebo, or western medicine
O (Outcomes)	Primary: the change of homeostatic model assessment (HOMA) of insulin resistance, total cholesterol (TC), triglyceride (TG), adiponectin, adverse events
	Secondary: body mass index (BMI), fasting insulin, fasting glucose, low density lipoprotein cholesterol (LDL-C), high density lipoprotein cholesterol (HDL-C), follicle stimulating hormone (FSH), luteotropic hormone (LH), total testosterone, sex hormone-binding globulin (SHBG)
S (Study type)	Randomized controlled trials (RCTs), which assess the effects of omega-3 fatty for the treatment of PCOS (with no limits on the manner by which randomization has been achieved, on blinding or on the language of publication)

A previous systemic review and meta-analysis which reviewed the research before 2015 have evaluated the effects of omega-3 fatty acids in PCOS women, and it reported that omega-3 fatty acids may not have a beneficial effect on improving insulin resistance in women with PCOS [16]. Over time, more randomized controlled trials (RCTs) about omega-3 fatty acid were published between 2015 and 2018. However, the new RCTs [17–20] showed that omega-3 fatty acid had a beneficial effect on serum adiponectin levels, insulin resistance, serum lipid levels and so on in PCOS patients, which is contrary to the result of the previous meta-analysis [16]. Therefore, the results of systematic review and meta-analysis need to be updated. This systemic review and meta-analysis is a registered

review with protocol (CRD42017065859) in PROS-PERO, which aims to evaluate the effects of omega-3 fatty acid on women with PCOS.

Methods
Protocol
Study selection, assessment of eligibility criteria, data extraction, and statistical analysis were performed based on a predefined protocol registered on PROSPERO (CRD42017065859).

Search strategy and selection criteria
A search strategy was designed to search all the available literature. We searched the Pubmed, Clinical-Trials, Embase, Medline Complete, Web of Science,

Table 2 Search Strategy for Pubmed

Database	Search Strategy
Pubmed	(n-3 Fatty Acids OR n 3 Fatty Acids OR n-3 Polyunsaturated Fatty Acid OR n 3 Polyunsaturated Fatty Acid OR n-3 PUFA OR PUFA, n-3 OR n 3 PUFA OR Omega 3 Fatty Acids OR n3 PUFA OR PUFA, n3 OR n3 Polyunsaturated Fatty Acid OR n3 Oils OR n-3 Oils OR n 3 Oils OR Omega-3 Fatty Acids OR n3 Fatty Acid OR Fatty Acid, n3) AND (Ovary Syndrome, Polycystic OR Syndrome, Polycystic Ovary OR Stein-Leventhal Syndrome OR Stein Leventhal Syndrome OR Syndrome, Stein-Leventhal OR Sclerocystic Ovarian Degeneration OR Ovarian Degeneration, Sclerocystic OR Sclerocystic Ovary Syndrome OR Polycystic Ovarian Syndrome OR Ovarian Syndrome, Polycystic OR Polycystic Ovary Syndrome 1 OR Sclerocystic Ovaries OR Ovary, Sclerocystic OR Sclerocystic Ovary OR PCOS) AND (randomized controlled trial [pt] OR controlled clinical trial [pt] OR placebo [tiab] OR drug therapy [sh] OR trial [tiab] OR groups [tiab] OR clinical trials as topic [mesh: noexp] OR Clinical Trial OR random* [tiab] OR random allocation [mh] OR single-blind method [mh] OR double-blind method [mh] OR cross-over studies) NOT (animals [mh] NOT humans [mh])

Cochrane Library (Until Issue 12, 2017), the Chinese Science and Technology Periodical Database (VIP), the Chinese National Knowledge Infrastructure Databases (CNKI), WanFang Database (Chinese Ministry of Science & Technology), Chinese Biomedical Database (CBM), from their inception to January, 2018. The search terms included omega-3 fatty acid, ω-3 fatty acid, n-3 fatty acid, polycystic ovary syndrome, PCOS.

Studies meeting the inclusion criteria were included in this review (see Table 1).

Due to the ovarian aging in post-menopausal women, studies involving post-menopausal women (over 50 years of age) were excluded, which meet the exclusion criteria.

Data analysis

All studies were reviewed and selected independently by three reviewers (Kailin Yang, Liuting Zeng, Tingting Bao). The titles and abstracts were reviewed, and articles which did not fit the eligibility criteria were excluded. If the title or abstract appeared to meet the eligibility criteria or they could not determine its eligibility, the full texts of the articles were obtained for further evaluation. For example, the search strategy for Pubmed was present in Table 2; ten studies of twenty-one studies in Pubmed were extracted. The data were extracted independently by three reviewers (Kailin Yang, Liuting Zeng and Tingting Bao) using a standardized data extraction form. Any discrepancies between the reviewers were resolved by consensus among all four reviewers (Kailin Yang, Liuting Zeng, Tingting Bao and Jinwen Ge). The characteristics and general information were extracted and tabulated, including Authors, time of publication, intervention, comparison group, outcomes, AEs, and follow-up period.

If there was missing information in the paper, such as methodology, diagnosis, interventions and outcomes, reviewers would try to contact the original authors to clarify the data, or impute the missing standard deviations according to the Cochrane Handbook 5.1.0—if there were missing standard deviations, if several candidate standard deviations are available, reviewers would to use their average to impute it.

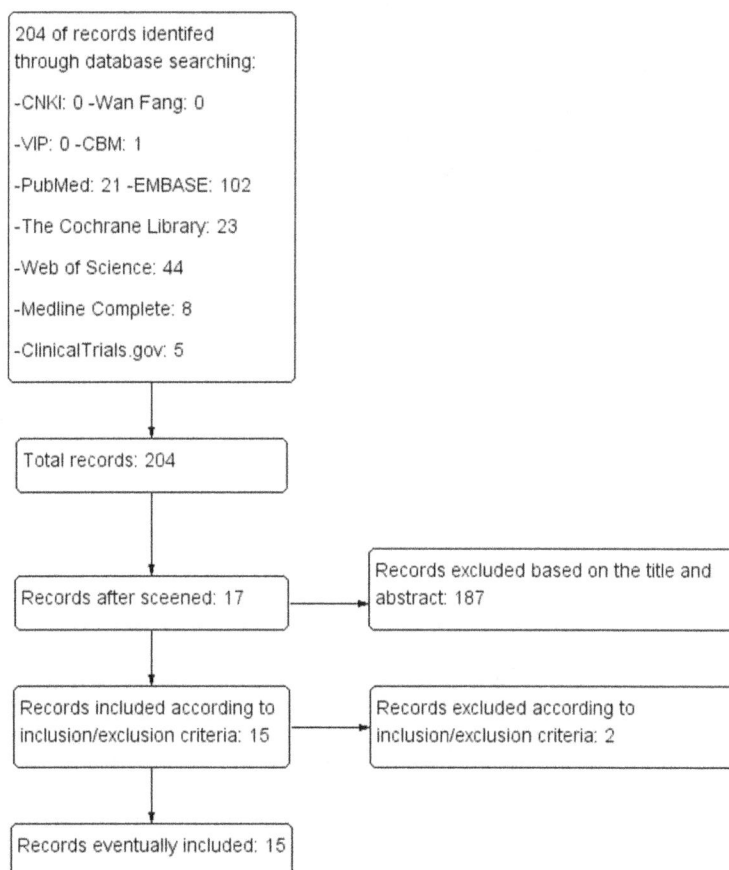

Fig. 1 Flow diagram of searching and article selection

Table 3 The characteristics of the included studies

Study	Sample size		Intervention		Relevant outcomes	Mean age (years)		Mean BMI (baseline)		Duration
	Trial group	Control group	Trial group	Control group		Trial group	Control group	Trial group	Control group	
Mohammadi 2012 [25]	30	31	Omega-3 fatty acids 4000 mg	Paraffin oil (placebo) 2000 mg	BMI, TG, TC, LDL-C, HDL-C, Adiponectin, fasting insulin, fasting glucose, the change of HOMA	27.33 ± 4.27	27.73 ± 4.53	28.67 ± 3.21	28.77 ± 2.92	8 weeks
Karakas 2016 [17]	34	17	Omega-3 fatty acids (including fish oils and flaxseed oils)	Soybean oil (placebo)	BMI, TG, TC, LDL-C, HDL-C, fasting insulin, fasting glucose, the change of HOMA	Fish oils: 31.7 ± 7.8; Flaxseed oils: 29.4 ± 6.6	28.9 ± 4.1	Fish oils: 36.3 ± 7.8; Flaxseed oils: 35.0 ± 10.3	33.2 ± 7.4	6 weeks
Nadjarzadeh 2015 [18]	39	39	Omega-3 fatty acids 900 mg	Paraffin oil (placebo) 3000 mg	BMI, Adiponectin, FSH, LH	26.9 ± 5.9	26.9 ± 5.0	31.46 ± 5.74	31.88 ± 3.86	12 weeks
Nadjarzadeh 2013 [26]	39	39	Omega-3 fatty acids 900 mg	Paraffin oil (placebo) 3000 mg	Total testosterone, SHGB	26.9 ± 5.9	26.9 ± 5.0	31.46 ± 5.74	31.88 ± 3.86	12 weeks
Rahmani 2017 [19]	34	34	Omega-3 fatty acids 1000 mg + Vitamin E 400 IU + Metformin	Placebos + Metformin	BMI, TG, TC, LDL-C, HDL-C, FSH, LH	24.9 ± 5.5	26.6 ± 5.6	28.4 ± 4.4	29.0 ± 6.5	12 weeks
Ebrahimi 2017 [20]	34	34	Omega-3 fatty acids 1000 mg + vitamin E 400 IU	Placebos	BMI, SHGB, fasting insulin, fasting glucose, the change of HOMA, total testosterone	23.8 ± 4.6	25.2 ± 5.2	28.0 ± 4.3	28.5 ± 6.6	12 weeks
Khani 2017 [8]	43	44	Omega-3 fatty acids 2000 mg	Olive oil (placebo) 2000 mg	BMI, TG, TC, LDL-C, HDL-C, fasting glucose	31.04 ± 5.04	29.23 ± 6.73	31.8 ± 3.61	31.79 ± 3.6	24 weeks
Mirmasoumi 2017 [27]	30	30	Omega-3 fatty acids 2000 mg + Metformin 500 mg	Paraffin oil (placebo) 1000 mg + Metformin 500 mg	BMI, TG, TC, LDL-C, HDL-C, fasting insulin, fasting glucose, the change of HOMA, total testosterone, SHBG, adverse events	28.4 ± 6.4	27.0 ± 3.2	26.9 ± 5.1	26.7 ± 5.3	12 weeks
Jamilian 2018 [28]	20	20	Omega-3 fatty acids 1000 mg + Vitamin E 400 IU	Paraffin oil (placebo)	BMI, the change of HOMA	22.3 ± 4.7	24.4 ± 4.7	28.8 ± 5.1	26.5 ± 5.9	12 weeks

(P=NS or $P > 0.05$), or reviewers imputed them by P-value ($P < 0.05$) [21].

The risk of bias was assessed using the risk of bias assessment tool by the Cochrane Handbook for Systematic Reviews of Interventions, version 5.1.0 [22]. The criteria consist of 7 items related to selection bias (random sequence generation and allocation concealment), performance bias (blinding of participants and personnel), detection bias (blinding of outcome assessment), attrition bias (incomplete outcome data), reporting bias (selective outcome reporting), and other sources of bias. Three reviewers (Liuting Zeng, Kailin Yang, Tingting Bao) independently performed this, and

any discrepancies between the two reviewers were resolved by consensus among all four reviewers (Kailin Yang, Liuting Zeng, Tingting Bao and Jinwen Ge).

The data were analyzed using RevMan 5.3 software. The dichotomous variable measure was summarized by risk ratio (RR) with a 95% confidence interval (CI). The continuous outcomes underwent meta-analysis using mean differences (MD) and 95% CI. Heterogeneity among studies was assessed using Cochrane's Q and I^2 statistic [23]. When $P > 0.1$, $I2 < 50\%$, we used a fixed effect model; when $P < 0.1$, $I2 > 50\%$, we would explore the reasons for heterogeneity, perform the subgroup analysis and use a random effect model.

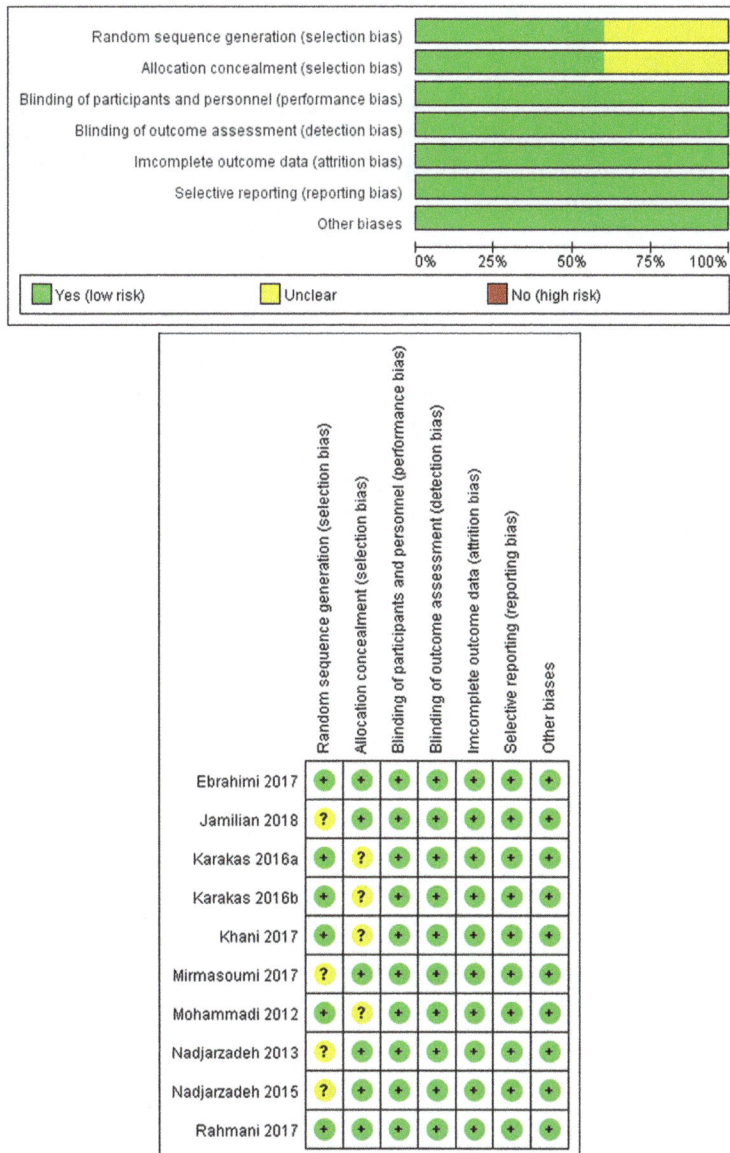

Fig. 2 The risk of bias

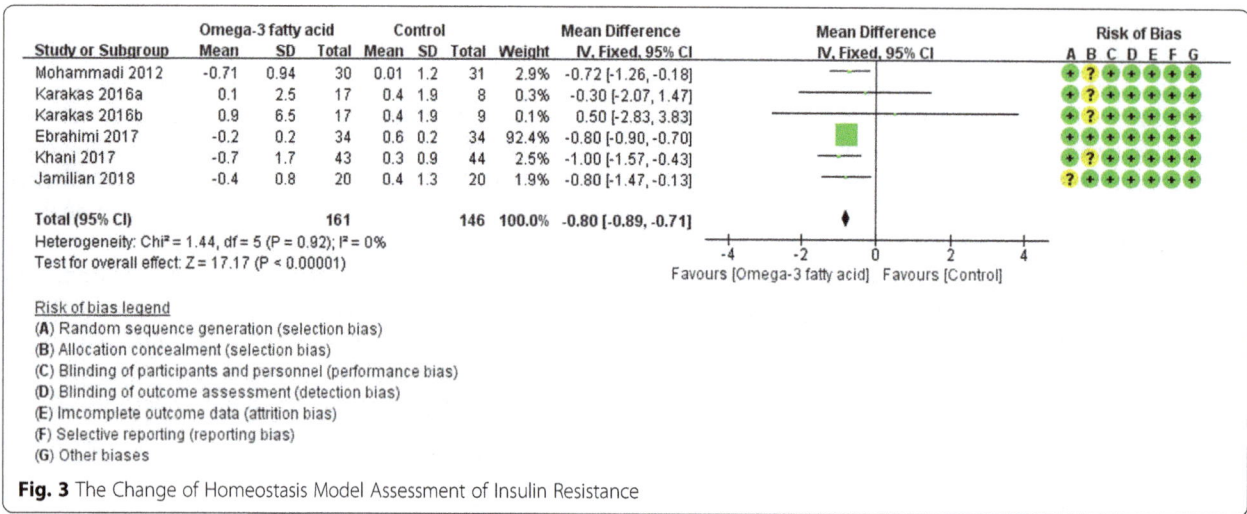

Fig. 3 The Change of Homeostasis Model Assessment of Insulin Resistance

Primary outcomes, secondary outcomes, and adverse events (AEs) would be reported. Except menstrual cycle regulation (no research reported the outcome), all outcomes were prespecified in the study protocol.

Results

Results of the search

Our initial search identified and screened 204 articles. We excluded 187 articles based on the title and abstract and retrieved 17 articles for more detailed evaluation. From these, we excluded 2 publications and included 15 studies in our review (Fig. 1).

Description of included trials and risk of Bias in included studies

Nine RCTs with 591 participants met the inclusion criteria. There are four records whose data [7, 12, 24, 25]

derived from the same clinical trial, so we counted them as one RCT (Mohammadi 2012 [25]). All of them were parallel-group RCTs. Because there are three groups in Karakas's research [17], two of them are trial groups, while one is control group; according to the Cochrane Handbook 5.1.0, we split the shared control group into two groups with smaller sample size [21], and include the two reasonably independent comparisons (Karakas 2016 a and Karakas 2016 b). Study characteristics are presented in Table 3.

Among the 9 included RCTs, four studies [18, 26–28] adopted unclear randomization procedures, while the others described adequate methods of random sequence generation: the block randomization procedure [25], website [17], random-maker software "random allocation" [8] or computer-generated randomization list [19, 20]; we rated the five studies

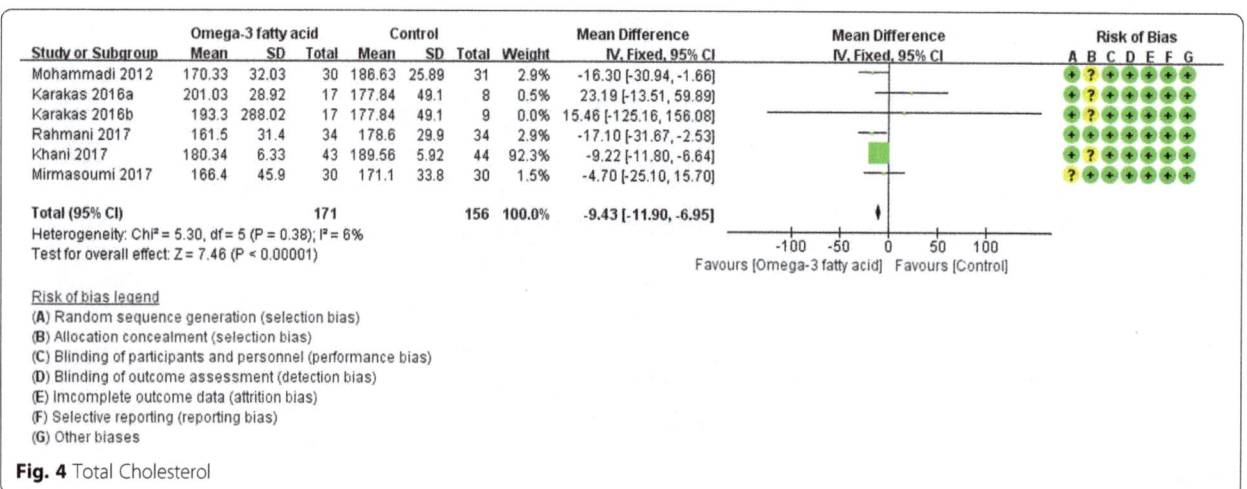

Fig. 4 Total Cholesterol

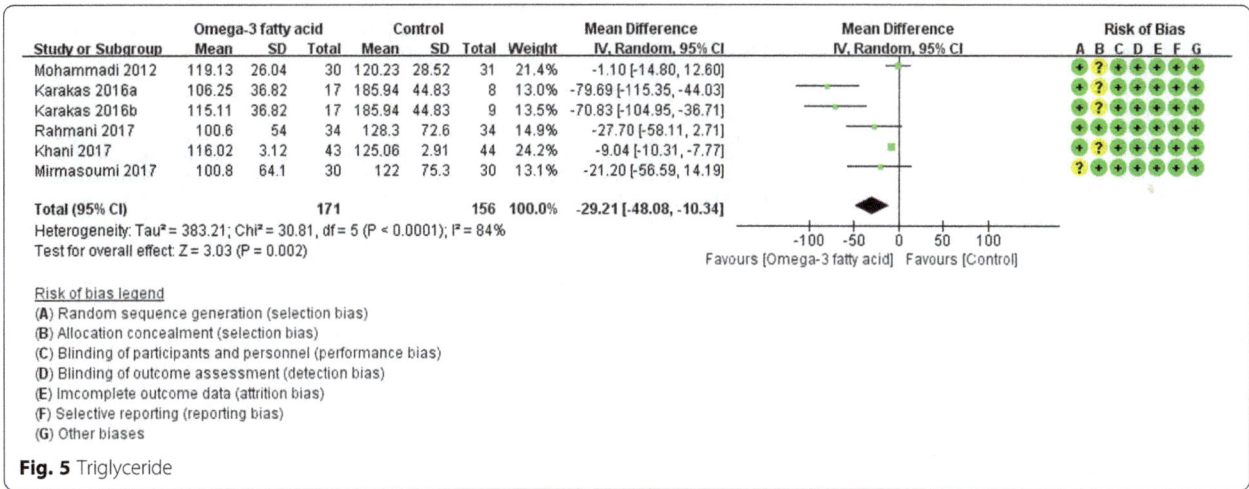

Fig. 5 Triglyceride

as having an unclear risk of bias, while the others trials were at low risk of bias. We rated three trials [8, 17, 25] as having an unclear risk of bias because they did not describe an acceptable method of allocation concealment; because of that the others [19, 20, 26–28] described that drugs in trial groups and control groups were similar in shape, size and so on that the patients and researcher were not aware until the end of the analysis, we rated them as having a low risk of bias. For participant and outcome assessment blinding, five trials were unclear [17–20, 26], but they used objective measures (e.g. TG, TC, adiponectin) and the outcome is not likely to be influenced by the lack of blinding, while the rest one studies used blinding; thus, we gave a low risk of bias for all. None of trials missed data and incompletely reported the outcomes, therefore we gave a low risk of bias.

Other sources of bias were at low risk in all of the included studies. A graphical summary of the risks of bias assessment is presented in Fig. 2.

Primary outcomes

Five RCTs [8, 17, 20, 25, 28] reported the change of HOMA at the end of treatment. Due to the low heterogeneity, we used fix effect model. In this index, it can be found that in improving insulin resistance, omega-3 fatty acid is better [the change of HOMA: (WMD -0.80; 95% CI -0.89, – 0.71; P<0. 00001)] (Fig. 3).

Five RCTs [8, 17, 19, 25, 27] reported total cholesterol. We used fix effect model. According to the result, compared with the control group, omega-3 fatty acid is better in decrease TC [TC: (WMD -9.43; 95% CI -11.90, – 6.95; P<0. 00001)] (Fig. 4).

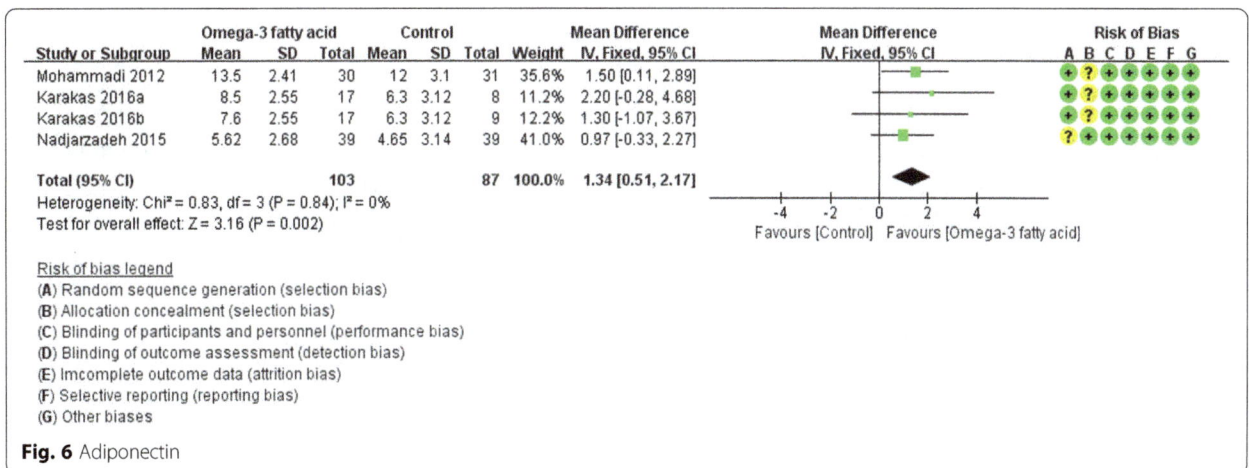

Fig. 6 Adiponectin

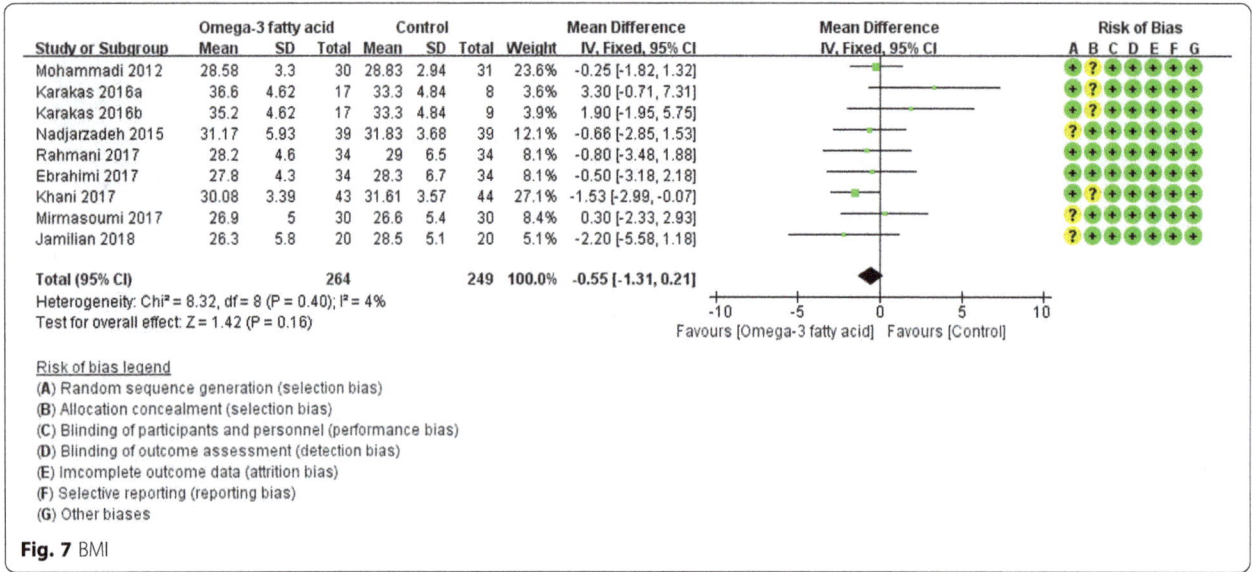

Study or Subgroup	Omega-3 fatty acid Mean	SD	Total	Control Mean	SD	Total	Weight	Mean Difference IV, Fixed, 95% CI
Mohammadi 2012	28.58	3.3	30	28.83	2.94	31	23.6%	-0.25 [-1.82, 1.32]
Karakas 2016a	36.6	4.62	17	33.3	4.84	8	3.6%	3.30 [-0.71, 7.31]
Karakas 2016b	35.2	4.62	17	33.3	4.84	9	3.9%	1.90 [-1.95, 5.75]
Nadjarzadeh 2015	31.17	5.93	39	31.83	3.68	39	12.1%	-0.66 [-2.85, 1.53]
Rahmani 2017	28.2	4.6	34	29	6.5	34	8.1%	-0.80 [-3.48, 1.88]
Ebrahimi 2017	27.8	4.3	34	28.3	6.7	34	8.1%	-0.50 [-3.18, 2.18]
Khani 2017	30.08	3.39	43	31.61	3.57	44	27.1%	-1.53 [-2.99, -0.07]
Mirmasoumi 2017	26.9	5	30	26.6	5.4	30	8.4%	0.30 [-2.33, 2.93]
Jamilian 2018	26.3	5.8	20	28.5	5.1	20	5.1%	-2.20 [-5.58, 1.18]
Total (95% CI)			**264**			**249**	**100.0%**	**-0.55 [-1.31, 0.21]**

Heterogeneity: Chi² = 8.32, df = 8 (P = 0.40); I² = 4%
Test for overall effect: Z = 1.42 (P = 0.16)

Risk of bias legend
(A) Random sequence generation (selection bias)
(B) Allocation concealment (selection bias)
(C) Blinding of participants and personnel (performance bias)
(D) Blinding of outcome assessment (detection bias)
(E) Imcomplete outcome data (attrition bias)
(F) Selective reporting (reporting bias)
(G) Other biases

Fig. 7 BMI

Five RCTs [8, 17, 19, 25, 27] reported triglyceride (TG) level. Due to the heterogeneity (Tau² = 383.21, I² = 84%, P<0.0001), we used random effect model. It seems like that compared with the control group, omega-3 fatty acid can decrease the TG level in PCOS patients [TG: (WMD -29.21; 95% CI -48.08, − 10.34; P = 0. 002)] (Fig. 5).

Three RCTs [17, 18, 25] reported adiponectin level. We used fix effect model. According to the results, compared with the control group, omega-3 fatty acid can increase the adiponectin level in PCOS patients [Adiponectin: (WMD 1.34; 95% CI 0.51, 2.17; P = 0. 002)] (Fig. 6).

Secondary outcomes
Eight RCTs [8, 17–20, 25, 27, 28] reported BMI. We used fix effect model. In this index, there is not strong

evidence that the omega-3 fatty acid has an effect on BMI because there was no statistical difference [BMI: (WMD -0.55; 95% CI -1.31, 0.21; P = 0. 16)] (Fig. 7).

Four RCTs [17, 19, 20, 27] reported fasting insulin and five RCTs reported fasting glucose [8, 17, 19, 20, 27] at the end of treatment. Due to the heterogeneity [Fasting insulin: (Tau² = 159.92, I² = 53%, P = 0.07); Fasting glucose: (Tau² = 17.20, I² = 70%, P = 0.005)], we used random effect model. For fasting insulin, compared with the control group, there is not strong evidence that the omega-3 fatty acid has an effect on hyperinsulinemia because there was no statistical difference (WMD -8.28; 95% CI -24.35, 7.79; P = 0. 31) (Fig. 8). And for fasting glucose, there is also not strong evidence that the omega-3 fatty acid has an

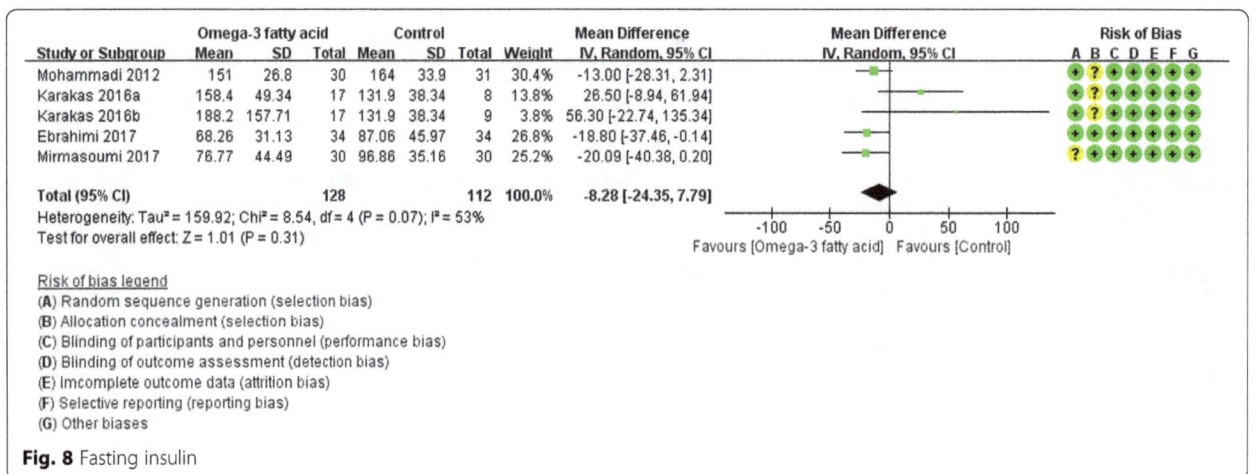

Study or Subgroup	Omega-3 fatty acid Mean	SD	Total	Control Mean	SD	Total	Weight	Mean Difference IV, Random, 95% CI
Mohammadi 2012	151	26.8	30	164	33.9	31	30.4%	-13.00 [-28.31, 2.31]
Karakas 2016a	158.4	49.34	17	131.9	38.34	8	13.8%	26.50 [-8.94, 61.94]
Karakas 2016b	188.2	157.71	17	131.9	38.34	9	3.8%	56.30 [-22.74, 135.34]
Ebrahimi 2017	68.26	31.13	34	87.06	45.97	34	26.8%	-18.80 [-37.46, -0.14]
Mirmasoumi 2017	76.77	44.49	30	96.86	35.16	30	25.2%	-20.09 [-40.38, 0.20]
Total (95% CI)			**128**			**112**	**100.0%**	**-8.28 [-24.35, 7.79]**

Heterogeneity: Tau² = 159.92; Chi² = 8.54, df = 4 (P = 0.07); I² = 53%
Test for overall effect: Z = 1.01 (P = 0.31)

Risk of bias legend
(A) Random sequence generation (selection bias)
(B) Allocation concealment (selection bias)
(C) Blinding of participants and personnel (performance bias)
(D) Blinding of outcome assessment (detection bias)
(E) Imcomplete outcome data (attrition bias)
(F) Selective reporting (reporting bias)
(G) Other biases

Fig. 8 Fasting insulin

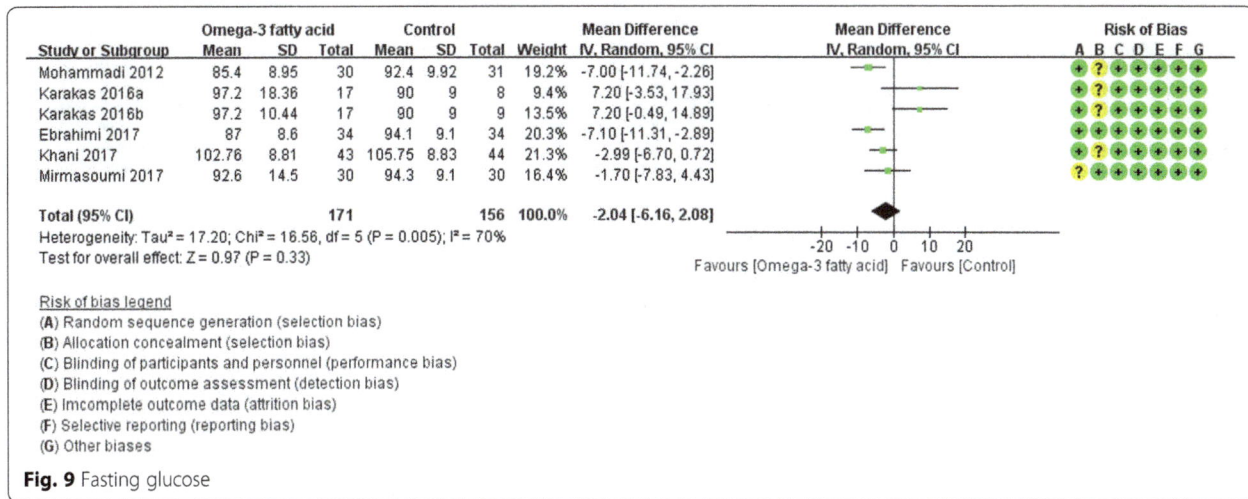

Fig. 9 Fasting glucose

effect on fasting glucose because there was no statistical difference (WMD -2.04; 95% CI -6.16, 2.08; P = 0. 33) (Fig. 9).

Five RCTs [8, 17, 19, 25, 27] reported LDL-C and HDL-C at the end of treatment. For LDL-C, we used fix effect model, and compared with the control group, the omega-3 is likely to decrease LDL-C (WMD -9.62; 95% CI -10.30, -8.94; P <0.00001) (Fig. 10). However, for HDL-C, we used random effect model because of its high heterogeneity (Tau^2 = 12.59, I^2 = 81%, P<0.0001), and there is also not strong evidence that the omega-3 fatty acid has an effect on fasting glucose because there was no statistical difference (WMD 1.32; 95% CI -2.16, 4.81; P = 0. 46) (Fig. 11).

Only two RCTs [19, 26] reported FSH and LH, and three RCTs [19, 20, 27] reported SHGB and total testosterone. For FSH, LH and SHBG, we used fix effect model; while for total testosterone, due to the heterogeneity (Tau^2 = 0.02, I^2 = 45%, P = 0.16), we used

random effect model. However, for all of these indexes, there is also not strong evidence that the omega-3 fatty acid has an effect on fasting glucose because there was no statistical difference. [FSH: (WMD -0.39; 95% CI -1. 32, 0.54; P = 0. 42); LH: (WMD -0.17; 95% CI -1.68, 1.33; P = 0. 82); SHGB: (WMD 0.55; 95% CI -7.07, 8.17; P = 0. 89); total testosterone: (WMD -0.08; 95% CI -0.29, 0.13; P = 0.49)] (Figs. 12, 13, 14 and 15).

Adverse events

Only one study [27] reported AEs and the rest of them did not mention AEs at all. And this study mentioned that there were no serious AEs reported.

Discussions

This systematic review and meta-analysis including 9 RCTs analyzes the effectiveness of omega-3 fatty acid for PCOS. Compared with the control group, omega-3 fatty acid may improve insulin resistance (improve HOMA

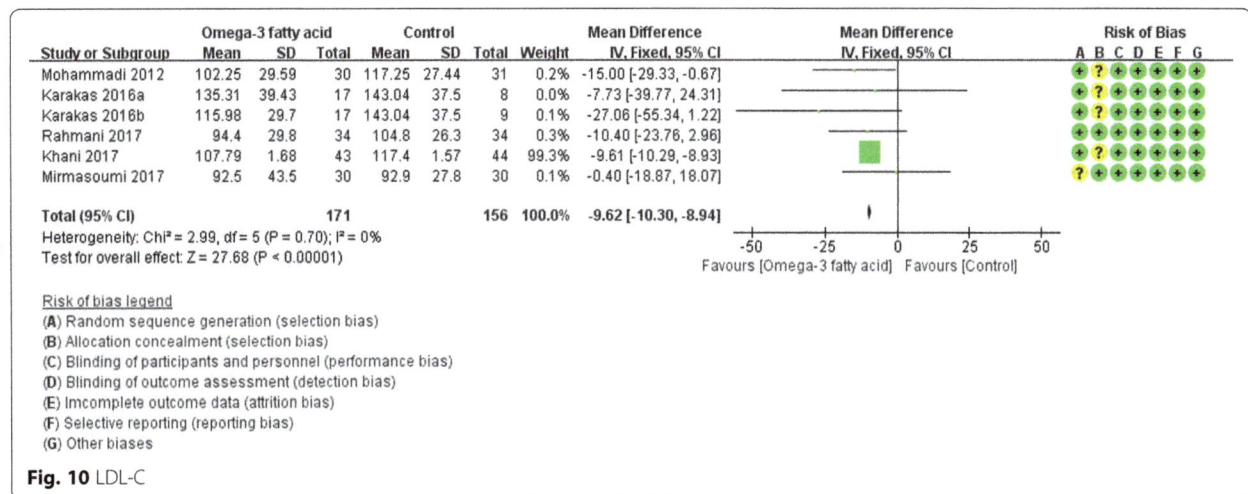

Fig. 10 LDL-C

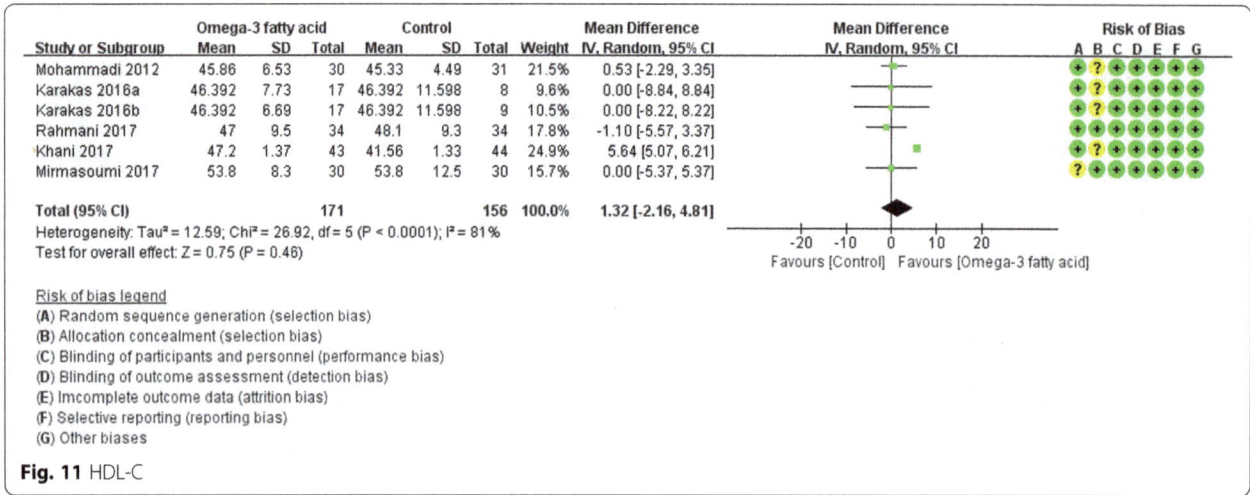

Fig. 11 HDL-C

index and increase adiponectin level), and decrease TC, TG, LDL-C. Meanwhile, there is not strong evidence that the omega-3 fatty acid has an effect on BMI, fasting insulin, fasting glucose, HDL-C, FSH, LH, SHGB and total testosterone. As PCOS is closely associated with insulin resistance and hyperandrogenism [29–31], based on current evidence, omega-3 fatty acid may be recommended for the treatment of PCOS with insulin resistance or/and high TC (especially LDL-C) and TG. While this finding seems promising, it should be interpreted with caution mainly due to the unclear risk of bias for selection bias (random sequence generation and allocation concealment) and a small number of participants. Although comparing with control group, there is not strong evidence that the omega-3 fatty acid has an effect on BMI, fasting insulin, fasting glucose, HDL-C, FSH, LH, SHGB and total testosterone, it does not mean there is no medical significance. Instead, it may

mean that omega-3 fatty acid may be the safer or cheaper treatment options.

Only one study [27] reported AEs and the rest of them did not mention AEs at all. This RCT reports that no relevant side effect was recorded during the therapy. However, the absence of information on AEs does not mean that the intervention is safe [32]. Thus, although based on current evidences, we consider that omega-3 fatty acid is a relatively safe treatment, we cannot assure it. Future clinical trials are required to report AEs with more explanations [33].

PCOS is one of the most common endocrine disorders that women suffer from [34], which is closely related to insulin resistance and hyperandrogenism [4–6]. The relationship between insulin resistance and hyperandrogenism is that insulin resistance can stimulate the production and secretion of androgens and ovarian failure [35–37]. Therefore, improving insulin resistance is considered to be of quit importance for

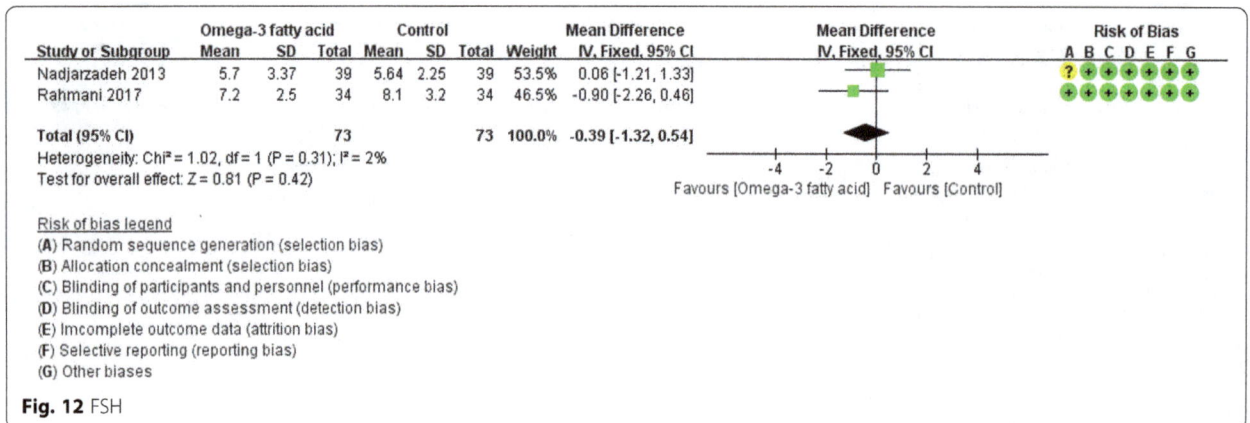

Fig. 12 FSH

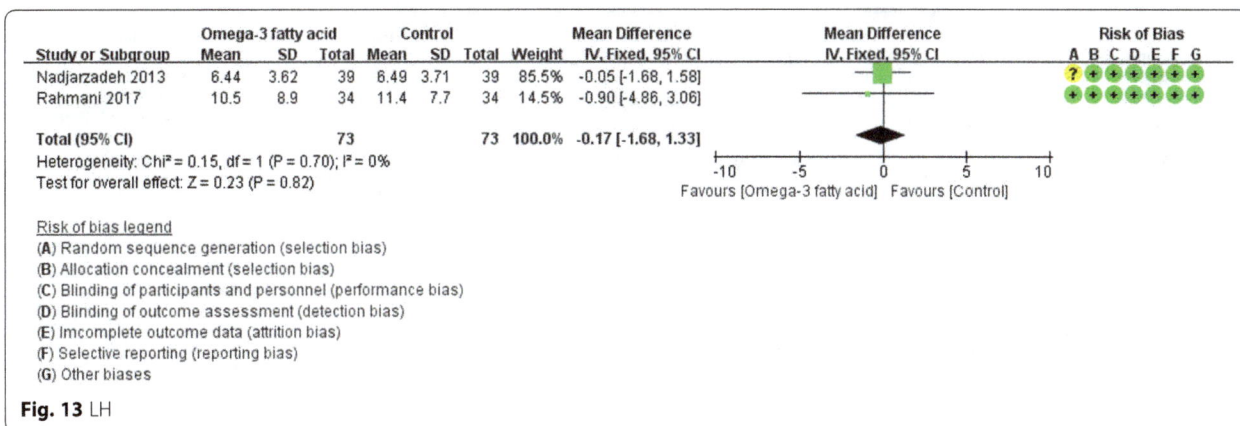

Study or Subgroup	Omega-3 fatty acid			Control			Weight	Mean Difference IV, Fixed, 95% CI	Mean Difference IV, Fixed, 95% CI	Risk of Bias A B C D E F G
	Mean	SD	Total	Mean	SD	Total				
Nadjarzadeh 2013	6.44	3.62	39	6.49	3.71	39	85.5%	-0.05 [-1.68, 1.58]		? + + + + + +
Rahmani 2017	10.5	8.9	34	11.4	7.7	34	14.5%	-0.90 [-4.86, 3.06]		+ + + + + + +
Total (95% CI)			73			73	100.0%	-0.17 [-1.68, 1.33]		

Heterogeneity: Chi² = 0.15, df = 1 (P = 0.70); I² = 0%
Test for overall effect: Z = 0.23 (P = 0.82)

Favours [Omega-3 fatty acid] Favours [Control]

Risk of bias legend
(A) Random sequence generation (selection bias)
(B) Allocation concealment (selection bias)
(C) Blinding of participants and personnel (performance bias)
(D) Blinding of outcome assessment (detection bias)
(E) Imcomplete outcome data (attrition bias)
(F) Selective reporting (reporting bias)
(G) Other biases

Fig. 13 LH

PCOS [35]. Omega-3 fatty acids are the very substance that increases the sensitivity to insulin by producing and secreting anti-inflammatory adipokine (such as adiponectin) and reducing inflammation and proinflammatory cytokines [25, 28–39], which has been revealed in our meta-analysis. Omega-3 fatty acids can also reduce cholesterol absorption and LDL-C synthesis, improve LDL receptor activity in liver, and increase fractional rate of catabolism of LDL-C [40, 41]. Therefore, omega-3 fatty acid supplementation had a beneficial effect on some cardiometabolic risk factors in women with PCOS [13].

Comparing with previous reviews [16], the strengths of this systematic review and meta-analysis are that it indicates that omega-3 fatty acid may be suitable for the treatments of PCOS with insulin resistance or/ and high TC (especially LDL-C) and TG. And this review included six recent (2016–2018) RCTs [8, 17, 19, 20, 27, 28]. A study concluded that publication bias is smaller in meta-analysis of more recent studies [42];

therefore, the risk of publication bias of this review may not be high. The limitations include the small number of trials, the small number of participants and the high heterogeneity for some outcomes (such as TG and HDL-C). The high level of heterogeneity was explored using sensitivity analysis for risk of bias, however, upon removal of the RCTs with medium risk of bias, there was no difference in the direction of effect or the heterogeneity. The heterogeneity may come from placebo effects or other places. Meanwhile, study duration is generally short-to-medium term (mostly 12 weeks), the long-term efficacy of omega-3 fatty acid is temporarily uncertain. Additionally, due to none of trials that reported AEs, the safety of omega-3 fatty acid should be interpreted with caution. Finally, the absolute treatment effects should also be interpreted with caution because the number of participants is small and it may not be generalizable to all types of PCOS. Further rigorously designed studies are needed to confirm the

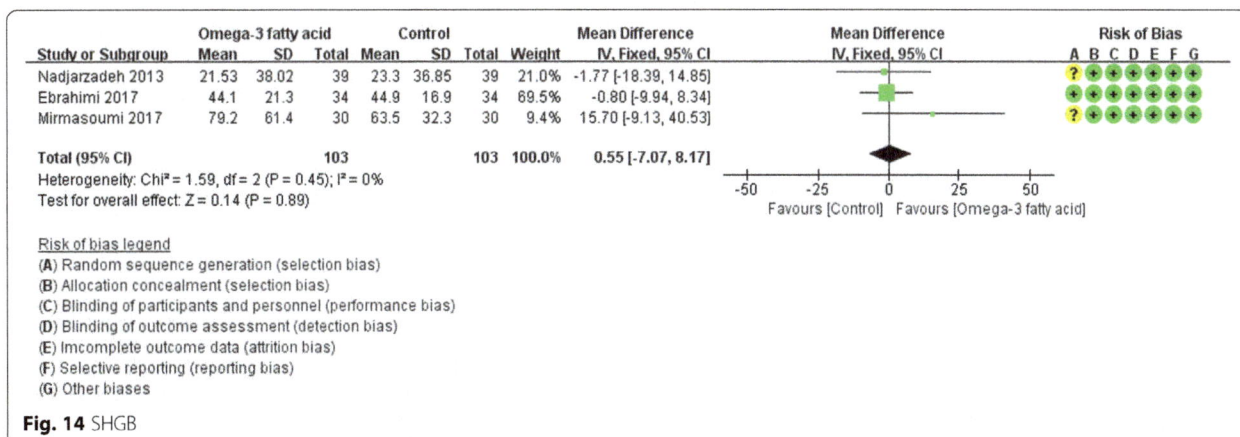

Study or Subgroup	Omega-3 fatty acid			Control			Weight	Mean Difference IV, Fixed, 95% CI	Mean Difference IV, Fixed, 95% CI	Risk of Bias A B C D E F G
	Mean	SD	Total	Mean	SD	Total				
Nadjarzadeh 2013	21.53	38.02	39	23.3	36.85	39	21.0%	-1.77 [-18.39, 14.85]		? + + + + + +
Ebrahimi 2017	44.1	21.3	34	44.9	16.9	34	69.5%	-0.80 [-9.94, 8.34]		+ + + + + + +
Mirmasoumi 2017	79.2	61.4	30	63.5	32.3	30	9.4%	15.70 [-9.13, 40.53]		? + + + + + +
Total (95% CI)			103			103	100.0%	0.55 [-7.07, 8.17]		

Heterogeneity: Chi² = 1.59, df = 2 (P = 0.45); I² = 0%
Test for overall effect: Z = 0.14 (P = 0.89)

Favours [Control] Favours [Omega-3 fatty acid]

Risk of bias legend
(A) Random sequence generation (selection bias)
(B) Allocation concealment (selection bias)
(C) Blinding of participants and personnel (performance bias)
(D) Blinding of outcome assessment (detection bias)
(E) Imcomplete outcome data (attrition bias)
(F) Selective reporting (reporting bias)
(G) Other biases

Fig. 14 SHGB

Study or Subgroup	Omega-3 fatty acid			Control			Weight	Mean Difference IV, Random, 95% CI
	Mean	SD	Total	Mean	SD	Total		
Nadjarzadeh 2013	0.3	0.63	39	0.25	0.5	39	36.1%	0.05 [-0.20, 0.30]
Ebrahimi 2017	0.7	0.6	34	1	0.6	34	31.6%	-0.30 [-0.59, -0.01]
Mirmasoumi 2017	0.8	0.6	30	0.8	0.5	30	32.3%	0.00 [-0.28, 0.28]
Total (95% CI)			103			103	100.0%	-0.08 [-0.29, 0.13]

Heterogeneity: Tau² = 0.02; Chi² = 3.61, df = 2 (P = 0.16); I² = 45%
Test for overall effect: Z = 0.71 (P = 0.48)

Risk of bias legend
(A) Random sequence generation (selection bias)
(B) Allocation concealment (selection bias)
(C) Blinding of participants and personnel (performance bias)
(D) Blinding of outcome assessment (detection bias)
(E) Imcomplete outcome data (attrition bias)
(F) Selective reporting (reporting bias)
(G) Other biases

Fig. 15 Total testosterone

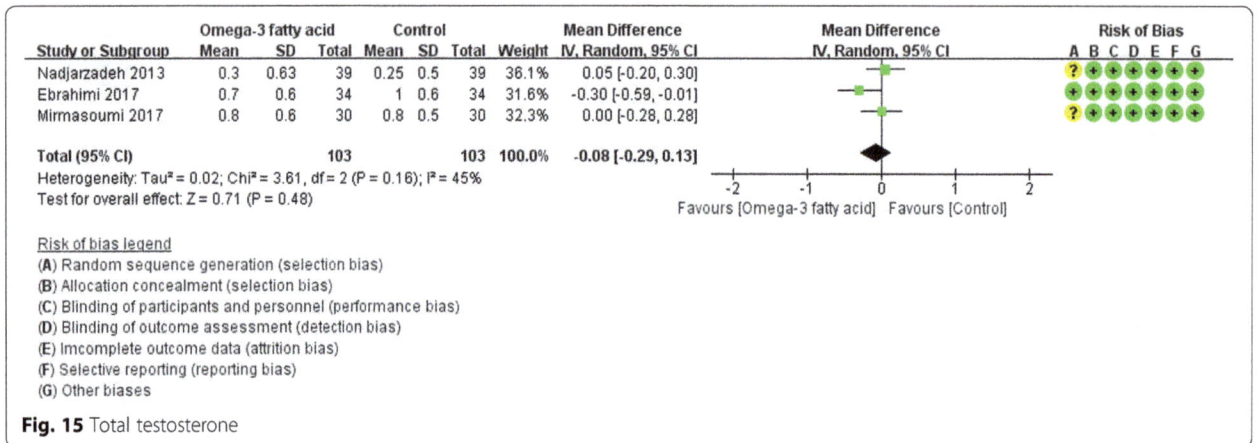

effectiveness and safety of omega-3 fatty acid in patients with PCOS. Furthermore, the individual patient data (IPD) meta-analysis, which would allow analysis to control for all types of heterogeneity due to differences in studies and/or patients and may be potentially more reliable than aggregate data meta-analysis, are also needed in the future [43, 44].

Conclusion

Our systematic review and meta-analysis provides evidence that omega-3 fatty acid may be a novel drug for PCOS patients. And based on current evidence, omega-3 fatty acid may be recommended for the treatment of PCOS with insulin resistance as well as high TC (especially LDL-C) and TG. However, current RCTs have limitations, including small sample sizes and short duration. The benefits from long term treatment of omega-3 fatty beyond 6 months remain to be defined by future studies. Meanwhile, more randomized, double-blind, large sample size trials of omega-3 fatty for PCOS are needed in the future to confirm or modify the result of this work.

Acknowledgments
This work is supported by the National Natural Science Foundation of China (No. 81274008).

Funding
The National Natural Science Foundation of China (No. 81274008).

Authors' contributions
KY and LZ contributed equally to this work. KY, LZ and JG are responsible for the study concept and design. KY, LZ and TB are responsible for the literature searching; KY, LZ, TB and JG are responsible for data analysis and interpretation; KY and JG drafted the paper; JG and TB supervised the study; all authors participated in the analysis and interpretation of data and approved the final paper.

Competing interests
The authors declare that they have no competing interests.

Author details
[1]Hunan University of Chinese Medicine, Changsha 410208, Hunan Province, China. [2]Beijing University of Chinese Medicine, Beijing 100029, Beijing, China.

References
1. Kelley CE, Brown AJ, Diehl AM, Setji TL. Review of nonalcoholic fatty liver disease in women with polycystic ovary syndrome. World J Gastroenterol. 2014;20:14172–84.
2. Baptiste CG, Battista MC, Trottier A, Baillargeon JP. Insulin and hyperandrogenism in women with polycystic ovary syndrome. J Steroid Biochem Mol Biol. 2010;122:42–52.
3. Chittenden BG, Fullerton G, Maheshwari A, Bhattacharya S. Polycystic ovary syndrome and the risk of gynaecological cancer: a systematic review. Reprod BioMed Online. 2009;19:398–405.
4. Ovalle F, Azziz R. Insulin resistance, polycystic ovary syndrome, and type 2 diabetes mellitus. Fertil Steril. 2002;77:1095–105.
5. Glueck CJ, Papanna R, Wang P, Goldenberg N, Sieve-Smith L. Incidence and treatment of metabolic syndrome in newly referred women with confirmed polycystic ovarian syndrome. Metabolism. 2003;52:908–15.
6. Phelan N, O'Connor A, Kyaw Tun T, Correia N, Boran G, Roche HM, et al. Hormonal and metabolic effects of polyunsaturated fatty acids in young women with polycystic ovary syndrome: results from a cross-sectional analysis and a randomized, placebo-controlled, crossover trial. Am J Clin Nutr. 2011;93:652–62.
7. Rafraf M, Mohammadi E, Asghari-Jafarabadi M, Farzadi L. Omega-3 fatty acids improve glucose metabolism without effects on obesity values and serum visfatin levels in women with polycystic ovary syndrome. J Am Coll Nutr. 2012;31:361–8.
8. Khani B, Mardanian F, Fesharaki SJ. Omega-3 supplementation effects on polycystic ovary syndrome symptoms and metabolic syndrome. J Res Med Sci. 2017;22:64. https://doi.org/10.4103/jrms.JRMS_644_16. eCollection 2017
9. Hurst S, Curtis CL, Rees SG, Harwood JL, Caterson B. Effects of n-3 polyunsaturated fatty acids on COX-2 and PGE2 protein levels in articular cartilage chondrocytes. Int J Exp Pathol. 2004;85:A22–3.
10. Sekhon LH, Gupta S, Kim Y, Agarwal A. Female infertility and antioxidants. Curr Womens Health Rev. 2010;6:84–95.
11. Ruder EH, Hartman TJ, Blumberg J, Goldman M. Oxidative stress and antioxidants: exposure and impact on female fertility. Hum Reprod Update. 2008;14:345–57.
12. Mohammadi E, Rafraf M. Benefits of omega-3 fatty acids supplementation on serum paraoxonase 1 activity and lipids ratios in polycystic ovary syndrome. Health Promot Perspect. 2012;2:197–204. https://doi.org/10.5681/hpp.2012.023. eCollection 2012

13. Cussons AJ, Watts GF, Mori TA, Stuckey BGA. Omega-3 fatty acid supplementation decreases liver fat content in polycystic ovary syndrome: a randomized controlled trial employing proton magnetic resonance spectroscopy. J Clin Endocrinol Metab. 2009;94:3842–8.

14. Sarbolouki SH, Djalali M, Dorosty AR, Djazayery SA, Eshraghian MR, SAR E, et al. Effects of EPA and vitamin E on serum enzymatic antioxidants and peroxidation indices in patients with type II diabetes mellitus. Iranian J Publ Health. 2010;39:82–91.

15. Tayyebi-Khosroshahi H, Houshyar J, Tabrizi A, Vatankhah AM, Razzaghi Zonouz N, Dehghan-Hesari R. Effect of omega-3 fatty acid on oxidative stress in patients on hemodialysis. Iran J Kidney Dis. 2010;4:322–6.

16. Sadeghi A, Djafarian K, Mohammadi H, Shab-Bidar S. Effect of omega-3 fatty acids supplementation on insulin resistance in women with polycystic ovary syndrome: meta-analysis of randomized controlled trials. Diabetes Metab Syndr. 2017;11:157–62. https://doi.org/10.1016/j.dsx.2016.06.025.

17. Karakas SE, Perroud B, Kind T, Palazoglu M, Fiehn O. Changes in plasma metabolites and glucose homeostasis during omega-3 polyunsaturated fatty acid supplementation in women with polycystic ovary syndrome. BBA Clin. 2016; 5: 179–185. doi: https://doi.org/10.1016/j.bbacli.2016.04.003. eCollection 2016 Jun.

18. Nadjarzadeh A, Dehghani-Firouzabadi R, Daneshbodi H, Lotfi MH, Vaziri N, Mozaffari-Khosravi H. Effect of Omega-3 supplementation on Visfatin, adiponectin, and anthropometric indices in women with polycystic ovarian syndrome. J Reprod Infertil. 2015;16:212–20.

19. Rahmani E, Samimi M, Ebrahimi FA, et al. The effects of omega-3 fatty acids and vitamin E co-supplementation on gene expression of lipoprotein(a) and oxidized low-density lipoprotein, lipid profiles and biomarkers of oxidative stress in patients with polycystic ovary syndrome. Mol Cell Endocrinol. 2016; 439:247–55.

20. Ebrahimi FA, Samimi M, Foroozanfard F, Jamilian M, Akbari H, Rahmani E, Ahmadi S, Taghizadeh M, Memarzadeh MR, Asemi Z. The effects of Omega-3 fatty acids and vitamin E co-supplementation on indices of insulin resistance and hormonal parameters in patients with polycystic ovary syndrome: a randomized, double-blind, Placebo-Controlled Trial. Exp Clin Endocrinol Diabetes. 2017;125:353–9. https://doi.org/10.1055/s-0042-117773. Epub 2017 Apr 13

21. Deeks JJ, Higgins JP, Altman DG. Chapter 16: special topics in statistics. In: Higgins JP, Green S, editors. Cochrane handbook for systematic reviews of interventions. UK: The Cochrane Collaboration; 2011.

22. Deeks JJ, Higgins JP, Altman DG. Chapter 8: assessing risk of bias in included studies. In: Higgins JP, Green S, editors. Cochrane Handbook or Systematic Reviews of Interventions Version 5.1.0. The Cochrane Collaboration: UK; 2011.

23. Deeks JJ, Higgins JP, Altman DG. Chapter 9: Analyzing data and undertaking meta-analyses. In: Higgins JP, Green S, editors. Cochrane handbook for systematic reviews of interventions. UK: The Cochrane Collaboration; 2011.

24. Rafraf M, Mohammadi E, Farzadi L. Asghari-Jafarabadi. Effects of omega-3 fatty acid supplement on serum lipid profile and markers of oxidative stress in women with polycystic ovary syndrome. Iran J Obstet Gynecol Infertil. 2012;15:1–10.

25. Mohammadi E, Rafraf M, Farzadi L, Asghari-Jafarabadi M, Sabour S. Effects of omega-3 fatty acids supplementation on serum adiponectin levels and some metabolic risk factors in women with polycystic ovary syndrome. Asia Pac J Clin Nutr. 2012;21:511–8.

26. Nadjarzadeh A, Dehghani Firouzabadi R, Vaziri N, Daneshbodi H, Lotfi MH, Mozaffari-Khosravi H. The effect of omega-3 supplementation on androgen profile and menstrual status in women with polycystic ovary syndrome: a randomized clinical trial. Iran J Reprod Med. 2013;11:665–72.

27. Mirmasoumi G, Fazilati M, Foroozanfard F, Vahedpoor Z, Mahmoodi S, Taghizadeh M, Esfeh NK, Mohseni M4 Karbassizadeh H, Asemi Z. The effects of flaxseed oil Omega-3 fatty acids supplementation on metabolic status of patients with polycystic ovary syndrome: a randomized, double-blind, placebo-controlled trial. Exp Clin Endocrinol Diabetes. 2017; https://doi.org/10.1055/s-0043-119751.

28. Jamilian M, Shojaei A, Samimi M, Afshar Ebrahimi F, Aghadavod E, Karamali M, Taghizadeh M, Jamilian H, Alaeinasab S, Jafarnejad S, Asemi Z. The effects of omega-3 and vitamin E co-supplementation on parameters of mental health and gene expression related to insulin and inflammation in subjects with polycystic ovary syndrome. J Affect Disord. 2018;229:41–7. https://doi.org/10.1016/j.jad.2017.12.049.

29. Azziz R, Carmina E, Dewailly D, Diamanti-Kandarakis E, Escobar-Morreale HF, Futterweit W, Janssen OE, Legro RS, Norman RJ, Taylor AE, Witchel SF. Task force on the phenotype of the polycystic ovary syndrome of the androgen excess PCOS society 2009. The androgen excess and PCOS society criteria for the polycystic ovary syndrome: the complete task force report. Fertil Steril. 2009;91:456–88.

30. Azziz R, Carmina E, Dewailly D, Diamanti-Kandarakis E, Escobar-Morreale HF, Futterweit W, Janssen OE, Legro RS, Norman RJ, Taylor AE, Witchel SF. Androgen excess society 2006.: positions statement: criteria for defining polycystic ovary syndrome as a predominantly hyperandrogenic syndrome: an androgen excess society guideline. J Clin Endocrinol Metab. 2006;91:4237–45.

31. Moran LJ, Misso ML, Wild RA, Norman RJ. Impaired glucose tolerance, type 2 diabetes and metabolic syndrome in polycystic ovary syndrome: a systematic review and meta-analysis. Hum Reprod Update. 2010;16:347–63.

32. Loke Y, Price D, Herxheimer A. Chapter 14: Adverse effects. In: JPT H, Green S, editors. Cochrane Handbook for Systematic Reviews of Interventions. chapter 14. Chichester: John Wiley & Sons; 2011.

33. Ioannidis JPA, Evans SJW, Gøtzsche PC, et al. Better reporting of harms in randomized trials: an extension of the CONSORT statement. Ann Intern Med. 2004;141:781–8.

34. Abbott D, Dumesic D, Franks S. Developmental origin of polycystic ovary syndrome-a hypothesis. J Endocrinol. 2002;174:1–5.

35. Oner G, Muderris II. Efficacy of omega-3 in the treatment of polycystic ovary syndrome. J Obstet Gynaecol. 2013;33:289–91.

36. Ardawi MSM, Rouzi AA. Plasma adiponectin and insulin resistance in women with polycystic ovary syndrome. Fertil Steril. 2005;83:1708–16.

37. Abbott DH, Bacha F. Ontogeny of polycystic ovary syndrome and insulin resistance in utero and early childhood. Fertil Steril. 2013;100:2–11.

38. González F, Kirwan JP, Rote NS, et al. Glucose ingestion stimulates atherothrombotic inflammation in polycystic ovary syndrome. Am J Physiol Endocrinol Metab. 2013;304:375–83.

39. Magee P, Pearson S, Whittingham-Dowd J, et al. PPARγ as a molecular target of EPA anti-inflammatory activity during TNF-α-impaired skeletal muscle cell differentiation. J Nutr Biochem. 2012;23:1440–8.

40. Davidson MH. Mechanisms for the hypotriglyceridemic effect of marine omega-3 fatty acids. Am J Cardiol. 2006;98:27i–33i.

41. Nestel PJ. Fish oil and cardiovascular disease: lipids and arterial function. Am J Clin Nutr. 2000;71:228S–31S.

42. Kicinski M, Springate DA, Kontopantelis E. Publication bias in meta-analyses from the Cochrane database of systematic reviews. Stat Med. 2015;34(20): 2781–93. https://doi.org/10.1002/sim.6525. Epub 2015 May 18

43. Riley RD, Lambert PC, Abo-Zaid G. Meta-analysis of individual participant data: rationale, conduct, and reporting. BMJ. 2010;340:c221. https://doi.org/ 10.1136/bmj.c221.

44. Kontopantelis E, Reeves D. A short guide and a forest plot command (ipdforest) for one-stage meta-analysis. Stata J. 2013;13(3):574–87.

## 2

A novel and compact review on the role of oxidative stress in female reproduction

Jiayin Lu, Zixu Wang, Jing Cao, Yaoxing Chen[*] and Yulan Dong[*]

Abstract

In recent years, the study of oxidative stress (OS) has become increasingly popular. In particular, the role of OS on female fertility is very important and has been focused on closely. The occurrence of OS is due to the excessive production of reactive oxygen species (ROS). ROS are a double-edged sword; they not only play an important role as secondary messengers in many intracellular signaling cascades, but they also exert indispensable effects on pathological processes involving the female genital tract. ROS and antioxidants join in the regulation of reproductive processes in both animals and humans. Imbalances between pro-oxidants and antioxidants could lead to a number of female reproductive diseases. This review focuses on the mechanism of OS and a series of female reproductive processes, explaining the role of OS in female reproduction and female reproductive diseases caused by OS, including polycystic ovary syndrome (PCOS), endometriosis, preeclampsia and so on. Many signaling pathways involved in female reproduction, including the Keap1-Nrf2, NF-κB, FOXO and MAPK pathways, which are affected by OS, are described, providing new ideas for the mechanism of reproductive diseases.

Keywords: ROS, Oxidative stress, Reproductive diseases, Antioxidants, Imbalance, Female fertility, Signaling pathways

Background

Oxygen is a necessary element of aerobic life, and oxidative metabolism represents a principal source of energy. Cells have a defense system against ROS under aerobic conditions, and in healthy biology, there is an appropriate balance between pro-oxidants and antioxidants. OS occurs with the generation of excessive ROS or when the antioxidants' defense mechanisms are weakened [1–3]. The most important biologically ROS are superoxide anion ($O_2^{-}\cdot$), hydroxyl radical ($\cdot OH$), peroxyl ($ROO^{\cdot}$), alkoxyl ($RO^{\cdot}$) and hydroperoxyl ($HO_2^{\cdot}$). Free radical species are unstable and highly reactive, but they can become stable by acquiring electrons from lipids, nucleic acids, proteins, carbohydrates or nearby molecules, causing a cascade of chain reactions and resulting in cellular damage and disease [4–6]. Therefore, OS can cause DNA damage, lipids peroxidation and protein damage. Under normal circumstances, there are two types of antioxidants in the body: non-enzymatic antioxidants and enzymatic antioxidants. Enzymatic antioxidants include superoxide dismutase (SOD), glutathione

peroxidase (GPx), catalase (CAT) and glutathione reductase (GSR), which can cause reduction of H_2O_2 to water and alcohol. Non-enzymatic antioxidants are known as synthetic antioxidants or dietary supplements, including vitamin C, vitamin E, β-carotene, selenium, zinc, taurine, glutathione and so on [7].

OS is considered to be responsible for the initiation or development of pathological processes affecting female reproductive processes [8, 9], such as embryonic resorption, recurrent pregnancy loss, preeclampsia, intrauterine growth restriction (IUGR) and fetal death [10]. However, the relationship between ROS-induced OS and diseases is unclear and cannot be adequately investigated in human pregnancies because of self-evident ethical reasons. Therefore, animal models of both normal and disturbed pregnancies are essential for filling these important gaps in our knowledge. The normal level of ROS plays an important regulatory role through various signaling transduction pathways in folliculogenesis, corpus luteum oocyte maturation and feto-placental development [11]. However, ROS can sometimes exert damaging effects when overabundant. They have a close relationship with reproductive events, so tightly controlled ROS generation is an important process. It is one

* Correspondence: yxchen@cau.edu.cn; ylbcdong@cau.edu.cn
Laboratory of Neurobiology, College of Animal Medicine, China Agricultural University, Haidian, Beijing 100193, People's Republic of China

of the central elements of cell signaling, gene expression, maintenance of redox homeostasis and signal transduction pathways involved in cell function, growth, differentiation and death [12]. When keywords were searched in the NCBI and Web of Science databases, there were more than 100,000 articles on reproduction and oxidative stress, but there were only approximately 20,000 articles on the relationship between female reproduction and oxidative stress. There were more than 3000 articles about the mechanism, but there were only approximately 800 articles on uterine and ovarian diseases and oxidative stress. There is very little research on the mechanism of uterine and ovarian diseases and oxidative stress, only 30 articles, and review articles are rare. This review not only sheds light on the mechanism of action of oxidative stress under normal physiological conditions, but it also explores and speculates on the mechanisms of joint reproductive diseases, providing readers with more comprehensive content. The 133 articles selected in this article have a greater impact on the fields of reproduction and stress. By summarizing previous studies, a convincing review is offered.

The previous discussion of reproduction and oxidative stress was limited to individual diseases. This review aims to provide a comprehensive discussion of the role of oxidative stress in female reproduction, and it speculates on new mechanisms of action. This review mainly examines the available evidence for the involvement of cellular ROS-induced OS in pregnancy-related diseases, and it explores the new signaling pathways between OS and female reproduction.

Reproductive processes

It is well known that the development of ovarian follicles is a continuous process (Fig. 1). There are five stages in female mammals. During these stages, the structure of the endometrium undergoes some changes. Estrogen and progesterone are secreted via the ovaries and uterus and undergo changes during the estrus cycle. In addition, the basal body temperature also changes, while the thickness of the endometrium undergoes the corresponding transformation [13] (Fig. 2).

The combination of sperm and egg consists of three steps: corona radiata dissolution; zona pellucida dissolution; and egg fertilization and cortical reaction (Fig. 3). The process occurs in the ampulla portion of the fallopian tube. Pregnancy starts when the fertilized egg is formed. Human chorionic gonadotropin (HCG) increases first and then decreases. Both estrogen and progesterone are increased during pregnancy (Fig. 4). It is noted that the process of implantation is significant in reproductive events. The process includes contact, dissolution, invasion, wrapping and repair (Fig. 5). Ovarian function and blastocyst development from ovulation to implantation are common in many mammalian species after ovulation (Fig. 5) [14].

Oxidative stress
Reactive oxygen species (ROS)

ROS are a double-edged sword: they not only play important roles as secondary messengers in many intracellular signaling cascades, but they also exert indispensable effects on pathological processes involving the generation of excessive ROS. The three major types of ROS are superoxide anion ($O_2^-\cdot$), hydrogen peroxide (H_2O_2), and hydroxyl ($\cdot OH$).

Most ROS are produced when electrons leak from the mitochondrial respiratory chain, also referred to as the electron transport chain (ETC) [15]. According to an estimate, up to 2% oxygen consumed can be diverted to the production of ROS formation by mitochondria, especially at complexes I and III [16]. The free radical superoxide anion ($O_2^-\cdot$) is formed by the addition of one electron to ground state dioxygen, but it is unstable in aqueous solutions due to its being able to react spontaneously with itself, producing hydrogen peroxide (H_2O_2) and molecular oxygen (O_2) (reaction 1). It can reduce Fe^{3+} to Fe^{2+} and transform into O_2 (reaction 2). H_2O_2 is not a free radical, but it is very harmful to cells because it is able to cross biological membranes and break down into the highly reactive hydroxyl radical ($\cdot OH$).

The main source of hydroxyl radical is the metal-catalyzed Haver-Weiss reaction (reaction 3), the second of which is the Fenton-type reaction (reaction 4).

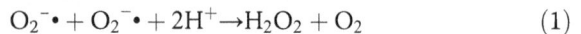

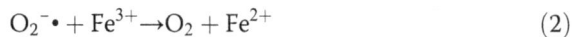

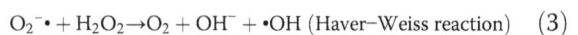

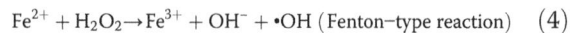

$$O_2^-\cdot + O_2^-\cdot + 2H^+ \rightarrow H_2O_2 + O_2 \tag{1}$$

$$O_2^-\cdot + Fe^{3+} \rightarrow O_2 + Fe^{2+} \tag{2}$$

$$O_2^-\cdot + H_2O_2 \rightarrow O_2 + OH^- + \cdot OH \,(\text{Haver–Weiss reaction}) \tag{3}$$

$$Fe^{2+} + H_2O_2 \rightarrow Fe^{3+} + OH^- + \cdot OH \,(\text{Fenton–type reaction}) \tag{4}$$

The defense mechanism against oxygen free radicals
Primary defenses

As we all know, SOD, CAT, GPx and GSR belong to the primary defense mechanism (Fig. 6). SOD catalyzes $O_2^-\cdot$ dismutation to produce H_2O_2 and O_2 at a rate 10^4 times higher than spontaneous dismutation at the physiological pH [17, 18]. CAT is the enzyme that removes H_2O_2 from the cell when the latter is at high concentrations (reaction 5) [19]. GPx is an enzyme that catalyzes the reduction of H_2O_2 and organic free hydroperoxides requiring glutathione as a co-substrate (reaction 6 and 7)

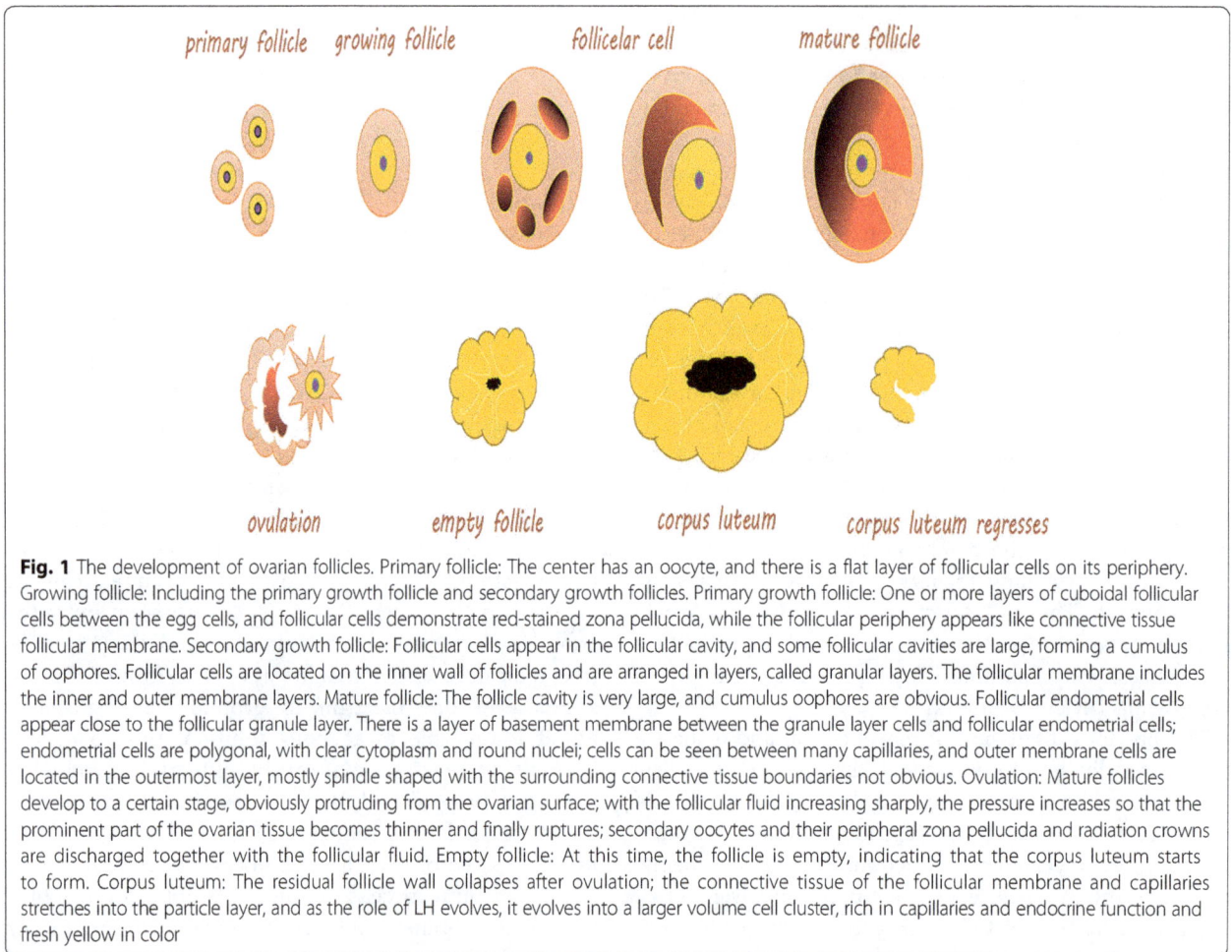

Fig. 1 The development of ovarian follicles. Primary follicle: The center has an oocyte, and there is a flat layer of follicular cells on its periphery. Growing follicle: Including the primary growth follicle and secondary growth follicles. Primary growth follicle: One or more layers of cuboidal follicular cells between the egg cells, and follicular cells demonstrate red-stained zona pellucida, while the follicular periphery appears like connective tissue follicular membrane. Secondary growth follicle: Follicular cells appear in the follicular cavity, and some follicular cavities are large, forming a cumulus of oophores. Follicular cells are located on the inner wall of follicles and are arranged in layers, called granular layers. The follicular membrane includes the inner and outer membrane layers. Mature follicle: The follicle cavity is very large, and cumulus oophores are obvious. Follicular endometrial cells appear close to the follicular granule layer. There is a layer of basement membrane between the granule layer cells and follicular endometrial cells; endometrial cells are polygonal, with clear cytoplasm and round nuclei; cells can be seen between many capillaries, and outer membrane cells are located in the outermost layer, mostly spindle shaped with the surrounding connective tissue boundaries not obvious. Ovulation: Mature follicles develop to a certain stage, obviously protruding from the ovarian surface; with the follicular fluid increasing sharply, the pressure increases so that the prominent part of the ovarian tissue becomes thinner and finally ruptures; secondary oocytes and their peripheral zona pellucida and radiation crowns are discharged together with the follicular fluid. Empty follicle: At this time, the follicle is empty, indicating that the corpus luteum starts to form. Corpus luteum: The residual follicle wall collapses after ovulation; the connective tissue of the follicular membrane and capillaries stretches into the particle layer, and as the role of LH evolves, it evolves into a larger volume cell cluster, rich in capillaries and endocrine function and fresh yellow in color

[20]. GSR is a cytosolic protein with a tissue distribution similar to that of GPx. The enzyme reduces oxidized glutathione, utilizing NADPH generated by various systems (reaction 8) [21].

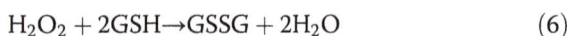

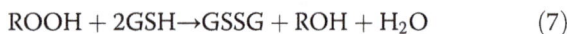

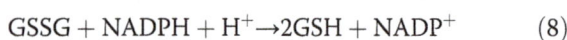

$$2H_2O_2 \rightarrow 2H_2O + O_2 \tag{5}$$

$$H_2O_2 + 2GSH \rightarrow GSSG + 2H_2O \tag{6}$$

$$ROOH + 2GSH \rightarrow GSSG + ROH + H_2O \tag{7}$$

$$GSSG + NADPH + H^+ \rightarrow 2GSH + NADP^+ \tag{8}$$

Secondary defense

The existence has been reported of an enzyme with peroxidase activity called phospholipid hydroperoxidase GPx, which is capable of reducing lipid hydroperoxides without the action of phospholipase A2 [22]. In addition, different oxidoreductases that catalyze reduction reactions of thiol and other protein groups when these molecules are oxidatively damaged are protective enzymes against oxygen free radicals. Nuclear enzymes for DNA repair are considered to be defense systems against oxidative injury by oxygen free radicals [23]. Vitamin E, the major lipid-soluble antioxidant present in all cellular membranes, protects against lipid peroxidation. The tocopheryl radical might also be directly reduced by the ascorbic acid-GSH redox couple. β-carotene exerts the most efficient scavenger action with vitamin E, while β-carotene acts at low oxygen pressures. However, vitamin E protects conjugated double bonds of β-carotene from oxidation.

In all, OS plays an important role in the pathophysiology of complicated pregnancies. OS was described as an imbalance in the generation of ROS [1]. These ROS are oxygen free radicals produced by the reduction in molecular oxygen and generated as byproducts of aerobic respiration and metabolism. These molecules are capable of activating and modulating various signaling pathways, including those involved in cell growth, differentiation and metabolism [24]. They can also induce cellular oxidative damage by interacting with DNA and intracellular macromolecules, such as protein and membrane lipids, so they can lead to cellular malfunction that can initiate pathological processes.

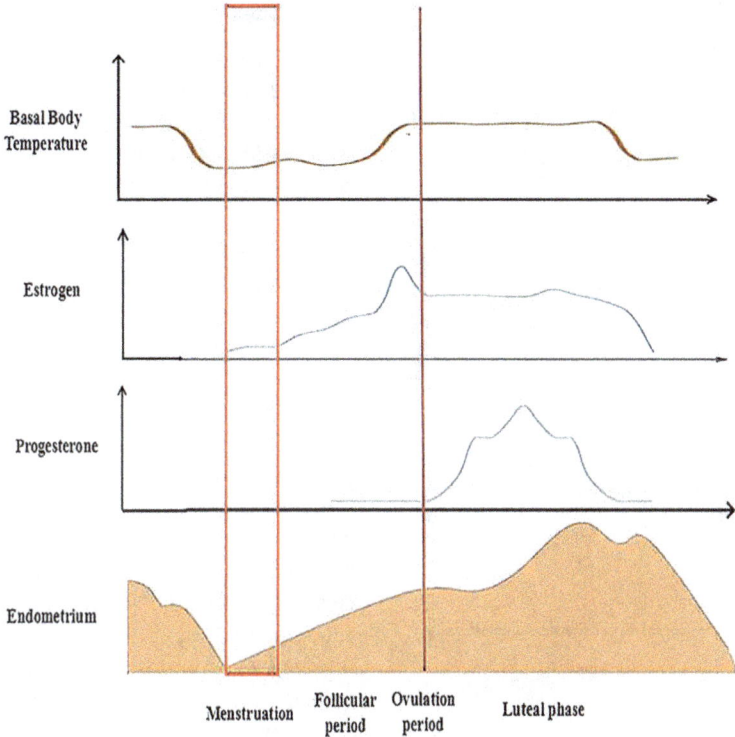

Fig. 2 The changes of biology during different estrus cycle. Estrogen and progesterone are secreted via the ovary or uterus and undergo changes during the estrus cycle. In addition, the basal body temperature also changes, while the thickness of the endometrium has corresponding transformations. After menstruation, the new estrus cycle starts to develop. During the follicular period, the level of the basal body temperature and estrogen gradually rise. The thickness of the endometrium also increases. The levels of basal body temperature and estrogen maintain certain concentrations until the ovulation period. Thus, progesterone starts to increase. With the appearance of the luteal phase, all changes are restored until the end of menstruation

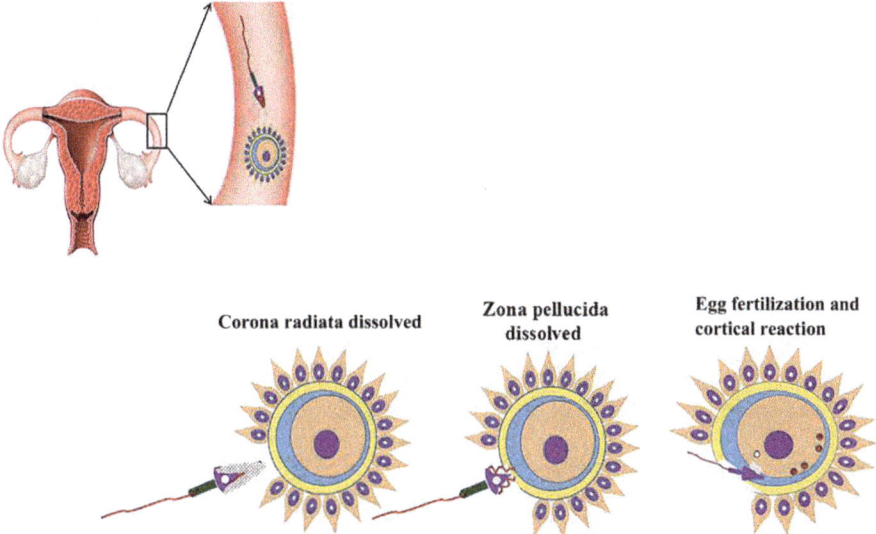

Fig. 3 Fertilization processes of most viviparous and ovoviviparous animals. In most viviparous and ovoviviparous animals, the sperm and oocyte combine at the fallopian tube ampulla. In the picture, the first zygote shows a radiation crown dissolving; the second zygote shows the zona pellucida dissolving; the last zygote shows fertilized eggs and cortical response

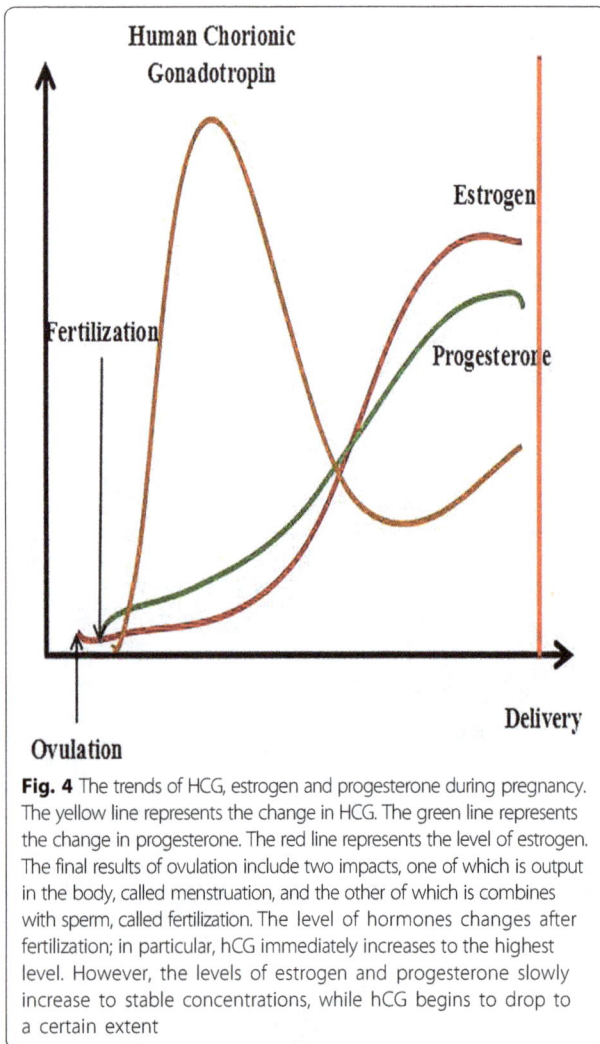

Fig. 4 The trends of HCG, estrogen and progesterone during pregnancy. The yellow line represents the change in HCG. The green line represents the change in progesterone. The red line represents the level of estrogen. The final results of ovulation include two impacts, one of which is output in the body, called menstruation, and the other of which is combines with sperm, called fertilization. The level of hormones changes after fertilization; in particular, hCG immediately increases to the highest level. However, the levels of estrogen and progesterone slowly increase to stable concentrations, while hCG begins to drop to a certain extent

Oxidative stress in ovary

ROS affect a variety of physiologic functions of the ovary, including ovarian steroid genesis, oocyte maturation, ovulation, formation of blastocysts, implantation, luteolysis and luteal maintenance in pregnancy. OS is an important modulator of ovarian germ cell and stromal cell physiology [25]. Concentrations of ROS could also play a major role in the implantation and fertilization of eggs, and a relevant study showed localization of SOD in the ovary and found that copper-zinc SOD (Cu-Zn SOD) was localized in the granulose cell of growing follicles and mature Graafian follicles, as well as manganese superoxide dismutase (MnSOD) being localized in luteal cells of the corpus luteum in rats [26].

ROS exert both negative and positive effects on mammalian ovaries [27]. ROS affect multiple physiological and pathological activities in the ovaries, from oocyte maturation to fertilization. In cycling ovaries, different markers of OS are negatively affected [28, 29]. Macrophages, leukocytes, and cytokines present in the

follicular fluid microenvironment are major sources of ROS. ROS in the follicular fluid join in follicular growth, oocyte maturation, and ovarian steroid biosynthesis [15]. At the same time, a critical process for ovarian folliculogenesis, dominant follicle selection, CL formation and embryo formation is angiogenesis [30, 31], which is a complex process. It is promoted by estrogens that regulates some cellular factors, such as VEGF [32]. ROS produced from NADP(H) oxidase were shown to be significant for angiogenesis in vivo and VEGF signaling in vitro [33]. Accordingly, ROS are involved in follicular growth in part by regulating angiogenesis.

The appropriate amount of ROS is required for ovulation. ROS produced by the preovulatory follicle are considered critical inducers of ovulation, and inhibition of ROS has been confirmed to disturb ovulation [27, 34]. Oxygen deprivation stimulates follicular angiogenesis, which is important for abundant growth and development of ovarian follicles [35]. The development of follicles from the primordial stage to antral follicles is accompanied by a marked increase in the metabolic function of granulosa cells, especially a large increase in cytochrome P450 activity with steroid biosynthesis [36]. Large amounts of ROS are produced during electron transport, indicating that functional granulosa cells are related to the pro-oxidant state in the follicles. ROS are induced in preovulatory follicles with oscillation of prostaglandins, cytokines, proteolytic enzymes, and steroids, resulting in blood flow alterations and eventual follicle rupture [37]. With the exception of dominant follicles, which are released for fertilization, the other growing follicles all undergo apoptosis, and this process is promoted by ROS. In parallel, follicle-stimulating hormone (FSH)-induced estrogen synthesis and upregulation of CAT and GSH in growing follicles resist the apoptotic process to maintain the balance during normal ovarian function [38]. ROS are generated in the CL and are involved in functional luteolysis. ROS and antioxidants are related to progesterone synthesis in the luteal phase [35] (Table 1).

However, excessive deprivation of oxygen will also cause some damage to follicles, as we discuss in the following. Cu/Zn-SOD is increased in the CL during the early to mid-luteal phase, but it is decreased during the regression phase, which could explain the increase in ROS concentrations during regression, and this change in activity is similar to that in progesterone concentrations. Other possible explanation for the decrease in Cu-Zn SOD during the regression phase is an increase in prostaglandin $PGF_{2\alpha}$ or macrophages; another reliable explanation is a decrease in ovarian blood flow [35]. Prostaglandin $F_{2\alpha}$ stimulates production of the SO anion by luteal cells and phagocytic leukocytes in the CL. The reduction of ovarian blood flow causes tissue damage by

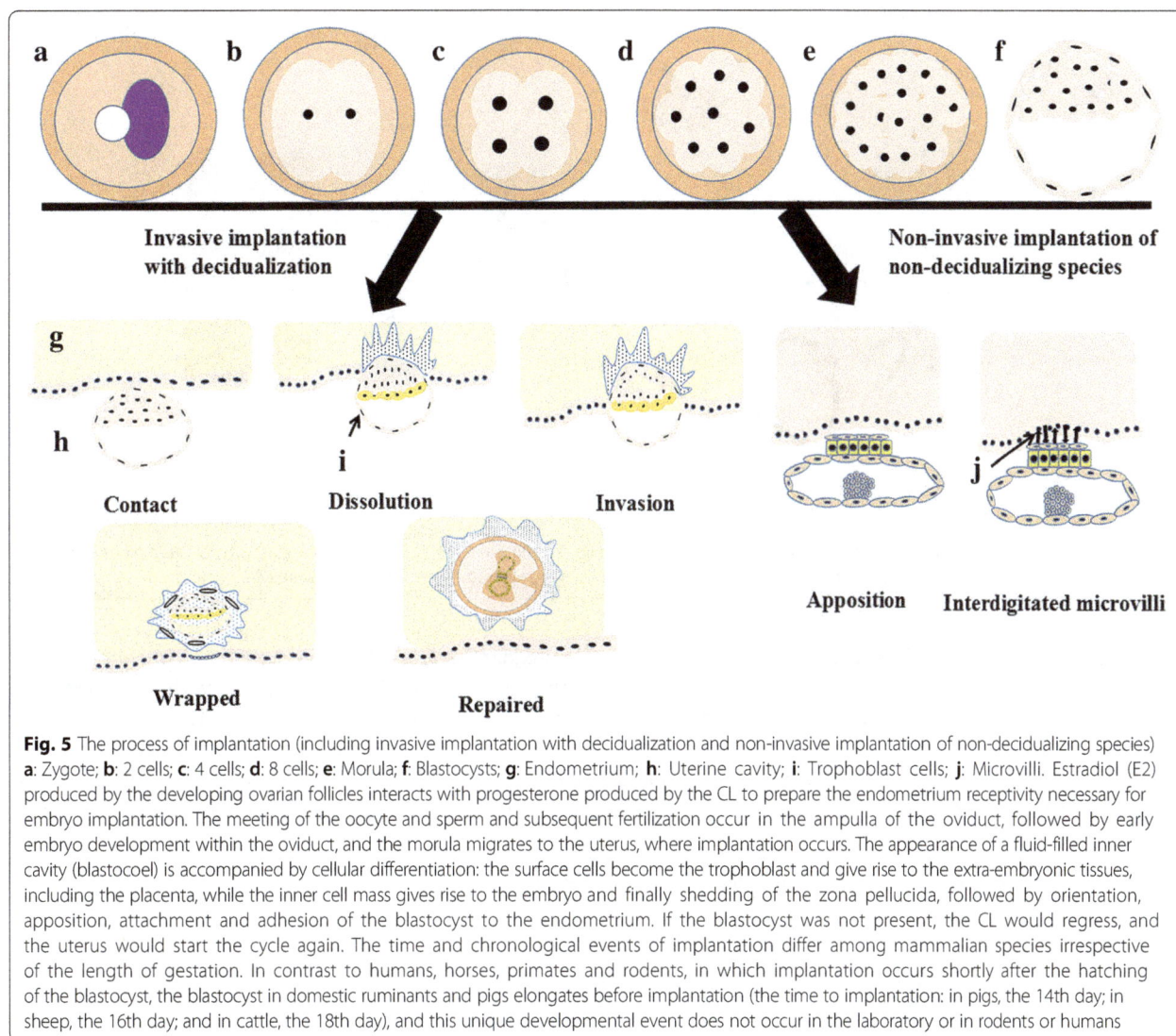

Fig. 5 The process of implantation (including invasive implantation with decidualization and non-invasive implantation of non-decidualizing species) **a**: Zygote; **b**: 2 cells; **c**: 4 cells; **d**: 8 cells; **e**: Morula; **f**: Blastocysts; **g**: Endometrium; **h**: Uterine cavity; **i**: Trophoblast cells; **j**: Microvilli. Estradiol (E2) produced by the developing ovarian follicles interacts with progesterone produced by the CL to prepare the endometrium receptivity necessary for embryo implantation. The meeting of the oocyte and sperm and subsequent fertilization occur in the ampulla of the oviduct, followed by early embryo development within the oviduct, and the morula migrates to the uterus, where implantation occurs. The appearance of a fluid-filled inner cavity (blastocoel) is accompanied by cellular differentiation: the surface cells become the trophoblast and give rise to the extra-embryonic tissues, including the placenta, while the inner cell mass gives rise to the embryo and finally shedding of the zona pellucida, followed by orientation, apposition, attachment and adhesion of the blastocyst to the endometrium. If the blastocyst was not present, the CL would regress, and the uterus would start the cycle again. The time and chronological events of implantation differ among mammalian species irrespective of the length of gestation. In contrast to humans, horses, primates and rodents, in which implantation occurs shortly after the hatching of the blastocyst, the blastocyst in domestic ruminants and pigs elongates before implantation (the time to implantation: in pigs, the 14th day; in sheep, the 16th day; and in cattle, the 18th day), and this unique developmental event does not occur in the laboratory or in rodents or humans

ROS production. However, the concentration of Mn-SOD in the CL during regression is increased, thus scavenging the ROS produced in the mitochondria by inflammatory reactions and cytokines. Therefore, complete disruption of the CL leads to a significant decrease in Mn-SOD in the regressed cells, and cell death is imminent [39]. In addition, ROS also participate in mammalian ovulation and follicular rupture. The generation of the two processes is the result of vascular changes or the proteolytic cascade. The crosstalk between these two cascades is mediated by ROS, cytokines, and vascular endothelial growth factor (VEGF) [40, 41]. Ad4BP, a zinc finger DNA-binding protein, was identified as a transcription factor regulating steroidogenic P-450 genes in a cAMP-dependent manner [42], and a recent study showed that the correlation between Ad4BP and SOD expression suggested an association between OS and ovarian steroid genesis. Both human granulosa

and luteal cells respond to hydrogen peroxide with extirpation of gonadotropin action and inhibition of progesterone secretion. Hydrogen peroxide lowers both cAMP-dependent and non-cAMP-dependent steroidogenesis [28, 43]. As we all know, OS influences the entire reproductive process of women's lives. ROS attacks the 8th carbon atom of guanine in DNA to generate 8-hydroxy-deoxyguanosine (8-OHDG), which is an oxidized derivative of deoxyguanosine, the levels of which are higher in aging oocytes [44]. 8-OHdG is the most familiar base modification in mutagenic damage. 8-OHdG causes base mutation and mismatches in DNA replication, resulting in G mutations to T and G:C to T:A transversion. Therefore, 8-OHdG has become a marker for OS.

OS has been implicated in different female diseases, including PCOS, which is the most common endocrine abnormality of reproductive-aged women and has a prevalence of approximately 18%. It is a disorder

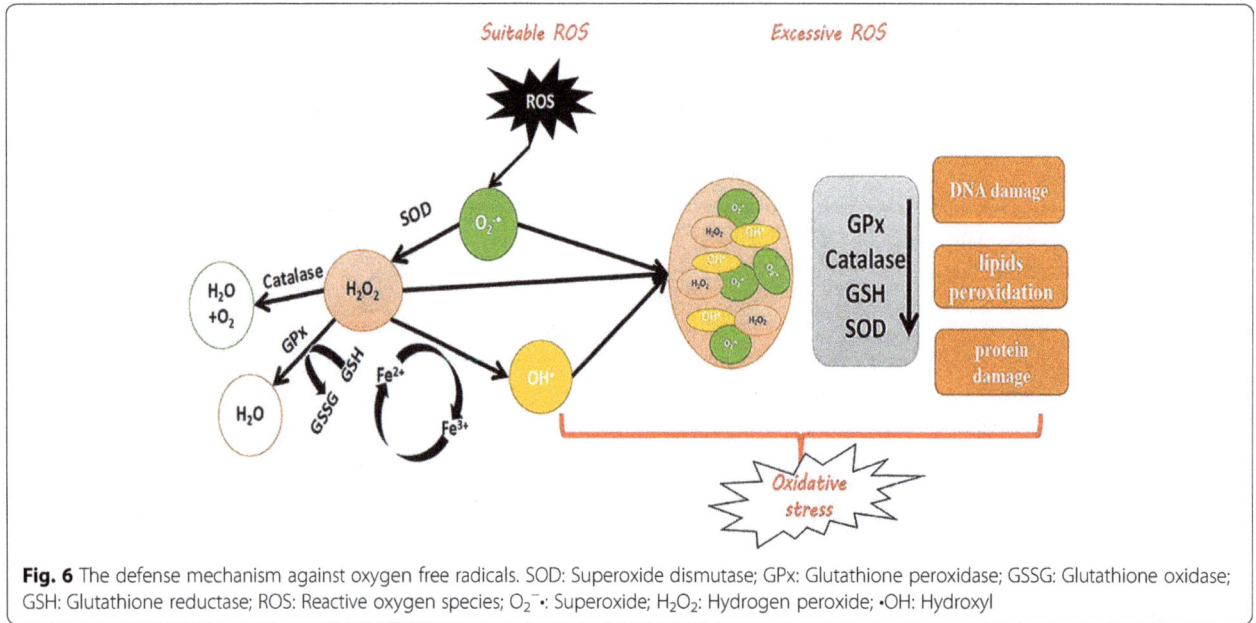

Fig. 6 The defense mechanism against oxygen free radicals. SOD: Superoxide dismutase; GPx: Glutathione peroxidase; GSSG: Glutathione oxidase; GSH: Glutathione reductase; ROS: Reactive oxygen species; $O_2^-\cdot$: Superoxide; H_2O_2: Hydrogen peroxide; $\cdot OH$: Hydroxyl

characterized by hyperandrogenism, ovulatory dysfunction, and polycystic ovaries [45]. Various studies have reflected the presence of OS in PCOS patients. In a study by Hilali et al., PCOS patients had increased serum prolidase activity, as well as higher total oxidant status and OS indices—the ratio of oxidants to total antioxidant status. The decrease in mitochondrial O_2 consumption and GSH levels, along with increased ROS production, explains the mitochondrial dysfunction in PCOS patients. Physiological hyperglycemia generates increased levels of ROS from mononuclear cells, which activate the release of tumor necrosis factor-α (TNF-α)

Table 1 The role of oxidative stress in the female reproductive process

Function	Reproductive process	Reference
Positive effect	Zn-Cu SOD↑ → Promotion of the development of follicles	[26]
	Biosynthesis of ovarian steroids → P450↑ → ROS↑ → Blood flow↑ → Rupture of follicles → Ovulation	[36, 37, 40, 41]
	ROS↑ → Promotion apoptosis of non-dominant follicles FSH↑ → E2↑ → CAT and GSH↑ → Protection of cells from apoptosis	[38]
	E2 and P ↓ → SOD↓ → OS↑ → Endometrial shedding and implant failure	[62]
	ROS↑ → NF-κB↑ → PGF$_{2\alpha}$↑ → Luteum dissolution	[35, 39, 61]
	Sperm-ovum binding → ROS↑ → Corpus luteus functional↑ ROS↑ → Antioxidants↑ → Synthesis of progesterone	[39]
Negative effect	PCOS: Serum proline activity↑, OS↑ Physiological hyperglycemia → ROS↑ (Monocytes) → TNF-α↑ → NF-κB↑ → Resistance of Insulin↑	[45, 46]
	Preeclampsia: Defective placenta → Hypoxia and reperfusion injury → OS↑ → Cytokines↑, Prostaglandins↑ → TAS↓, GPx of placenta↓ V$_C$↓ → Risk of preeclampsia↑ (MDA↑) ROS↑ → Vasoconstriction↑ → Coagulation activity↓ OS↑ → Vascular endothelial injury↑ → ROS↑ → TNF-α↑, ox-LDL↑ → Endothelial subtypes of activated NAD(P)H oxidase → SO anion↑ Auto-antibodies of AT1-AA↑ → NAD(P)H oxidase↑ → ROS↑ → SO anion↑	[67, 76–81, 83–85]
	Endometriosis: In the peritoneal fluid, MDA↑, IL-6↑,TNF-α↑, IL-8↑, VEGF↑, MCP-1↑, ox-LDL↑. In endometriotic lesions: OS↑ → NF-κB↑ → Inflammation↑ In endometriotic cells: MAPK↑ ROS↑ → IUGR, abortion, fetal malformation	[71–73, 75]

The '→' indicates that it has an effect on the next step. The '↑' represents an increase and the '↓'represents a decrease

and increase the inflammatory transcription factor nuclear factor-kappa B (NF-κB). As a result, concentrations of TNF-α, a known mediator of insulin resistance, are further increased. The resultant OS creates an inflammatory environment that further increases insulin resistance [46], causing abnormal ovarian extracellular remodeling, multiple cyst formation, and chronic anovulation, leading to infertility [47] (Table 1).

Recently, PCOS has been paid significant attention because it exerts severe effects on female reproduction. In this review, we collect some interesting evidence that implies a delicate relationship between stress and PCOS [48]. Its etio-pathogenesis and pathophysiology include roles for genetic, environmental and endocrine factors. Franks et al. defined PCOS as a gene-dependent ovarian pathology, characterized by the overproduction of androgens and not uniformly represented by the interaction of genetic "propensities" with other genetic and environmental factors [49]. Thus, PCOS seems to be a genetic disease, but after investigation by Escobar-Morreale HF et al. found that it is caused by the interaction of susceptibility and protective genetic variants, and these mutations could be chosen due to survival advantages in the evolution process, requiring an accurate study of environmental factors, including race, diet and lifestyle [50]. V. De Leo et al. reported that disruption of the delicate balance between intra-ovarian and extra-ovarian factors alters and impairs the formation of mature oocytes, leading to infertility. In addition, insulin plays a particular role in PCOS, and in vitro studies have demonstrated that insulin stimulates thecal cell proliferation, increases secretion of androgens mediated by LH and increases cytochrome P450 expression of LH and IGF-1 receptor [51]. As we all know, P450 can increase ROS. The above evidence indicates that ROS join in the pathological process of PCOS.

Oxidative stress in the uterus and placenta

Pregnancy itself is a state of OS, arising from the increased metabolic activity in the placental mitochondria and increased ROS production due to the higher metabolic demand of the growing fetus [52, 53]. Superoxide (SO) anions produced by the placental mitochondria appear to be a major source of ROS and lipid per-oxidation contributing to OS in the placenta [54], supported by mitochondrial production of lipid peroxides, free radicals, and vitamin E in the placenta, which increases as gestation progresses[55]. In the second trimester, the placenta gradually matures and increases in size, with less hairiness and wider blood vessels. The cytotrophoblast becomes a single cell and gradually replaces the endothelial layer covering the smooth muscle of the spiral artery. Slowly, maternal blood penetrates from the mother's spiral artery into the interstitial space [55–57]. During this process, placental tissue forms a large amount of free radicals, and oxidation occurs. Intense stress results, but the placenta gradually adapts to this environment and returns to normal under the action of antioxidant activity [58, 59]. While physiological concentrations of endogenous glucocorticoids are supportive of fetal development, excessive glucocorticoids in utero (i.e., maternal stress) adversely affect mammalian offspring by "programming" abnormalities that are primarily manifested postpartum [60]. ROS are also believed to play a role in the different phases of the endometrial cycle. The late luteal phase is characterized by elevated levels of lipid peroxide and a decrease in the antioxidant SOD. ROS stimulate the secretion of $PGF_{2\alpha}$ through activation of NF-κB [61]. Decreased levels of estrogen and progesterone lead to decreased SOD expression and hence generate OS in the uterus, resulting ultimately in endometrial shedding and lack of implantation. Controlled levels of ROS have, however, been associated with angiogenic activity in the endometrium, causing regeneration during every cycle. These studies showed that limited levels of ROS are necessary to maintain physiological function, but when present in higher concentrations, ROS can have deleterious effects [62]. In other words, although a physiological balance between ROS and antioxidant activity is maintained in normal pregnancies [63], an imbalance can increase OS. The placenta experiences a heightened level of OS in certain pathologic conditions of pregnancies, including gestational diabetes, fetal growth restriction, preeclampsia and miscarriage [64–66].

OS leads to endothelial cell dysfunction. In the uterus, endothelial cell dysfunction results in many diseases, such as preeclampsia and endometriosis. There are many causes that induced endothelial cell dysfunction. TNF-α, a plasma cytokine, has been demonstrated to cause endothelial cell injury, but the antioxidant Mn-SOD neutralizes SO anions generated by the cytokine TNF-α. This process is a self-protective mechanism against TNF-α-induced OS. In addition, defective placentation leads to placental hypoxia and reperfusion injury due to ischemia, and the resultant OS triggers the release of cytokines and prostaglandins, resulting in endothelial cell dysfunction and playing an important role in the development of preeclampsia [67]. In addition, ROS generated from NADP (H) oxidase are critical for VEGF signaling in vitro and angiogenesis in vivo [33]. Small amounts of ROS are produced from endothelial NADP (H) oxidase activated by growth factors and cytokines. ROS generated in and around the vascular endothelium could play a role in normal cellular signaling mechanisms. They might also be important causative factors in endothelial dysfunction.

Endometriosis is a benign, estrogen-dependent, chronic gynecological disorder characterized by the presence of endometrial tissue outside the uterus. There was a report suggested that the elevated ROS causing OS are produced by erythrocytes and apoptotic endometrioma cells, as well as the activated macrophages that are recruited to phagocytize apoptotic cells [10]. Additionally, the ROS producing enzyme xanthine oxidase, which is considered another contributor to excess ROS, are expressed in greater quantities in women with endometriosis [68]. OS plays a large role in infertility. Another way in which cells are damaged through OS is via lipid peroxidation, which is the oxidative destruction of polyunsaturated fatty acids in the plasma membrane [69]. This leads to "increased membrane permeability, degraded membrane integrity, inactivated enzymes and structural damage of the DNA; cell death rapidly follows" [70]. In addition, OS induces local inflammation, resulting in elevated levels of cytokines and other factors that promote endometriosis, as discussed later [8].

The peritoneal fluid of patients has been found to contain high concentrations of malondialdehyde (MDA), pro-inflammatory cytokines (IL-6, TNF-α, and IL-1β), angiogenic factors (IL-8 and VEGF), monocyte chemoattractant protein-1 (MCP-1) [71], and oxidized LDL (ox-LDL). Pro-inflammatory and chemotactic cytokines play central roles in the recruitment and activation of phagocytic cells, which are the main producers of ROS and RNS. Activation of NF-κB by OS has been detected in the endometriotic lesions and peritoneal macrophages of patients with endometriosis [72]. Signaling mediated by NF-κB stimulates inflammation, invasion, angiogenesis, and cell proliferation, and it also promotes the apoptosis of endometriotic cells. Additionally, N-acetylcysteine (NAC) and vitamin E are antioxidants that limit the proliferation of endometriotic cells, likely by inhibiting activation of NF-κB [73]. A study indicated a therapeutic effect of NAC and vitamin E supplementation on endometriotic growth [74]. Similar to tumor cells, increased ROS and subsequent cellular proliferation in endometriotic cells activate of mitogen-activated protein kinase (MAPK) and extracellular regulated kinase (ERK1/2) [75]. More seriously, the increase in ROS in endometriosis patients can lead to adverse effects on embryos, such as IUGR, spontaneous abortion, or fetal dysmorphogenesis [69] (Table 1).

Preeclampsia is a vascular pregnancy disorder that often involves impaired placental development. It is a complex multisystem disorder that can affect normotensive women. It can cause the poor implantation and growth restriction observed in preeclampsia because OS causes increased nitration of p38 MAPK, resulting in a reduction in its catalytic activity.

Increased ROS concentrations in patients with preeclampsia have been proved by the increased levels of MDA, an index of lipid peroxidation [76]. Under normal conditions, the impairment of circulatory homeostasis is caused chiefly by vascular endothelial dysfunction in preeclampsia. It is characterized by the tendency to cause vasoconstriction and low anticoagulant activity. ROS seem to play a critical role in the endothelial dysfunction associated with preeclampsia [77]. In other words, the pathologic event in preeclampsia is injury to the vascular endothelium regulated by OS from increased placental ROS [78] or decreased antioxidant activity [79].

There are many reasons for the increase in ROS. For instance, neutrophil modulation occurring in preeclampsia is an important source of ROS, resulting in increased production of the SO anion and decreased levels of NO, ultimately causing endothelial cell damage in patients with preeclampsia. Levels of TNF-α and oxLDL are increased in preeclampsia and have been shown to activate the endothelial isoform of NAD(P)H oxidase, ultimately resulting in increased levels of the SO anion. These results suggest that the consumption of antioxidants to counteract heightened lipid per-oxidation might injure the vascular endothelium and could be involved in the pathogenesis of preeclampsia [80].

In addition, autoantibodies against the angiotensin receptor AT1, particularly the second loop (AT1-AA), can stimulate NAD(P)H oxidase, leading to increased generation of ROS [81]. The AT1 receptor of preeclamptic women has been observed to promote both the generation of the SO anion and over-expression of NAD(P)H oxidase in cultured trophoblasts and smooth muscle cells. Therefore, early placental development can be affected by dysregulated vascular development and function secondary to NAD(P)H oxidase-mediated altered gene expression [82]. Preeclamptic women produce ROS and exhibit higher NAD(P)H expression than those without the disease [35]. More specifically, it has been reported that women with early-onset preeclampsia produce larger amounts of the SO anion than women with late-onset disease [83]. Affected women also have decreased total antioxidant status (TAS) and placental GPx [84] and low levels of vitamins C and E. Lack of vitamin C intake seems to be associated with an increased risk of preeclampsia, and some studies have shown that periconceptional supplementation with multivitamins can lower the risk of preeclampsia in normal or underweight women [85].

There have been studies focusing on the effects of restraint stress on uterine and embryo implantation in pregnant mice. In these studies, uterine local micro-environment changes and uterine histomorphology research were emphasized. Liu Guanhui et al. reported that the mice were subjected to restraint stress from embryonic day1 (E1). This study demonstrated that restraint stress increased the level of corticosterone (CORT) in plasma, and uterine natural killer (uNK) cells in the endometrium were significantly increased, accompanied by the decreased density of mast cells in the myometrium. In addition, restraint stress markedly decreased the CD3$^+$CD4$^+$ T/CD3$^+$CD8$^+$ T cell ratio. Additionally, antioxidant ability was compromised, and the concentration of MDA was increased [86]. Moreover, restraint stress reduced the weight of the uterus and ovary and the intake of food with reduction in weight, while the relative endometrial area and uterine gland area were reduced after restraint stress. In addition, restraint stress decreased micro-vessel density and VEGF expression [87].

The signaling molecules between oxidative stress and reproduction

OS has led to a variety of signaling pathways, resulting in crosstalk among many protein factors in the body. Especially in the female reproductive organs, OS leads to a series of abnormal events in egg production and ovulation. During pregnancy, implantation will be impaired, leading to loss of embryos and changes in local immune function in the uterus. Research on these signals is currently the most important concept in this field and is of great significance to the reproduction of female animals.

Before this review, there were a number of reviews discussing the contact between reproduction and OS. For example, Perucci et al. proposed a hypothesis that the ADAMs pathway protects women from the inflammatory lesions of preeclampsia [88]. Wu et al. elaborated on potential therapeutic approaches to placental stress by exploring the relationship between OS and apoptosis and between OS and cellular autophagy, resulting in speculation about a comprehensive therapeutic target [89]. Sultana et al. fully summarized the adverse pregnancy outcomes caused by aging placentas, explaining the mechanisms of telomerase and placental disorders [59]. Wojsiat et al. explained the effects of OS on oocyte and fertilization outcomes and the effect of overproduction of active substances on in vitro fertilization [90]. Nevertheless, our review not only summarizes the above discussion but also makes reasonable assumptions about the signaling pathways in reproductive diseases.

Hypoxia and inflammation lead to the production of TNF-α, which induces the release of large amounts of ROS from the mitochondria in cells. Excessive ROS cause an imbalance between oxidation and antioxidation, leading to OS. The body's signaling pathway will evince a series of changes following to exposure to the dual impact of OS and inflammation. This article focuses on the collection of OS-induced reproductive disease-related signaling pathways, including the p38 MAPK pathway,

the Kelch-like ECH-associated protein 1 (Keap1)-Nuclear factor erythroid 2-related factor 2 (Nrf2) pathway, the Jun N-terminal kinase (JNK) pathway, the forkhead transcription factors of the O class (FOXO) family, and apoptosis.

Nrf2 is a key molecule activated in response to OS, and it regulates antioxidant response to protect cell function [91]. Normally, Nrf2 binds to Keap1, is sequestered in the cytoplasm, and then is degraded by a proteasome pathway [92]. After activation, it transfers to the nucleus to activate a large number of antioxidant genes [93]. In other words, transcriptional activation of antioxidant defense genes and restoration of vascular redox homeostasis are necessary when OS occurs. Importantly, the redox-sensitive Keap1-Nrf2 pathway plays a key role in the process [94]. These studies also implied that Nrf2 deficiency caused fetal DNA damage and neurological deficits, and inactivation of Nrf2 has also been shown to underlie inflammation-induced trophoblastic apoptosis. As studies have progressed, the literature has increasingly revealed that Nrf2 plays a significant role in pregnancy and has highlighted the important role of Nrf2 in protecting the fetus in utero OS [95]. Nrf2 is sensitive to maternal immunological status. In normal pregnancy, Nrf2 is only decreased after term vaginal delivery. However, notably, the expression of Nrf2 is significantly reduced when the uterus is infected [96]. Furthermore, the mechanism of Nrf2 antioxidant defense plays an important role in adverse pregnancy priming. Nrf2 is a regulator of antioxidant defense in vascular dysfunction and oxidative damage [95]. Many studies have shown that suitable OS increased Nrf2 and the expression of downstream targets, such as heme oxygenase 1 (HO-1), NAD(P)H: quinoneoxidoreductase (NQO1), and glutamate-cysteine ligase subunit catalysis (GCLC), etc., to resist OS [97]. However, as described above, we speculate that the activity of Nrf2 significantly decreases, and Keap1 binds to Nrf2 more strongly when excessive OS causes severe inflammation in the uterus. Related studies have shown that FOXO3 participates in the interaction between Keap1 and Nrf2. Loss of FOXO3 leads to severe inactivation of Keap1, which in turn cannot prevent the activation of Nrf2, which is a very important finding in tumors. Research also revealed the important role of FOXO3 in the Keap1-Nrf2 axis. At the same time, it is not denied that, in the absence of FOXO3, Nrf2 is activated under the induction of AKT and protects cells from damage due to OS by this form [98]. Therefore, we hypothesize that, if OS induces inflammation in the reproductive system, the changes in FOXO3 affect the interaction between Keap1 and Nrf2, which could be a marker of damaging OS in our study (Table 2).

NF-κB is an active molecule in the immune system. In mammals, the NF-κB family is composed of five related transcription factors: c-Rel, p50, p52, RelB and RelA

Table 2 The important proteins in reproductive mechanisms

Protein	Function and role in reproductive process	Interaction between proteins	Reference
Keap1-Nrf2 pathway	Keap1: Keap1 binds to Nrf2 in cytoplasm. Nrf2: Protects cells under moderate oxidative stress A regulator of antioxidant defense in vascular dysfunction and oxidative damage. Deletion of Nrf2 → Fetal DNA damage and nervous system defects (the basis of trophoblast cell apoptosis). Vaginal delivery and Uterine infection: Nrf2↓	The right amount of OS → Nrf2↑ → HO-1↑,NQO1↑,GCLC↑ Excessive OS → FOXO3↑ → Ability of Keap1 to bind to Nrf2↑ Deletion of FOXO3: OS↑ → AKT↑ → Nrf2↑	[91–93, 95–98]
NF-κB pathway	An active molecule in the immune system; Redox-Sensitive transcription factors Placental stress: OS → NF-κB↑ → Pro-inflammatory Cytokines↑ → Placental apoptotic process is activated Endometriosis: OS↑ → TNF-α↑ → NF-κB↑ In vitro: IL-1β → NF-κB↑ → MIF↑, TNF-α↑	Inhibitory IκB protein family binds to NF-κB in cytoplasm IKKB protein is degraded (IKKα, IKKβ, NEMO mediate) → NF-κB enters nuclear to regulate target gene. IKKβ↑ → p-FOXO3↑ Deletion of FOXO3 → NF-κB↓ FOXO3↑ → BCL10↑ → IKKβ↓ → NF-κB↑ → Anti-apoptosis gene↑	[2, 99–104, 108, 109]
FOXO family	FOXO1(all tissues): Deletion of FOXO1, embryonic cell death due to incomplete blood vessel development FOXO3(all tissues): Deletion of FOXO1, lymphocyte proliferation, extensive organ inflammation FOXO4 (muscle, kidney, colorectal): Deletion of FOXO4, inflammation of the colon in response to inflammatory stimuli FOXO6(brain, liver): Deletion of FOXO6, shows normal learning, but memory consolidation is impaired FOXO1↑ → Apoptotic pathway in decidual stromal cells, and Inhibits endometrial epithelial cell growth	FOXO1↑ → WNT4↑,PRL↑,IGFBP1↑ JNK↑ → FOXO1↑ → MnSOD↑, CAT↑ → Protecting cells	[111, 112, 115–120]
MAPK family	JNK: Activated by stress and inflammation P38 MAPK: Activated by stress and inflammation ERK: Activated by inflammation and growth factors OS↑ → p38 MAPK↑ → Aging and premature aging of fetal tissue Endometriosis: ERK↑ Endometrial stromal cells: time of p-ERK↑; OS↑ → ERK↑,H_2O_2↑ → p-ERK↑	JNK↑ → FOXO1↑ → MnSOD↑, CAT↑ → Protecting cells P450↑ → ROS↑ → ASK1-P-p38 MAPK	[118, 121, 123–126, 129, 130]

The '→' indicates that it has an effect on the next step. The '↑' represents an increase and the '↓'represents a decrease

(a.k.a. p65) [99]. NF-κB is the nodal point of a primary inflammation-stimulated signaling pathway that plays a significant role in the immune response [100], while NF-κB is also a redox-sensitive transcription factor [101]. Therefore, its effect is self-evident in OS, including embryonic stresses. The NF-κB pathway is activated when embryonic stresses occurs, and a variety of pro-inflammatory cytokines is increased. Then, the apoptotic process of the placenta is activated [2]. Therefore, this study indicated that NF-κB controls cell survival through the enhancement of anti-apoptotic gene transcription. In most cells, the NF-κB complex is inactive, and it is mainly present in the cytoplasm by binding to the inhibitory IκB protein family. When the NF-κB pathway is activated, the IκB protein is degraded, NF-κB complex enters the nucleus to modulate the expression of target genes, and the degradation of IκB protein is mediated through the IκB kinase (IKK) complex, which consists of two catalytically active kinases (IKKα and IKKβ) and the regulatory scaffold protein NEMO. In the activation pathway, IKKβ and NEMO are very necessary for activation of the complex [102], while IKKβ also acts on other factors, such as Forkhead box O3, a transcription regulator. A study showed that FOXO3 is subject to IKKβ-mediated phosphorylation, leading to the nuclear exclusion and degradation of FOXO3 [103]. In addition, a study reported that FOXO3 was a positive regulator of NF-κB signaling and found that over-expression of FOXO3 increased and knockdown of FOXO3 repressed NF-κB activities. The study indicated that FOXO3 activated NF-κB by inducing expression of B-cell lymphoma/leukemia 10 (BCL10), an upstream regulator of inhibitor of kappa B kinase (IKK)/NF-κB signaling [104]. In reproductive stress diseases, for example, endometriosis, increased expression of NF-κB has been confirmed in cultured endometriotic stromal cells [105] and peritoneal macrophages isolated from women with endometriomas [106]. In any case, changes in NF-κB are strongly associated with inflammation. Endometriosis is a disease caused by OS during reproductive. OS leads to an increase in TNF-α, which in turn causes inflammation, and the NF-κB pathway is activated. Additionally, in vitro evidence raised the possibility that the changes might be due to the endometriotic microenvironment. IL-1β stimulates NF-κB with subsequent increased production of inflammatory cytokines [107], including macrophage migration inhibitory factor (MIF) in endometrial stromal cells [108] and TNF-α in the immortalized epithelial (12Z) cell line [109]. In conclusion, the NF-κB pathway is activated when reproductive OS occurs (Table 2).

FOXO1, the same family as FOXO3, is also involved in the processes of OS and pregnancy. The FOXO subfamily of Forkhead transcription factors is a direct downstream target of the PI3K/Akt pathway [110]. The mammalian forkhead transcription factors of the O class

(FOXOs) number four: FOXO1, FOXO3, FOXO4, and FOXO6. Further, FOXO1 and FOXO3 exist in nearly all tissues. FOXO4 is highly expressed in the muscle and kidneys, and FOXO6 is primarily expressed in the brain and liver. They are involved in the processes of proliferation, apoptosis, autophagy, metabolism, inflammation, differentiation and stress tolerance [111]. However, FOXO1 plays a significant role in reproduction. It regulates cyclic differentiation and apoptosis in the normal endometrium [112]. Additionally, genome-wide expression profiling demonstrated that FOXO1 knockdown perturbs the expression of more than 500 types of genes in decidualizing human endometrial stromal cells [113]. In the past, many studies of human endometrium provided reliable evidence for this ability of FOXO transcription factors to regulate diverse genes in response to change hormones [114]. However, the interaction between progesterone and FOXO1 is even more striking. It is well known that progesterone exerts inhibitory effects on endometrial epithelial growth, and a study revealed this mechanism and showed that siRNA inhibition of FOXO1 significantly attenuated the effects of progestin in inhibiting endometrial epithelial cell growth. Therefore, FOXO1 is essential for the anti-proliferative effects of progesterone on both endometrial stromal and epithelial cells [115].

Further, FOXO1 is indispensable for the induction of the most highly responsive decidual marker genes, including WNT4, prolactin (PRL) and insulin-like growth factor-binding protein 1 (IGFBP1) [116]. It has been found that FOXO1 activates apoptotic pathways in decidual stromal cells. The pro-apoptotic Bcl-2 homology 3 domain-only protein BIM is a major intermediate in this pathway [117]. It was validated that BIM is a FOXO1 target gene and is induced under the stimulation of cAMP. Both cAMP and progestin promote increases in FOXO1, but BIM is only increased and cell death occurs when progestin disappears [120]. Additionally, targeted phosphorylation of cytoplasmic FOXO factors by JNK promotes nuclear import and increases cellular protection against OS via the transcriptional activation of MnSOD and CAT [118]. Thus, FOXO1 has emerged as a major regulator of progesterone-dependent differentiation of human endometrium and subsequent process (Fig. 7) [119]. Thoughtfully, FOXO1 is markedly induced upon decidualization both in vivo and in vitro, whereas FOXO3 expression is suppressed [120]. At any rate, FOXO1 plays a unique role either in reproduction or in OS (Table 2).

The extracellular environment activates three pathways, with ERK predominantly activated by inflammation and growth factors, while JNK and p38 MAPK are predominantly activated by stress and inflammation [121]. Additionally, studies by Lee et al. showed that ROS generated by dysfunctional electron transport in

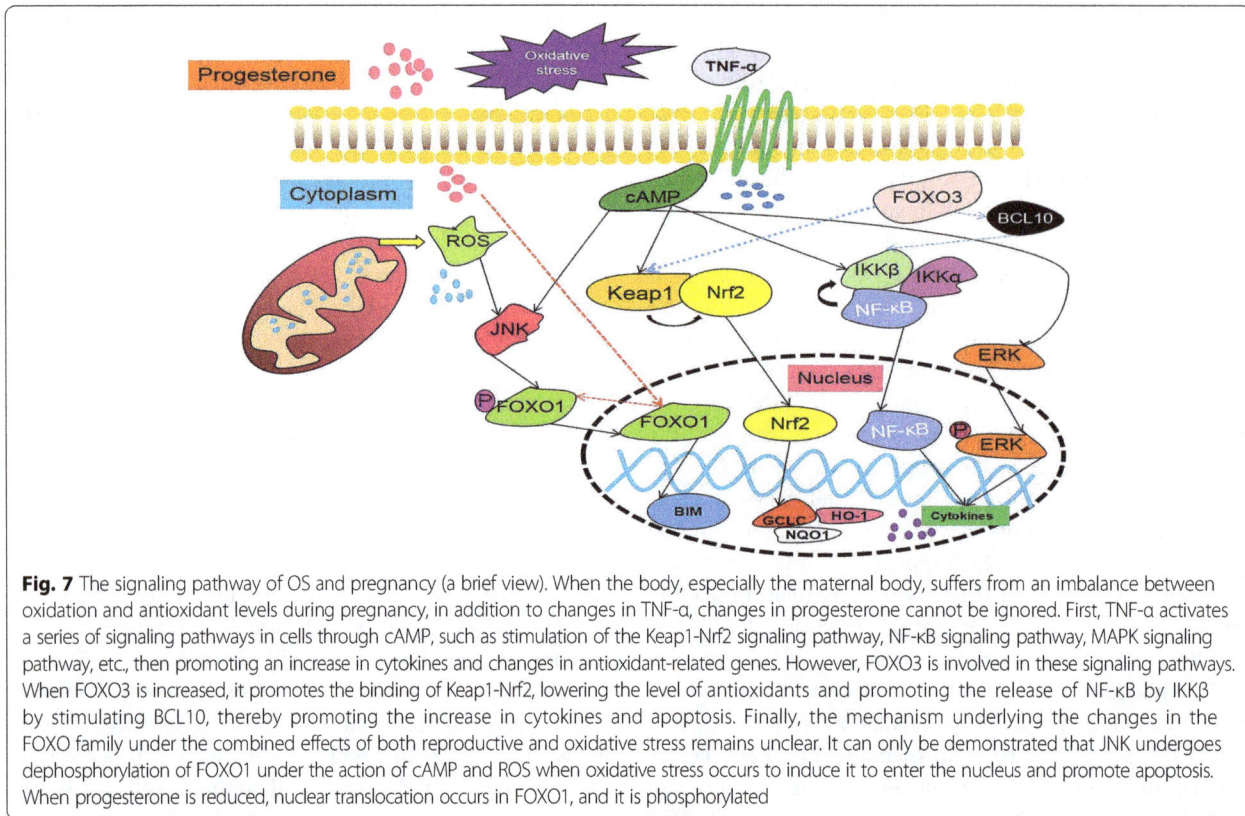

Fig. 7 The signaling pathway of OS and pregnancy (a brief view). When the body, especially the maternal body, suffers from an imbalance between oxidation and antioxidant levels during pregnancy, in addition to changes in TNF-α, changes in progesterone cannot be ignored. First, TNF-α activates a series of signaling pathways in cells through cAMP, such as stimulation of the Keap1-Nrf2 signaling pathway, NF-κB signaling pathway, MAPK signaling pathway, etc., then promoting an increase in cytokines and changes in antioxidant-related genes. However, FOXO3 is involved in these signaling pathways. When FOXO3 is increased, it promotes the binding of Keap1-Nrf2, lowering the level of antioxidants and promoting the release of NF-κB by IKKβ by stimulating BCL10, thereby promoting the increase in cytokines and apoptosis. Finally, the mechanism underlying the changes in the FOXO family under the combined effects of both reproductive and oxidative stress remains unclear. It can only be demonstrated that JNK undergoes dephosphorylation of FOXO1 under the action of cAMP and ROS when oxidative stress occurs to induce it to enter the nucleus and promote apoptosis. When progesterone is reduced, nuclear translocation occurs in FOXO1, and it is phosphorylated

mitochondria activate the inflammatory ASK1-P-p38 MAPK pathway [122]. The recent literature has identified the physiologic aging of fetal tissues as a potential mechanistic feature of normal parturition. This process is affected by telomere-dependent and p38 MAPK-induced senescence activation (Fig. 7). Pregnancy-associated risk factors can cause pathologic activation of this pathway, causing OS-induced p38 MAPK activation and leading to senescence and premature aging of fetal tissues [123, 124].

It has been reported that the activation of ERK was increased in endometriotic tissue, suggesting that ERK might play a role in endometriosis pathogenesis, and phosphorylated ERK is increased in primary eutopic epithelial cells [125, 126]. Prolonged phosphorylation of ERK in endometrial stromal cells occurs in women with endometriosis, compared with women without endometriosis [127]. Therefore, the endometriotic microenvironment could induce increased ERK activity in ectopic cells. Although only IL-1β-induced cyclo-oxygenase 2 (COX2) production and IL-8 secretion could be attenuated by the ERK1/2-specific inhibitor PD98059, both TNF-α and IL-1β activate ERK and induce the expression of IL-8 and IL-6 [128]. However, another study found that the IL-1β-mediated COX2 expression was not affected when ERK inhibition occurs in endometriotic stromal cells, but it occurred rather through p38 MAPK activation [129]. OS may also contribute to ERK

activation. H_2O_2 induces ERK phosphorylation in endometriotic stromal cells with a more serious induction compared with stromal cells from women who do not have endometriosis [130]. Today, although, no direct relationship between phosphorylated ERK (p-ERK) activation and OS is confirmed, an increase in OS markers is discovered in epithelial and stromal cells derived from women with endometriosis in a similar pattern to p-ERK level (Table 2).

Conclusion

Based on the above, OS influences the entire reproductive process of woman. The production of excessive ROS leads to OS events. ROS, including superoxide ($O_2^-\bullet$), hydrogen peroxide (H_2O_2) and hydroxyl ($\bullet OH$), cause DNA damage, lipid per-oxidation and protein damage. The antioxidative system is activated when slight OS occurred, such as SOD and GPx. In addition, when ROS levels exceed the scavenging capacity of the system, the redox system can repair oxidized and damage molecules using NADPH as an original electron source in such situations. Thus, the maintenance of high redox potential is a prerequisite for maintaining the reproductive systems in a healthy state [15].

In this review, we mainly introduced the relative reproductive diseases caused by OS and a series of signaling pathways, including in PCOS, endometriosis, preeclampsia and so on. They switch on a variety of molecules, including NF-κB, MAPK, FOXO and Keap1-Nrf2. In the above descriptions, we found that the role of each molecule is not independent and that they will form networks and interactions between them, leading to the complexity of signal molecule research. The OS that occurs during reproduction activates many molecules, but the interaction among them is not very clear, requiring us to determine the signaling cues in other organs or other diseases.

It is speculated that we know that the FOXO protein family is involved in the signaling pathways of Keap1-Nrf2 and NF-κB. There are also subtle relationships between the various subtypes of the MAPK family. Therefore, regarding OS in the reproductive process, we can verify these viewpoints to better address the relationship between OS and reproductive harm. A large part of reproductive disease is caused by inflammation in the reproductive organs, leading to changes in the inflammatory factors that promote the body's protection or, in severe cases, promote cell death.

Compared to other diseases, disease research in the reproductive system is complicated, especially in humans or females during pregnancy. This complexity requires us to concretize the experimental period and break it down. In this discussion, we summarize the following. First, OS is involved in the development of diseases of the reproductive system, and it plays the role of a double-edged sword. Second, to a large extent, OS impairs the reproductive organs, including the placenta. Third, the inflammatory environment caused by OS causes a series of signal activations in the uterus. Fourth, the connection between OS and progesterone causes the reproductive process to become obstructed. Finally, we can re-examine the future development trends in reproductive system diseases by speculating on the relationship between these signaling molecules.

Female animals also undergo complex reproductive changes during the course of their illnesses and their deaths. In this review, the follicular development of animals, the development of fertilized eggs, and the processes of hormone changes are demonstrated. OS-related reproductive diseases have also been elucidated. By speculating on the changes in other diseases and on the factors related to reproductive diseases in cells in the face of reproductive system diseases, this article provides some institutional recommendations. This common point of these signals is that they are activated during inflammatory processes induced by OS. Under the influence of TNF-α, cAMP messengers are activated, causing massive release of ROS in the mitochondria and deposition in the cytoplasm. Further, NF-κB, FOXO, and the MAPK family are induced. IKKβ releases NF-κB into the nucleus, resulting in a large number of cytokines

increasing and promoting apoptosis. Further, FOXO3 directs the activation of BCL10, thus controlling NF-κB activity, but it is also activated through AKT pathway. ROS activate JNK to target phosphorylated FOXO1 in the cytoplasm to promote transcription into the nucleus. Progesterone's antiproliferative effect on uterine epithelial cells is affected by FOXO1, and an increase in progesterone activates FOXO1 to release into the nucleus. Under the influence of TNF-α and IL-1β, the MAPK family is activated. When ERK is inhibited, p38 MAPK joins the battle, playing the same role as ERK.

In addition, Nrf2 plays an important role in mitigating OS-induced cellular dysfunction and developmental defects. Continued exposure to OS in postnatal and later life periods can further exacerbate the loss of Nrf2-regulated antioxidant defenses established in utero and thereby enhance susceptibility to disease in offspring. The Nrf2 antioxidant defense pathway might therefore provide a therapeutic target for ameliorating OS associated with adverse pregnancies and could provide an opportunity to modulate developmental priming via OS.

Although Nrf2 is a master regulator of cellular redox homeostasis following stress, Nrf2 activity in vascular and other cell types is known to decline [131] and could play an important role in age-related cellular dysfunction and disease onset. As highlighted by Zhang et al. in a special issue [132], the molecular mechanisms underlying the loss of response to OS by the Keap1-Nrf2 defense pathway in aging remain to be elucidated. Keap1-Nrf2 is the most classical pathway in OS, and it has also been shown in recent studies to play an important role in fetal development.

In conclusion, FOXO, as a key node of the signaling pathway, plays an important role in the signaling network and is a factor worth studying.

Future directions

In the future, a strategy to reinforce the antioxidant defense system and target the mitochondria will be a huge step. To increase the antioxidant capacity of the body, we must decrease the production of ROS from the mitochondrial electron transport chain that occurs in response to high glucose and fatty acid levels and decrease ROS production without significantly affecting ATP production. At the same time, we should increase the degradation of intracellular ROS and increase the bioavailability of antioxidants, and their passage through the barriers must be considered. Targeting the mitochondria and increase its overall antioxidant defense system will be a challenge. It is now considered certain that the pharmacological effects of antioxidants depend on their targeting. The delivery of antioxidants to mitochondria is a field of active research [133].

In addition, if these signaling molecules were studied completely, we would develop many blocking agents to prevent the occurrence of damage. ROS-activated JNK molecules and their downstream FOXO transcription factors (also involved in reproductive events) are worth exploring. In addition, OS-induced NF-κB signaling molecules should be linked to the molecules of the reproductive process, and for the future better study of reproductive diseases, drugs have very important research value. As we all know, an increasing number of social diseases attack our bodies, and some aging questions also perplex us. The mechanisms described in this review have important implications for these diseases, and the silence of certain factors in the FOXO family can cause activation of the antioxidant mechanism, the role of which in tumor diseases cannot be underestimated, so the study of OS in the study of cell protection mechanisms is unique and critical for the mechanism of disease.

Abbreviations

8-OHDG: 8-hydroxy-deoxyguanosine; BCL10: B-cell lymphoma/leukemia 10; CAT: Catalase; CL: Corpus luteum; CORT: Corticosterone; COX2: Cyclo-oxygenase 2; Cu-Zn SOD: Copper-zinc SOD; ERK1/2: Extracellular regulated kinase 1/2; ETC: Electron transport chain; FSH: Follicle-stimulating hormone; GCLC: Glutamate-cysteine ligase subunit catalysis; GPx: Glutathione peroxidase; GSR: Glutathione reductase; HCG: Human chorionic gonadotropin; HO-1: Heme oxygenase 1; IGFBP1: Insulin-like growth factor-binding protein 1; IKK: Inhibitor of nuclear factor kappa-B kinase; IUGR: Intrauterine growth restriction; JNK: Jun N-terminal kinase; Keap1: Kelch-like ECH-associated protein 1; MAPK: Mitogen-activated protein kinase; MCP-1: Monocyte chemoattractant protein-1; MDA: Malondialdehyde; MIF: Migration inhibitory factor; MnSoD: Manganese superoxide dismutase; NAC: N-acetylcysteine; NADP(H): Nicotinamide adenine dinucleotide phosphate; NF-κB: Nuclear factor-kappa B; NQO1: NAD(P)H dehydrogenase (quinone 1); OS: Oxidative stress; ox-LDL: Oxidized LDL; PCOS: Polycystic ovary syndrome; $PGF_{2\alpha}$: Prostaglandin-F-2α; PRL: Prolactin; SO: Superoxide; SOD: Superoxide dismutase; TAS: Total antioxidant status; TNF-α: Tumor necrosis factor-α; uNK: Uterine natural killer; VEGF: Vascular endothelial growth factor

Acknowledgements
The finalization of this article relies on the opinions of the authors of all of the papers. We are very grateful for their contributions to this article. In addition, the present study was supported by the National Natural Science Foundation of China (grant nos. 31572476, 31272483, 31372332) and National Natural Science Foundation of Beijing (grant no. 6172022).

Funding
The present study was supported by the National Natural Science Foundation of China (grant nos. 31572476, 31272483, 31372332) and the National Natural Science Foundation of Beijing (grant no. 6172022).

Authors' contributions
JYL and YLD contributed to the initial literature search, acquisition of data, analysis and design of the first draft of the article. YXC and ZXW were included in reviewing the manuscript and further revision of it. JC was mainly responsible for designing illustrations and graphs, and YLD proofread the final manuscript before submission. All of the authors read and approved the final manuscript.

Competing interests
The authors declare that they have no competing interests.

References
1. Burton GJ, Jauniaux E. Oxidative stress. Best Practice & Research Clinical Obstetrics & Gynaecology. 2011;25:287–99.
2. Cindrova-Davies T, Yung HW, Johns J, Spasic-Boskovic O, Korolchuk S, Jauniaux E, Burton GJ, Charnock-Jones DS. Oxidative stress, gene expression, and protein changes induced in the human placenta during labor. Am J Pathol. 2007;171:1168–79.
3. Ruder EH, Hartman TJ, Goldman MB. Impact of oxidative stress on female fertility. Current Opinion in Obstetrics & Gynecology. 2009;21:219–22.
4. Attaran M, Pasqualotto E, Falcone T, Goldberg JM, Miller KF, Agarwal A, Sharma RK. The effect of follicular fluid reactive oxygen species on the outcome of in vitro fertilization. International Journal of Fertility and Womens Medicine. 2000;45:314–20.
5. Szczepanska M, Kozlik J, Skrzypczak J, Mikolajczyk M. Oxidative stress may be a piece in the endometriosis puzzle. Fertil Steril. 2003;79:1288–93.
6. Van Langendonckt A, Casanas-Roux F, Donnez J. Oxidative stress and peritoneal endometriosis. Fertil Steril. 2002;77:861–70.
7. Pierce JD, Cackler AB, Arnett MG. Why should you care about free radicals? Rn. 2004;67:38–42.
8. Agarwal A. Role of oxidative stress in endometriosis. Reprod BioMed Online. 2006;13:126–34.
9. Agarwal A, Allamaneni SSR. Role of free radicals in female reproductive diseases and assisted reproduction. Reprod BioMed Online. 2004;9:338–47.
10. Gupta S, Agarwal A, Banerjee J, Alvarez JG. The role of oxidative stress in spontaneous abortion and recurrent pregnancy loss: a systematic review. Obstetrical & Gynecological Survey. 2007;62:335–47.
11. Agarwal A, Gupta S, Sekhon L, Shah R. Redox considerations in female reproductive function and assisted reproduction: from molecular mechanisms to health implications. Antioxid Redox Signal. 2008;10:1375–403.
12. Valko M, Leibfritz D, Moncol J, Cronin MTD, Mazur M, Telser J. Free radicals and antioxidants in normal physiological functions and human disease. Int J Biochem Cell Biol. 2007;39:44–84.
13. Banks WJ. Applied veterinary histology. 2nd ed. Baltimore, MD: William and Wilkins; 1981.
14. Al-Gubory KH, Fowler PA, Garrel C. The roles of cellular reactive oxygen species, oxidative stress and antioxidants in pregnancy outcomes. Int J Biochem Cell Biol. 2010;42:1634–50.
15. Fujii J, Iuchi Y, Okada F: Fundamental roles of reactive oxygen species and protective mechanisms in the female reproductive system. Reproductive Biology and Endocrinology 2005, 3:10%18 Sep %19 review %! Fundamental roles of reactive oxygen species and protective mechanisms in the female reproductive system.
16. Murphy MP. How mitochondria produce reactive oxygen species. Biochem J. 2009;417:1–13.
17. Dhaunsi GS, Gulati S, Singh AK, Orak JK, Asayama K, Singh I. Demonstration of cu-ZN superoxide-dismutase in rat-liver peroxisomes - biochemical and immunochemical evidence. J Biol Chem. 1992;267:6870–3.
18. Oberley LW. Mechanism of the tumor suppressive effect of MnSOD overexpression. Biomed Pharmacother. 2005;59:143–8.
19. Harris ED. Regulation of antioxidant enzymes. FASEB J. 1992;6:2675–83.
20. Spallholz JE, Roveri A, Yan L, Boylan LM, Kang CR, Ursini F. Glutathione-peroxidase and phospholipid HYDROPEROXIDE glutathione-peroxidase in tissues of BALB/c mice. FASEB J. 1991;5:A714.
21. Proctor PH, Reynolds ES. Free-radicals and disease in man. Physiol Chem Phys Med NMR. 1984;16:175–95.
22. Davies KJA, Wiese AG, Sevanian A, Kim EH: REPAIR SYSTEMS IN OXIDATIVE STRESS. Finch, C E and T E Johnson (Ed) Ucla (University of California-Los Angeles) Symposia on Molecular and Cellular Biology New Series, Vol 123 Molecular Biology of Aging; Colloquium, Sante Fe, New Mexico, USA, March 4-10, 1989 Xvii+430p Wiley-Liss: New York, New York, USA Illus 1990:123–142.
23. Ketterer B, Meyer DJ. Glutathione TRANSFERASE - a possible role in the DETOXICATION and repair of DNA and lipid HYDROPEROXIDES. Mutat Res. 1989;214:33–40.
24. Kurlak LO, Green A, Loughna P, Pipkin FB. Oxidative stress markers in hypertensive states of pregnancy: preterm and term disease. Front Physiol. 2014;5:310.
25. Sharma RK, Agarwal A. Role of reactive oxygen species in gynecologic diseases. Reproductive Medicine and Biology. 2004;3:177–99.

26. Ishikawa M. Oxygen radicals-superoxide dismutase system and reproduction medicine. Nihon Sanka Fujinka Gakkai zasshi. 1993;45:842–8.

27. Shkolnik K, Tadmor A, Ben-Dor S, Nevo N, Galiani D, Dekel N. Reactive oxygen species are indispensable in ovulation. Proc Natl Acad Sci U S A. 2011;108:1462–7.

28. Suzuki T, Sugino N, Fukaya T, Sugiyama S, Uda T, Takaya R, Yajima A, Sasano H. Superoxide dismutase in normal cycling human ovaries: immunohistochemical localization and characterization. Fertil Steril. 1999;72:720–6.

29. Tamate K, Sengoku K, Ishikawa M. The role of superoxide dismutase in the human ovary and fallopian tube. J Obstet Gynaecol (Tokyo 1995). 1995;21:401–9.

30. Geva E, Jaffe RB. Role of angiopoietins in reproductive tract angiogenesis. Obstetrical & Gynecological Survey. 2000;55:511–9.

31. Gordon JD, Mesiano S, Zaloudek CJ, Jaffe RB. Vascular endothelial growth factor localization in human ovary and fallopian tubes: possible role in reproductive function and ovarian cyst formation. J Clin Endocrinol Metab. 1996;81:353–9.

32. Albrecht ED, Babischkin JS, Lidor Y, Anderson LD, Udoff LC, Pepe GJ. Effect of estrogen on angiogenesis in co-cultures of human endometrial cells and microvascular endothelial cells. Hum Reprod. 2003;18:2039–47.

33. Ushio-Fukai M, Alexander RW. Reactive oxygen species as mediators of angiogenesis signaling - role of NAD(P)H oxidase. Mol Cell Biochem. 2004;264:85–97.

34. Miyazaki T, Sueoka K, Dharmarajan AM, Atlas SJ, Bulkley GB, Wallach EE. Effect of inhibition of oxygen free-radical on ovulation and progesterone production by the INVITRO perfused rabbit ovary. J Reprod Fertil. 1991;91:207–12.

35. Behrman HR, Kodaman PH, Preston SL, Gao SP. Oxidative stress and the ovary. J Soc Gynecol Investig. 2001;8:S40–2.

36. Richards JS. Hormonal control of gene expression in the ovary. Endocr Rev. 1994;15:725–51.

37. Du BT, Takahashi K, Ishida GM, Nakahara K, Saito H, Kurachi H. Usefulness of intralovarian artery pulsatility and resistance indices measurement on the day of follicle aspiration for the assessment of oocyte quality. Fertil Steril. 2006;85:366–70.

38. Sugino N. Roles of reactive oxygen species in the corpus luteum. Anim Sci J. 2006;77:556–65.

39. Agarwal A, Aponte-Mellado A, Premkumar BJ, Shaman A, Gupta S. The effects of oxidative stress on female reproduction: a review. Reprod Biol Endocrinol. 2012;10:31.

40. Ahmed A, Cudmore MJ. Can the biology of VEGF and haem oxygenases help solve pre-eclampsia? Biochem Soc Trans. 2009;37:1237–42.

41. Szpera-Gozdziewicz A, Breborowicz GH. Endothelial dysfunction in the pathogenesis of pre-eclampsia. Frontiers in Bioscience-Landmark. 2014;19:734–46.

42. Morohashi K, Iida H, Nomura M, Hatano O, Honda S, Tsukiyama T, Niwa O, Hara T, Takakusu A, Shibata Y, Omura T. Functional difference between AD4BP and ELP, and their distributions in STEROIDOGENIC tissues. Mol Endocrinol. 1994;8:643–53.

43. Vega M, Carrasco I, Castillo T, Troncoso JL, Videla LA, Devoto L. Functional LUTEOLYSIS in response to hydrogen-peroxide in human luteal cells. J Endocrinol. 1995;147:177–82.

44. Tamura H, Takasaki A, Miwa I, Tanoguchi K, Maekawa R, Asada H, Taketani T, Matsuoka A, Yamagata Y, Shimamura K, et al. Oxidative stress impairs oocyte quality and melatonin protects oocytes from free radical damage and improves fertilization rate. J Pineal Res. 2008;44:280–7.

45. Fauser B, Chang J, Azziz R, Legro R, Dewailly D, Franks S, Tarlatzis BC, Fauser B, Balen A, Bouchard P, et al. Revised 2003 consensus on diagnostic criteria and long-term health risks related to polycystic ovary syndrome (PCOS). Hum Reprod. 2004(19):41–7.

46. Costello MF, Shrestha B, Eden J, Johnson NP, Sjoblom P. Metformin versus oral contraceptive pill in polycystic ovary syndrome: a Cochrane review. Hum Reprod. 2007;22:1200–9.

47. Hilali N, Vural M, Camuzcuoglu H, Camuzcuoglu A, Aksoy N. Increased prolidase activity and oxidative stress in PCOS. Clin Endocrinol. 2013;79:105–10.

48. Cimino I, Casoni F, Liu X, Messina A, Parkash J, Jamin SP, Catteau-Jonard S, Collier F, Baroncini M, Dewailly D, et al. Novel role for anti-Mullerian hormone in the regulation of GnRH neuron excitability and hormone secretion. Nat Commun. 2016;7:10055.

49. Franks S, Mc Carthy M, Hardy K. Development of polycystic ovary syndrome: involvement of genetic and environmental factors. Int J Androl. 2006;29:278–85.

50. Escobar-Morreale HF, Luque-Ramírez M, San Millán JL. The molecular-genetic basis of functional hyperandrogenism and the polycystic ovary syndrome. Endocr Rev. 2005;26:251–82.

51. Bremer AA, Miller WL. The serine phosphorylation hypothesis of polycystic ovary syndrome: a unifying mechanism of hyperandrogenemia and insulin resistance. Fertil Steril. 2008;89:1039–48.

52. Myatt L, Cui XL. Oxidative stress in the placenta. Histochem Cell Biol. 2004;122:369–82.

53. Wisdom SJ, Wilson R, McKillop JH, Walker JJ. Antioxidant systems in normal-pregnancy and in pregnancy-induced hypertension. Am J Obstet Gynecol. 1991;165:1701–4.

54. Wang Y, Walsh SW. Placental mitochondria as a source of oxidative stress in pre-eclampsia. Placenta. 1998;19:581–6.

55. Jauniaux E, Gulbis B, Burton GJ. The human first trimester gestational sac limits rather than facilitates oxygen transfer to the foetus--a review. Placenta. 2003;24(Suppl A):S86–93.

56. Lim KH, Zhou Y, Janatpour M, McMaster M, Bass K, Chun SH, Fisher SJ. Human cytotrophoblast differentiation/invasion is abnormal in pre-eclampsia. Am J Pathol. 1997;151:1809–18.

57. Jaffe R, Jauniaux E, Hustin J. Maternal circulation in the first-trimester human placenta - myth or reality? Am J Obstet Gynecol. 1997;176:695–705.

58. Jauniaux E, Watson AL, Hempstock J, Bao YP, Skepper JN, Burton GJ. Onset of maternal arterial blood flow and placental oxidative stress - a possible factor in human early pregnancy failure. Am J Pathol. 2000;157:2111–22.

59. Sultana Z, Maiti K, Aitken J, Morris J, Dedman L, Smith R. Oxidative stress, placental aging-related pathologies and adverse pregnancy outcomes. Am J Reprod Immunol. 2017;77: e12653.

60. Witorsch RJ. Effects of elevated glucocorticoids on reproduction and development: relevance to endocrine disruptor screening. Crit Rev Toxicol. 2016;46:420–36.

61. Preutthipan S, Chen SH, Tilly JL, Kugu K, Lareu RR, Dharmarajan AM. Inhibition of nitric oxide synthesis potentiates apoptosis in the rabbit corpus luteum. Reprod BioMed Online. 2004;9:264–70.

62. Ghafourifar P, Richter C. Nitric oxide synthase activity in mitochondria. FEBS Lett. 1997;418:291–6.

63. Wang YP, Walsh SW, Guo JD, Zhang JY. Maternal levels of prostacyclin, thromboxane, vitamin-E, and lipid peroxides throughout normal-pregnancy. Am J Obstet Gynecol. 1991;165:1690–4.

64. Menon R, Fortunato SJ, Yu J, Milne GL, Sanchez S, Drobek CO, Lappas M, Taylor RN. Cigarette smoke induces oxidative stress and apoptosis in normal term fetal membranes. Placenta. 2011;32:317–22.

65. Sbrana E, Suter MA, Abramovici AR, Hawkins HK, Moss JE, Patterson L, Shope C, Aagaard-Tillery K. Maternal tobacco use is associated with increased markers of oxidative stress in the placenta. Am J Obstet Gynecol. 2011;205:7.

66. Smith R, Maiti K, Aitken RJ. Unexplained antepartum stillbirth: a consequence of placental aging? Placenta. 2013;34:310–3.

67. Oner-Iyidogan Y, Kocak H, Gurdol F, Korkmaz D, Buyru F. Indices of oxidative stress in eutopic and ectopic endometria of women with endometriosis. Gynecol Obstet Investig. 2004;57:214–7.

68. Ota H, Igarashi S, Tanaka T. Xanthine oxidase in eutopic and ectopic endometrium in endometriosis and adenomyosis. Fertil Steril. 2001;75:785–90.

69. Agarwal A, Gupta S, Sikka S. The role of free radicals and antioxidants in reproduction. Current Opinion in Obstetrics & Gynecology. 2006;18:325–32.

70. Bedaiwy MA, Falcone T, Sharma RK, Goldberg JM, Attaran M, Nelson DR, Agarwal A. Prediction of endometriosis with serum and peritoneal fluid markers: a prospective controlled trial. Hum Reprod. 2002;17:426–31.

71. Mier-Cabrera J, Jimenez-Zamudio L, Garcia-Latorre E, Cruz-Orozco O, Hernandez-Guerrero C. Quantitative and qualitative peritoneal immune profiles, T-cell apoptosis and oxidative stress-associated characteristics in women with minimal and mild endometriosis. BJOG. 2011;118:6–16.

72. Kajihara H, Yamada Y, Kanayama S, Furukawa N, Noguchi T, Haruta S, Yoshida S, Sado T, Oi H, Kobayashi H. New insights into the pathophysiology of endometriosis: from chronic inflammation to danger signal. Gynecol Endocrinol. 2011;27:73–9.

73. Li YQ, Zhang ZX, Xu YJ, Ni W, Chen SX, Yang Z, Ma D. N-acetyl-L-cysteine and pyrrolidine dithiocarbamate inhibited nuclear factor-kappa B activation in alveolar macrophages by different mechanisms. Acta Pharmacol Sin. 2006;27:339–46.

74. Ngo C, Chereau C, Nicco C, Weill B, Chapron C, Batteux F. Reactive oxygen

species controls endometriosis progression. Am J Pathol. 2009;175:225–34.

75. McCubrey JA, LaHair MM, Franklin RA. Reactive oxygen species-induced activation of the MAP kinase signaling pathways. Antioxid Redox Signal. 2006;8:1775–89.

76. Madazli R, Benian A, Aydin S, Uzun H, Tolun N. The plasma and placental levels of malondialdehyde, glutathione and superoxide dismutase in pre-eclampsia. J Obstet Gynaecol. 2002;22:477–80.

77. Matsubara K, Higaki T, Matsubara Y, Nawa A. Nitric oxide and reactive oxygen species in the pathogenesis of preeclampsia. Int J Mol Sci. 2015;16:4600–14.

78. Roberts JM, Taylor RN, Musci TJ, Rodgers GM, Hubel CA, McLaughlin MK. Preeclampsia - an endothelial-cell disorder. Am J Obstet Gynecol. 1989;161: 1200–4.

79. Hubel CA, Roberts JM, Taylor RN, Musci TJ, Rogers GM, McLaughlin MK. Lipid-peroxidation in pregnancy - new perspectives on preeclampsia. Am J Obstet Gynecol. 1989;161:1025–34.

80. Uzun H, Benian A, Madazli R, Topcuoglu MA, Aydin S, Albayrak M. Circulating oxidized low-density lipoprotein and paraoxonase activity in preeclampsia. Gynecol Obstet Investig. 2005;60:195–200.

81. Wallukat G, Homuth V, Fischer T, Lindschau C, Horstkamp B, Jupner A, Baur E, Nissen E, Vetter K, Neichel D, et al. Patients with preeclampsia develop agonistic autoantibodies against the angiotensin AT(1) receptor. J Clin Investig. 1999;103:945–52.

82. Griendling KK, Sorescu D, Lassegue B, Ushio-Fukai M. Modulation of protein kinase activity and gene expression by reactive oxygen species and their role in vascular physiology and pathophysiology. Arterioscler Thromb Vasc Biol. 2000;20:2175–83.

83. Raijmakers MTM, Peters WHM, Steegers EAP, Poston L. NAD(P)H oxidase associated superoxide production in human placenta from normotensive and pre-eclamptic women. Placenta. 2004;25:S85–9.

84. Walsh SW. Eicosanoids in preeclampsia. Prostaglandins Leukotrienes and Essential Fatty Acids. 2004;70:223–32.

85. Klemmensen AK, Tabor A, Osterdal ML, Knudsen VK, Halldorsson TI, Mikkelsen TB, Olsen SF. Intake of vitamin C and E in pregnancy and risk of pre-eclampsia: prospective study among 57 346 women. BJOG. 2009;116:964–74.

86. Liu GH, Dong YL, Wang ZX, Cao J, Chen YX. Restraint stress delays endometrial adaptive remodeling during mouse embryo implantation. Stress-the International Journal on the Biology of Stress. 2015;18:699–709.

87. Liu GH, Dong YL, Wang ZX, Cao J, Chen YX. Restraint stress alters immune parameters and induces oxidative stress in the mouse uterus during embryo implantation. Stress-the International Journal on the Biology of Stress. 2014;17:494–503.

88. Perucci LO, Correa MD, Dusse LM, Gomes KB, Sousa LP. Resolution of inflammation pathways in preeclampsia-a narrative review. Immunol Res. 2017;65:774–89.

89. Wu F, Tian FJ, Lin Y. Oxidative stress in placenta: health and diseases. Biomed Res Int. 2015;2015:293271.

90. Wojsiat J, Korczynski J, Borowiecka M, Zbikowska HM. The role of oxidative stress in female infertility and in vitro fertilization. Postepy Hig Med Dosw (Online). 2017;71:359–66.

91. Itoh K, Chiba T, Takahashi S, Ishii T, Igarashi K, Katoh Y, Oyake T, Hayashi N, Satoh K, Hatayama I, et al. An Nrf2/small Maf heterodimer mediates the induction of phase II detoxifying enzyme genes through antioxidant response elements. Biochem Biophys Res Commun. 1997;236:313–22.

92. Itoh K, Wakabayashi N, Katoh Y, Ishii T, Igarashi K, Engel JD, Yamamoto M. Keap1 represses nuclear activation of antioxidant responsive elements by Nrf2 through binding to the amino-terminal Neh2 domain. Genes Dev. 1999;13:76–86.

93. Cho HY, Reddy SP, Debiase A, Yamamoto M, Kleeberger SR. Gene expression profiling of NRF2-mediated protection against oxidative injury. Free Radic Biol Med. 2005;38:325–43.

94. Ishii T, Itoh K, Takahashi S, Sato H, Yanagawa T, Katoh Y, Bannai S, Yamamoto M. Transcription factor Nrf2 coordinately regulates a group of oxidative stress-inducible genes in macrophages. J Biol Chem. 2000;275:16023–9.

95. Cheng XH, Chapple SJ, Patel B, Puszyk W, Sugden D, Yin XK, Mayr M, Siow RCM, Mann GE. Gestational diabetes mellitus impairs Nrf2-mediated adaptive antioxidant defenses and redox signaling in fetal endothelial cells in utero. Diabetes. 2013;62:4088–97.

96. Lim R, Barker G, Lappas M. The transcription factor Nrf2 is decreased after spontaneous term labour in human fetal membranes where it exerts anti-inflammatory properties. Placenta. 2015;36:7–17.

97. Kansanen E, Kuosmanen SM, Leinonen H, Levonen AL. The Keap1-Nrf2 pathway: mechanisms of activation and dysregulation in cancer. Redox Biol.

2013;1:45–9.

98. Guan L, Zhang L, Gong ZC, Hou XN, Xu YX, Feng XH, Wang HY, You H. FoxO3 inactivation promotes human Cholangiocarcinoma tumorigenesis and Chemoresistance through Keap1-Nrf2 signaling. Hepatology. 2016;63: 1914–27.

99. Gilmore TD. Introduction to NF-kappaB: players, pathways, perspectives. Oncogene. 2006;25:6680–4.

100. Hayden MS, West AP, Ghosh S. NF-kappa B and the immune response. Oncogene. 2006;25:6758–80.

101. Haddad JJ. Oxygen-sensing mechanisms and the regulation of redox-responsive transcription factors in development and pathophysiology. Respir Res. 2002;3:27.

102. Scheidereit C. IkappaB kinase complexes: gateways to NF-kappaB activation and transcription. Oncogene. 2006;25:6685–705.

103. Hu MCT, Lee DF, Xia WY, Golfman LS, Fu OY, Yang JY, Zou YY, Bao SL, Hanada N, Saso H, et al. I kappa B kinase promotes tumorigenesis through inhibition of forkhead FOXO3a. Cell. 2004;117:225–37.

104. Li Z, Zhang H, Chen Y, Fan L, Fang J. Forkhead transcription factor FOXO3a protein activates nuclear factor kappaB through B-cell lymphoma/leukemia 10 (BCL10) protein and promotes tumor cell survival in serum deprivation. J Biol Chem. 2012;287:17737–45.

105. Sakamoto Y, Harada T, Horie S, Iba Y, Taniguchi F, Yoshida S, Iwabe T, Terakawa N. Tumor necrosis factor-alpha-induced interleukin-8 (IL-8) expression in endometriotic stromal cells, probably through nuclear factor-kappa P activation: gonadotropin-releasing hormone agonist treatment reduced IL-8 expression. J Clin Endocrinol Metab. 2003;88: 730–5.

106. Lousse JC, Van Langendonckt A, Gonzalez-Ramos R, Defrere S, Renkin E, Donnez J. Increased activation of nuclear factor-kappa B (NF-kappa B) in isolated peritoneal macrophages of patients with, endometriosis. Fertil Steril. 2008;90:217–20.

107. Veillat V, Lavoie CH, Metz CN, Roger T, Labelle Y, Akoum A. Involvement of nuclear factor-kappa B in macrophage migration inhibitory factor gene transcription up-regulation induced by interleukin-1 beta in ectopic endometrial cells. Fertil Steril. 2009;91:2148–56.

108. Cao WG, Morin M, Sengers V, Metz C, Roger T, Maheux R, Akoum A. Tumour necrosis factor-alpha up-regulates macrophage migration inhibitory factor expression in endometrial stromal cells via the nuclear transcription factor NF-kappa B. Hum Reprod. 2006;21:421–8.

109. Grund EM, Kagan D, Obst CA, Zeitvogel A, Starzinski-Powitz A, Nataraja S, Palmer SS. Tumor necrosis factor-alpha regulates inflammatory and mesenchymal responses via mitogen-activated protein kinase kinase, p38, and nuclear factor kappa B in human endometriotic epithelial cells. Mol Pharmacol. 2008;73:1394–404.

110. Brunet A, Bonni A, Zigmond MJ, Lin MZ, Juo P, Hu LS, Anderson MJ, Arden KC, Blenis J, Greenberg ME. Akt promotes cell survival by phosphorylating and inhibiting a Forkhead transcription factor. Cell. 1999;96:857–68.

111. Van Der Vos KE, Coffer PJ. The extending network of FOXO transcriptional target genes. Antioxid Redox Signal. 2011;14:579–92.

112. Goto T, Takano M, Albergaria A, Briese J, Pomeranz KM, Cloke B, Fusi L, Feroze-Zaidi F, Maywald N, Sajin M, et al. Mechanism and functional consequences of loss of FOXO1 expression in endometrioid endometrial cancer cells. Oncogene. 2008;27:9–19.

113. Kajihara T, Brosens JJ, Ishihara O. The role of FOXO1 in the decidual transformation of the endometrium and early pregnancy. Med Mol Morphol. 2013;46:61–8.

114. Kajihara T, Jones M, Fusi L, Takano M, Feroze-Zaidi F, Pirianov G, Mehmet H, Ishihara O, Higham JM, Lam EW, Brosens JJ. Differential expression of FOXO1 and FOXO3a confers resistance to oxidative cell death upon endometrial decidualization. Mol Endocrinol. 2006;20:2444–55.

115. Kyo S, Sakaguchi J, Kiyono T, Shimizu Y, Maida Y, Mizumoto Y, Mori N, Nakamura M, Takakura M, Miyake K, et al. Forkhead transcription factor FOXO1 is a direct target of progestin to inhibit endometrial epithelial cell growth. Clin Cancer Res. 2011;17:525–37.

116. Gellersen B, Brosens J. Cyclic AMP and progesterone receptor cross-talk in human endometrium: a decidualizing affair. J Endocrinol. 2003;178:357–72.

117. Dijkers PF, Medema RH, Lammers JW, Koenderman L, Coffer PJ. Expression of the pro-apoptotic Bcl-2 family member Bim is regulated by the forkhead transcription factor FKHR-L1. Curr Biol. 2000;10:1201–4.

118. Eijkelenboom A, Burgering BM. FOXOs: signalling integrators for homeostasis maintenance. Nat Rev Mol Cell Biol. 2013;14:83–97.

119. Leitao B, Jones MC, Fusi L, Higham J, Lee Y, Takano M, Goto T, Christian M, Lam EWF, Brosens JJ. Silencing of the JNK pathway maintains progesterone receptor activity in decidualizing human endometrial stromal cells exposed to oxidative stress signals. Faseb Journal. 2010;24:1541–51. %1548 May %1549 Article %! Silencing of the JNK pathway maintains progesterone receptor activity in decidualizing human endometrial stromal cells exposed to oxidative stress signals

120. Labied S, Kajihara T, Madureira PA, Fusi L, Jones MC, Higham JM, Varshochi R, Francis JM, Zoumpoulidou G, Essafi A, et al. Progestins regulate the expression and activity of the forkhead transcription factor FOXO1 in differentiating human endometrium. Mol Endocrinol. 2006;20:35–44.

121. Dhillon AS, Hagan S, Rath O, Kolch W. MAP kinase signalling pathways in cancer. Oncogene. 2007;26:3279–90.

122. Lee CH, Ying TH, Chiou HL, Hsieh SC, Wen SH, Chou RH, Hsieh YH. Alpha-mangostin induces apoptosis through activation of reactive oxygen species and ASK1/p38 signaling pathway in cervical cancer cells. Oncotarget. 2017;8: 47425–39.

123. Bredeson S, Papaconstantinou J, Deford JH, Kechichian T, Syed TA, Saade GR, Menon R. HMGB1 promotes a p38MAPK associated non-infectious inflammatory response pathway in human fetal membranes. PLoS One. 2014;9:18.

124. Menon R, Papaconstantinou J. p38 mitogen activated protein kinase (MAPK): a new therapeutic target for reducing the risk of adverse pregnancy outcomes. Expert Opin Ther Targets. 2016;20:1397–412.

125. Matsuzaki S, Darcha C. Co-operation between the AKT and ERK signaling pathways may support growth of deep endometriosis in a fibrotic microenvironment in vitro. Hum Reprod. 2015;30:1606–16.

126. Yotova IY, Quan P, Leditznig N, Beer U, Wenzl R, Tschugguel W. Abnormal activation of Ras/Raf/MAPK and RhoA/ROCKII signalling pathways in eutopic endometrial stromal cells of patients with endometriosis. Hum Reprod. 2011;26:885–97.

127. Velarde MC, Aghajanova L, Nezhat CR, Giudice LC. Increased mitogen-activated protein kinase kinase/extracellularly regulated kinase activity in human endometrial stromal fibroblasts of women with endometriosis reduces 3′,5′-cyclic adenosine 5′-monophosphate inhibition of cyclin D1. Endocrinology. 2009;150:4701–12.

128. Yoshino O, Osuga Y, Hirota Y, Koga K, Hirata T, Harada M, Morimoto C, Yano T, Nishii O, Tsutsumi O, Taketani Y. Possible pathophysiological roles of mitogen-activated protein kinases (MAPKs) in endometriosis. Am J Reprod Immunol. 2004;52:306–11.

129. Huang F, Cao J, Liu Q, Zou Y, Li H, Yin T. MAPK/ERK signal pathway involved expression of COX-2 and VEGF by IL-1beta induced in human endometriosis stromal cells in vitro. Int J Clin Exp Pathol. 2013;6:2129–36.

130. Andrade SS, Azevedo Ade C, Monasterio IC, Paredes-Gamero EJ, Goncalves GA, Bonetti TC, Albertoni G, Schor E, Barreto JA, Luiza Oliva M, et al. 17beta-estradiol and steady-state concentrations of H2O2: antiapoptotic effect in endometrial cells from patients with endometriosis. Free Radic Biol Med. 2013;60:63–72.

131. Rahman MM, Sykiotis GP, Nishimura M, Bodmer R, Bohmann D. Declining signal dependence of Nrf2-MafS-regulated gene expression correlates with aging phenotypes. Aging Cell. 2013;12:554–62.

132. Zhang HQ, Davies KJA, Forman HJ. Oxidative stress response and Nrf2 signaling in aging. Free Radic Biol Med. 2015;88:314–36.

133. Sheu SS, Nauduri D, Anders MW. Targeting antioxidants to mitochondria: a new therapeutic direction. Biochimica Et Biophysica Acta-Molecular Basis of Disease. 2006;1762:256–65.

## 3

Identification and characterization of microRNAs in the pituitary of pubescent goats

Jing Ye[1,3†], Zhiqiu Yao[1,3†], Wenyu Si[1,3], Xiaoxiao Gao[1], Chen Yang[1], Ya Liu[1,2,3], Jianping Ding[1,2,3], Weiping Huang[1,2,3], Fugui Fang[1,2,3*] 🅙 and Jie Zhou[1,3]

Abstract

Background: Puberty is the period during a female mammal's life when it enters estrus and ovulates for the first time; this indicates that a mammal is capable of reproduction. The onset of puberty is a complex and tightly coordinated biological event; it has been reported that microRNAs (miRNAs) are involved in regulating the initiation of puberty.

Methods: We performed miRNA sequencing on pituitary tissue from prepubescent and pubescent goats to investigate differences in miRNA expression during the onset of puberty in female goats. The target genes of these miRNAs were evaluated by GO enrichment and KEGG pathway analysis to identify critical pathways regulated by these miRNAs during puberty in goats. Finally, we selected four known miRNA and one novel miRNAs to evaluate expression patterns in two samples via qRT-PCR to validate the RNA-seq data.

Results: In this study, 476 miRNAs were detected in goat pituitary tissue; 13 of these were specifically expressed in the pituitary of prepubescent goats, and 17 were unique to the pituitary of pubescent goats. Additionally, 73 novel miRNAs were predicted in these two libraries. 20 differentially expressed miRNAs were identified in this study. KEGG pathway enrichment analysis revealed that the differentially expressed miRNA target genes were enriched in pathways related to ovary development during puberty, including the GABAergic synapse, oxytocin signaling pathway, the cAMP signaling pathway, progesterone-mediated oocyte maturation. In this study, differential miRNA expression in the pituitary tissue of prepubescent and pubescent goats were identified and characterized.

Conclusion: These results provide important information regarding the potential regulation of the onset of goat puberty by miRNAs, and contribute to the elucidation of miRNA regulated processes during maturation and reproduction.

Keywords: Goat, MicroRNA, Pubescent, Pituitary

Background

MicroRNAs (miRNAs) are a class of non-coding RNAs that play a key roles in regulating gene expression during transcription and post-transcriptionally regulating protein expression [1]. MiRNAs are short, single-stranded RNA molecules that are approximately19–23 nucleotides in length [2]. Genes that are regulated by miRNAs account for 10–30% of all protein-coding gene [3]. MiRNAs have two canonical activities to implement gene regulation: the first way which is most effective useful in plants, is a miRNA to bind to a fully complementary sequence on a target mRNA and induces its cleavage [4, 5]. Another method of miRNA gene targeting is through incomplete matching of a miRNA to a partial complementary sequence on the 3′ untranslated region (3' UTR) of its target mRNA, resulting in degradation of the mRNA and/or inhibition of protein translation [6]. MiRNAs play an important role in regulating many biological processes,

* Correspondence: fgfang@163.com
†Jing Ye and Zhiqiu Yao contributed equally to this work.
[1]Anhui Provincial Laboratory of Animal Genetic Resources Protection and Breeding, College of Animal Science and Technology, Anhui Agricultural University, 130 Changjiang West Road, Hefei 230036, Anhui, China
[2]Anhui Provincial Laboratory for Local Livestock and Poultry Genetic Resource Conservation and Bio-Breeding, 130 Changjiang West Road, Hefei 230036, Anhui, China
Full list of author information is available at the end of the article

including cell proliferation [7], apoptosis [8], cell differentiation [9], metabolism [10], hematopoiesis, and development [8]. Recent studies have shown that miRNAs play a direct role in apoptosis of bovine luteal regulation [11], suggesting that miRNAs are involved in reproductive regulation.

The pituitary is an important mammalian endocrine gland that composed of the adenohypophysis and neurohypophysis. Hormones produced and released by the pituitary affect many biological processes including animal growth, bone metabolism, and cell cycle activity [12]. Recently, studies have found that miR-26b plays an important role in pituitary development [13]. miR-15 and miR-16 are down-regulated in pituitary adenomas and are associated with secretion of p43 protein [14], suggesting a relationship between miRNAs and pituitary function.

Puberty is a critical stage of female goat development. It marks the first occurrence of ovulation and the onset of reproductive capability [15]. The mechanism of puberty onset is complex and thought to be associated with environmental factors, neuroendocrine factors, genetic factors, and interactions between these factors. The strongest factor that contributes to the onset of puberty is thought to be inheritable, as the development and timing of puberty are highly heritable. Genome wide association studies (GWAS) have identified many loci which may affect the timing and development of puberty [16]. GWAS have disclosed that variants in/near LIN28b influence both adult height and onset of menarche [17]. LIN28 and LIN28b are related RNA-binding proteins, they bind to the terminal loops of let-7 miRNA family, inhibiting the processing of let-7 family members into mature miRNA [18]. These reports indicate that puberty is likely closely regulated by miRNAs, and that miRNA are likely involved in the onset of puberty in mammals.

We hypothesized that the onset of goat puberty is also regulated by miRNAs, and that critical pituitary functions during puberty may be regulated by miRNA. The expression profile of miRNAs in the pituitary of pubescent goat remains unknown. In this study, we applied Solexa sequencing and investigated the expression of miRNAs in prepubescent and pubescent goats to explore the relation of miRNAs with the onset of puberty.

Methods
Pituitary collection and total RNA isolation
Three pubescent Anhuai female goats, aged 4.5–5 months and weighing 17.43 ± 1.63 kg, and three prepubescent aged 2.5–3 months and weighing 9.6 ± 2.36 kg, were used in this study. Pubescent goat was identified via the change in vaginal and ovarian physiology (Additional file 1), hormone profiles (Additional file 2) and rams test conditions [19]. Briefly, rams test conditions is use a healthy ram to test that whether female goats were in estrus. A piece of

cloth was tied on the abdomen of the ram to prevent mating while testing. Mount behaviour would occur when the female goats were in estrus. Rams test conditions were performed twice daily at 08:00 and 16:00. The cunnus of pubescent goats became inflamed, and histological observation identified some mature follicles in the ovaries(Additional file 1). Pituitary glands were collected from pubescent ($n = 3$) and prepubescent ($n = 3$) goats [20, 21] after animals were anesthetized with injection of 0.1 ml xylazine hydrochloride (Muhua China, Lot number 150804) before sacrificed. And the surgery for removing the pituitary is feferred the study of Bjarkam et al. [22]. The collected tissues were immediately placed in liquid nitrogen and stored at − 80 °C. Total RNA was isolated using TRIzol (Invitrogen, Carlsbad, CA, USA) according to the manufacturer's protocol. RNA integrity for sequencing was assessed using the RNA Nano 6000 Assay Kit and a Agilent Bioanalyzer 2100 system (Agilent Technologies, CA, USA). The concentration of total RNA for qRT-PCR was quantifiedc at 260 nm with a NanoDrop spectrophotometer (ND-2000, USA). The quality of total RNA for qRT-PCR was assessed by agarose gel electrophoresis.

Small RNA library construction and sequencing
A total of 3 μg total RNA per sample was used as input material for the small RNA (sRNA) library construction. Sequencing libraries were generated using NEBNext® Multiplex Small RNA Library Prep Set for Illumina® (NEB, USA.) following manufacturer's recommendations. Total RNA was used as the starting sample, the sRNA ends are directly connected with the adapter, followed by reverse transcription synthesis into cDNA. DNA fragments of 140-160 bp were separated by PAGE gel electrophoresis, and the cDNA library was recovered. Finally, library quality was assessed on the Agilent Bioanalyzer 2100 system using DNA High Sensitivity Chips.

Sequence analysis
Clean sequencing reads were obtained by removing from the raw data reads containing poly-N, with 5′ adapter contaminants, without 3′ adapters or the insert tag, containing poly A, T, G, or C, low quality reads, and reads shorter than 18 nt. After read clean up, the high-quality reads were mapped to a reference sequence by Bowtie [23] without mismatch to analyze their expression and distribution on the reference sequence.

To remove tags originating from protein-coding genes, repeat sequences, rRNA, tRNA, snRNA, and snoRNA, sRNA tags were mapped to the RepeatMasker, Rfam database. The clean reads were compared to the miRNA precursor/mature miRNA of all animals in miRBase 21.0, and show the sequence and count of miRNA families (not species-specific) that can be found in the samples. The characteristics of the hairpin structure of miRNA precursors was evaluated to predict novel miRNAs.

Differential expression analysis

In order to find out the differentially expressed miRNAs between pituitary tissue from prepubescent and pubescent goats, expression data were Log2-transformed ratio figure and plotted on a scatter plot. Briefly, the procedures were as follow: (1) miRNA expression from the two libraries was normalized to obtain the expression of transcript per million reads (TPM). Normalization formula: Normalized expression = mapped readcount/Total reads*1×10^6; (2) Calculate fold-change and P-value from the normalized expression. P-value was adjusted using qvalue. Qvalue< 0.01 and |log2(foldchange)| > 1 was set as the threshold for significantly differential expression by default. Finally, generate the Log2-ratio figure and Scatter Plot.

When the normalized expression of a miRNA was zero between two libraries, its expression value was adjusted to 0.01 (as 0 cannot be plotted on a log plot). If the normalized expression of a certain miRNA in two libraries was all lower than 1, further differential expression analysis was conducted without this miRNA.

GO enrichment and KEGG pathway analyses

Gene Ontology (GO; http://www.geneontology.org) is an international standard classification system for gene function. After selecting miRNA target genes, the distribution of the target genes among biological pathways/functions in Gene Ontology will clarify the biological differences between the samples based on gene function. Using this method, first candidate target genes are mapped to the GO terms (biological functions) in the database (http://www.geneontology.org), the number of genes in every term is calculated, and a hypergeometric test is performed to identify significantly enriched GO terms in the target gene candidate list out of the background of the reference gene list.

The Kyoto Encyclopedia of Genes and Genomes (KEGG) database is a public database of pathway data, and is a resource for understanding high-level functions and processes active in a biological system [24]. KEGG pathway analysis identifies significantly enriched metabolic pathways or signal transduction pathways enriched in target gene candidates compared to a reference gene background, using the hypergeometric test.

Quantitative real-time PCR

We extracted the total RNA from the pituitary, then, the quality and concentration of the total RNA was assessed. Samples demonstrating satisfactory RNA quality were selected for further analysis. That is, in the agarose gel electrophoresis, the RNA showed three bands, they are 28 s, 18 s and 5 s, respectively (Additional file 3). And the concentration of total RNA for each example was over 555 ng/µl (Additional file 4), which showed low degradation.

In order to validate the RNA-seq data, we randomly selected four known miRNA and one novel miRNAs to evaluate expression patterns in prepuberty and puberty via qRT-PCR. Another three goats were used in each group and the qRT-PCR experiments were repeated three times per sample, and all of the reactions were carried out in triplicate. We used Primer 5 software to design primers online and evaluated specificity using BLAST at NCBI. The list of the forward primer and universal miRNA qPCR primer sequences are shown in Table 1 and U6 was housekeeping gene. We used Trans-Script° Green miRNA Two-Step qRT-PCR SuperMix(-TransScript, AQ202, China) to perform reverse transcription and qRT-PCR. The reverse transcription reaction system and program are shown as below: (1)Mixed 500 ng total RNA, 1 µl TransScript° miRNA reverse transcription(RT) enzyme mix, 2× TS miRNA reaction mix and RNase-free water to 20 µl, and then incubated the mixture at 37 °C for 1 h followed inactivated the RT enzyme mix at 85 °C for 5 s. The cDNA obtained after reverse transcription is diluted 10-fold before qPCR. The PCR mixture included 2 µl of cDNA for every miRNA, 0.4 µl forward primer(10Um), 0.4 µl universal miRNA qPCR primer(10uM), 10 µl 2 × TransScript° tip g reen qPCR supermix, 0.4 µl passive reference dye(50×) and ddH$_2$O to 20 µl. The PCR conditions were as follows: initial denaturation at 94 °C for 30 s, followed by 40 cycles of 94 °C for 5 s, 60 °C for 15 s, and 72 °C for 10 s, and a terminal hold at 4 °C. We collected the cycle threshold (Ct) from each reaction, and the expression level of each gene was evaluated using the $2^{-\Delta\Delta CT}$ method.

Statistical analysis

We used the statistical package R statistical software (R, Auckland, NZL) for further analysis of RNA-seq data. R was used for graphical representations, as well as to

Table 1 Primer sequences for qRT-PCR

The name of primer	Sequence,5′-3′
chi-miR-543-3p	AAACATTCGCGGTGCACTTCT
chi-miR-493-5p	TTGTACATGGTAGGCTTTCATT
chi-miR-335-3p	TTTTTCATTATTGCTCCTGACC
chi-miR-411a-3p	TATGTAACACGGTCCACTAAC
novel_128	TAATCTCAGCTGGCAACTGTGA
U6	GGCAAGGATGACACGC
Universal miRNA qPCR Primer	GATCGCCCTTCTACGTCGTAT

correct for to multiple testing and *P*-value corrections. We analyzed the qRT-PCR data by SPSS 17.0 software package (SPSS, Chicago, IL, USA). Data were expressed as mean ± standard error, with $P < 0.05$ indicating significant difference. Graphpad 5.0 was used to draw figures.

Results

Overview of RNA sequencing data

In order to identify miRNAs that are differentially expressed the pituitary of pubescent and prepubescent goats, two sRNA libraries were constructed by Solexa sequencing. The error rate of the sequencing data from these two libraries is 0.01%, and the Q30 ≥ 97.8%, indicating that the sequencing data is high quality and suitable for this study. A total of 11,793,577 reads and 10,676,789 reads were acquired from the pituitary libraries of pubescent and prepubescent goats, respectively. After discarding the sequences that are below background, over 86% sRNAs were mapped to the reference genome in the two libraries (Table 2). Subsequently, all identical sequence reads were classified as groups, and 365,515 and 296,547 unique sequences were obtained. We then chose a specific sRNA length range from the clean reads and calculated the length distribution of sRNA (Fig. 1). The majority of the sRNAs are between 21 and 24 nt in size. Sequences of 22 nt in length, the traditional size of Dicer-derived products [25], accounted for 39.25 and 37.3% of the total sequence reads in the pituitary libraries from pubescent and prepubescent goats, respectively.

In order to analyze the sRNA expression and distribution based on the reference sequence, the sRNAs were mapped to the reference sequence by Bowtie [23] without mismatch, and 8,823,349 and 9,765,115 sRNAs were obtained. The remaining reads were compared with the RepeatMasker, Rfam database to remove possible mRNA, rRNA, tRNA, snRNA, snoRNA and repeat sequences. However, some sRNA tags may be mapped to more than one category. To make every unique sRNAs mapped to only one annotation, we followed the

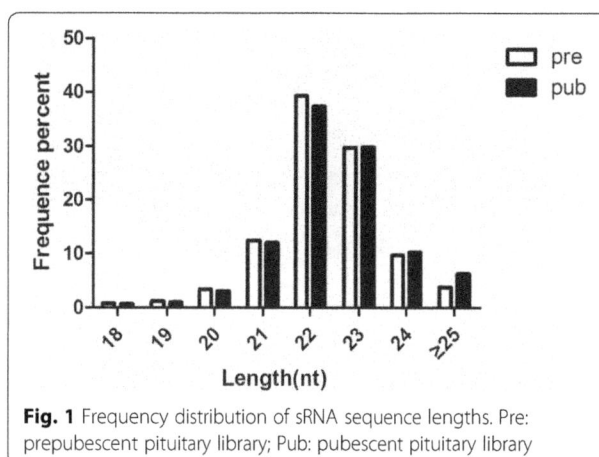

Fig. 1 Frequency distribution of sRNA sequence lengths. Pre: prepubescent pituitary library; Pub: pubescent pituitary library

following priority rule: rRNAetc (Genbank > Rfam) > known miRNA > repeat > exon > intron [26]. All of the clean reads were divided into the following categories: exon_sense, exon_antisense, intron_sense, intron_antisense, miRNA, rRNA, repeat, scRNA, snRNA, snoRNA, srpRNA, tRNA, unknown (sequences not mapped to any known reference databases). The composition of the RNA classes in each library is shown in Fig. 2. The proportion of total rRNA is indicative of sample quality; for a high quality sample it should be less than 60% in plant samples [27] and 40% in animal samples (unpublished data by BGI). The proportion of total rRNA was 1.16 and 0.87% in the pituitary libraries of pubescent and prepubescent goats, respectively, indicating that the pituitary RNA samples collected were of high quality. In the clean reads from the pituitary libraries of pubescent and prepubescent goats, 8,823,349 reads (account for 86.84%) and 9,765,115 reads (account for 86.64%), respectively were mapped to the goat reference genome (Additional file 5). Known miRNAs accounted for 62.57 and 59.16% of the total clean reads, and accounted for 2.23 and 1.76% of the unique reads in the pituitary sRNA libraries of pubescent and prepubescent goats, respectively (Fig. 2). The analysis of these two libraries suggests that miRNA sequences are enriched among the sRNA libraries.

Known miRNAs

In order to identify known miRNAs in goat pituitary, the dataset was compared to known miRNAs (miRNA precursors and mature miRNAs) in miRBase21.0. A total of 3669 and 3781 unique sequences in the pituitary libraries of pubescent and prepubescent goats,were mapped to known miRNAs in miRBase 21.0, respectively. Our results showed a total of 403 mature miRNAs, 253 miRNA hairpins, 7450 unique sRNA, and 11,297,037 total sRNA were obtained (Table 3).

Table 2 The quality of library sequences by Solexa sequencing

Type	Pub		Pre	
	Counts	Percent	Counts	Percent
Total reads	11,793,577	100%	10,676,789	100%
N% > 10%	124	0.00%	125	0.00%
Low quality	3434	0.03%	2956	0.03%
5′ adapter contamine	165	0.00%	93	0.00%
3 adapter null or insert null	234,299	1.99%	184,344	1.73%
With polyA/T/G/C	5158	0.04%	4261	0.04%
Clean reads	11,550,397	97.94%	10,485,010	98.20%

Pre preuberty; *Pub* puberty

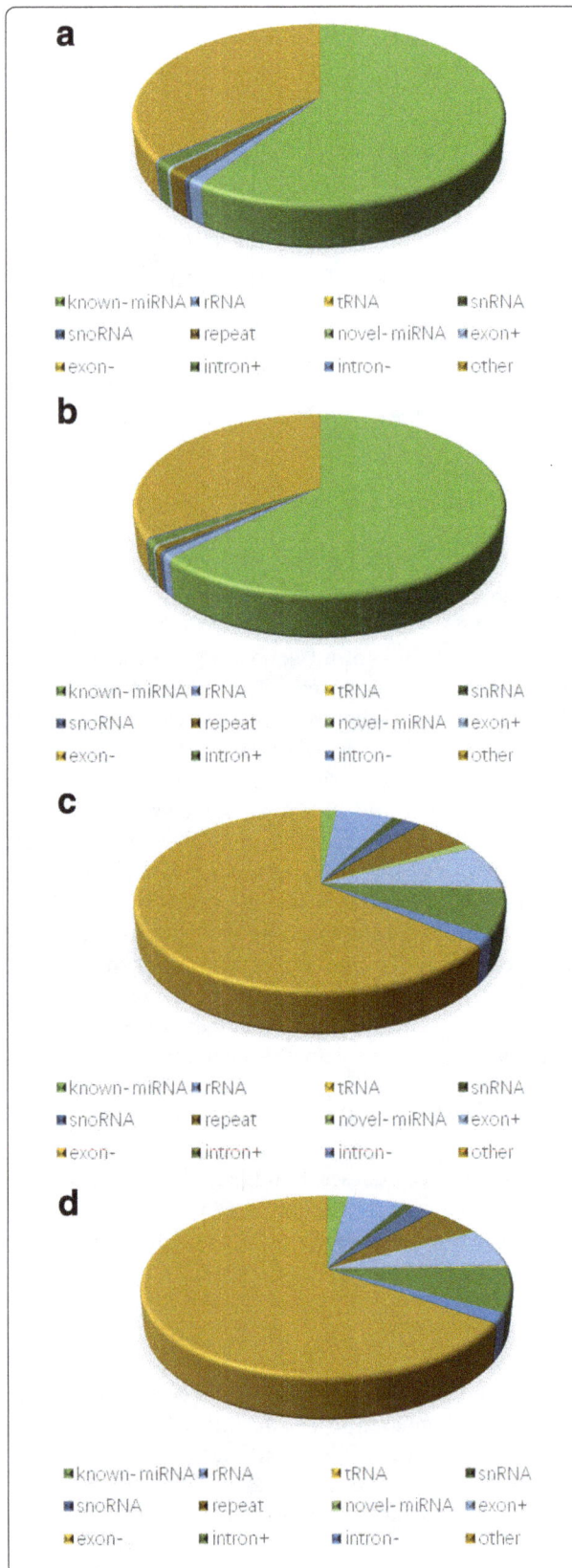

Fig. 2 Composition of small RNA classes from Solexa sequencing. **a** Total number of reads in the pubescent goat pituitary library. **b** Total number of reads in the prepubescent goat pituitary library. **c** Total number of unique sequences in the pubescent goat pituitary library. **d** Total number of reads in the prepubescent goat pituitary library. Pre: prepubescent pituitary library; Pub: pubescent pituitary library

Identification of potential novel miRNAs

The presence of a hairpin RNA structure, characteristic of a miRNA precursor, can be used to predict novel miRNAs. Novel miRNAs were predicted by mapping precursor sequences to goat the genome by integrated miREvo [28] and miRDeep2 [29] miRNA prediction software. We detected 73 potential novel miRNAs (Table 4). Novel miRNAs were predicted by exploring the secondary structure, predicting the Dicer cleavage site and binding energy.

Differential expression of miRNA in the pituitary of pubescent and prepubescent goats

As shown in Fig. 3, 476 unique miRNA were analyzed from the pituitary libraries of pubescent and prepubescent goats (Additional file 6). Among them, 446 miRNAs were co-expressed in both libraries, while 17 miRNAs were specifically expressed in pubescent goat pituitary and 13 miRNAs were specifically expressed prepubecent goat pituitary.

Using a volcano plot, the overall distribution of the miRNAs can be determined. Significatly differentially expressed miRNAs are screened based on two factors: Fold change and corrected level (*padj* / *qvalue*). After repetition of the biological samples, differentially expressed miRNAs were screened as: *padj* < 0.05. Twenty miRNA were significantly differentially expressed, including ten over-expressed miRNAs, and ten under-expressed miRNA (Additional file 7).

miRNA target gene prediction

Prediction of miRNA target genes performed by miRanda. In the two libraries, 653,807 target sites in 25,619 target genes were predicted for the 403 known miRNAs 126,299 target sites in 25,015 target genes were predicted for the 73 novel miRNAs (Additional file 8).

Table 3 Statistics of known miRNA identified in pituitary of prepubescent and pubescent goats

Types	Total	Pub	Pre
Mapped mature	403	397	396
Mapped hairpin	253	253	254
Mapped unique sRNA	7450	3669	3781
Mapped total sRNA	11,297,037	5,776,657	5,520,380

Pre preuberty; *Pub* puberty

Table 4 Statistics of the predicted novel miRNAs mapping to small RNAs

Types	Total	Pub	Pre
Mapped mature	73	66	63
Mapped star	33	28	29
Mapped hairpin	79	72	71
Mapped unique sRNA	603	302	301
Mapped total sRNA	23,994	13,624	10,370

Pre preuberty; *Pub* puberty

Gene ontology (GO) enrichment and KEGG pathway analysis of miRNA target genes

In this study, the candidate target genes for differentially expressed miRNAs was used for the GO enrichment assessment to predict biological functions. Statistical analysis of the significantly enriched number of genes in each term are indicated in Fig. 4.

KEGG pathway analysis showed that 273 pathways were involved in the candidate genes of miRNAs present in the pituitary tissue of prepubescent and pubescent goats. The enriched terms were mainly focused on the olfactory transduction signaling pathway. The results of KEGG pathway analysis also indicated seveal enriched terms were involved in puberty, such as Vasopressin-regulated water reabsorption, Glutamatergic synapse, Oxytocin signaling pathway, cAMP signaling pathway, Progesterone-mediated oocyte maturation, and the GnRH signaling pathway (Fig. 4, Table 5).

Quantitative RT-PCR validation of miRNA expression

The expression of 5 different miRNA from the pituitary of pubescent and prepubescent goats were selected

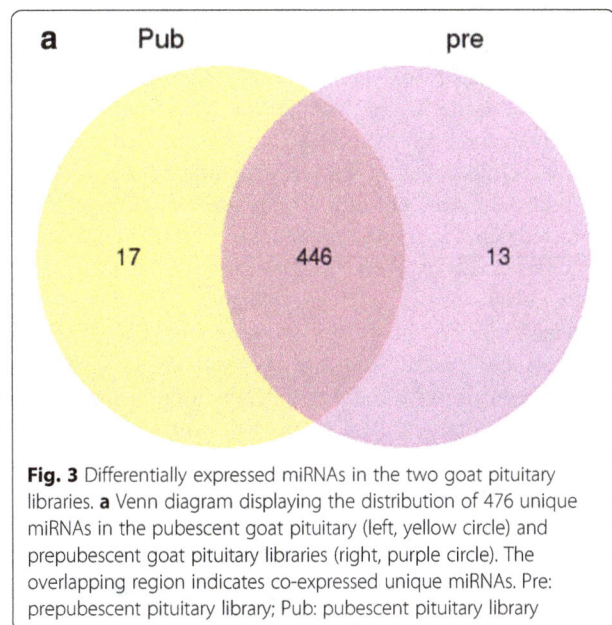

Fig. 4 The vertical axis represents the pathway name, and the horizontal axis represents the enrichment factor. The size of the dot indicates the number of candidate target genes in the pathway, and the color of the dot corresponds to the different Q value range. Pre: prepubescent pituitary library; Pub: pubescent pituitary library

randomly for expression validation using qRT-PCR. qRT-qPCR analysis with U6 as housekeeping gen indicated that the expression of chi-miR-335-3p, chi-miR-493-5p, chi-miR-543-3p and chi-miR-411a-3p had decreasing trends ($P < 0.05$), and the expression of novel_128 was increased ($P < 0.05$) in the pubescent goats compared to prepubescent goats (Fig. 5); these data were consistent with the Solexa sequencing results, which indicates that these miRNAs may be involved in regulating the onest of puberty.

Discussion

The normal and regular onset of puberty and sexual maturation is of critical importance to the reproductive performance of goats. Breeding goats early in pubescence can not only reduce feeding costs and enhance the utilization of females, but also can shorten the interval between female generations and can accelerate selective breeding methods. Therefore, there are a focus on molecular-assisted breeding techniques and miRNAs in breeding research [30–34].

When we initially reported on miRNA expression in the pituitary of pubescent goats, samples from individual animals were mixed, according to previous papers [21, 32]. Mixing of samples for sequencing can impair the detection of low abundance genes [20, 21]. Nevertheless,

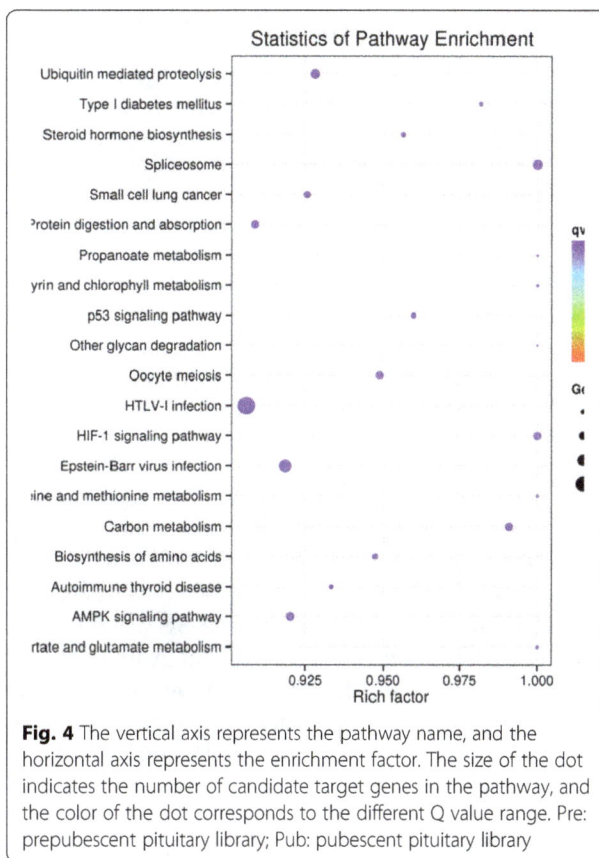

Fig. 3 Differentially expressed miRNAs in the two goat pituitary libraries. **a** Venn diagram displaying the distribution of 476 unique miRNAs in the pubescent goat pituitary (left, yellow circle) and prepubescent goat pituitary libraries (right, purple circle). The overlapping region indicates co-expressed unique miRNAs. Pre: prepubescent pituitary library; Pub: pubescent pituitary library

Table 5 List of the candidate target genes with significantly enriched pathways and functions

Term	Sample number	Background number	P-value	Corrected P-value
Vasopressin-regulated water reabsorption	14	45	0.412	0.951
Glutamatergic synapse	35	114	0.342	0.951
Oxytocin signaling pathway	53	155	0.117	0.951
cAMP signaling pathway	66	213	0.249	0.951
Progesterone-mediated oocyte maturation	24	84	0.498	0.951
GnRH signaling pathway	24	88	0.578	0.951

the qRT-PCR validation of differential miRNA expression from pituitary tissue of individual animals that we report here indicates results of the Solexa sequencing are reliable.

In the present study, sRNAs in the pituitary tissues of prepubescent and pubescent goats were sequenced by Illumina Solexa technology. We analyzed the differentially expressed miRNAs, predicted the novel miRNAs, and performed GO enrichment and KEGG pathway analysis of target genes from these two miRNA libraries.

Sequencing revealed that the sRNA sequence lengths in the sRNA libraries were between 20 and 24 nt; the most abundant sRNA length from the total sRNA sequences was at 22 nt, which is the classical length of goat miRNAs. The distribution of length in sRNAs of goats was similar to previous studies indicating the distribution of sRNA in cattle, pigs, and chickens [34–37]. The peak length of what sRNA that was obtained by high-throughput sequencing was at 24 nt [38], indicating that there are significant differences in the distribution of miRNA between species. The localization of miRNAs may be associated with miRNA function, and studies of miRNA localization can provide a rich blueprint for the

elucidating the architecture of the goat genome [39, 40]. In this study, 403 known mature miRNAs were found by mapping sRNAs to the known miRbase. According to the pre-miRNA structure in the reference genome sequence, 73 new miRNAs were predicted; this greatly enriches our understanding of the goat miRNA transcription, and lays a foundation for further study on the role of mRNA and miRNA regulatory networks in goats.

Using Solexa sequencing, we identified 463 and 459 unique miRNAs in the pituitary RNA libraries from pubescent and prepubescent goats, respectively. Compared with previous studies [41], we identified more goat miRNA using our method. This may be influenced by the fact that we compared the sequences of our clean reads to miRBase 21.0, which has additional miRNA species compared to earlier miRBase releases. We also we compared sRNA sequences to all animal miRNAs, including all species of miRNAs, thereby increasing the number of miRNA sequences that was available to compare.

The known miRNA and novel miRNA were analyzed for differential expression levels: twenty miRNA genes were significantly differentially expressed, evaluated both by fold change and corrected significance level (q < 0.05); these differential miRNA genes were novel_128, which was over-expressed, and chi-miR-335-3p, chi-miR-411a-3p, chi-miR-493-5p, and chi-miR-543-3p, which were under-expressed. These four known miRNA were also found in Saanen dairy goat [42], but the function in reproductive or physiological still remain unknown until now. Chi-miR-9-5p and chi-miR-30f-5p are two differentially expressed genes in the present study, and similarly, they are also differentially expressed in the ovaries of Jining gray and Laiwu black goats [43]. Homologues of differentially expressed miRNAs play a role in various cellular activities. For instance, chi-miR-9-3p has been shown to be an important regulator of osteoblast differentiation in mouse iPS cells and also targets β1 integrin to sensitize claudin-low breast cancer cells to MEK inhibition [44, 45]. The chi-miR-9-5p processed by the same precursor may be involved in the regulation of puberty initiation in this study. Two highly expressed differential miRNAs (miR-10b and miR-99a) identified in the present study are also highly expressed in the ovaries of goats, pigs and other animal

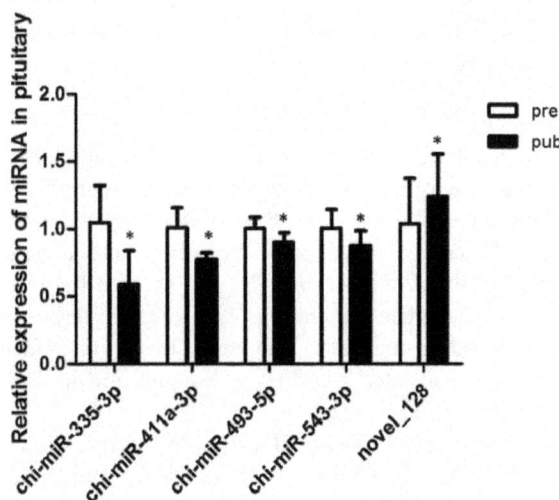

Fig. 5 qRT-PCR validation of Solexa sequencing. Pre: prepubescent pituitary; Pub: pubescent pituitary

species as reviewed by Li et al. [46]. MiR-99a is one of the most important miRNA populations in the ovary of mammals [32, 43, 47]; it induces G1-phase cell cycle arrest and inhibits tumorigenesis, which may play a decisive part in normal ovarian function [48, 49]. MiR-335 is involved in rat epididymal development via regulation of the RAS p21 protein activator 1 [50]. In human stem cells, miR-335 regulates cell proliferation, migration and differentiation [51, 52] and is involved in the inhibition of tumor reinitiation [53]. In this study, we found that miR-335 is under-expressed in pubescent goat pituitary, which indicates that miR-335 may be related to the regulation of goat empathema. There are few other reports on the relationship between miRNA expression and puberty. KEGG pathway annotations of miR-34c show that most of its target genes are involved in cancer signaling pathways and in actin cytoskeleton KEGG terms. MiR-34c was reported to be important for self-renewal of spermatogonial stem cell and spermatogenesis [54], was found to regulate differentiation of mouse embryonic stem cells into male germinal cells through RARg [55], was shown to operate downstream of p53 to induce apoptosis in germ line stem cells (mGSCs) of male dairy goats [56]. In this study, we found that miR-34c is a up-regulated in puberty, indicating that miR-34c may be involved in the regulation and control of goat empathema.

MiRNA also plays an important part in central neuroendocrine control of the reproductive system. MiRNAs active in the hypothalamic GnRH network. For instance, previous study shows that miRNA-155 and miRNA-200/429 are key components of a complex developmental switch that control the GnRH promoter activity, and its function is necessary for initiation of puberty and reproduction in animals [57]. Blocking the expression of miR-132/212 impairs the up-regulation of FSH secretion by GnRH [58]. These findings indicates that miRNA could participate in the process of GnRH-regulated gonadotropin secretion, which directly affect the onset of puberty in animals.

We used TargetScan to predict the gene targets of known and novel miRNAs, and we evaluated these target genes with GO enrichment and KEGG functional analysis. In the KEGG functional enrichment, candidate target genes are involved in pathways related to puberty, including Vasopressin-regulated water reabsorption, Glutamatergic synapse, Oxytocin signaling pathway, cAMP signaling pathway, Progesterone-mediated oocyte maturation, and the GnRH signaling pathway. It is worth to noting that some target genes of miRNAs that were not differentially expressed in the pituitary of prepubescent and pubescent goats are also involved in puberty development-related networks. In summary, the enrichment of these target gene pathways may provide a reference for future research in this field.

In summary, we identified 446 miRNA that were co-expressed, and 13 and 17 miRNA that were specifically expressed in the pituitary of prepubescent and pubescent goats, respectively. We predicted 73 novel miRNA were from the two pituitary RNA libraries. We identified four miRNAs that were differentially expressed between prepubescent and pubescent goat pituitary, including three that were over-expressed and one that was under-expressed. KEGG pathway enrichment analysis showed that the target of miRNAs were significantly enriched in pathways related to puberty. These results provide important information regarding the potential regulation of the onset of goat puberty by miRNAs, and contribute to the elucidation of miRNA regulated processes during maturation and reproduction.

Conclusion
Our results demonstrate that different expression of miRNA occur from prepuberty to puberty in goat. The results provide important information for the potential regulation of the onset of goat puberty and contribute to elucidate the processes of miRNA regulation during maturation and reproduction.

Additional files

Additional file 1: Character of prepuberty and puberty goat. A: Vulva of goat in prepuberty. B: Vulva of goat in puberty. C: Ovarian of goat in prepuberty. D: Ovarian of goat in puberty. (DOCX 1429 kb)

Additional file 2: Serum E2 and P4 levels the development of puberty in Anhuai goat (Mean ± SE). Note:Means with the different superscripts within the same column differ significantly($P < 0.05$) (DOCX 15 kb)

Additional file 3: RNA quality. (DOCX 56 kb)

Additional file 4: The concentration of total RNA. Pre: prepubescent sample; Pub: pubescent sample. (DOCX 14 kb)

Additional file 5: Reads mapped to the goat reference genome in pubescent and prepubescent goat pituitary libraries. (XLS 75 kb)

Additional file 6: Unique sequences from the pituitary libraries of pubescent and prepubescent goat pituitary. (XLSX 10 kb)

Additional file 7: Significantly differentially expressed miRNAs in pubescent and prepubescent goat pituitary. (XLSX 10 kb)

Additional file 8: 73 novel miRNAs identified from pubescent and prepubescent goat pituitary. (XLS 30 kb)

Abbreviations
GO: Gene ontology; GWAS: Genome wide association studies; KEGG: Kyoto encyclopedia of genes and genomes

Acknowledgments
We would like to thank the members of Anhui Provincial Laboratory of Animal Genetic Resources Protection and Breeding, Anhui Provincial Laboratory for Local Livestock and Poultry Genetic Resource Conservation and Bio-Breeding for their abundant discussions and valuable sggestions.

Funding

This work was supported by grants from the National Natural Science Foundation of China [grant number 31472096] and the Anhui Provincial Natural Science Foundation [grant number 1408085MKL40].

Authors' contributions

JY, ZQY, FGF, JZ and WYS designed the experiments. JY, YL, JPD, YHZ and ZQY collected the samples and performed the experiments. JY, ZQY, XXG, WPH and CY analysed the data and wrote the manuscript. All authors discussed the study results and reviewed and approved the final manuscript.

Competing interests

The authors declare that they have no competing interests.

Author details

[1]Anhui Provincial Laboratory of Animal Genetic Resources Protection and Breeding, College of Animal Science and Technology, Anhui Agricultural University, 130 Changjiang West Road, Hefei 230036, Anhui, China. [2]Anhui Provincial Laboratory for Local Livestock and Poultry Genetic Resource Conservation and Bio-Breeding, 130 Changjiang West Road, Hefei 230036, Anhui, China. [3]Department of Animal Veterinary Science, College of Animal Science and Technology, Anhui Agricultural University, 130 Changjiang West Road, Hefei 230036, Anhui, China.

References

1. Kunej T, Godnic I, Horvat S, Zorc M, Calin GA. Cross talk between MicroRNA and coding Cancer genes. Cancer J. 2012;18:223–31.
2. Bartel DP. MicroRNAs: genomics, biogenesis, mechanism, and function. Cell. 2004;116:281–97.
3. Filipowicz W, Bhattacharyya SN, Sonenberg N. Mechanisms of post-transcriptional regulation by microRNAs: are the answers in sight? Nat Rev Genet. 2008;9:102–14.
4. Reinhart BJ, Weinstein EG, Rhoades MW, Bartel B, Bartel DP. MicroRNAs in plants. Genes Dev. 2002;16:1616–26.
5. Yekta S, Shih IH, Bartel DP. MicroRNA-directed cleavage of HOXB8 mRNA. Science. 2004;304:594–6.
6. Williams AE. Functional aspects of animal microRNAs. Cell Mol Life Sci. 2008; 65:545–62.
7. Hwang HW, Mendell JT. MicroRNAs in cell proliferation, cell death, and tumorigenesis. Br J Cancer. 2006;94:776–80.
8. Ambros V. The functions of animal microRNAs. Nature. 2004;431:350–5.
9. Ivey KN, Srivastava D. MicroRNAs as regulators of differentiation and cell fate decisions. Cell Stem Cell. 2010;7:36–41.
10. Rottiers V, Naar AM. MicroRNAs in metabolism and metabolic disorders (vol 13, pg 239, 2012). Nat Rev Mol Cell Biol. 2012;13:281.
11. Arainga M, Takeda E, Aida Y. Identification of bovine leukemia virus tax function associated with host cell transcription, signaling, stress response and immune response pathway by microarray- based gene expression analysis. BMC Genomics. 2012;13
12. Wierinckx A, Roche M, Legras-Lachuer C, Trouillas J, Raverot G, Lachuer J. MicroRNAs in pituitary tumors. Mol Cell Endocrinol. 2017;456:51-61.
13. Li XH, Wang EL, Zhou HM, Yoshimoto K, Qian ZR. MicroRNAs in human pituitary adenomas. Int J Endocrinol. 2014;2014:435171.
14. Cimmino A, Calin GA, Fabbri M, Iorio MV, Ferracin M, Shimizu M, Wojcik SE, Aqeilan RI, Zupo S, Dono M, et al. miR-15 and miR-16 induce apoptosis by targeting BCL2 (vol 102, pg 13944, 2005). Proc Natl Acad Sci U S A. 2006; 103:2464.
15. Cao GL, Feng T, Chu MX, Di R, Zhang YL, Huang DW, Liu QY, Hu WP, Wang XY: Subtraction suppressive hybridisation analysis of differentially expressed genes associated with puberty in the goat hypothalamus. Reproduction, Fertility and Development 2015:Epub ahead of print.
16. Corre C, Shinoda G, Zhu H, Cousminer DL, Crossman C, Bellissimo C, Goldenberg A, Daley GQ, Palmert MR. Sex-specific regulation of weight and puberty by the Lin28/let-7 axis. J Endocrinol. 2016;228:179–91.
17. Elks CE, Perry JRB, Sulem P, Chasman DI, Franceschini N, He CY, Lunetta KL, Visser JA, Byrne EM, Cousminer DL, et al. Thirty new loci for age at menarche identified by a meta-analysis of genome-wide association studies. Nat Genet. 2010;42:1077–U1073.
18. Viswanathan SR, Daley GQ. Lin28: a MicroRNA regulator with a macro role. Cell. 2010;140:445–9.
19. Dantas A, Siqueira ER, Fernandes S, Oba E, Castilho AM, Meirelles PRL, Sartori MMP, Santos PTR. Influence of feeding differentiation on the age at onset of puberty in Brazilian Bergamasca dairy ewe lambs. Arquivo Brasileiro De Medicina Veterinaria E Zootecnia. 2016;68:22–8.
20. Ran ML, Chen B, Wu MS, Liu XC, He CQ, Yang AQ, Li Z, Xiang YJ, Li ZH, Zhang SW. Integrated analysis of miRNA and mRNA expression profiles in development of porcine testes. RSC Adv. 2015;5:63439–49.
21. Fu Y, Lan JC, Wu XH, Yang DY, Zhang ZH, Nie HM, Hou R, Zhang RH, Zheng WP, Xie Y, et al. Identification of Dirofilaria immitis miRNA using illumina deep sequencing. Vet Res. 2013;44:3.
22. Bjarkam CR, Orlowski D, Tvilling L, Bech J, Glud AN, Sorensen JH. Exposure of the pig CNS for histological analysis: a manual for decapitation, skull opening, and brain removal. J Vis Exp. 2017;122:e55511.
23. Langmead B, Trapnell C, Pop M, Salzberg SL. Ultrafast and memory-efficient alignment of short DNA sequences to the human genome. Genome Biol. 2009;10:R25.
24. Kanehisa M, Araki M, Goto S, Hattori M, Hirakawa M, Itoh M, Katayama T, Kawashima S, Okuda S, Tokimatsu T, Yamanishi Y. KEGG for linking genomes to life and the environment. Nucleic Acids Res. 2008;36:D480–4.
25. Xie SS, Li XY, Liu T, Cao JH, Zhong QA, Zhao SH. Discovery of porcine microRNAs in multiple tissues by a Solexa deep sequencing approach. PLoS One. 2011;6:e16235.
26. Calabrese JM, Seila AC, Yeo GW, Sharp PA. RNA sequence analysis defines Dicer's role in mouse embryonic stem cells (vol 104, pg 18097, 2007). Proc Natl Acad Sci U S A. 2007;104:21021.
27. Hao DC, Yang L, Xiao PG, Liu M. Identification of Taxus microRNAs and their targets with high-throughput sequencing and degradome analysis. Physiol Plant. 2012;146:388–403.
28. Wen M, Shen Y, Shi SH, Tang T. miREvo: an integrative microRNA evolutionary analysis platform for next-generation sequencing experiments. Bmc Bioinformatics. 2012;13:140.
29. Friedlander MR, Mackowiak SD, Li N, Chen W, Rajewsky N. miRDeep2 accurately identifies known and hundreds of novel microRNA genes in seven animal clades. Nucleic Acids Res. 2012;40:37–52.
30. Hu SJ, Ren G, Liu JL, Zhao ZA, Yu YS, Su RW, Ma XH, Ni H, Lei W, Yang ZM. MicroRNA expression and regulation in mouse uterus during embryo implantation. J Biol Chem. 2008;283:23473–84.
31. Hawkins SM, Buchold GM, Matzuk MM. Minireview: the roles of small RNA pathways in reproductive medicine. Mol Endocrinol. 2011;25:1257–79.
32. Zhang XD, Zhang YH, Ling YH, Liu Y, Cao HG, Yin ZJ, Ding JP, Zhang XR. Characterization and differential expression of microRNAs in the ovaries of pregnant and non-pregnant goats (Capra hircus). BMC Genomics. 2013;14:157.
33. McBride D, Carre W, Sontakke SD, Hogg CO, Law A, Donadeu FX, Clinton M. Identification of miRNAs associated with the follicular-luteal transition in the ruminant ovary. Reproduction. 2012;144:221–33.
34. Huang JM, Ju ZH, Li QL, Hou QL, Wang CF, Li JB, Li RL, Wang LL, Sun T, Hang SQ, et al. Solexa sequencing of novel and differentially expressed MicroRNAs in testicular and ovarian tissues in Holstein cattle. Int J Biol Sci. 2011;7:1016–26.
35. Chen X, Li QB, Wang J, Guo X, Jiang XR, Ren ZJ, Weng CY, Sun GX, Wang XQ, Liu YP, et al. Identification and characterization of novel amphioxus microRNAs by Solexa sequencing. Genome Biol. 2009;10:R78.
36. Li GX, Li YJ, Li XJ, Ning XM, Li MH, Yang GS. MicroRNA identity and abundance in developing swine adipose tissue as determined by Solexa sequencing. J Cell Biochem. 2011;112:1318–28.
37. Li TT, Wu RM, Zhang Y, Zhu DH. A systematic analysis of the skeletal muscle miRNA transcriptome of chicken varieties with divergent skeletal muscle growth identifies novel miRNAs and differentially expressed miRNAs. BMC Genomics. 2011;12:186.
38. Wei B, Cai T, Zhang RZ, Li AL, Huo NX, Li S, Gu YQ, Vogel J, Jia JZ, Qi YJ, Mao L. Novel microRNAs uncovered by deep sequencing of small RNA transcriptomes in bread wheat (Triticum aestivum L.) and Brachypodium distachyon (L.) Beauv. Funct Integr Genomics. 2009;9:499–511.
39. Bao N, Lye KW, Barton MK. MicroRNA binding sites in Arabidopsis class III HD-ZIP mRNAs are required for methylation of the template chromosome. Dev Cell. 2004;7:653–62.

40. Guo XJ, Su B, Zhou ZM, Sha JH. Rapid evolution of mammalian X-linked testis microRNAs. BMC Genomics. 2009;10:97.

41. Yuan C, Wang XL, Geng RQ, He XL, Qu L, Chen YL. Discovery of cashmere goat (Capra hircus) microRNAs in skin and hair follicles by Solexa sequencing. BMC Genomics. 2013;14:511.

42. Wu J, Zhu H, Song W, Li M, Liu C, Li N, Tang F, Mu H, Liao M, Li X, et al. Identification of conservative MicroRNAs in Saanen dairy goat testis through deep sequencing. Reprod Domest Anim. 2014;49:32–40.

43. Miao XY, Luo QM, Zhao HJ, Qin XY. Genome-wide analysis of miRNAs in the ovaries of Jining Grey and Laiwu black goats to explore the regulation of fecundity. Sci Rep. 2016;6:37983.

44. Okamoto H, Matsumi Y, Hoshikawa Y, Takubo K, Ryoke K, Shiota G. Involvement of MicroRNAs in regulation of osteoblastic differentiation in mouse induced pluripotent stem cells. PLoS One. 2012;7:e43800.

45. Zawistowski JS, Nakamura K, Parker JS, Granger DA, Golitz BT, Johnson GL. MicroRNA 9-3p targets beta1 integrin to sensitize claudin-low breast cancer cells to MEK inhibition. Mol Cell Biol. 2013;33:2260–74.

46. Li Y, Fang Y, Liu Y, Yang XK. MicroRNAs in ovarian function and disorders. J Ovarian Res. 2015;8:51.

47. Hossain MM, Sohel MMH, Schellander K, Tesfaye D. Characterization and importance of microRNAs in mammalian gonadal functions. Cell Tissue Res. 2012;349:679–90.

48. Cui L, Zhou H, Zhao H, Zhou YJ, Xu RF, Xu XL, Zheng L, Xue Z, Xia W, Zhang B, et al. MicroRNA-99a induces G1-phase cell cycle arrest and suppresses tumorigenicity in renal cell carcinoma. BMC Cancer. 2012;12:546.

49. Zi XD, Lu JY, Ma L. Identification and comparative analysis of the ovarian microRNAs of prolific and non-prolific goats during the follicular phase using high-throughput sequencing. Sci Rep. 2017;7:1921.

50. Wang J, Ruan K. miR-335 is involved in the rat epididymal development by targeting the mRNA of RASA1. Biochem Biophys Res Commun. 2010;402:222–7.

51. Chen C, Wu CQ, Zhang ZQ, Yao DK, Zhu L. Loss of expression of miR-335 is implicated in hepatic stellate cell migration and activation. Exp Cell Res. 2011;317:1714–25.

52. Tome M, Lopez-Romero P, Albo C, Sepulveda JC, Fernandez-Gutierrez B, Dopazo A, Bernad A, Gonzalez MA. miR-335 orchestrates cell proliferation, migration and differentiation in human mesenchymal stem cells. Cell Death Differ. 2011;18:985–95.

53. Png KJ, Yoshida M, Zhang XH, Shu W, Lee H, Rimner A, Chan TA, Comen E, Andrade VP, Kim SW, et al. MicroRNA-335 inhibits tumor reinitiation and is silenced through genetic and epigenetic mechanisms in human breast cancer. Genes Dev. 2011;25:226–31.

54. Bouhallier F, Allioli N, Lavial F, Chalmel F, Perrard MH, Durand P, Samarut J, Pain B, Rouault JP. Role of miR-34c microRNA in the late steps of spermatogenesis. Rna-a Publication of the Rna Society. 2010;16:720–31.

55. Zhang SS, Yu M, Liu C, Wang L, Hu Y, Bai YF, Hua JL. MIR-34c regulates mouse embryonic stem cells differentiation into male germ-like cells through RARg. Cell Biochem Funct. 2012;30:623–32.

56. Li M, Yu M, Liu C, Zhu H, He X, Peng S, Hua J. miR-34c works downstream of p53 leading to dairy goat male germline stem-cell (mGSCs) apoptosis. Cell Prolif. 2013;46:223–31.

57. Messina A, Langlet F, Chachlaki K, Roa J, Rasika S, Jouy N, Gallet S, Gaytan F, Parkash J, Tena-Sempere M, et al. A microRNA switch regulates the rise in hypothalamic GnRH production before puberty (vol 19, pg 835, 2016). Nat Neurosci. 2016;19:1115.

58. Lannes J, L'Hote D, Garrel G, Laverriere JN, Cohen-Tannoudji J, Querat B. Rapid communication: a microRNA-132/212 pathway mediates GnRH activation of FSH expression. Mol Endocrinol. 2015;29:364–72.

## 4

PAPP-A2 deficiency does not exacerbate the phenotype of a mouse model of intrauterine growth restriction

Julian K. Christians[*]⬤, Kendra I. Lennie, Maria F. Huicochea Munoz and Nimrat Binning

Abstract

Background: Pregnancy-associated plasma protein-A2 (PAPP-A2) is consistently upregulated in the placentae of pregnancies complicated by preeclampsia and fetal growth restriction. The causes and significance of this upregulation remain unknown, but it has been hypothesized that it is a compensatory response to improve placental growth and development. We predicted that, if the upregulation of PAPP-A2 in pregnancy complications reflects a compensatory response, then deletion of *Pappa2* in mice would exacerbate the effects of a gene deletion previously reported to impair placental development: deficiency of matrix metalloproteinase-9 (MMP9).

Methods: We crossed mice carrying deletions in *Pappa2* and *Mmp9* to produce pregnancies deficient in one, both, or neither of these genes. We measured pregnancy rates, number of conceptuses, fetal and placental growth, and the histological structure of the placenta.

Results: We found no evidence of reduced fertility, increased pregnancy loss, or increased fetal demise in $Mmp9^{-/-}$ females. In pregnancies segregating for *Mmp9*, $Mmp9^{-/-}$ fetuses were lighter than their siblings with a functional *Mmp9* allele. However, deletion of *Pappa2* did not exacerbate or reveal any effects of *Mmp9* deficiency. We observed some effects of *Pappa2* deletion on placental structure that were independent of *Mmp9* deficiency, but no effects on fetal growth. At G16, male fetuses were heavier than female fetuses and had heavier placentae with larger junctional zones and smaller labyrinths.

Conclusions: Effects of *Mmp9* deficiency were not exacerbated by the deletion of *Pappa2*. Our results do not provide evidence that upregulation of placental PAPP-A2 represents a mechanism to compensate for impaired fetal growth.

Keywords: Placenta, Pregnancy, Preeclampsia, Intrauterine growth restriction, Pregnancy associated plasma protein, Matrix metalloproteinase, Insulin-like growth factor

Background

Intrauterine growth restriction and preeclampsia threaten the health and wellbeing of both the fetus and the mother, affecting 5–7% of pregnancies and constituting leading causes of perinatal and maternal mortality [1]. These conditions are thought to be caused, at least in part, by abnormal placental development and function [2]. There have been enormous efforts to identify the molecular mechanisms responsible for placental dysfunction in preeclampsia and intrauterine growth restriction, with numerous studies examining placental gene expression at delivery. Pregnancy-associated plasma protein-A2 (PAPP-A2) is one of the genes most consistently found to be upregulated in preeclampsia [3–7] and is also associated with fetal growth restriction [8]. Furthermore, elevated levels of PAPP-A2 in the maternal circulation in the first trimester have also been associated with preeclampsia [9, 10]. PAPP-A2 is a protease of insulin-like growth factor binding protein 5 (IGFBP-5) [11] and is thought to regulate insulin-like growth factor (IGF) availability, although it may also function through other pathways [12]. IGFs play key roles in placental development [13], and their availability is regulated by six IGF binding proteins (IGFBPs). IGFs are released primarily through cleavage of the IGFBPs by proteases [14].

* Correspondence: julian_christians@sfu.ca
Department of Biological Sciences, Simon Fraser University, Burnaby, BC, Canada

PAPP-A2 deficiency would therefore be expected to reduce IGF availability, and indeed loss-of-function mutations in humans reduce stature [15] while *Pappa2* deletion in mice reduces body size [16–18] and increases IGFBP-5 levels [19].

Despite the high expression of PAPP-A2 in mouse placenta [20], *Pappa2* deletion has no effect on pregnancy outcomes, apart from slightly reduced birthweight, which may be due to deletion in the fetus itself [16, 21]. We therefore hypothesized that the upregulation of PAPP-A2 in human pregnancy complications represents a compensatory response to increase IGF signaling to promote placental growth and development [10, 22, 23]. To test this hypothesis, we deleted *Pappa2* in a mouse model of preeclampsia and intrauterine growth restriction: deficiency of matrix metalloproteinase-9 (MMP9) [24]. We selected this model since *Mmp9* deletion impairs early placental development [24], and thus reflects "canonical" preeclampsia, rather than preeclampsia of other etiologies [25]. Deficiencies in early placental development would be expected to be ameliorated by increased IGF availability and, therefore, by increased PAPP-A2 expression. We predicted that, if the elevated expression of PAPP-A2 in preeclampsia in humans reflects a compensatory response, then deletion of *Pappa2* in mice would exacerbate effects of *Mmp9* deletion, i.e., mice null for both *Pappa2* and *Mmp9* would show a more severe phenotype than mice null for *Mmp9* only. We focused on the number and size of fetuses, as well as placental histology since these were traits expected to be affected by *Mmp9* deficiency [24] and potentially ameliorated by PAPP-A2 and increased IGF availability.

Methods

All work was carried out in accordance with the guidelines of the Canadian Council on Animal Care and approved by the SFU University Animal Care Committee (protocol 1188B). *Pappa2* deletion mice with a C57BL/6 background were generated as previously described [16, 19]. Females homozygous for *Pappa2* deletion ($Pappa2^{-/-}$) were crossed with a male homozygous for *Mmp9* deletion ($Mmp9^{-/-}$) obtained from the Jackson Laboratory (stock number 007084) to produce offspring heterozygous at both genes. The first generation (F1) offspring were crossed to produce an F2 population that included mice with all nine possible genotypes (three *Mmp9* genotypes x three *Pappa2* genotypes). Females and males from the F2 population were selected based on *Mmp9* and *Pappa2* genotype for breeding experiments, and were mated as described in Table 1. Rather than using only homozygous mice, we performed a variety of crosses to make use of as many mice as possible (Table 1). Furthermore, mating type 1 with $Mmp9^{+/-}$ males was previously reported to show a reduction in litter size and placental abnormalities

Table 1 *Mmp9* crosses performed in experiments

Mating type	Female MMP9 genotype	Male MMP9 genotype
0	−/−	−/−
1	−/−	+/−
2	+/−	−/−
3	+/−	+/−
4	+/+	+/+

Each type of *Mmp9* cross included either no functional *Pappa2* alleles ($Pappa2^{-/-}$ x $Pappa2^{-/-}$) or at least one functional *Pappa2* (achieved with various combinations of female and male genotype)

[24]. Beginning at approximately 8 weeks of age, females were placed with a male for one night, checked for vaginal plugs, and removed from the male whether or not a plug was observed. If no vaginal plug was observed and/or if female weight had not increased by ~ 1 g 1 week after mating, females were paired again. F2 females were collected at day 16 of gestation (G16; where the day after mating = day 0). To obtain mice for a further cohort, some females heterozygous at both genes ($Mmp9^{+/-}$; $Pappa2^{+/-}$) were paired with males homozygous for both deletions ($Mmp9^{-/-}$; $Pappa2^{-/-}$) and not collected during pregnancy. We produced a backcross (BC) population, rather than crossing heterozygotes, to increase the number of mice homozygous for *Mmp9* and/or *Pappa2* deletion. Females and males from the BC population were mated in the same manner as the F2 population, except that females were collected at day 18 of gestation (G18). Pregnancies were sampled at G18 in case effects were apparent only after G16. 63 F2 females were mated, yielding 43 G16 pregnancies (although one was mistakenly not collected during pregnancy) whereas 24 BC females were mated, yielding 20 G18 pregnancies.

At collection, females were blood sampled by cardiac puncture and the entire uterus was placed in 4% formaldehyde solution in phosphate buffered saline for 3 days before it was dissected to count and weigh individual fetuses and placentae, and to count putative fetal resorptions (green or green/brown masses). Maternal serum vascular endothelial growth factor (VEGF) was measured by enzyme-linked immunosorbent assay (R&D Systems, MMV00). Fixed placentae were stored in 70% ethanol until embedded in paraffin. A subset of placentae were selected for sectioning, attempting to include one male and one female placenta for each female, and excluding heterozygous genotypes. Because previous work reported that both embryonic and maternal *Mmp9* deficiency affect placental development [24], we selected $Mmp9^{-/-}$ placentae from both $Mmp9^{-/-}$ and $Mmp9^{+/-}$ dams, as well as $Mmp9^{+/+}$ placentae from $Mmp9^{+/+}$ dams. For each placenta, multiple sections (6 μm) were obtained ~ 440 μm apart, up to a maximum of 10 sections per placenta. Sections were stained with haematoxylin and eosin and the areas of the labyrinth, junctional zone and decidua were measured using ImageJ 1.48v. Damaged sections, and sections close to the edge of the placenta (i.e., where the labyrinth was mostly surrounded by junctional zone) were excluded, yielding 454 sections from 62 placentae (average: 7.3 sections per placenta). To obtain a single value for each of the labyrinth, junctional zone and decidua for each placenta, we analysed the areas from all 454 sections using a general linear model (proc GLM, SAS, Version 9.4) including terms for placenta identity and section location (i.e., close to the centre vs. further from the centre; sections further from the centre had smaller areas). From this analysis, we obtained the least squares mean for each placenta for each of the labyrinth, junctional zone and decidua.

To obtain tissue for genotyping, mice were ear-clipped at weaning or a small section of fetal tail was collected. *Pappa2* genotype [19] and fetal sex [26] were determined as previously described. *Mmp9* genotype was determined by PCR as recommended by the Jackson Laboratory (primers used: 5'-CTGAATGAACTGCA GGACGA-3'; 5'-ATACTTTCTCGGCAGGAGCA-3'; 5'-GTGGGACCATCATAACATCACA-3'; 5'-CTCG CGGCAAGTCTTCAGAGTA-3';).

All statistical analyses were performed using general linear models (proc GLM) or repeated measures analyses (proc MIXED) in SAS, Version 9.4 (SAS Institute Inc., Cary, NC). Repeated measures analyses (with dam as a random factor) were used for placental and fetal traits where there were multiple offspring per dam, since the dam was the unit of replication.

Results

The genotype ratios and postnatal growth of the F2 and BC populations are presented in the Additional file 1. Combining F2 and BC females, we found no evidence of reduced fertility or increased pregnancy loss in $Mmp9^{-/-}$ females. The proportion of females that became pregnant did not differ between $Mmp9^{-/-}$ females and other females, whether all females were analysed together (Fisher's Exact Test $P = 0.47$) or separately based on

whether at least one wild-type *Pappa2* allele was present (Fisher's Exact Test $P = 1.00$) or not (Fisher's Exact Test $P = 0.27$) (Table 2). Similarly, the proportion of females that had at least one failed mating (i.e., a vaginal plug was detected following mating, but pregnancy did not develop) did not differ between $Mmp9^{-/-}$ females and other females. This was true whether all females were analysed together (Fisher's Exact Test $P = 0.47$) or separately based on whether at least one wild-type *Pappa2* allele was present (Fisher's Exact Test $P = 0.33$) or not (Fisher's Exact Test $P = 1.00$) (Table 2). The number of times a female was paired with a male before becoming pregnant did not differ between $Mmp9^{-/-}$ and other females ($F_{1,59} = 0.18$; $P = 0.67$), and was not affected by whether at least one wild-type *Pappa2* allele was present ($F_{1,59} = 2.22$; $P = 0.14$), or by the interaction between these two factors ($F_{1,59} = 0.10$; $P = 0.76$) (Table 2). Since the number of times a female was paired with a male varied only from 1 to 6, we also analysed these data using a non-parametric Wilcoxon test. Again there was no difference between $Mmp9^{-/-}$ and other females ($P = 0.71$), pooling matings with and without at least one wild-type *Pappa2* allele present.

We also found no evidence of reduced fecundity or increased fetal loss in $Mmp9^{-/-}$ females. Including females collected at either G16 or G18, the number of fetuses did not differ between $Mmp9^{-/-}$ and other females ($F_{1,58} = 0.28$; $P = 0.60$), and was not affected by whether at least one wild-type *Pappa2* allele was present ($F_{1,58} = 0.00$; $P = 0.99$) or the interaction between these two factors ($F_{1,58} = 0.17$; $P = 0.68$) (Fig. 1). The number of putative embryo resorptions ranged from 0 to 4, and tended to be slightly lower in $Mmp9^{-/-}$ females (mean = 0.6) than in other females (mean = 0.9; Wilcoxon test $P = 0.25$). The proportion of females that had at least one resorption did not differ between $Mmp9$ genotypes (11/30 $Mmp9^{-/-}$ females vs. 16/32 other females; Fisher's Exact Test $P = 0.32$).

At G16, the average fetal mass and average placental mass did not differ between $Mmp9^{-/-}$ and other females,

Table 2 Effects of *Mmp9* and *Pappa2* deletion on fertility including F2 and BC females, i.e., females collected at G16 or G18

	No wild-type *Pappa2* alleles *Mmp9* mating type		At least one wild-type *Pappa2* allele *Mmp9* mating type	
	0–1	2–4	0–1	2–4
# matings for pregnancy[a]	2.3 ± 0.4	2.3 ± 0.3	2.7 ± 0.3	2.9 ± 0.3
# females that became pregnant	11	16	19	17
# females that did not become pregnant	2	9	7	6
# females with no failed matings[b]	9	18	18	19
# females with failed mating[b]	4	7	8	4

[a]Least-squares means ± standard error from a general linear model including *Mmp9* mating type, whether mating had any wild-type *Pappa2* alleles, and the interaction between these two terms
[b]A failed mating was defined as when a vaginal plug was detected following mating, but pregnancy did not develop; this analysis includes females that subsequently became pregnant, and those that never became pregnant

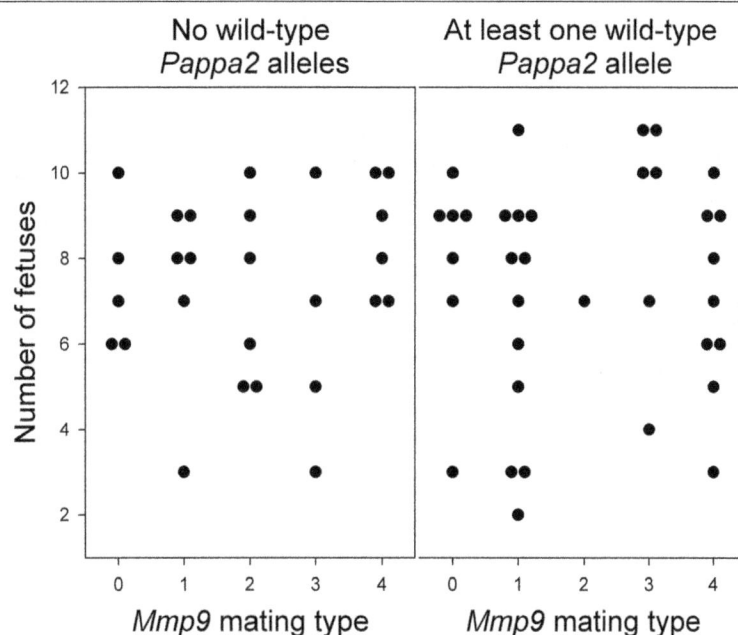

Fig. 1 Effect of *Mmp9* and *Pappa2* deletion on the number of fetuses, including females collected at either G16 or G18

and was not affected by whether at least one wild-type *Pappa2* allele was present or the interaction between these two factors (controlling for the number of fetuses, which was negatively related to fetal and placental mass; Table 3). There was no excess of very small or runted pups in *Mmp9*$^{-/-}$ pregnancies (Fig. 2). There was a tendency for *Mmp9*$^{-/-}$ females to have heavier placentae, but this was marginally non-significant ($P = 0.07$, Table 3). Considering only pregnancies with both *Mmp9*$^{+/-}$ and *Mmp9*$^{-/-}$ fetuses, *Mmp9*$^{-/-}$ fetuses and their placentae were significantly lighter than their *Mmp9*$^{+/-}$ siblings, but there was no effect of whether a wild-type *Pappa2* allele was present in the pregnancy, and no interaction between *Mmp9* and *Pappa2* (Table 4; Fig. 3). Male fetuses were heavier than female fetuses and had heavier placentae. The number of *Mmp9*$^{-/-}$ to *Mmp9*$^{+/-}$ conceptuses did not differ from the

expected 1:1 ratio (76 *Mmp9*$^{-/-}$ vs. 73 *Mmp9*$^{+/-}$; $\chi^2_1 = 0.06$; $P = 0.81$).

We also studied fetuses at G18, in case growth restriction was more apparent later in pregnancy. As at G16, the average fetal mass and average placental mass did not differ between *Mmp9*$^{-/-}$ and other females, and was not affected by whether at least one wild-type *Pappa2* allele was present or the interaction between these two factors, controlling for the number of fetuses (Table 3; Fig. 2). Average fetal mass tended to be lighter in *Mmp9*$^{-/-}$ females but this was marginally non-significant ($P = 0.08$, Table 3). Considering only pregnancies segregating at *Mmp9*, *Mmp9*$^{-/-}$ fetuses were lighter than their *Mmp9*$^{+/-}$ and *Mmp9*$^{+/+}$ siblings, but there was no effect of whether a wild-type *Pappa2* allele was present in the pregnancy, and no interaction

Table 3 Effects of *Mmp9* and *Pappa2* deletion on average fetal mass and average placental mass

	Term in model							
	Mmp9		*Pappa2*		*Mmp9*Pappa2* interaction		Number of fetuses	
G16								
	$F_{1,36}$	P	$F_{1,36}$	P	$F_{1,36}$	P	$F_{1,36}$	P
Average fetal mass	0.89	0.35	0.44	0.51	0.04	0.84	6.51	0.02
Average placental mass	3.50	0.07	0.82	0.37	0.01	0.94	10.76	0.002
G18								
	$F_{1,15}$	P	$F_{1,15}$	P	$F_{1,15}$	P	$F_{1,15}$	P
Average fetal mass	3.41	0.08	1.13	0.31	0.03	0.86	2.08	0.17
Average placental mass	0.61	0.45	1.00	0.33	0.00	0.98	1.11	0.31

Statistics are from general linear models including effects of *Mmp9* deletion (mating types 0 and 1 compared with others), *Pappa2* deletion (whether the cross included at least one functional *Pappa2* allele or not), the interaction between these two factors, and the number of fetuses as a covariate

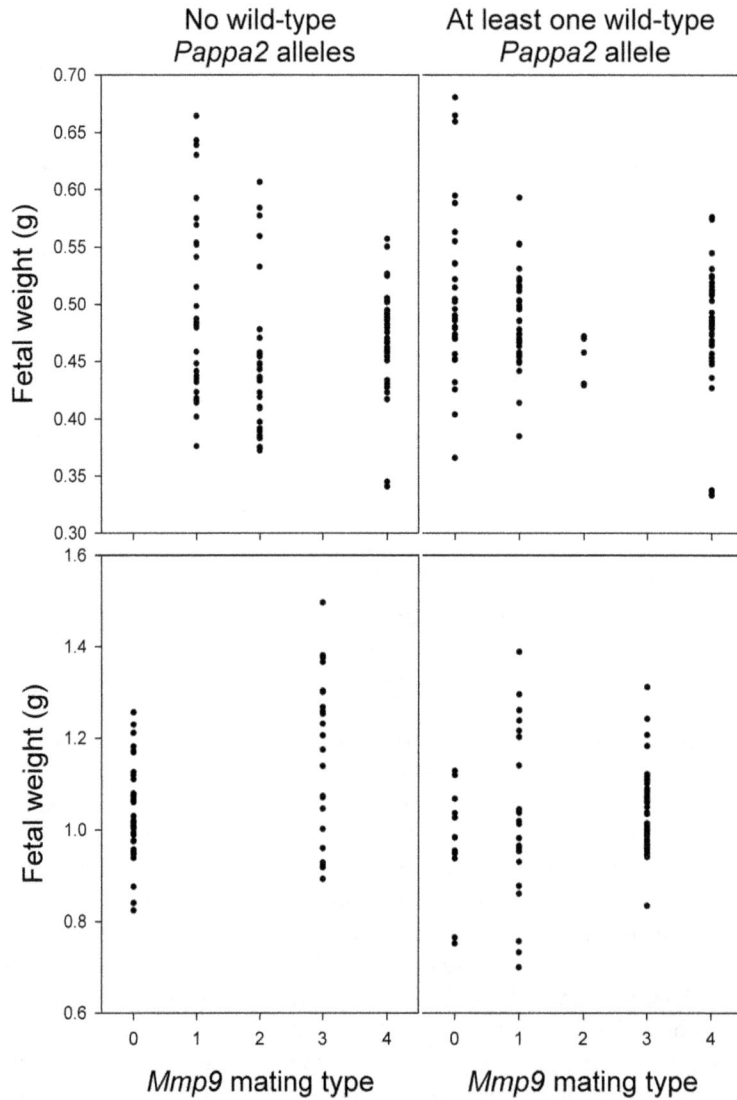

Fig. 2 Effect of *Mmp9* and *Pappa2* deletion on fetal weight at G16 (upper panels) and G18 (lower panels)

Table 4 Effects of *Mmp9* and *Pappa2* deletion on fetal mass and placental mass in pregnancies segregating for *Mmp9*

	Term in model									
	Mmp9		*Pappa2*		*Mmp9*Pappa2* interaction		Number of fetuses		Sex of fetus	
G16										
	$F_{1,16}$	P	$F_{1,18}$	P	$F_{1,16}$	P	$F_{1,18}$	P	$F_{1,15}$	P
Fetal mass	9.69	0.007	0.07	0.80	0.40	0.54	2.97	0.10	14.72	0.002
Placental mass	12.63	0.003	0.06	0.80	0.01	0.91	5.12	0.04	31.08	0.0001
G18										
	$F_{1,10}$	P	$F_{1,11}$	P	$F_{1,10}$	P	$F_{1,11}$	P	$F_{1,11}$	P
Fetal mass	9.53	0.012	0.59	0.46	0.03	0.88	7.24	0.02	1.06	0.32
Placental mass	0.81	0.39	1.13	0.31	1.26	0.29	4.49	0.06	17.82	0.0014

These analyses included multiple conceptuses per dam, and so statistics are from repeated measures analyses (with dam as a random factor), including effects of *Mmp9* genotype of conceptus (*Mmp9*$^{-/-}$ vs. *Mmp9*$^{+/-}$ and *Mmp9*$^{+/+}$), *Pappa2* deletion (whether the cross included at least one functional *Pappa2* allele or not), the interaction between these two factors, fetal sex, and the number of fetuses as a covariate

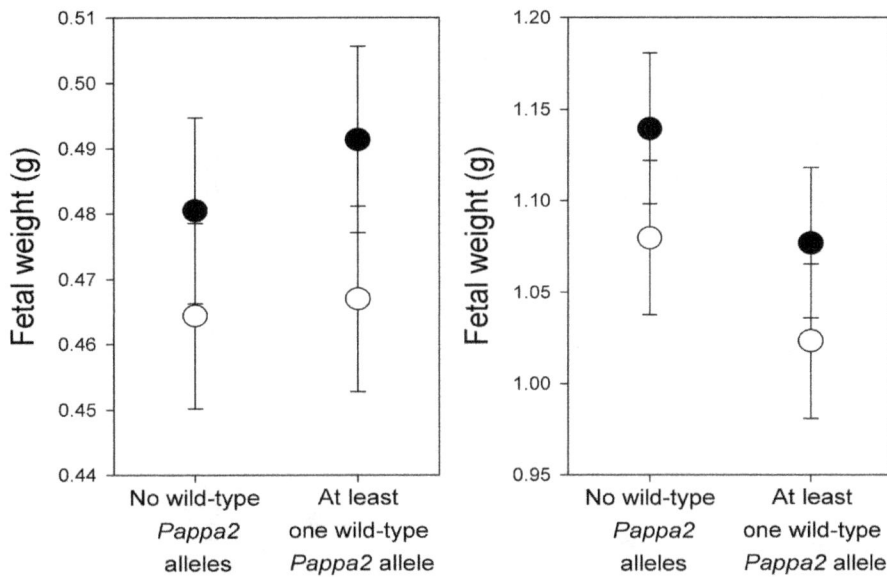

Fig. 3 Effect of *Mmp9* and *Pappa2* deletion on fetal weight at G16 (left) and G18 (right) in pregnancies segregating at *Mmp9*. Open symbols are $Mmp9^{-/-}$ fetuses and solid symbols are their $Mmp9^{+/-}$ and $Mmp9^{+/+}$ siblings. Error bars are pooled per *Mmp9* genotype (i.e., pooling *Pappa2* genotype)

between *Mmp9* and *Pappa2* (Table 4; Fig. 3). There was no effect of *Mmp9* genotype on placental weight. As at G16, male fetuses had heavier placentae than female fetuses. The genotype ratios did not differ from the expected Mendelian ratios in litters segregating for 2 genotypes (16 $Mmp9^{-/-}$: 9 $Mmp9^{+/-}$; $\chi^2_1 = 1.96$; $P = 0.16$) or three genotypes (26 $Mmp9^{-/-}$: 40 $Mmp9^{+/-}$: 12 $Mmp9^{+/+}$; $\chi^2_1 = 5.08$; $P = 0.08$). Though non-significant, the trend was for an excess of $Mmp9^{-/-}$ conceptuses.

At G16, we observed little effect of *Mmp9* deficiency on the areas of the labyrinth, junctional zone or decidua, either in absolute terms or in terms of each component as a percentage of the total area (Table 5; Figs. 4 and 5). There was generally no interaction between *Mmp9* deficiency and whether at least one wild-type *Pappa2* allele was present (Table 5; Fig. 4), although $Mmp9^{-/-}$ placentae from $Mmp9^{-/-}$ dams with no *Pappa2* had slightly smaller decidua area, when measured as a percentage of the total area (Table 5; Fig. 4). Pregnancies with no *Pappa2* had smaller deciduas in absolute terms, and had larger labyrinths and smaller deciduas as a percentage of the total area, compared to pregnancies where at least one wild-type *Pappa2* allele was present (Table 5; Fig. 4). Placentae of male fetuses had larger junctional zone

Table 5 Effects of *Mmp9* and *Pappa2* deletion on the areas of the labyrinth, junctional zone and decidua, either in absolute terms, or as a percentage of total area

	Term in model							
	$Mmp9^a$		*Pappa2*		*Mmp9*Pappa2* interaction		Sex of fetus	
	$F_{2,28}$	P	$F_{1,28}$	P	$F_{2,28}$	P	$F_{1,20}$	P
Absolute								
Labyrinth	0.20	0.82	0.00	0.98	1.64	0.21	0.10	0.75
Junctional Zone	0.38	0.69	1.93	0.18	0.69	0.51	14.76	0.001[b]
Decidua	3.17	0.06	7.89	0.01	2.62	0.09	2.90	0.10
Percentage of total								
Labyrinth	1.15	0.33	6.89	0.01	1.80	0.18	15.01	0.001[b]
Junctional Zone	1.41	0.26	0.79	0.38	0.04	0.96	11.63	0.003[b]
Decidua	4.10	0.03	6.97	0.01	3.96	0.03	0.00	0.98

These analyses included multiple conceptuses per dam, and so statistics are from repeated measures analyses (with dam as a random factor), including effects of *Mmp9* group, *Pappa2* deletion (whether the cross included at least one functional *Pappa2* allele or not), the interaction between these two factors, and fetal sex
[a]In these analyses, there were three *Mmp9* groups: $Mmp9^{-/-}$ placentae from $Mmp9^{-/-}$ dams, $Mmp9^{-/-}$ placentae from $Mmp9^{+/-}$ dams, and $Mmp9^{+/+}$ placentae from $Mmp9^{+/+}$ dams
[b]Area of the junctional zone, both absolute and as a percentage of the total area, was larger in males than females, while the area of the labyrinth as a percentage of the total was smaller in males

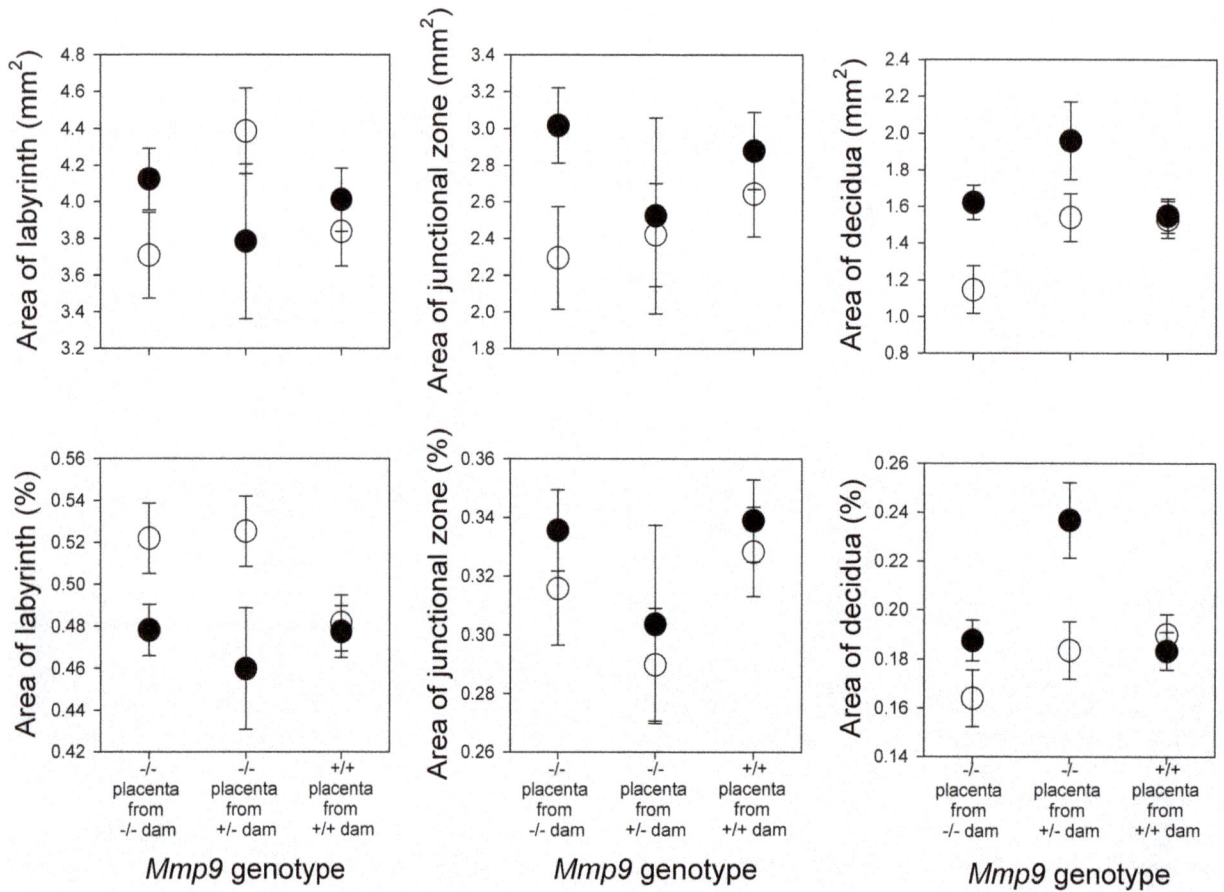

Fig. 4 Effect of *Mmp9* and *Pappa2* deletion on the areas of the labyrinth, junctional zone and decidua in absolute terms (upper panels) and as a percentage of the total area (lower panels). Open symbols are pregnancies without a functional *Pappa2* allele and solid symbols are pregnancies with at least one functional *Pappa2* allele. Error bars are from repeated measures analyses (with dam as a random factor), including effects of *Mmp9* group, *Pappa2* deletion, the interaction between these two factors, and fetal sex

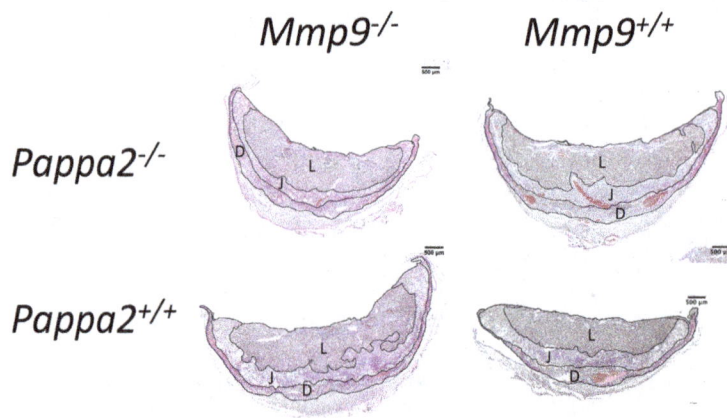

Fig. 5 Representative images of G16 placental sections from *Mmp9*^{−/−} placentae from *Mmp9*^{−/−} dams and *Mmp9*^{+/+} placentae from *Mmp9*^{+/+} dams, with and without *Pappa2*, showing the outlined labyrinth (L), junctional zone (J) and decidua (D). All placentae are from female fetuses

areas in absolute terms and, as a percentage of the total area, had larger junctional zones and smaller labyrinths.

The previous report of *Mmp9* deletion mice [24] described reduced serum VEGF levels in *Mmp9*$^{-/-}$ females. We analysed VEGF levels at G16 in a subset of pregnancies of *Mmp9*$^{-/-}$ and *Mmp9*$^{+/+}$ females, all with at least one wild-type *Pappa2* allele. VEGF levels did not differ between *Mmp9*$^{-/-}$ and *Mmp9*$^{+/+}$ females ($F_{1,10} = 0.12$; $P = 0.73$), but were positively related with the number of conceptuses ($F_{1,10} = 13.70$; $P = 0.004$; Fig. 6).

Discussion

In humans, placental PAPP-A2 is upregulated in preeclampsia [3–7] and fetal growth restriction [8]. However, deletion of *Pappa2* in mice has little effect on pregnancy outcome [16, 21], suggesting that the upregulation of PAPP-A2 in human pregnancy complications may represent a compensatory response [10, 22, 23]. If PAPP-A2 is important in compensating for placental insufficiency, it would be expected that its absence would exacerbate the effects of placental dysfunction. Previously, *Mmp9* deficiency has been reported to cause placental abnormalities resulting in growth restriction [24]. We observed that *Mmp9*$^{-/-}$ fetuses were lighter than *Mmp9*$^{+/-}$ siblings, but this difference was not exacerbated by deletion of *Pappa2*. Therefore, our results do not provide evidence that PAPP-A2 contributes to placental mechanisms that compensate for poor fetal growth.

Surprisingly, we found no effect of *Mmp9* deletion, with or without deletion of *Pappa2*, on fertility, fecundity, pregnancy loss, fetal loss or placental structure. While the publication describing *Mmp9* deletion as a model of preeclampsia and intrauterine growth

restriction reported "as much as a 50% reduction in litter size" [24], no data were presented, and the original report of *Mmp9* deletion described a much more modest reduction in litter size (1.6 pups) [27]. In our experiments, *Mmp9*$^{-/-}$ females were compared with control siblings, and no experimental females were daughters of *Mmp9*$^{-/-}$ females. It is therefore possible that by avoiding maternal effects of *Mmp9* deletion, the severity of the deletion was reduced; whether previous reports [24, 27] used our breeding scheme is not clear.

The previous report of the effects of *Mmp9* deficiency on pregnancy also reported reduced levels of VEGF in the maternal circulation [24]. VEGF influences placental angiogenesis, and maternal circulating VEGF levels are reduced in preeclamptic human pregnancies [28]. While there was no effect of *Mmp9* deficiency on circulating maternal VEGF in the present study, we found a positive association between VEGF levels and the number of conceptuses. The previous report of reduced VEGF in *Mmp9*$^{-/-}$ females [24] may therefore have been due to reduced numbers of conceptuses, rather than to placental pathology.

In addition to some modest effects of *Mmp9* and *Pappa2* deletion, we observed more robust differences between the sexes in fetal mass, placental mass, and placental structure at G16, as well as placental mass at G18. These differences may reflect sex-specific strategies for fetal growth and placental function [29] with potential long term effects on offspring health [30].

Conclusions

Previous work reported that deletion of *Mmp9* reduced pregnancy rates and implantation success following embryo transfer, decreased litter size, and increased rates of fetal demise and growth restriction [24]. In contrast, we found only modest effects of *Mmp9* deletion on fetal growth, and found no effects on the number of fetuses, the number of putative embryo resorptions, or female fertility (number of matings required to achieve pregnancy, the proportion of females that became pregnant, or the number of females with failed matings). The difference in results between our study and previous work may have been due to our experimental design, which compared *Mmp9*$^{-/-}$ females with control siblings and thus avoided confounding maternal effects. The effects of *Mmp9* deficiency were not exacerbated by the deletion of *Pappa2*, and therefore our results do not support the hypothesis that PAPP-A2 upregulation in human pregnancy complications represents a compensatory response to ameliorate placental growth and development. Our results provide insight into the role of PAPP-A2 dysregulation in devastating pregnancy complications, which may inform the use of this protein as an early biomarker of placental health [9, 10]. Our work also serves as a caution regarding the use of *Mmp9* deficiency as a model of these complications.

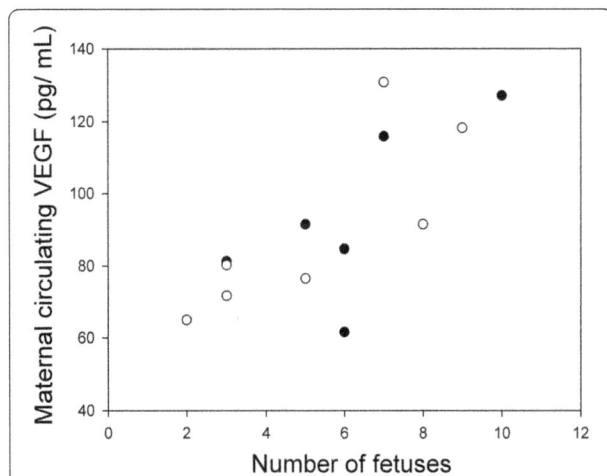

Fig. 6 Relationship between number of fetuses and VEGF levels in the maternal circulation of *Mmp9*$^{-/-}$ dams (open symbols) and *Mmp9*$^{+/+}$ dams (solid symbols) at G16. All pregnancies have at least one functional copy of *Pappa2*

Abbreviations
BC: Backcross; F1: First generation; F2: Second generation; G16, G18: day 16 or 18 of gestation, where the day after mating = day 0; IGF: Insulin-like growth factor; IGFBP: Insulin-like growth factor binding protein; MMP9: Matrix metalloproteinase-9; PAPP-A2: Pregnancy-associated plasma protein-A2; VEGF: Vascular endothelial growth factor

Acknowledgements
We are grateful for assistance from Alex Fraser (training in histological techniques), Danielle Mara and Alex Beristain (imaging placental sections), Rajan Sidhu (measuring placental areas), Monika Rogowska (genotyping), and the Animal Care staff at Simon Fraser University (animal maintenance and timed matings). We thank two anonymous reviewers for constructive comments on the manuscript.

Funding
This study was funded by an NSERC (Canada) Discovery Grant to JKC, a Simon Fraser University Vice President, Research Undergraduate Student Research Award (USRA) to KIL, and an NSERC USRA to NB. The funding bodies had no role in study design, collection, analysis, and interpretation of data or in manuscript preparation.

Authors' contributions
JKC conceived of the study, contributed to laboratory work, carried out statistical analyses, and wrote the manuscript. KIL performed the laboratory work and helped draft the manuscript. NB contributed to laboratory work, analysed the placental images, and helped draft the manuscript. MFHM analysed the placental images and helped draft the manuscript. All authors approve and are accountable for the final version.

Competing interests
The authors declare that they have no competing interests.

References
1. Huppertz B. Placental origins of preeclampsia - challenging the current hypothesis. Hypertension. 2008;51:970–5.
2. Pijnenborg R, Vercruysse L, Brosens I. Deep placentation. Best Pract Res Clin Obstet Gynaecol. 2011;25:273–85.
3. Vaiman D, Miralles F. An integrative analysis of preeclampsia based on the construction of an extended composite network featuring protein-protein physical interactions and transcriptional relationships. PLoS One. 2016;11: e0165849.
4. Brew O, Sullivan MHF, Woodman A. Comparison of normal and pre-eclamptic placental gene expression: a systematic review with meta-analysis. PLoS One. 2016;11:e0161504.
5. Kleinrouweler CE, van Uitert M, Moerland PD, Ris-Stalpers C, van der Post JAM, Afink GB. Differentially expressed genes in the pre-Eclamptic placenta: a systematic review and meta-analysis. PLoS One. 2013;8:e68991.
6. Kramer AW, Lamale-Smith LM, Winn VD. Differential expression of human placental PAPP-A2 over gestation and in preeclampsia. Placenta. 2016;37:19–25.
7. Macintire K, Tuohey L, Ye L, Palmer K, Gantier M, Tong S, et al. PAPPA2 is increased in severe early onset pre-eclampsia and upregulated with hypoxia. Reprod Fertil Dev. 2014;26:351–7.
8. Whitehead CL, Walker SP, Ye L, Mendis S, Kaitu'u-Lino TJ, Lappas M, et al. Placental specific mRNA in the maternal circulation are globally dysregulated in pregnancies complicated by fetal growth restriction. J Clin Endocrinol Metab. 2013;98:E429–36.
9. Hansen YB, Myrhøj V, Jørgensen FS, Oxvig C, Sørensen S. First trimester PAPP-A2, PAPP-A and hCGβ in small-for-gestational-age pregnancies. Clin Chem Lab Med. 2016;54:117–23.
10. Crosley EJ, Durland U, Seethram K, Macrae S, Gruslin A, Christians JK. First-trimester levels of pregnancy-associated plasma protein A2 (PAPP-A2) in the maternal circulation are elevated in pregnancies that subsequently develop preeclampsia. Reprod Sci. 2014;21:754–60.
11. Overgaard MT, Boldt HB, Laursen LS, Sottrup-Jensen L, Conover CA, Oxvig C. Pregnancy-associated plasma protein-A2 (PAPP-A2), a novel insulin-like growth factor-binding protein-5 proteinase. J Biol Chem. 2001;276:21849–53.
12. Kjaer-Sorensen K, Engholm DH, Jepsen MR, Morch MG, Weyer K, Hefting LL, et al. Papp-a2 modulates development of cranial cartilage and angiogenesis in zebrafish embryos. J Cell Sci. 2014;127:5027–37.
13. Sferruzzi-Perri AN, Owens JA, Pringle KG, Roberts CT. The neglected role of insulin-like growth factors in the maternal circulation regulating fetal growth. J Physiol. 2011;589:7–20.
14. Bunn RC, Fowlkes JL. Insulin-like growth factor binding protein proteolysis. Trends Endocrinol Metab. 2003;14:176–81.
15. Dauber A, Munoz-Calvo MT, Barrios V, Domene HM, Kloverpris S, Serra-Juhe C, et al. Mutations in pregnancy-associated plasma protein A2 cause short stature due to low IGF-I availability. EMBO Mol Med [Internet]. 2016;8:363–74. Available from: http://embomolmed.embopress.org/cgi/doi/10.15252/emmm.201506106
16. Christians JK, de Zwaan DR, Fung SHY. Pregnancy associated plasma protein A2 (PAPP-A2) affects bone size and shape and contributes to natural variation in postnatal growth in mice. PLoS One. 2013;8:e56260.
17. Amiri N, Christians JK. PAPP-A2 expression by osteoblasts is required for normal postnatal growth in mice. Growth Horm IGF Res. 2015;25:274–80.
18. Conover CA, Boldt HB, Bale LK, Clifton KB, Grell JA, Mader JR, et al. Pregnancy-associated plasma protein-A2 (PAPP-A2): tissue expression and biological consequences of gene knockout in mice. Endocrinology. 2011;152:2837–44.
19. Christians JK, Bath AK, Amiri N. Pappa2 deletion alters IGFBPs but has little effect on glucose disposal or adiposity. Growth Horm IGF Res. 2015;25:232–9.
20. Wang J, Qiu Q, Haider M, Bell M, Gruslin A, Christians JK. Expression of pregnancy-associated plasma protein A2 during pregnancy in human and mouse. J Endocrinol. 2009;202:337–45.
21. Christians JK, King AY, Rogowska MD, Hessels SM. Pappa2 deletion in mice affects male but not female fertility. Reprod Biol Endocrinol. 2015;13:109.
22. Wagner PK, Otomo A, Christians JK. Regulation of pregnancy-associated plasma protein A2 (PAPPA2) in a human placental trophoblast cell line (BeWo). Reprod Biol Endocrinol. 2011;9:48.
23. Christians JK, Gruslin A. Altered levels of insulin-like growth factor binding protein proteases in preeclampsia and intrauterine growth restriction. Prenat Diag. 2010;30:815–20.
24. Plaks V, Rinkenberger J, Dai J, Flannery M, Sund M, Kanasaki K, et al. Matrix metalloproteinase-9 deficiency phenocopies features of preeclampsia and intrauterine growth restriction. Proc Natl Acad Sci U S A. 2013;110:11109–14.
25. Leavey K, Benton SJ, Grynspan D, Kingdom JC, Bainbridge SA, Cox BJ. Unsupervised placental gene expression profiling identifies clinically relevant subclasses of human preeclampsia. Hypertension. 2016;68:137–47.
26. McFarlane L, Truong V, Palmer JS, Wilhelm D. Novel PCR assay for determining the genetic sex of mice. Sex Dev. 2013;7:207–11.
27. Dubois B, Arnold B, Opdenakker G. Gelatinase B deficiency impairs reproduction. J Clin Invest. 2000;106:627–8.
28. Andraweera PH, Dekker GA, Roberts CT. The vascular endothelial growth factor family in adverse pregnancy outcomes. Hum Reprod Update. 2012;18:436–57.
29. Clifton VL. Review: Sex and the human placenta: mediating differential strategies of fetal growth and survival. Placenta. 2010;31:S33–9.
30. Chin EH, Christians JK. When are sex-specific effects really sex-specific? J Dev Orig Health Dis. 2015;6:438–42.

## 5

Three-dimensional evaluation of murine ovarian follicles using a modified CUBIC tissue clearing method

Kyosuke Kagami[1,2], Yohei Shinmyo[2], Masanori Ono[1], Hiroshi Kawasaki[2*] and Hiroshi Fujiwara[1*] (iD)

Abstract

Background: Recently, we demonstrated the three-dimensional (3D) localization of murine trophoblast giant cells in the pregnant uterus using a modified Clear Unobstructed Brain Imaging Cocktails and Computational analysis (CUBIC) tissue-clearing method and hybrid construct consisting of the cytomegalovirus enhancer fused to the chicken beta-actin promoter (CAG) conjugated enhanced green fluorescent protein (EGFP) transgenic mice. In this study, we applied this method to obtain a transparent whole-image of the ovary and observed the 3D localization of individual oocytes in the developing follicles.

Methods: Ovarian samples were obtained from EGFP transgenic mice and subjected to nuclear staining with propidium iodide (PI) and CUBIC treatment. The detection of double fluorescence signals (green and red) and subsequent reconstruction of 3D images of the whole ovary were performed by light-sheet microscopy and computer programs, respectively.

Results: The ovary became transparent using the CUBIC method and each nucleus of the follicle component cells was uniformly fluoro-stained by PI perfusion. In contrast, EGFP signals were strong in oocytes, whereas those of surrounding granulosa cells were faint. These signal differences in EGFP expression among oocytes, granulosa cells, and theca-interstitial cells produce well-contrasted images of the growing follicles, providing clear information of the 3D localization of individual oocytes.

Conclusion: These results indicate that this procedure is one of the effective approaches to analyze the 3D structure of follicles in the whole ovary.

Keywords: Clear unobstructed brain imaging cocktails and computational analysis (CUBIC), Three-dimensional visualization, Tissue clearing, Ovary, Enhanced green fluorescent protein transgenic mice

Background

The ovary is a specific reproductive organ that contains oocytes. Each oocyte individually matures within its own follicular unit, which contains granulosa cells during folliculogenesis and theca cells from secondary stage onward. The follicle is also an important endocrine unit that produces sex steroid hormones, such as androgen and estrogen. During the development process, follicles become enlarged to prepare for ovulation, accumulating follicular fluid in the cavity concomitant with the proliferation of granulosa and theca cells [1].

It has been established that close interactions among oocytes, granulosa cells, and theca cells are critical for the development of follicles [2]. In order to analyze the relationship between adjacent cell populations, histological evaluation by immunohistochemistry has been one of the useful methods contributing to clarifying the underlying mechanisms. However, it is sometimes difficult to histologically investigate the relationship between oocytes and granulosa cells in well-developed follicles since the oocyte is not centrally located in the follicular cavity, being surrounded by granulosa cells of the cumulus oophorus. These granulosa cells are connected with

* Correspondence: kawasaki-labo@umin.ac.jp; fuji@med.kanazawa-u.ac.jp
[2]Department of Medical Neuroscience, Graduate School of Medical Sciences, Kanazawa University, Takara-machi 13-1, Kanazawa, Ishikawa 920-8640, Japan
[1]Department of Obstetrics and Gynecology, Graduate School of Medical Sciences, Kanazawa University, Takara-machi 13-1, Kanazawa, Ishikawa 920-8640, Japan

mural granulosa cells that line the basement membrane throughout the follicular wall [1]. Consequently, the three-dimensional (3D) detection of oocytes in well-developed follicles will provide valuable information in both physiological and pathological conditions.

As a conventional method to obtain 3D images, sequential tissue sections are prepared and subjected to various staining methods, and then 3D images are reconstructed from these images [3–7]. Although these classical techniques are useful to analyze precise structures of various tissues, the preparation of thin and sequential sections of the follicular fluid-containing large follicles is often difficult while maintaining fine structures, and the reconstruction of 3D images, especially around the oocyte, is complex.

To overcome this disadvantage, we used a tissue-clearing technology that can provide 3D images of the entire structure of the follicle without having to make tissue sections. Several groups have developed useful tissue-clearing methods to visualize 3D structures of entire organs, such as Scale, See Deep Brain (SeeDB), CLARITY, 3D Imaging of Solvent-Cleared Organs (3DISCO), and Clear Unobstructed Brain Imaging Cocktails and Computational analysis (CUBIC) [8–12]. Among them, ScaleA2 was recently applied to the murine fetal ovary and the cleared transparent ovary was subjected to whole-mount immunofluorescence staining, observing the numbers of germ cells in intact ovaries using confocal microscopy and three-dimensional software analyses [13]. We recently reported that CUBIC is an effective method to make the pregnant uterus and placenta transparent. Using hybrid construct consisting of the cytomegalovirus enhancer fused to the chicken beta-actin promoter (CAG) conjugated enhanced green fluorescent protein (EGFP) transgenic mice, we also demonstrated the 3D localization of murine trophoblast giant cells within the maternal uterine muscle layer [14]. Consequently, in this study, we applied this method to the adult ovary to obtain transparent whole images and observed the 3D localization of the individual oocytes in the developing follicles.

Methods
Preparation of reagents
CUBIC reagents were prepared as described [12]. CUBIC-1 reagent was prepared as a mixture of 25% weight/weight (w/w) urea (Nacalai Tesque, 35,904–45, Japan), 25% weight/volume (w/v) N, N, N', N'-tetrakis (2-hydroxypropyl) ethylenediamine (Tokyo Chemical Industry, T0781, Japan), and 15% (w/v) polyethylene glycol mono-pisooctylphenyl ether (Triton X-100) (Nacalai Tesque, 25,987–85, Japan). CUBIC-2 reagent was prepared as a mixture of 50 wt% sucrose (Nacalai Tesque, 30,403–55, Japan), 25% (w/v) urea, 10% (w/v) 2, 20,

20'-nitrilotriethanol (Wako, 145–05605, Japan), and 0.1% volume/volume (v/v) Triton X-100. Both reagents were prepared just prior to use. Before adding Triton X-100, all other chemicals were dissolved with a hot stirrer at 60 °C. Because water evaporation will make it difficult for highly concentrated chemicals to be dissolved, the weight of the solution was monitored frequently, and distilled water was added during a mixing step. After all chemicals except Triton X-100 were dissolved, the solution was cooled to room temperature, and finally Triton X-100 was added.

Animals
We used nine transgenic female mice expressing EGFP under the control of the CAG promoter (C57BL/6-Tg) [15] and eight wild-type female mice (CD-1/ICR). These mice were sacrificed at the age of 6–12 months. Wild-type mice were purchased from SLC (Hamamatsu, Japan), and all mice were reared under a normal 12-h light/dark schedule. All experimental procedures and housing conditions were approved by the Animal Care and Use Committee of the Kanazawa University Animal Experiment Committee (Approval Number, AP-163714), and all of the animals were cared for and treated humanely in accordance with the Institutional Guidelines for Experiments using animals.

The CUBIC protocol for the ovary
CUBIC was performed as described previously with modifications [12, 14] (Fig. 1a). Eight female wild-type mice and six female CAG-EGFP mice were sacrificed by deep anesthesia and transcardial perfusion by 4% paraformaldehyde (PFA) in PBS with or without propidium iodide (PI, Life Technologies), and the bilateral reproductive organs including the uterus, Fallopian tube and ovary were removed. Isolated organs were further immersed in 4% PFA at 4 °C overnight and then incubated in CUBIC-1 reagent at 37 °C for 5 days with gentle shaking. After washing 3 times by PBS with gentle shaking at room temperature for 30 min, the organs were immersed in 20% sucrose in PBS at 4 °C for one day, and incubated in CUBIC-2 regent at room temperature for 2 days.

Immunostaining
Three adult female CAG-EGFP mice were deeply anesthetized and transcardially perfused with 4% PFA in PBS. To make sections, the ovary was partially dissected, post-fixed by overnight immersion in the same fixative, cryoprotected by overnight immersion in sucrose-containing PBS, and embedded in Optimal Cutting Temperature (OCT) compound (Sakura Finetek, Japan). Sections of 14-μm thickness were made using a cryostat, permeabilized with 0.5% Triton X-100 in PBS, and incubated at 4 °C overnight with rabbit anti-green fluorescent protein (GFP) antibody (Molecular Probe A-11122, 1:500). After being incubated

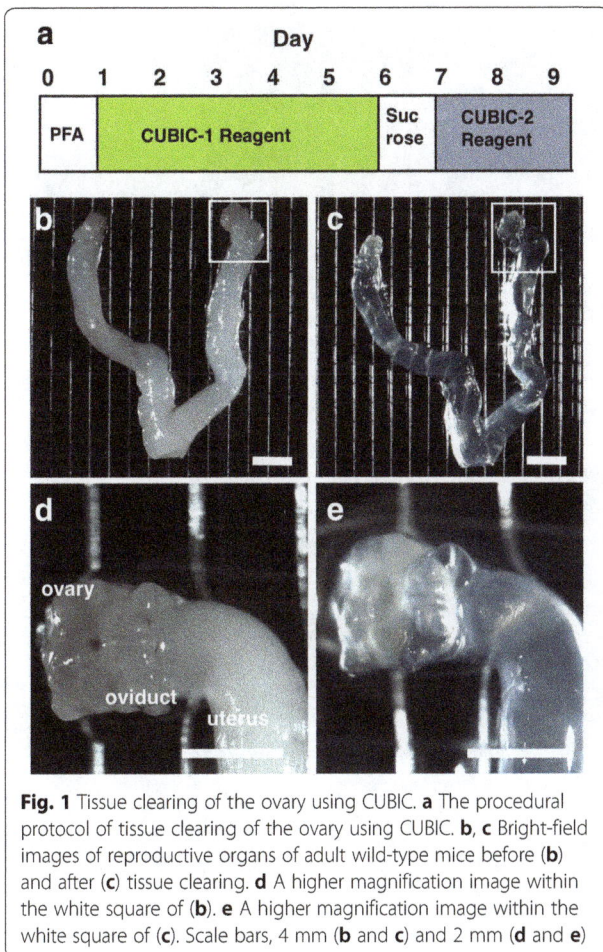

Fig. 1 Tissue clearing of the ovary using CUBIC. **a** The procedural protocol of tissue clearing of the ovary using CUBIC. **b, c** Bright-field images of reproductive organs of adult wild-type mice before (**b**) and after (**c**) tissue clearing. **d** A higher magnification image within the white square of (**b**). **e** A higher magnification image within the white square of (**c**). Scale bars, 4 mm (**b** and **c**) and 2 mm (**d** and **e**).

at 37 °C for 2 h with Cy3-conjugated secondary antibody (EMD Millipore AP132C, 1:500) and 1 μg/mL Hoechst 33,342, the sections were washed and mounted.

Microscopy and image analysis

Bright-field images of the ovaries were taken using a stereomicroscope (MZ16F, Leica). Immunohistochemically stained tissue sections were observed with an epifluorescence microscope (AxioImager A1, Carl Zeiss). Three-dimensional images of transparent organs were acquired using a light-sheet microscope (Lightsheet Z.1, Carl Zeiss) and an epifluorescence confocal microscope (LSM510, Carl Zeiss). Images of the whole ovary were obtained using a 5×/0.16 NA objective lens, and detailed single-cell resolution images were acquired using a 20×/1.0 NA objective lens for the clearing method. Three-dimensional images were analyzed using ZEN software (Carl Zeiss).

Results

Tissue clearing of reproductive organs using CUBIC

After tissue-clearing treatment (Fig. 1a), reproductive organs including the ovary became transparent using CUBIC (Fig. 1c and e). Fortunately, the sizes of reproductive organs were not affected by CUBIC (Compare Fig. 1b and d), although it was often reported that the size of organs became larger after tissue clearing [9]. These results suggest that CUBIC is an appropriate method for making the ovary transparent.

Imaging of the ovary using CUBIC and nuclear staining

To visualize fine structures in the ovary, we combined CUBIC with PI nuclear staining and observed PI images by light-sheet microscopy. We successfully detected fluorescence PI signals deep in the ovary and obtained sequential 2D images of the entire ovary with single-cell resolution without having to make tissue sections (Fig. 2b and c). Using the sequential 2D images of PI signals, we were able to reconstruct 3D images of the entire ovary (Fig. 2a). Then, using 3D images of the entire ovary, we were able to reconstruct 2D images of angle-free cross-sections (Fig. 2d). We also clearly observed theca-interstitial structures around antral follicles (Fig. 2c). These results indicate that PI nuclear staining is useful to observe structures in the ovary after CUBIC.

Imaging of the ovary using CUBIC and EGFP transgenic mice

Although PI staining enabled us to visualize the distribution of the nucleus of each cell, we could barely distinguish the oocytes from other cells. Accordingly, we then used transgenic mice (CAG-EGFP mice) expressing GFP under the control of the CAG promoter, which contains the chicken beta-actin promoter and cytomegalovirus enhancer. The ovary of CAG-EGFP mice with PI treatment was subjected to CUBIC, and 3D images were reconstructed by light-sheet microscopy (Fig. 3a). We clearly observed strong EGFP fluorescence in the oocytes, theca cells, epithelial cells, and stromal cells in 2D images of X-Y cross-sections, whereas the fluorescence signal of EGFP was very weak in granulosa cells surrounding oocyte (Figs. 3b, c, d and e). These differences in EGFP signals among the follicular component cells facilitate contrast imaging that can clearly show the whole shape of oocytes (Fig. 3b and c). In addition, we also obtained high quality images of the preantral and mature antral follicles using confocal microscopy without manual tissue sectioning (Fig. 3d and e, Additional files 1 and 2). Although confocal microscopy unfits the wide-field capturing, these images confirmed that the structure of antral follicle was maintained even though the tissue clearing method was performed (Fig. 3e).

Since a previous study reported that almost all kinds of cells express EGFP in this mouse line [15], we additionally performed immunohistochemistry using anti-GFP antibody to confirm the expression of GFP protein. We detected EGFP protein in granulosa cells

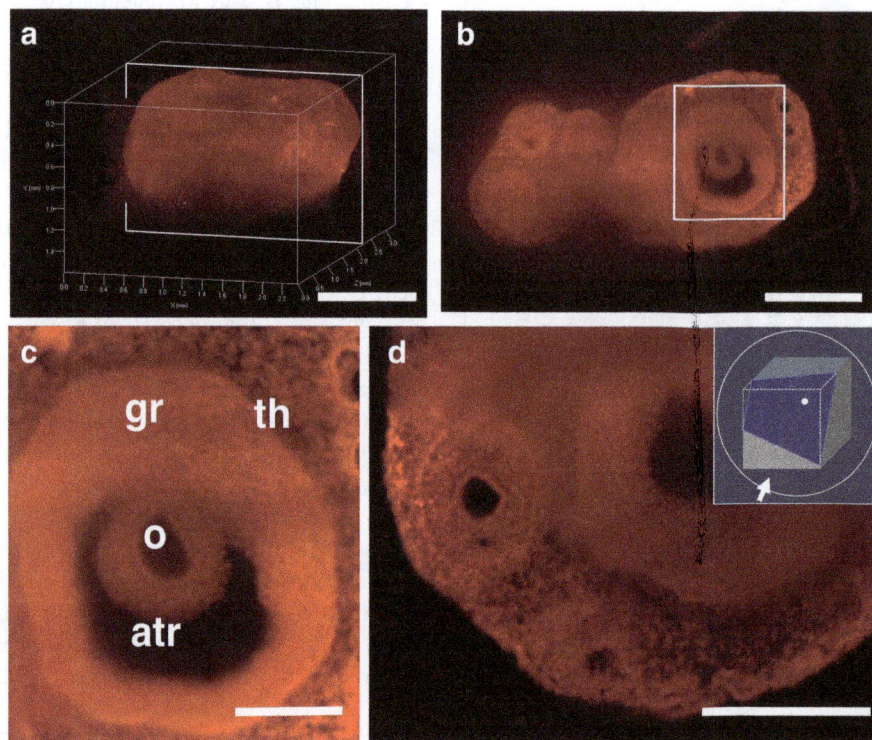

Fig. 2 Three-dimensional and cross-sectional images of the ovary stained with PI. **a–d** Female mice were transcardially perfused with 4% PFA containing PI, and the isolated ovaries were subjected to CUBIC. Three-dimensional images were taken by light-sheet microscopy. **a** A 3D image of PI signals of the whole ovary. **b** A sectional image within the white square of (**a**). **c** A higher magnification image within the white square of (**b**). **d** A free-angle cross sectional image. gr, granulosa cells; atr, antrum; o, oocyte; th, thecal cells. Scale bars, 1 mm (**a**), 500 μm (**b**, **d**), and 200 μm (**c**)

even though its expression level was relatively low (Additional file 3).

Moreover, using datasets of 3D images, we produced a stereoscopic image, with which 3D locations of EGFP-positive oocytes at various stages could be clearly identified (Fig. 4 and Additional file 4).

Discussion

Here, we have shown that 3D images of the whole ovary can be successfully obtained by CUBIC and light-sheet microscopy using EGFP transgenic mice. Previous pioneering studies demonstrated that two key factors of tissue clearing are the homogenization of refractive indices and removal of lipids [16]. Most tissue-clearing methods have been successfully applied to the brain, which is a lipid-rich organ [8–12]. In contrast to the brain, since the ovary does not contain such high lipid levels, it was unclear whether the CUBIC tissue-clearing method was suitable for the mature ovary. Although a recent report demonstrated that ScaleA2 was applicable to the small and immature ovaries before birth [13], in our preliminary experiments using mature ovarian organs, CUBIC provided more transparent than Sca/eA2. Therefore, we applied CUBIC to the mature ovarian organs. Fortunately, the present study clearly indicates that CUBIC is useful to make the ovary transparent.

Conventional histological techniques require a large number of thin tissue sections to create 3D images of the whole ovary. In addition, thin tissue sections of the ovarian tissues are often deformed during experiments because the growing follicles contain follicular fluid. Based on this background, this study indicates that the combination of tissue clearing techniques and light-sheet microscopy can be applied to understand the 3D structure of the whole ovary without having to cut the tissue sections. Especially when CAG-EGFP transgenic mice were used, 3D images of the ovary clearly demonstrated follicles and the corpus luteum at various developmental stages and provided precise information on volumes, numbers, and locations of follicles with single cell resolution. However, since structural information of granulosa cells around oocytes is insufficient in our 3D images, it is relatively difficult to distinguish a primordial or a healthy follicle from a primary or an atretic follicle, respectively, compared with traditional hematoxylin and eosin staining.

Interestingly, although a previous study reported that EGFP is expressed in almost all kinds of cells in

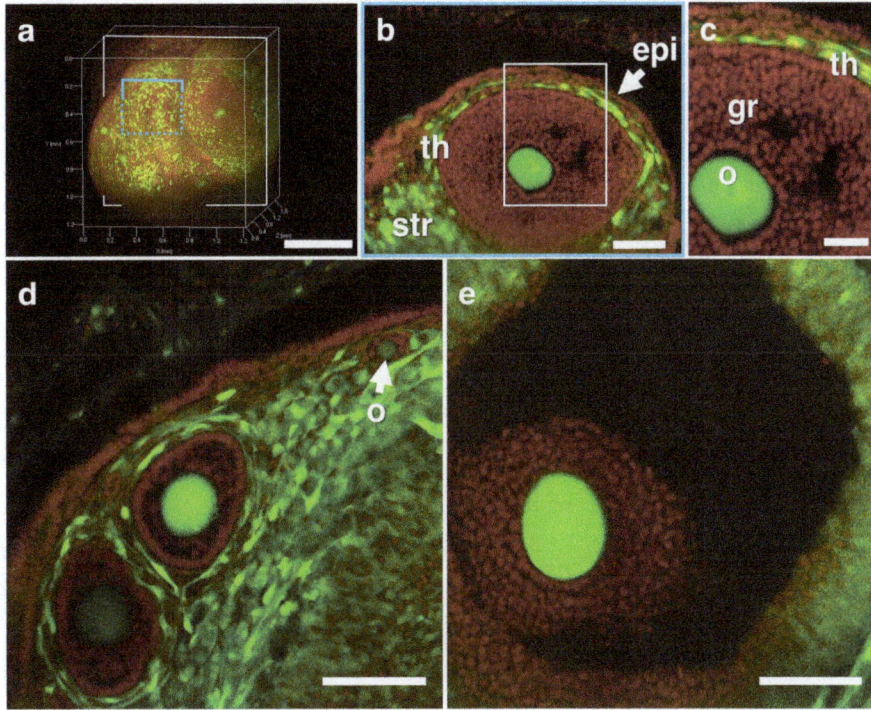

Fig. 3 Three-dimensional image of the EGFP-positive mouse ovary. Female EGFP-transgenic mice were transcardially perfused with 4% PFA containing PI. After the isolated ovaries were subjected to CUBIC, 3D and cross-sectional images were taken by light-sheet microscopy (**a**, **b** and **c**) or confocal microscopy (**d** and **e**). **a** A 3D image of EGFP and PI signals of the whole ovary. **b** A sectional image within the blue square of (**a**). **c** A higher-magnification image within the white square of (**b**). **d** Preantral follicles. **e** Mature antral follicle. Note that EGFP fluorescence was strongly visible in the oocyte and ovarian stromal cells, but not in granulosa cells around oocytes. gr, granulosa cells; o, oocyte; th, thecal cells; epi, surface epithelial cells; str, stromal cells. Scale bars, 500 μm (**a**), 100 μm (**b**, **d** and **e**), and 50 μm (**c**)

CAG-EGFP mice [15], GFP fluorescence in granulosa cells was very weak in CAG-EGFP mice. To clarify the reason for the reduction of EGFP fluorescence in granulosa cells, we immunohistochemically confirmed that immunoreactive EGFP protein was expressed in granulosa cells. Although the precise mechanisms to explain the discrepancy between EGFP fluorescence and EGFP protein expression or differences in EGFP fluorescence intensity among the follicular component cells are still unclear, we consider that there are some differences

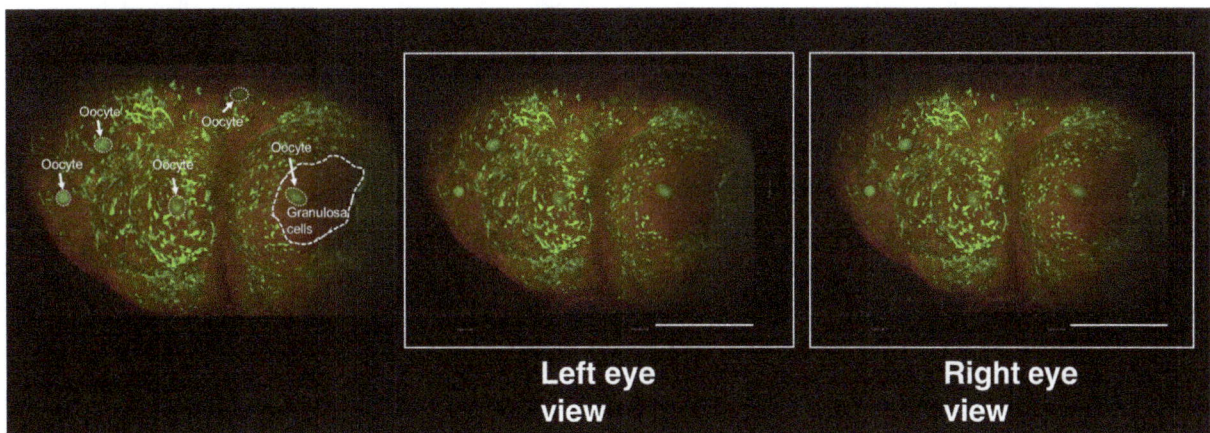

Fig. 4 Stereoscopic image of the ovaries of EGFP transgenic mice. Female CAG-EGFP transgenic mice were transcardially perfused with 4% PFA containing PI. After the isolated ovaries were subjected to CUBIC, 3D images were taken by light-sheet microscopy, and then stereoscopic images were reconstructed. Note that the distribution and sizes of EGFP-positive oocytes could be clearly identified. Scale bars, 500 μm

in the expressing efficiency of the GFP gene under the control of the CAG promoter in reproductive organs. To support this, we observed that there are similar differences in intensity of GFP fluorescence among endometrial epithelial cells, endometrial stromal cells, and myometrial cells within the uterus of CAG-EGFP mice (in preparation). Regardless of the reasons, this characterization of CAG-EGFP mice results in enhancing tissue contrast between various cell types. Since a GFP-positive oocyte is surrounded by granulosa cells bearing faint GFP fluorescence, the size and shape of the oocyte were clearly distinguishable with this method. Since several fluorescent agents such as Cy3 and FITC were reported to be tolerant to CUBIC, we can immunocytologically stain the ovarian cells by fluorescent agents-labeled-antibody during tissue clearing method [17]. Consequently, it is also possible that this method is successfully applied to human ovarian tissues.

Taken together with our previous report using the pregnant uterus and placenta [14], we here propose that CUBIC is appropriate for tissue clearing of reproductive organs. Using 3D images of the whole ovary, 2D images of angle-free cross-sections can easily be reconstructed (Fig. 2d). As described in our previous report [14], we can perform additional immunohistochemical experiments using real tissue sections freshly prepared from the transparent ovary, which correspond to adequate cross-sections that were selected by stereoscopic imaging and the subsequent computed 3D imaging analysis. This advantage offers enormous potential for elucidating the mechanisms of ovarian development and disorders.

Conclusion

This study successfully demonstrates that the combination of CUBIC, light-sheet microscopy, and EGFP-transgenic mice is useful to observe 3D structures of the whole ovary with single cell resolution. From the 3D images of the whole ovary, we can reconstruct 2D images of angle-free cross-sections without having to make tissue sections. Since the component cells of the ovarian follicles showed different EGFP fluorescence intensities, we also obtained well-contrasted and stereoscopic images and observed 3D localization of oocytes within the individual follicles. Furthermore, a site-specific Cre-loxP recombination system enables us to visualize specific-gene-expressing cells by inserting reporter genes for fluorescent proteins. Consequently, combining our method and a Cre-loxP recombination system, we can theoretically obtain 3D-images of specific-gene-expressing cells in the whole transparent ovary. Based on these advantages, this procedure has the potential to markedly contribute to identifying the mechanisms of ovarian development and disorders in the future.

Additional files

Additional file 1: Sequential 2D images of X-Y cross-sections of the EGFP-positive preantral follicles. Female EGFP-transgenic mice were transcardially perfused with 4% PFA containing PI. After the isolated ovaries were subjected to CUBIC, sequential 2D images of X-Y cross-sections containing primordial and preantral follicles corresponding to Fig. 3d were taken using a confocal microscope. (MOV 918 kb)

Additional file 2: Sequential 2D images of X-Y cross-sections of the EGFP-positive antral follicle. Female EGFP-transgenic mice were transcardially perfused with 4% PFA containing PI. After the isolated ovaries were subjected to CUBIC, sequential 2D images of X-Y cross-sections containing an antral follicle corresponding to Fig. 3e were taken using a confocal microscope. (MOV 710 kb)

Additional file 3: GFP immunohistochemistry using ovaries of CAG-EGFP mice. Female CAG-EGFP mice were fixed with the transcardial perfusion of 4% PFA. Sections were stained with Hoechst 33,342 and anti-GFP antibody to reveal the expression of EGFP protein. Note that although GFP fluorescence was undetectable in granulosa cells, the expression of immunoreactive EGFP protein was detected. Scale bars, 100 μm. (668 kb)

Additional file 4: A 3D movie of the EGFP-positive mouse ovary. Female EGFP-transgenic mice were transcardially perfused with 4% PFA containing PI. After the isolated ovaries were subjected to CUBIC, 3D images were obtained using a light-sheet microscope. (MOV 2096 kb)

Abbreviations

3D: Three-dimensional; 3DISCO: 3D Imaging of Solvent-Cleared Organs; CAG: Hybrid construct consisting of the cytomegalovirus enhancer fused to the chicken beta-actin promoter; CUBIC: Clear Unobstructed Brain Imaging Cocktails and Computational analysis; EGFP: Enhanced green fluorescent protein; GFP: Green fluorescent protein; O.C.T.: Optimal Cutting Temperature; PFA: Paraformaldehyde; PI: Propidium iodide; SeeDB: See Deep Brain; v/v: Volume/volume; w/v: Weight/volume; w/w: Weight/weight

Acknowledgments

We thank Yasuhiko Sato, Kazuyoshi Hosoya, Hiroyasu Oshima (Carl Zeiss), Dr. Makoto Sato (Kanazawa University), Zachary Blalock, Fujiwara lab. Members, and Kawasaki lab. Members for their helpful support.

Funding

This work was supported by a Grant-in-Aid for Scientific Research from the Ministry of Education, Culture, Sports, Science and Technology-Japan (MEXT), the Japan Agency for Medical Research and Development (AMED), and the Uehara Memorial Foundation and Takeda Science Foundation.

Authors' contributions

KK and HK designed the experiments. KK conducted most experiments. YS and MO helped with some experiments. KK, MO, HK, and HF wrote the manuscript. All authors read and approved the final manuscript.

Competing interests

The authors declare that they have no competing interests.

References

1. Strauss JF, William CJ. The ovarian life cycle. In: Strauss JF, Barbieri RL, editors. Yen & Jaffe's reproductive endocrinology: physiology, pathophysiology, and clinical management. 7th ed. Philadelphia: Elsevier Sounders; 2014. p. 157–92.

2. Komatsu K, Masubuchi S. Observation of the dynamics of follicular development in the ovary. Reprod Med Biol. 2017;16:21–7.

3. Takemori K, Okamura H, Kanzaki H, Koshida M, Konishi I. Scanning electron microscopy study on corrosion cast of rat uterine vasculature during the first half of pregnancy. J Anat. 1984;138:163–73.

4. Gundersen HJ, Bagger P, Bendtsen TF, Evans SM, Korbo L, Marcussen N, Moller A, Nielsen K, Nyengaard JR, Pakkenberg B, et al. The new stereological tools: disector, fractionator, nucleator and point sampled intercepts and their use in pathological research and diagnosis. APMIS. 1988;96:857–81.

5. Gundersen HJ, Bendtsen TF, Korbo L, Marcussen N, Moller A, Nielsen K, Nyengaard JR, Pakkenberg B, Sorensen FB, Vesterby A, et al. Some new, simple and efficient stereological methods and their use in pathological research and diagnosis. APMIS. 1988;96:379–94.

6. Mayhew TM. The new stereological methods for interpreting functional morphology from slices of cells and organs. Exp Physiol. 1991;76:639–65.

7. Mayhew TM. A stereological perspective on placental morphology in normal and complicated pregnancies. J Anat. 2009;215:77–90.

8. Hama H, Kurokawa H, Kawano H, Ando R, Shimogori T, Noda H, Fukami K, Sakaue-Sawano A, Miyawaki A. Scale: a chemical approach for fluorescence imaging and reconstruction of transparent mouse brain. Nat Neurosci. 2011; 14:1481–8.

9. Ke MT, Fujimoto S, Imai T. SeeDB: a simple and morphology-preserving optical clearing agent for neuronal circuit reconstruction. Nat Neurosci. 2013;16:1154–61.

10. Chung K, Wallace J, Kim SY, Kalyanasundaram S, Andalman AS, Davidson TJ, Mirzabekov JJ, Zalocusky KA, Mattis J, Denisin AK, et al. Structural and molecular interrogation of intact biological systems. Nature. 2013;497:332–7.

11. Erturk A, Becker K, Jahrling N, Mauch CP, Hojer CD, Egen JG, Hellal F, Bradke F, Sheng M, Dodt HU. Three-dimensional imaging of solvent-cleared organs using 3DISCO. Nat Protoc. 2012;7:1983–95.

12. Susaki EA, Tainaka K, Perrin D, Kishino F, Tawara T, Watanabe TM, Yokoyama C, Onoe H, Eguchi M, Yamaguchi S, et al. Whole-brain imaging with single-cell resolution using chemical cocktails and computational analysis. Cell. 2014;157:726–39.

13. Malki S, Tharp ME, Bortvin A. A Whole-mount approach for accurate quantitative and spatial assessment of fetal oocyte dynamics in mice. Biol Reprod. 2015;93:113.

14. Kagami K, Shinmyo Y, Ono M, Kawasaki H, Fujiwara H. Three-dimensional visualization of intrauterine conceptus through the uterine wall by tissue clearing method. Sci Rep. 2017;7:5964.

15. Okabe M, Ikawa M, Kominami K, Nakanishi T, Nishimune Y. 'Green mice' as a source of ubiquitous green cells. FEBS Lett. 1997;407:313–9.

16. Lee E, Kim HJ, Sun W. See-through Technology for Biological Tissue: 3-dimensional visualization of macromolecules. Int Neurourol J. 2016;20(Suppl 1):15–22.

17. Tainaka K, Kubota SI, Suyama TQ, Susaki EA, Perrin D, Ukai-Tadenuma M, Ukai H, Ueda HR. Whole-body imaging with single-cell resolution by tissue decolorization. Cell. 2014;159:911–24.

## 6

Apa-I polymorphism in *VDR* gene is related to metabolic syndrome in polycystic ovary syndrome

Betânia Rodrigues Santos[1,2], Sheila Bunecker Lecke[1,3] and Poli Mara Spritzer[1,2*] (iD)

Abstract

Background: Polycystic ovary syndrome (PCOS) is a common endocrine disorder determined by polygenic traits as well as environmental factors. Lower vitamin D levels have been detected in PCOS women and related to hormone and metabolic disturbances. Vitamin D acts in tissues through the vitamin D receptor (VDR). *VDR* gene variants have been associated with worse metabolic profile in the general population. We investigated the genotype and haplotype distribution of the Bsm-I (rs1544410), Apa-I (rs7975232), and Taq-I (rs731236) *VDR* gene polymorphisms in PCOS and non-hirsute women from southern Brazil. We further investigated the associations of these gene variants and their haplotypes with PCOS, vitamin D levels, and metabolic abnormalities, including the metabolic syndrome (MetS).

Methods: A group of 191 women with PCOS (Rotterdam criteria) and 100 non-hirsute controls with regular ovulatory cycles were genotyped for all polymorphisms by real-time PCR, with allelic discrimination assays. MetS and the cutoffs for its isolated components were defined in accordance with the Joint Scientific Statement.

Results: Women with PCOS were younger and had significantly higher BMI and total testosterone levels than controls ($p < 0.05$). The frequency of MetS in PCOS and controls was 26.5% and 4.8% respectively. The CC genotype of Apa-I entailed higher risk of MetS in PCOS (OR: 2.133; 95% CI 1.020–4.464, $p = 0.042$), and was associated with higher systolic blood pressure ($p = 0.009$), total cholesterol ($p = 0.040$), and LDL-cholesterol ($p = 0.038$) in both PCOS and control groups (two-way ANOVA). The frequencies of *VDR* haplotypes were similar in PCOS and control women.

Conclusions: The present results suggest that the Apa-I variant in *VDR* gene may be associated with MetS in southern Brazilian women with PCOS, and with blood pressure, total cholesterol, and LDL-c in women with and without PCOS.

Keywords: PCOS, Vitamin D receptor, Gene polymorphisms, Metabolic syndrome

Background

Polycystic ovary syndrome (PCOS) is a common endocrine disorder affecting 9 to 18% of women of reproductive age according to different diagnostic criteria [1–3]. While its etiology remains unclear, PCOS is considered a polygenic and multifactorial disease, with metabolic, endocrine, and reproductive alterations [4]. In PCOS women, evidence suggests that vitamin D levels may be decreased and related to hormone and metabolic disturbances [5, 6].

The vitamin D receptor (VDR) is expressed in many tissues and organs (such as those involved in calcium homeostasis mechanisms), in glucose metabolism, and in the reproductive system [7], and modulates vitamin D action in these systems. *VDR* gene (ID: 7421) polymorphisms have been investigated in PCOS as well as in

* Correspondence: spritzer@ufrgs.br
[1]Division of Endocrinology, Gynecological Endocrinology Unit, Hospital de Clínicas de Porto Alegre, Rua Ramiro Barcelos, 2350, Porto Alegre, RS 90035-003, Brazil
[2]Department of Physiology, Laboratory of Molecular Endocrinology, Universidade Federal do Rio Grande do Sul (UFRGS), Porto Alegre, Brazil
Full list of author information is available at the end of the article

disturbances of androgen secretion. A previous study has suggested an association between *VDR* gene variants and precocious pubarche (PP) [8]; in turn, data on PCOS risk are controversial, with a relationship between *VDR* gene variants and PCOS detected by some [9–12] but not all studies [13–15]. Regarding endocrine characteristics, *VDR* gene polymorphism has been associated with total testosterone in PCOS and PP populations [8, 13], with estradiol levels in PP girls [8], and with metabolic abnormalities in different non-PCOS populations [16–23].

Therefore, the aims of the present study were to assess the genotypic and allelic distribution of Bsm-I (rs1544410), Apa-I (rs7975232) and Taq-I (rs731236) polymorphisms of the *VDR* gene and to determine whether these gene variants are associated with 25-hydroxyvitamin D [25(OH)D] levels and with metabolic abnormalities, including MetS, in women with PCOS in comparison to non-hirsute, ovulatory control women.

Methods

Patients

This is a cross-sectional study including 191 patients with PCOS and 100 non-hirsute women with regular, ovulatory cycles, recruited by advertisement in the local media. The characteristics of the study sample have been described elsewhere [24]. PCOS was diagnosed according to Rotterdam criteria [25]. Neither PCOS nor control participants had received any drugs known to interfere with hormone levels (such as oral contraceptive pills, antiandrogens, metformin, fibrates, or statins) for at least 3 months before the study. The exclusion criteria were pregnancy and liver or kidney disease. Approval for this study was obtained from the Institutional Review Board and the local Ethics Committee at Hospital de Clínicas de Porto Alegre. Written informed consent was obtained from every subject.

Study protocol

Anthropometric measurements included body mass index (BMI) and waist circumference (measured at the midpoint between the lower rib margin and the iliac crest). Blood pressure was measured after a 10-min rest, with the patient seated, with both feet on the floor and the arm supported at heart level. Two measurements were obtained 10 min apart using an Omron HEM-742INT automatic blood pressure monitor (Rio de Janeiro, Brazil) with the correct cuff size for the arm diameter [26–29]. MetS and the cutoffs for its isolated components were defined in accordance with the Joint Scientific Statement [30].

Laboratory measurements

All samples were obtained between the 2nd and 10th days of the menstrual cycle, or on any day if the patient was amenorrheic, between 8:00 and 10:00 am, after a 12-h overnight fast. Blood samples were drawn from an antecubital vein for determination of hormone levels. Blood samples were also collected for genomic DNA extraction.

Total cholesterol, high-density lipoprotein cholesterol (HDL-c), triglycerides, and glucose levels were determined by colorimetric-enzymatic methods (Bayer 1650 Advia System). LDL-cholesterol (LDL-c) was determined indirectly with the formula total cholesterol – HDL-c – triglycerides/5. Total testosterone levels were measured by chemiluminescence (Siemens Advia Centaur XP), with a sensitivity of 0.10 ng/mL and intra- and interassay coefficients of variation (CVs) of 3.3 and 7.5% respectively. Plasma insulin and sex hormone–binding globulin (SHBG) levels were measured by chemiluminescence (Siemens Advia Centaur XP), with a sensitivity of 0. 50 U/mL and 0.035 nmol/L, respectively, with intra-assay CV < 3% and interassay CV < 5%. The free androgen index (FAI) was calculated as testosterone (nmol/L)/SHBG (nmol/L) × 100. The homeostasis model assessment index (HOMA index) was calculated by multiplying insulin (μIU/mL) by glucose (mmol/L) and dividing this product by 22.5 [31]. 25(OH)D levels were measured in a subset of 102 women (54 PCOS and 48 controls) by chemiluminescence (Liaison, DiaSorin), with intra-assay and interassay CV of 7.7 and 10.9% respectively.

Genotype analysis

Genomic DNA was extracted from peripheral blood leukocytes [32]. The DNA samples were diluted to 2 ng/mL. Molecular genotyping was performed through real-time polymerase chain reaction (7500 Fast Real-Time Polymerase Chain Reaction System, Applied Biosystems, CA, USA), using the allelic discrimination assay with TaqMan MGB primers and probes (Applied Biosystems, CA, USA).

For genotyping the single nucleotide polymorphisms (SNPs) Apa-I and Taq-I, the following were added: TaqMan Master mix (2.5 μL), TaqMan assay (0.25 μL), and H2O (1.25 μL), for a final volume of 4 μL per sample, followed by addition of 1μLof DNA for a total reaction volume of 5 μL. To genotype SNP Bsm-I, TaqMan Master mix (5.0 μL), TaqMan assay (0.50 μL), and H2O (3. 5 μL) were added for a final volume of 9 μL per sample, and 1 μL of DNA was added for a total reaction volume of 10 μL. Reaction conditions for all polymorphisms were: 10 min at 95 °C after 50 cycles of denaturation at 95 °C (15 s) and annealing at 60 °C (1 min). Endpoint fluorescent readings were performed in the 7500 Fast System Sequence Detection Software version 1.4 environment. The internal quality of genotype data was assessed by typing 10% of blinded samples in duplicate.

Statistical analysis

Sample size estimation was based on the study by Al-Daghri et al. [16], which found an association between Apa-I variants of the *VDR* gene and higher blood pressure in MetS in female and male control subjects. Therefore, considering a difference of 3.9 mmHg in blood pressure between Apa-I genotypes [CC or CA + AA], an alpha of 5%, and a beta of 80%, the sample size was estimated as 91 PCOS women for each genotype.

The Shapiro-Wilk normality test and descriptive statistics were used to evaluate the distribution of data. Results are presented as means ± standard deviation or percentages. Non-Gaussian variables were log-transformed for statistical analysis and reported after being back-transformed into their original units of measure. Comparisons between means were analyzed by the unpaired two-tailed Student's t-test. Two-way ANOVA was used for testing the interaction between diagnosis and genotype groups. Categorical variables and the agreement of genotype frequencies with Hardy-Weinberg equilibrium for each SNP were analyzed using the Pearson chi-square test (χ^2). Odds ratios (OR) and 95% confidence intervals (95%CI) were obtained using χ^2 risk estimate. Lewontin's D' statistic for linkage disequilibrium was calculated for each pair of polymorphisms. Haplotypes were inferred using the Phase 2.1 program, which uses Bayesian statistics. Data were considered as statistically significant at $p < 0.05$. The Statistical Package for the Social Sciences v. 24 (SPSS, Chicago, IL) was used for the analyses.

Results

Clinical, hormonal, and metabolic features

The clinical, hormonal and metabolic characteristics of the studied population have been previously described [24]. Women with PCOS were younger than controls (22.9 ± 6.7 vs. 25.2 ± 7.7 years, $p = 0.013$), and presented higher BMI (29.7 ± 6.4 vs. 27.0 ± 6.1 kg/m^2, $p = 0.001$) and higher frequency of overweight/obesity ($p = 0.002$) and of MetS ($p < 0.001$). PCOS participants also had significantly higher total testosterone and FAI, as well as lower SHBG ($p < 0.001$), than controls (Table 1). Vitamin D levels were similar in PCOS and controls ($p = 0.985$).

When only the PCOS group was analyzed, the presence of MetS ($p = 0.018$), glucose ≥100 mg/dL ($p = 0.025$), waist circumference ≥ 88 cm ($p = 0.040$) and triglycerides ≥150 mg/dL ($p = 0.011$) were linked to lower vitamin D levels (Table 2).

VDR gene polymorphisms

All the three studied polymorphisms were in Hardy-Weinberg equilibrium, and over 98% ($n = 287$) of the sample were effectively genotyped. Genotype and allele frequencies of *VDR* gene variants are presented in

Table 1 Clinical and endocrine features of PCOS and control women

Variable	PCOS (191)	Controls (100)	P value
Age (years)	22.89 ± 6.66	25.18 ± 7.72	0.013
BMI ≥ 25(kg/m^2)	72.6%	53.4%	0.002
Metabolic syndrome	26.5%	4.8%	< 0.001
TT (ng/mL)	0.90 ± 0.41	0.54 ± 0.17	< 0.001
FAI	16.52 ± 15.81	5.28 ± 3.41	< 0.001
SHBG (nmol/L)	29.18 ± 20.35	43.37 ± 19.37	< 0.001
25(OH)D (ng/mL)	21.47 ± 7.61	21.50 ± 6.90	0.985

Data are expressed as means ± SD (Student t test) or percentages (Pearson chi-square test). *BMI* body mass index, *TT* total testosterone, *FAI* free androgen index, *SHBG* sex hormone–binding globulin, *25(OH)D* 25-hydroxyvitamin D

Table 3. The genotype and allele distribution of all three polymorphisms was similar in PCOS and control groups.

Figure 1 shows the frequency of MetS in PCOS participants according to Apa-I genotypes. Individuals with the CC genotype had higher risk of MetS vs. the CA + AA genotype (OR: 2.133; 95% CI 1.020–4.464, $p = 0.042$). The CC genotype was also associated with higher systolic blood pressure ($p = 0.009$), total cholesterol ($p = 0.040$) and LDL-c ($p = 0.038$) in both PCOS and control groups. There was no interaction between genotypes and PCOS or control groups ($p > 0.05$) (Table 4).

The Bsm-I (G → A) polymorphism was in almost complete linkage disequilibrium with the Apa-I (C → A) polymorphism (|D'| = 1.00; r^2 = 1.00), and in partial linkage disequilibrium with Taq-I (A → G) (|D'| = 0.75; r^2 = 0.21). Apa-I (C → A) was also in partial linkage disequilibrium with Taq-I (A → G) (|D'| = 0.87; r^2 = 0.35). Eight haplotypes were inferred in the sample: AAA, AAG, ACA, ACG, GAA, GAG, GCA, and GCG, with frequencies of 0.022, 0.340, 0.015, 0.004, 0.192, 0.019, 0.393, and 0.015 respectively. The first letter of each haplotype refers to Bsm-I, the second to Apa-I, and the third to Taq-I. Taking into consideration the results of individual polymorphism analyses, haplotypes were grouped according to the presence of the C allele of Apa-I (ACA + ACG + GCA + GCG vs. AAA + AAG + GAA + GAG). The frequency of combined haplotypes was similar in PCOS and control groups ($p = 0.332$).

Discussion

In the present study, despite the similar vitamin D levels detected in PCOS and control participants, the CC genotype of Apa-I SNP of the *VDR* gene was specifically related to higher risk of MetS in PCOS participants. Moreover, this same genotype was associated with higher blood pressure, total cholesterol, and LDL-c in both PCOS and control participants. To the best of our knowledge, this is the first report to show an association

Table 2 25(OH)D levels according to the presence of metabolic syndrome and its components in PCOS women

Status of MetS/components	25(OH)D levels (ng/mL)					
	MetS	Glu ≥100 mg/dL	BP ≥130/85 mmHg	WC ≥88 cm	HDL-c < 50 mg/dL	Trig ≥150 mg/dL
Yes	17.17 ± 5.46	14.83 ± 6.24	23.25 ± 7.80	19.28 ± 5.92	21.50 ± 7.66	17.84 ± 4.37
No	22.83 ± 7.74	22.22 ± 7.47	20.78 ± 7.61	23.46 ± 8.47	21.42 ± 7.74	22.71 ± 7.85
p value	0.018	0.025	0.318	0.040	0.974	0.011

Data are expressed as means ± SD. P value by Student t test. Glu: glucose; BP: blood pressure; WC: waist circumference; HDL-c: high-density lipoprotein cholesterol. Trig: triglycerides

between Apa-I *VDR* gene polymorphism and MetS in a PCOS population. This observation is relevant because it may help explain the meaning of vitamin D level variation, which may not play a role per se, but rather reflect a putative gene-environment interaction in different populations.

The few available studies analyzing the influence of Apa-I *VDR* gene polymorphisms on metabolic variables in PCOS women have reported no association with insulin resistance [10, 13] or glucose and lipid abnormalities [10]. However, data from non-PCOS populations suggest that metabolic abnormalities, such as obesity, insulin resistance, low HDL-c, and type 2 diabetes are associated with the *VDR* gene [16–21]. In this sense, a recent meta-analysis comprising 9232 participants showed that the association between insulin resistance-related diseases and Apa-I and Bsm-I

Table 3 Genotype and allele frequencies of *VDR* gene variants in PCOS and control women

SNP	PCOS n (%)	Controls n (%)	p
Bsm-I			
GG	74 (39.6)	41 (41.0)	0.147
GA	76 (40.6)	48 (48.0)	
AA	37 (19.8)	11 (11.0)	
G	224 (60.0)	130 (65.0)	0.231
A	150 (40.0)	70 (35.0)	
Apa-I			
AA	61 (32.1)	36 (36.0)	0.516
AC	88 (46.3)	48 (48.0)	
CC	41 (21.6)	16 (16.0)	
A	210 (55.3)	120 (60.0)	0.275
C	170 (44.7)	80 (40.0)	
Taq-I			
AA	70 (37.2)	40 (40.4)	0.493
AG	87 (46.3)	48 (48.5)	
GG	31 (16.5)	11 (11.1)	
A	227 (60.4)	128 (64.6)	0.318
G	149 (39.6)	70 (35.4)	

Data are expressed as percentages; p value by Pearson's χ^2 test

VDR gene variants was more pronounced in dark-pigmented Caucasians and Asians than in Caucasians with white skin. In the sub-group analysis, Bsm-I (GG genotype) was associated with MetS, and the Apa-I variant (CC genotype) was associated with insulin resistance-related diseases in a population living in a mid-latitude zone (30°–60°) [23], which is also the case of the present population (30°01′59″S).

While a functional role of *VDR* gene polymorphisms has not yet been established, the association between Apa-I gene variant and MetS observed in the present study could be assumed to be linked to disturbed *VDR* gene expression [33]. The Apa-I polymorphism is located at the 3′ untranslated region (3′ UTR) of the *VDR* gene, which has been recognized as being involved in the modulation of gene expression, especially through the regulation of mRNA stability and efficiency of protein translation [34]. Moreover, the methylation levels of the *VDR* gene appear to be altered according to race and presence of the polymorphisms of the 3'UTR region of the gene [35]. Additionally, Apa-I is in strong linkage disequilibrium with other *VDR* gene polymorphisms in different populations [22, 36], which may be contributing to the general transcriptional activity of *VDR* in different biological processes. Importantly, the *VDR* gene regulates more than 200 genes, and mediates most effects of vitamin D on gene expression via formation of a heterodimer with the retinoid X receptor molecule, which binds to promoter regions of many target genes [37, 38].

In our study, lower 25(OH)D levels were associated with MetS and with its isolated components in PCOS women, such as higher glucose, waist circumference and triglycerides. In this sense, the present results are in agreement with a meta-analysis reporting that women with PCOS and vitamin D deficiency are more likely to have dysglycemia compared to those without vitamin D deficiency [5], and that in women with both PCOS and MetS, vitamin D levels are lower than in women with PCOS and without MetS [39].

Similar vitamin D levels were detected in the present study in PCOS and control participants regardless of the presence of Apa-I SNP. Interestingly,

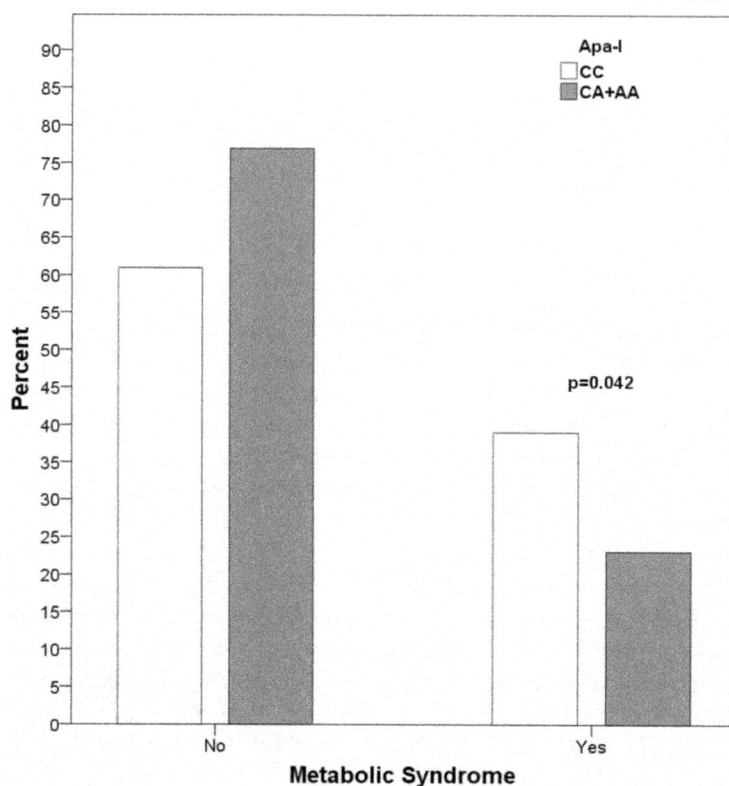

Fig. 1 Frequency of metabolic syndrome in PCOS women according to Apa-I genotypes. Data are expressed as percentages (Pearson chi-square test). Frequency values: Apa-I: No – CC: 61.0%; CA + AA: 76.9% / Yes – CC: 39.0%; CA + AA: 23.1%. OR: 2.133; 95% CI: 1.020–4.464

Table 4 Clinical, endocrine, and metabolic features of PCOS and control women according to presence or absence of Apa-I SNP

Variable	PCOS (n = 190)		Controls (n = 100)		
	CC (41)	CA + AA (149)	CC (16)	CA + AA (84)	p gen
WC (cm)[#]	91.97 ± 15.45	88.56 ± 14.96	81.42 ± 13.08	77.41 ± 11.20	0.149
SBP (mmHg)[#]	127.02 ± 19.79 [a]	119.49 ± 13.69 [b]	113.83 ± 11.35 [a]	108.60 ± 13.10 [b]	0.009
DBP (mmHg)[#]	81.30 ± 13.46	77.21 ± 10.84	72.77 ± 10.17	70.41 ± 9.24	0.079
Glucose (mg/dL)	87.88 ± 13.18	89.14 ± 15.92	90.47 ± 7.13	88.08 ± 7.65	0.805
Insulin (μUI/mL)[#]	20.28 ± 12.85	22.41 ± 21.27	11.64 ± 5.78	12.03 ± 6.71	0.846
HOMA-IR[#]	4.45 ± 3.07	5.12 ± 5.86	2.56 ± 1.45	2.50 ± 1.60	0.654
TC (mg/dL)	180.95 ± 37.35 [a]	172.73 ± 38.55 [b]	183.80 ± 36.87 [a]	167.26 ± 28.76 [b]	0.040
HDL-c (mg/dL)[#]	46.12 ± 10.73	49.59 ± 10.86	53.73 ± 11.21	52.65 ± 12.55	0.529
LDL-c (mg/dL)	111.05 ± 31.97 [a]	102.52 ± 31.69 [b]	111.99 ± 32.73 [a]	99.56 ± 24.48 [b]	0.038
Trig (mg/dL)[#]	118.90 ± 99.18	104.29 ± 62.18	90.40 ± 55.15	75.28 ± 41.89	0.149
25(OH)D (ng/mL)	19.41 ± 5.23	22.12 ± 8.17	21.31 ± 6.15	21.52 ± 7.16	0.399

WC waist circumference, *SBP* systolic blood pressure, *DBP* diastolic blood pressure, *HOMA* homeostasis model assessment index, *TC* total cholesterol, *HDL-c* high-density lipoprotein cholesterol, *LDL-c* low-density lipoprotein cholesterol, *Trig* triglycerides, 25(OH)D 25-hydroxyvitamin D
Values are expressed as means ± SD (two-way ANOVA). Different superscript letters indicate statistical difference for comparisons between genotypes, grouped by the absence or presence of the polymorphic allele, in PCOS and control groups. [#] $p < 0.005$ for comparisons between PCOS (CC and CA + AA) and control (CC and CA + AA) groups

while two meta-analyses [5, 6] comprising 3182 and 2262 women respectively showed that serum 25(OH) D concentrations were lower in PCOS compared to controls, the reported standardized mean difference between the groups in both studies seems of little clinical relevance – only 0.74 ng/mL (95%IC: -1.26 to – 0.22) [5] and 0.64 ng/mL (95%IC: -1.12 to – 0.15) [6]. In turn, the fact that our PCOS patients with MetS had lower vitamin D levels and higher frequency of CC polymorphism compared to those without MetS suggests that the Apa-I gene variant might impact vitamin D levels in PCOS with MetS. In fact, vitamin D status is influenced by many factors, especially dietary pattern, season, and genetic traits [40]. A better understanding of the genetic factors that may be involved in vitamin D level variation and metabolic disturbances could shed some light on hypothetical gene-environment interactions of vitamin D. Further studies with larger PCOS populations and higher proportion of MetS are needed in order to confirm this hypothesis.

We did not find any association between genotypes or haplotypes of VDR gene variants in PCOS participants. Only a few studies are available in the literature assessing VDR gene polymorphism and risk of PCOS, with uncertain conclusions, which vary according to the studied sample. While some studies show an association between at least one VDR gene polymorphism and PCOS [9–12, 41], others report similar distributions of Bsm-I, Apa-I and Taq-I polymorphisms in PCOS and control women [13–15]. Also, regarding haplotypes of VDR gene variants, no definitive data are available, with few reports of distinct haplotypes of VDR gene polymorphisms presenting slightly higher frequency in PCOS women when compared to controls [10, 12, 14]. These unclear data may be, at least in part, attributed to ethnic differences in the studied populations and to the polygenic condition of PCOS. Yet, other studies have reported an association of VDR gene polymorphisms with PP [8] and diabetes [42–45].

One strength of our study is the focus on a less well represented ethnic group, PCOS women from southern Brazil, with assessment of gene variants which may be contributing to this polygenic and multifactorial disease. Furthermore, we evaluated polymorphisms found in a genomic position that plays an important role in the modulation of gene expression. Limitations of the present study are the relatively small sample size of 291 participants (191 PCOS and 100 controls) and the low frequency of MetS in the control group, precluding complementary analyses correlating VDR gene polymorphisms and MetS in that group. In addition, further studies on functional evaluation of VDR SNPs are needed in order to deepen the understanding of findings.

Conclusions

Our results indicate that Bsm-I, Apa-I, and Taq-I polymorphisms in VDR gene are not related to PCOS. However, there seems to be an association of the CC genotype of Apa-I with MetS in PCOS women, and with blood pressure, total cholesterol, and LDL-c in women with and without PCOS. Despite the similarity in the vitamin D levels of PCOS and control participants, our study suggests that Apa-I impacts vitamin D levels in PCOS with MetS.

Abbreviations
25(OH)D: 25-hydroxyvitamin D; BMI: Body mass index; BP: Blood pressure; CV: Coefficient of variation; DBP: Diastolic blood pressure; FAI: Free androgen index; Glu: Glucose; HDL-c: High-density lipoprotein cholesterol; HOMA: Homeostasis model assessment index; LDL-c: Low-density lipoprotein cholesterol; MetS: Metabolic syndrome; PCOS: Polycystic ovary syndrome; PCR: Polymerase chain reaction; PP: Precocious pubarche; SBP: Systolic blood pressure; SHBG: Sex hormone–binding globulin; SNP: Single nucleotide polymorphism; TC: Total cholesterol; Trig: Triglyceride; TT: Total testosterone; VDR: Vitamin D receptor; WC: Waist circumference

Funding
This work was supported by grants from Conselho Nacional de Desenvolvimento Científico e Tecnológico/Brazilian National Institute of Hormones and Women's Health (CNPq/INCT 465482/2014–7) and Coordenacão de Aperfeiçoamento de Pessoal de Nível Superior (CAPES, Post-doc grant to BRS). The funders had no role in study design, data collection and analysis, decision to publish, or preparation of the manuscript.

Authors' contributions
BRS and PMS were involved in the conception and design of the study, BRS, SBL and PMS were involved in data collection and analysis. BRS and PMS drafted the article. All the authors read and approved the final manuscript.

Competing interests
The authors declare that they have no competing interests.

Author details
[1]Division of Endocrinology, Gynecological Endocrinology Unit, Hospital de Clínicas de Porto Alegre, Rua Ramiro Barcelos, 2350, Porto Alegre, RS 90035-003, Brazil. [2]Department of Physiology, Laboratory of Molecular Endocrinology, Universidade Federal do Rio Grande do Sul (UFRGS), Porto Alegre, Brazil. [3]Department of Diagnostic Methods, Universidade Federal de Ciências Médicas de Porto Alegre (UFCSPA), Porto Alegre, Brazil.

References
1. Azziz R, Woods KS, Reyna R, Key TJ, Knochenhauer ES, Yildiz BO. The prevalence and features of the polycystic ovary syndrome in an unselected population. J Clin Endocrinol Metab. 2004;89:2745–9.

2. Asuncion M, Calvo RM, San Millan JL, Sancho J, Avila S, Escobar-Morreale HF. A prospective study of the prevalence of the polycystic ovary syndrome in unselected Caucasian women from Spain. J Clin Endocrinol Metab. 2000; 85:2434–8.

3. March WA, Moore VM, Willson KJ, Phillips DIW, Norman RJ, Davies MJ. The prevalence of polycystic ovary syndrome in a community sample assessed under contrasting diagnostic criteria. Hum Reprod. 2010;25:544–51.

4. De Leo V, Musacchio MC, Cappelli V, Massaro MG, Morgante G, Petraglia F. Genetic, hormonal and metabolic aspects of PCOS: an update. Reprod Biol Endocrinol. 2016;14:38.

5. He CL, Lin ZM, Robb SW, Ezeamama AE. Serum vitamin D levels and polycystic ovary syndrome: a systematic review and meta-analysis. Nutrients. 2015;7:4555–77.

6. Bacopoulou F, Kolias E, Efthymiou V, Antonopoulos CN, Charmandari E. Vitamin D predictors in polycystic ovary syndrome: a meta-analysis. Eur J Clin Investig. 2017;47:746–55.

7. Palomer X, Gonzalez-Clemente JM, Blanco-Vaca F, Mauricio D. Role of vitamin D in the pathogenesis of type 2 diabetes mellitus. Diabetes Obes Metab. 2008;10:185–97.

8. Santos BR, Mascarenhas LP, Satler F, Boguszewski MC, Spritzer PM. Vitamin D receptor gene polymorphisms and sex steroid secretion in girls with precocious pubarche in southern Brazil: a pilot study. J Endocrinol Investig. 2012;35:725–9.

9. Mahmoudi T. Genetic variation in the vitamin D receptor and polycystic ovary syndrome risk. Fertil Steril. 2009;92:1381–3.

10. El-Shal AS, Shalaby SM, Aly NM, Rashad NM, Abdelaziz AM. Genetic variation in the vitamin D receptor gene and vitamin D serum levels in Egyptian women with polycystic ovary syndrome. Mol Biol Rep. 2013;40:6063–73.

11. Mahmoudi T, Majidzadeh-A K, Farahani H, Mirakhorli M, Dabiri R, Nobakht H, et al. Association of vitamin D receptor gene variants with polycystic ovary syndrome: a case control study. Int J Reprod Biomed (Yazd). 2015; 13(12):793–800.

12. Siddamalla S, Reddy TV, Govatati S, Erram N, Deenadayal M, Shivaji S, et al. Vitamin D receptor gene polymorphisms and risk of polycystic ovary syndrome in south Indian women. Gynecol Endocrinol. 2017;3:1–5.

13. Wehr E, Trummer O, Giuliani A, Gruber HJ, Pieber TR, Obermayer-Pietsch B. Vitamin D-associated polymorphisms are related to insulin resistance and vitamin D deficiency in polycystic ovary syndrome. Eur J Endocrinol. 2011; 164:741–9.

14. Dasgupta S, Dutta J, Annamaneni S, Kudugunti N, Battini MR. Association of vitamin D receptor gene polymorphisms with polycystic ovary syndrome among Indian women. Indian J Med Res. 2015;142:276–85.

15. Jedrzejuk D, Laczmanski L, Milewicz A, Kuliczkowska-Plaksej J, Lenarcik-Kabza A, Hirnle L, et al. Classic PCOS phenotype is not associated with deficiency of endogenous vitamin D and VDR genepolymorphisms rs731236 (Taqı), rs7975232 (Apaı), rs1544410 (Bsmı), rs10735810 (Fokı): a case-control study of lower Silesian women. Gynecol Endocrinol. 2015;31:976–9.

16. Al-Daghri NM, Al-Attas OS, Alkharfy KM, Khan N, Mohammed AK, Vinodson B, et al. Association of VDR-gene variants with factors related to the metabolic syndrome, type 2 diabetes and vitamin D deficiency. Gene. 2014; 542:129–33.

17. Hitman GA, Mannan N, McDermott MF, Aganna E, Ogunkolade BW, Hales CN, et al. Vitamin D receptor gene polymorphisms influence insulin secretion in Bangladeshi Asians. Diabetes. 1998;47:688–90.

18. Bienertová-Vašků J, Zlámal F, Pohořalá A, Mikeš O, Goldbergová-Pávková M, Novák J, Šplíchal Z, Pikhart H. Allelic variants in vitamin D receptor gene are associated with adiposity measures in the central-European population. BMC Medical Genetics. 2017;18:90–99.

19. Alvarez JA, Ashraf A. Role of vitamin D in insulin secretion and insulin sensitivity for glucose homeostasis. Int J Endocrinol. 2010;92:1344–9.

20. Oh JY, Barrett-Connor E. Association between vitamin D receptor polymorphism and type 2 diabetes or metabolic syndrome in community-dwelling older adults: the rancho Bernardo study. Metabolism. 2002; 51:356–9.

21. Ortlepp JR, Metrikat J, Albrecht M, von Korff A, Hanrath P, Hoffmann R. The vitamin D receptor gene variant and physical activity predicts fasting glucose levels in healthy young men. Diabet Med. 2003;20:451–4.

22. Santos BR, Mascarenhas LPG, Satler F, Boguszewski MCS, Spritzer PM. Vitamin D deficiency in girls from South Brazil: a cross-sectional study on prevalence and association with vitamin D receptor gene variants. BMC Pediatr. 2012;12:62–8.

23. Han FF, Lv YL, Gong LL, Liu H, Wan ZR, Liu LH. VDR gene variation and insulin resistance related diseases. Lipids Health Dis. 2017;16(1):157.

24. Santos BR, Lecke SB, Spritzer PM. Genetic variant in vitamin D-binding protein is associated with metabolic syndrome and lower 25-hydroxyvitamin D levels in polycystic ovary syndrome: a cross-sectional study. PLoS One. 2017;12:e0173695.

25. Group REA-SPCW. Revised 2003 consensus on diagnostic criteria and long-term health risks related to polycystic ovary syndrome. Fertil Steril. 2004; 81:19–25.

26. Toscani M, Mighavacca R, Sisson de Castro JA, Spritzer PM. Estimation of truncal adiposity using waist circumference or the sum of trunk skinfolds: a pilot study for insulin resistance screening in hirsute patients with or without polycystic ovary syndrome. Metabolism. 2007;56:992–7.

27. Graff SK, Mario FM, Alves BC, Spritzer PM. Dietary glycemic index is associated with less favorable anthropometric and metabolic profiles in polycystic ovary syndrome women with different phenotypes. Fertil Steril. 2013;100:1081–8.

28. Di Domenico K, Wiltgen D, Nickel FJ, Magalhaes JA, Moraes RS, Spritzer PM. Cardiac autonomic modulation in polycystic ovary syndrome: does the phenotype matter? Fertil Steril. 2013;99:286–92.

29. Ramos RB, Spritzer PMFTO. Gene variants are not associated with polycystic ovary syndrome in women from southern Brazil. Gene. 2015;560:25–9.

30. Alberti K, Eckel RH, Grundy SM, Zimmet PZ, Cleeman JI, Donato KA, et al. Harmonizing the metabolic syndrome a joint interim statement of the international diabetes federation task force on epidemiology and prevention; National Heart, Lung, and Blood Institute; American Heart Association; world heart federation; international atherosclerosis society; and International Association for the Study of obesity. Circulation. 2009; 120:1640–5.

31. Wallace TM, Levy JC, Matthews DR. Use and abuse of HOMA modeling. Diabetes Care. 2004;27:1487–95.

32. Miller SA, Dykes DD, Polesky HF. A simple salting out procedure for extracting DNA from human nucleated cells. Nucleic Acids Res. 1988; 16:1215.

33. La Marra F, Stinco G, Buligan C, Chiriacò G, Serraino D, Di Loreto C, et al. Immunohistochemical evaluation of vitamin D receptor (VDR) expression in cutaneous melanoma tissues and four VDR gene polymorphisms. Cancer Biol Med. 2017;14:162–75.

34. Ogunkolade BW, Boucher BJ, Prahl JM, Bustin SA, Burrin JM, Noonan K, et al. Vitamin D receptor (VDR) mRNA and VDR protein levels in relation to vitamin D status, insulin secretory capacity, and VDR genotype in Bangladeshi Asians. Diabetes. 2002;51:2294–300.

35. Meyer V, Saccone DS, Tugizimana F, Asani FF, Jeffery TJ, Bornman L. Methylation of the vitamin D receptor (VDR) gene, together with genetic variation, race, and environment influence the signaling efficacy of the toll-like receptor 2/1-VDR pathway. Front Immunol. 2017;8:1048.

36. Uitterlinden AG, Fang Y, Van Meurs JB, Pols HA, Van Leeuwen JP. Genetics and biology of vitamin D receptor polymorphisms. Gene. 2004;338:143–56.

37. Pike JW, Meyer MB. The vitamin D receptor: new paradigms for the regulation of gene expression by 1,25-Dihydroxyvitamin D-3. Endocrinol Metab Clin N Am. 2010;39:255–69.

38. Dilworth FJ, Chambon P. Nuclear receptors coordinate the activities of chromatin remodeling complexes and coactivators to facilitate initiation of transcription. Oncogene. 2001;20:3047–54.

39. Joham AE, Teede HJ, Cassar S, Stepto NK, Strauss BJ, Harrison CL, et al. Vitamin D in polycystic ovary syndrome: relationship to obesity and insulin resistance. Mol Nutr Food Res. 2016;60:110–8.

40. Bahrami A, Sadeghnia HR, Tabatabaeizadeh SA, Bahrami-Taghanaki H, Behboodi N, Esmaeili H, Ferns GA, Mobarhan MG, Avan A. Genetic and epigenetic factors influencing vitamin D status. J Cell Physiol. 2018;233: 4033–43.

41. Bagheri M, Abdi Rad I, Hosseini Jazani N, Nanbakhsh F. Vitamin D receptor Taqı gene variant in exon 9 and polycystic ovary syndrome risk. Int J Fertil Steril. 2013;7:116–21.

## 7

Altered miRNA profile in testis of post-cryptorchidopexy patients with non-obstructive azoospermia

Dongdong Tang[1,2,3†], Zhenyu Huang[4†], Xiaojin He[1,2,3], Huan Wu[1,2,3], Dangwei Peng[4], Li Zhang[4*] and Xiansheng Zhang[4*]

Abstract

Background: Cryptorchidism is one of the most common causes of non-obstructive azoospermia (NOA) leading to male infertility. Despite various medical approaches been utilised, many patients still suffer from infertility. MicroRNAs (miRNAs) play vital roles in the progress of spermatogenesis; however, little is known about the miRNA expression profile in the testes. Therefore, the miRNA profile was assessed in the testis of post-cryptorchidopexy patients.

Methods: Three post-cryptorchidopexy testicular tissue samples from patients aged 23, 26 and 28 years old and three testis tissues from patients with obstructive azoospermia (controls) aged 24, 25 and 36 years old were used in this study. Next-generation sequencing (NGS) was used to perform the miRNA expression profiling. Quantitative real-time reverse transcription polymerase chain reaction (qRT-PCR) assays were subsequently used to confirm the results of several randomly-selected and annotated miRNAs.

Results: A series of miRNAs were found to be altered between post-cryptorchidopexy testicular tissues and control tissues, including 297 downregulated and 152 upregulated miRNAs. In the subsequent qRT-PCR assays, the expression levels of most of the selected miRNAs (9/12, $P < 0.05$) were consistent with the results of NGS technology. Furthermore, signal transduction, adaptive immune response and biological regulation were associated with the putative target genes of the differentially-expressed miRNAs via GO analysis. In addition, oxidative phosphorylation, Parkinson's disease and ribosomal pathways were shown to be enriched using KEGG pathway analysis of the differentially-expressed genes.

Conclusions: This study provides a global view of the miRNAs involved in post-cryptorchidopexy testicular tissues as well as the altered expression of miRNAs compared to control tissues, thus confirming the vital role of miRNAs in cryptorchidism.

Keywords: miRNA, Cryptorchidism, Cryptorchidopexy, Spermatogenesis, Next-generation small RNA sequencing

Background

Male factors account for approximately 50% of infertility cases, which affect 10–15% of couples around the world [1]. Although most cases of male infertility are idiopathic with no known etiological factor, some causes (i.e. varicocele, sexual dysfunction etc.) are known [2]. Among these causes, cryptorchidism is a relatively common anomaly in the male genitalia that affects approximately 2–4% of male infants. Despite various medical approaches (i.e. surgical operations and hormone administration) being applied for years, many patients still suffer from infertility [3, 4], and little is known about the clear mechanism of spermatogenesis arrest in these patients.

Spermatogenesis is a complex process consisted of three phases including mitotic, meiotic and haploid processes [5]. These cellular events require highly regulated spatiotemporal expression of specific protein-coding genes,

* Correspondence: tensionzl@126.com; xiansheng-zhang@163.com
†Dongdong Tang and Zhenyu Huang contributed equally to this work.
4Department of Urology, The First Affiliated Hospital of Anhui Medical University, Hefei, Anhui, People's Republic of China
Full list of author information is available at the end of the article

especailly at the post-transcriptional levels [6]. MicroRNAs (miRNAs) are a series of small noncoding RNAs that negatively regulate gene expression after transcription [7]. Research has shown that miRNAs play crucial roles in spermatogenesis [5, 6, 8–13]; for example, Lian et al. identified a series of altered miRNAs in patients with non-obstructive azoospermia (NOA) using microarray technology. These identified 154 significantly downregulated and 19 upregulated miRNAs indicated the important role of miRNAs in spermatogenesis [10]. It was reported that during mouse testicular development, up-regulation of miR-449 coincided with initiation of meiotic, and miR-449 was predominantly expressed in spermatocytes and spermatids during adult spermatogenesis. Furthermore, Cdc20b/miR-449 cluster activity was documented to be cooperatively mediated by CREMT and SOX5 during postnatal testes development [5]. Later on, Comazzetto et al. have identified the miR-34 family consisted of miR-34b/c and miR-449a/b/c as upregulated from late meiosis to sperm stage. miR-34b/c and miR-449 deletion led to sterility due to abnormal spermatozoa production with reduced motility [11]. With regards to the effects of miRNAs in cryptorchidism, Duan et al. found that miR-210, a significantly upregulated miRNA in patients with NOA, was also highly expressed in patients with cryptorchidism [12]. In addition, Moritoki et al. demonstrated that miR-135a was downregulated in unilateral undescended testes in a rat model of cryptorchidism [13].

Although some miRNAs were shown to be involved in the regulation of spermatogenesis in patients with cryptorchidism, no studies have yet investigated miRNA expression in the testis of post-cryptorchidopexy patients with NOA. Therefore this study investigated the miRNA profile in the testis of post-cryptorchidopexy patients and aimed to provide a platform to expound the mechanism of spermatogenesis arrest in post-cryptorchidopexy patients with NOA.

Methods

Ethics statement
Three patients (23, 26 and 28 years old) who underwent cryptorchidopexy but were still experiencing NOA, as well as three patients (24, 25 and 36 years old) suffering from obstructive azoospermia (OA) signed informed consent and approved the use of their tissues for research purposes. The local medical ethics committee approved this study.

Clinical specimen collection
Testes tissues were collected by testicular biopsy from all six subjects between July 2017 and January 2018 at the Reproductive Medicine Center, First Affiliated Hospital of Anhui Medical University (Hefei, Anhui, China). For post-cryptorchidopexy patients, all cases

were bilateral. Case one was 23 years old and underwent the operation 1 year ago, case two was 26 years old and underwent the operation 18 years ago and case three was 28 years old and underwent the operation 12 years ago. Testes samples were frozen at – 80 °C in RNAlater (Ambion, USA) immediately after surgery. Haematoxylin and eosin (HE) staining and the Johnson score system were used to assess testicular spermatogenic function.

Construction of a smRNA library and next-generation sequencing (NGS)
Total RNA was extracted from the six samples using TRIzol (Life Technologies, USA) and was used to construct miRNA libraries using the NEBNext® Multiplex Small RNA Library Prep Set (Illumina®) according to the manufacturer's instructions. Sequencing was performed on a Hiseq X (Illumina) using the HiSeq X Reagent Kit v2.

Data analyses and novel miRNA exploration
Data were analysed according to previously-reported methods. Known miRNAs were identified by mapping reads to miRBase (version 21.0) in *Homo sapiens*, whilst nonmatched reads were subsequently aligned against other noncoding RNAs within the Ensembl database [14]. The remaining nonannotated sequences were selected for alignment with the integrated human transcriptome to explore novel miRNAs. All hairpin-like structures containing unclassified smRNA reads (no less than 45 reads) were predicted using miRDeep2 [15] following the criteria described previously [16].

Bioinformatic analyses for miRNAs with differential expression patterns
The target genes of the differentially-expressed miRNAs in the two groups were predicted using TargetScan [17] and miRanda [18]. Enriched GO terms and KEGG pathway analysis was subsequently applied to predict the target genes of miRNAs with differential expression patterns in the two groups of specimens.

QRT-PCR verification for altered miRNA expression
cDNA synthesis was performed using a PrimeScript RT reagent kit following the manufacturer's instructions (Takara, Japan). The abundance of individual miRNAs was subsequently assessed via an Applied Biosystems 7500 PCR System (Applied Biosystems) using SYBR Premix Ex Taq II (Tli RNaseH Plus, Takara) under optimised reaction conditions. The specific reverse transcription and qPCR primers for all miRNAs are listed in Additional file 1. The processes were performed in accordance with the protocols supplied by the manufacturers. Briefly, for qPCR, triplicate

reactions were performed at 95 °C for 10 min, and the subsequent 40 amplification cycles were conducted at 95 °C for 15 s and 60 °C for 60 s. Meanwhile, 18S rRNA was used as an internal normalised control. Relative miRNA abundances were calculated using $2^{-\triangle\triangle Ct}$ (threshold cycle) formula, where $\triangle Ct = Ct_{miRNA} - Ct_{18S rRNA}$ and $\triangle\triangle Ct = (\triangle Ct_{post-cryptorchidopexy} - \triangle Ct_{obstructive azoospermia})$. The miRNA concentration differences between post-cryptorchidopexy and control tissues were analysed using unpaired t-tests. $P < 0.05$ indicated a statistically significant difference.

Results

Histopathological characteristics of post-cryptorchidopexy testicular tissue and control tissue

To clarify the histopathological characteristics of the post-cryptorchidopexy testicular tissue (hereafter referred to as 'cryptorchid tissue') and control tissue (hereafter referred to as 'normal tissue'), HE staining and the Johnson scoring system were used to assess the function of spermatogenesis (Fig. 1). The Johnson scores were 3, 3 and 3 in cryptorchid tissues, which indicated maturation arrest, and 9, 9 and 10 in normal control tissues, which indicated normal spermatogenesis.

Comprehensive overview of whole genome smRNAs in cryptorchid and normal tissues

All smRNAs [18–32 nucleotides (nt)] acquired from cryptorchid and normal tissues were deep sequenced by NGS. A total of 19,931,698 (out of 21,212,215) and 20,243,124 (out of 21,524,351) sequence reads that aligned to the human genome sequence dataset were obtained in the cryptorchid and normal tissues, respectively. MiRNAs accounted for 85.5% and 71.19% in cryptorchid and normal tissues, respectively (Fig. 2).

The most abundant of these smRNAs in cryptorchid tissue were 21 nt in length, and these smRNAs were more abundant than the 22-nt and 23-nt RNAs which

were in second and third place, respectively. However, the most abundant smRNAs in normal tissue were 22 nt in length, and these were more abundant than the 21-nt and 23-nt RNAs which were in second and third place, respectively (see Additional file 2).

Understanding the distribution pattern of miRNA genes may help to elucidate their roles, therefore the chromosomal locations of miRNA genes were evaluated. In cryptorchid tissue, most miRNA genes were located on chromosomes X, 9, 3 and 21. Similarly, in normal tissues, most miRNA genes were located on chromosome X, 15, 9 and 5 (see Additional file 3).

Features of the most abundant miRNAs in cryptorchid and normal tissues

The NGS results were used to compile a list of the 20 most abundant and known miRNAs in cryptorchid tissue and the 10 most abundant and novel miRNAs in normal tissue. In cryptorchid tissue, miR-514a-3p, miR-143-3p, miR-26a-5p, miR-99a-5p, miR-202-5p, miR-509-3-5p, miR-10b-5p, miR-508-3p, let-7 g-5p and let-7f-5p were the most abundant known miRNAs. In normal tissue, miR-514a-3p, miR-143-3p, miR-26a-5p, miR-509-3-5p, miR-99a-5p, miR-202-5p, miR-10b-5p, let-7f-5p, miR-508-3p and let-7 g-5p were the most abundant known miRNAs (Table 1). Detailed information is shown in Table 1. Of the 10 most abundant novel miRNAs, only one was different between cryptorchid and normal tissues. Detailed information is shown in Table 2.

Differential expression of miRNAs between cryptorchid and normal tissues

As described previously by Zhang et al. [16], miRNAs were considered to be significantly differentially expressed between cryptorchid and normal tissues if they were altered by at least two-fold with $P < 0.05$ on the t-test. The results showed that 449 miRNAs were significantly

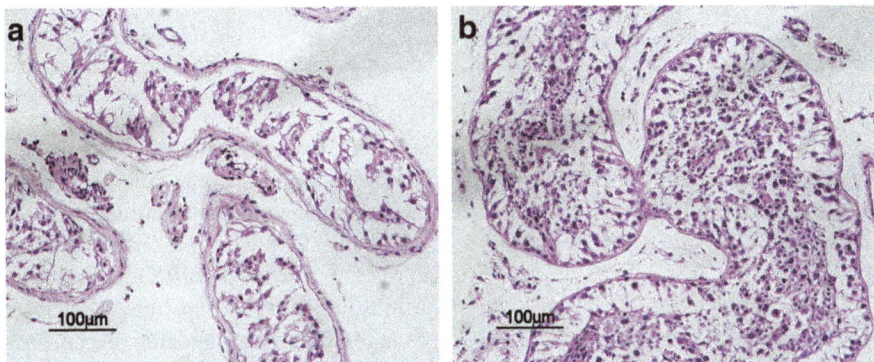

Fig. 1 HE-staining of cryptorchid tissue and control tissue, which clarify the histopathological characteristics of cryptorchid tissues (**a**) and control tissues (**b**).

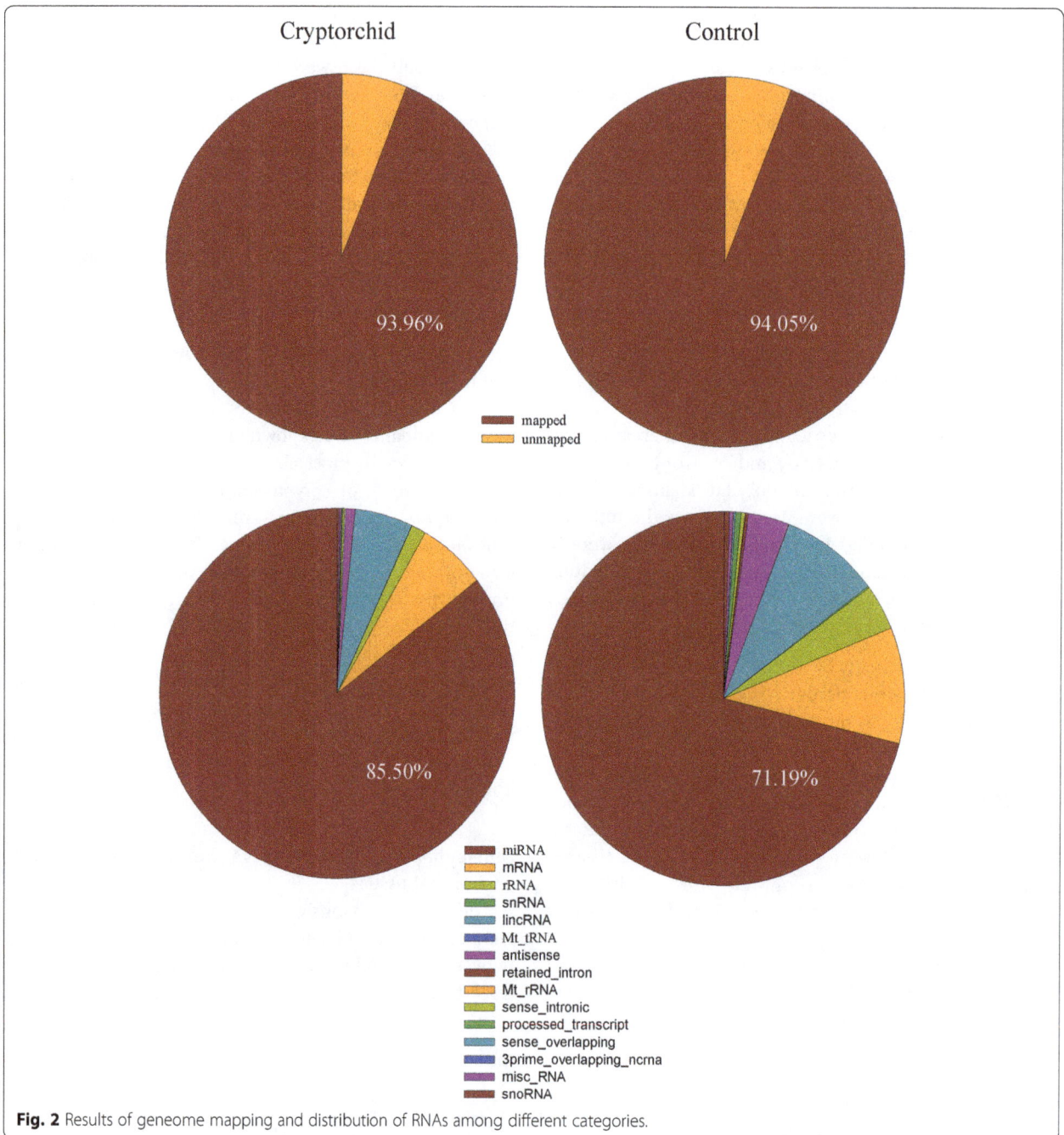

Fig. 2 Results of geneome mapping and distribution of RNAs among different categories.

differentially expressed in cryptorchid tissue (Fig. 3). Of these, 297 were downregulated and 152 were upregulated compared to normal tissue. The 30 most downregulated and upregulated known miRNAs are listed in Tables 3 and 4, respectively.

Validating the altered expression level of miRNAs by qRT-PCR

QRT-PCR was performed to validate the altered miRNA expression. Among these deregulated miRNAs, we firstly selected two well-established spermatogenesis-associated miRNAs, miR-449a and miR-34c-5p [5, 11]. Additionally, to better proving the accuracy of NGS, the other validated miRNAs were picked from the non-top 30 most deregulated known miRNAs (see Additional file 4 and Additional file 5), so that the relatively small fold changes could be validated. According to the previous studies, ten miRNAs were picked for qRT-PCR validation randomly [16, 19]. Eventually, a total of 12 differentially-expressed miRNAs (seven upregulated

Table 1 The top 20 most abundant known miRNAs expressed in cryptorchid and normal tissues

miRNA name	Cryptorchid		miRNA name	Control	
	Reads count	Normalized reads count		Reads count	Normalized reads count
hsa-miR-514a-3p	2,313,282	109,499	hsa-miR-514a-3p	1,008,914	98,435
hsa-miR-143-3p	864,140	45,306	hsa-miR-143-3p	677,433	65,245
hsa-miR-26a-5p	829,953	46,035	hsa-miR-26a-5p	407,763	39,613
hsa-miR-99a-5p	705,575	38,041	hsa-miR-509-3-5p	392,074	37,711
hsa-miR-202-5p	616,580	30,770	hsa-miR-99a-5p	346,310	33,871
hsa-miR-509-3-5p	593,363	28,054	hsa-miR-202-5p	258,855	25,790
hsa-miR-10b-5p	428,806	24,984	hsa-miR-10b-5p	248,352	24,218
hsa-miR-508-3p	303,445	14,625	hsa-let-7f-5p	154,806	15,116
hsa-let-7 g-5p	296,741	15,472	hsa-miR-508-3p	153,631	15,059
hsa-let-7f-5p	266,118	14,707	hsa-let-7 g-5p	151,745	14,851
hsa-let-7a-5p	265,013	14,644	hsa-let-7a-5p	137,886	13,412
hsa-miR-21-5p	248,959	12,378	hsa-miR-21-5p	132,197	12,931
hsa-miR-509-5p	194,212	9293	hsa-miR-148a-3p	119,576	11,671
hsa-miR-148a-3p	188,828	10,645	hsa-miR-100-5p	103,191	10,071
hsa-miR-125b-5p	172,432	9013	hsa-miR-125b-5p	93,627	9134
hsa-miR-100-5p	169,375	9160	hsa-miR-27b-3p	92,637	8927
hsa-miR-199a-3p	154,971	8592	hsa-miR-509-5p	81,898	8124
hsa-miR-27b-3p	144,132	7610	hsa-miR-126-3p	79,980	7687
hsa-let-7i-5p	140,689	7772	hsa-miR-125a-5p	72,130	7013
hsa-let-7b-5p	112,327	6040	hsa-miR-34c-5p	69,568	6885
hsa-miR-125a-5p	107,449	5594	hsa-let-7i-5p	66,915	6560

and five downregulated) were selected for qRT-PCR analysis. The results showed that the expression levels of most miRNAs (9/12; $P < 0.05$) were consistent with the results of NGS technology. Detailed information is shown in Fig. 4.

GO enrichment analysis of differentially-expressed genes in cryptorchid and normal tissues

After predicting the target genes of differentially-expressed miRNAs in cryptorchid and normal tissues, GO enrichment analysis was conducted. The 10 most enriched GO terms, including signal transduction and adaptive immune response, are shown in Table 5.

KEGG pathway analysis of differentially-expressed genes in cryptorchid and normal tissues

After GO analysis, KEGG pathway enrichment analysis was performed. A total of five KEGG pathways were enriched, including oxidative phosphorylation, Parkinson's disease, Ribosomal pathways, Huntington's disease and Alzheimer's disease. The results are presented in Table 6.

Discussion

As one of the most common congenital defects in newborn boys, cryptorchidism influences male fertility and increases the risk of testicular cancer. Reductions in seminiferous tubules and germ cells are common histological changes in cryptorchid testis [20]. Despite surgery being recommended for many patients with cryptorchidism, the success of orchidopexy depends on the timing of the procedure and the position of the testis: some may not benefit from cryptorchidopexy [21, 22]. Although research has identified some biological processes involved in spermatogenic arrest in cryptorchid testis (i.e. significant apoptotic changes in germ cells), the causative roles of genes in spermatogenic arrest or apoptosis remain unclear [23–26]. This is the first study to investigate the possible mechanisms of spermatogenic arrest in cryptorchid testes by assessing the miRNA profiles in post-cryptorchidopexy testes.

Many rodent and primate models were developed to identify altered miRNAs in cryptorchid testis. For example, Duan et al. established a mouse model of cryptorchidism and showed that miR-210 was highly expressed in cryptorchid testes compared with control testes. Moreover, they showed that this miRNA regulated spermatogenesis by inhibiting the expression of NR1D2 [12]. Moritoki et al. compared the miRNA expression profiles of unilateral undescended testes with contralateral descended testes in a rat model of cryptorchidism using microarray analysis.

Table 2 The list of top 10 most abundant novel miRNAs expressed in cryptorchid and normal tissues

Cryptorchid tissues

miRNA ID	Mature Sequence	Reads count	Location of novel miRNA precursor
chrX_47246	AUUGACACU UCUGUGAGU AGA	2,280,438	chrX:146366172..146366230:-
chr12_27425	UUCAAGUAA UCCAGGAUAG GCU	826,714	chr12:58218403..58218462:-
chr3_5958	UUCAAGUAA UCCAGGAUAG GCU	826,558	chr3:38010903..38010964:+
chr21_44054	AACCCGUAG AUCCGAUCUU GU	693,017	chr21:17911420..17911480:+
chrX_47235	UACUGCAGA CGUGGCAAUC AUG	592,879	chrX:146341178..146341235:-
chr10_23103	UUCCUAUGC AUAUACUUCU UU	586,995	chr10:135061041..135061097:-
chr5_9937	UGAGAUGAA GCACUGUAGC UC	534,462	chr5:148808506..148808561:+
chr2_3766	UACCCUGUA GAACCGAAUU UGU	428,617	chr2:177015056..177015117:+
chrX_47228	UGAUUGUAG CCUUUUGGAG UAGA	298,225	chrX:146318462..146318520:-
chr3_7283	UGAGGUAGU AGUUUGUACA GUU	295,643	chr3:52302295..52302373:-

Normal tissues

miRNA ID	Mature Sequence	Reads count	Location of novel miRNA precursor
chrX_47246	AUUGACACU UCUGUGAGU AGA	996,346	chrX:146366172..146366230:-
chr5_9937	UGAGAUGAA GCACUGUAGC UC	419,103	chr5:148808506..148808561:+
chr12_27425	UUCAAGUAA UCCAGGAUAG GCU	405,817	chr12:58218403..58218462:-
chr3_5958	UUCAAGUAA UCCAGGAUAG GCU	405,621	chr3:38010903..38010964:+
chrX_47235	UACUGCAGA CGUGGCAAUC AUG	391,755	chrX:146341178..146341235:-
chr21_44054	AACCCGUAG AUCCGAUCUU GU	340,009	chr21:17911420..17911480:+
chr2_3766	UACCCUGUA GAACCGAAU UUGU	248,236	chr2:177015056..177015117:+

Table 2 The list of top 10 most abundant novel miRNAs expressed in cryptorchid and normal tissues *(Continued)*

Cryptorchid tissues

chr10_23103	UUCCUAUGC AUAUACUUC UUU	246,558	chr10:135061041..135061097:-
chr9_18744	UGAGGUAGU AGAUUGUAUA GUU	154,925	chr9:96938634..96938712:+
chr3_7283	UGAGGUAGU AGUUUGUACA GUU	151,154	chr3:52302295..52302373:-

These authors found that only miR-135a expression was lower in unilateral undescended testes and that its target, FoxO1, played essential roles in stem cell maintenance [13]. Furthermore, Duan et al., also found that miR-210 was upregulated in human cryptorchidism, thus suggesting a vital role for miRNAs in humans [12]. In this study, 297 downregulated and 152 upregulated miRNAs were identified in post-cryptorchidopexy testicular tissue compared with normal testis tissue. However, miR-210 was not significantly altered, which may be due to the different types of human cryptorchid tissue. For example, Duan et al. used cryptorchid testis tissue obtained during the cryptorchidopexy, whilst this study used post-cryptorchidopexy testicular tissue. Some miRNA expression levels may change after the operation.

Despite the insights gained into cryptorchidism over the years, the mechanism of spermatogenesis arrest in patients with this disease remains largely elusive. Germ cell apoptosis is commonly seen at the histological level in cryptorchid testes. Yin et al. revealed

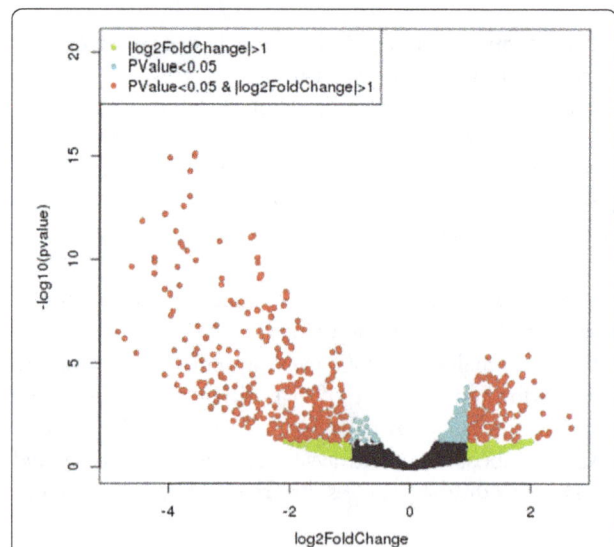

Fig. 3 The overview of the volcano plot generated by miRNAs profile in cryptorchid tissues and control tissues.

Table 3 A collection of the top 30 most downregulated known miRNAs detected by deep sequencing in cryptorchid tissues

MiRNA name	baseMean	log2FoldChange	lfcSE	stat	p	Adjust p
hsa-miR-3663-5p	41.936	−4.426	0.624	−7.089	1.35E-12	2.39E-10
hsa-miR-1233-3p	25.216	−4.227	0.679	−6.225	4.79E-10	1.84E-08
hsa-miR-552-5p	66.556	−4.055	0.563	−7.195	6.24E-13	1.21E-10
hsa-miR-449b-5p	392.523	−3.972	0.496	−8.001	1.23E-15	5.26E-13
hsa-miR-7153-5p	108.897	− 3.812	0.634	−6.010	1.84E-09	5.18E-08
hsa-miR-122-5p	525.785	−3.790	0.562	−6.741	1.57E-11	1.60E-09
hsa-miR-552-3p	65.189	−3.760	0.562	−6.680	2.38E-11	2.31E-09
hsa-miR-449a	5575.001	−3.740	0.511	−7.317	2.52E-13	5.97E-11
hsa-miR-122-3p	4.738	−3.722	1.011	−3.679	0.00023	0.0016
hsa-miR-34b-5p	123.524	−3.688	0.558	−6.610	3.84E-11	3.56E-09
hsa-miR-449c-5p	2234.173	−3.637	0.465	−7.816	5.42E-15	1.93E-12
hsa-miR-34c-5p	39,328.272	−3.553	0.440	−8.060	7.58E-16	5.26E-13
hsa-miR-449c-3p	7.961	−3.441	0.902	−3.812	0.00014	0.0011
hsa-miR-375	491.449	−3.408	0.362	−9.416	4.68E-21	9.99E-18
hsa-miR-3663-3p	37.612	−3.385	0.676	−5.001	5.68E-07	9.63E-06
hsa-miR-7159-5p	20.897	−3.259	0.705	−4.618	3.87E-06	5.29E-05
hsa-miR-449b-3p	142.460	−3.212	0.610	−5.262	1.42E-07	2.75E-06
hsa-miR-4700-5p	4.985	−3.208	0.951	−3.370	0.00075	0.0043
hsa-miR-522-3p	121.036	−3.153	0.465	−6.768	1.30E-11	1.46E-09
hsa-miR-1273a	38.566	−3.118	0.508	−6.135	8.47E-10	2.44E-08
hsa-miR-1295a	11.735	−3.075	0.760	−4.041	5.31E-05	0.0005
hsa-miR-34b-3p	1137.731	−2.970	0.516	−5.753	8.72E-09	2.16E-07
hsa-miR-1283	139.436	−2.798	0.488	−5.731	9.95E-09	2.41E-07
hsa-miR-3150b-3p	3.547	−2.768	0.991	−2.791	0.0052	0.020
hsa-miR-4423-3p	16.582	−2.702	0.755	−3.578	0.00035	0.0023
hsa-miR-6507-5p	7.696	−2.698	0.811	−3.325	0.00088	0.0049
hsa-miR-7154-5p	406.827	−2.646	0.981	−2.697	0.0070	0.025
hsa-miR-517c-3p	95.074	−2.639	0.386	−6.832	8.37E-12	9.92E-10
hsa-miR-3925-3p	10.324	−2.613	0.735	−3.553	0.00038	0.0025
hsa-miR-515-5p	84.007	−2.600	0.379	−6.856	7.04E-12	8.84E-10

that cryptorchidism induced germ cell apoptosis in an experimental mouse model via p53-dependent and p53-independent pathways [23]. Liu et al. also found that the Hsf1/Phlda1 pathway participated in primary spermatocyte apoptosis in surgery-induced cryptorchid testes of rats [27]. The expression of many apoptosis-related miRNAs was also shown to be altered in post-cryptorchidopexy testicular tissues. It was reported that miR-299-5p could modulate apoptosis through autophagy in neurons and ameliorate the cognitive capacity of APPswe/PS1dE9 mice [28]. In addition, miR-299-5p was significantly upregulated in post-cryptorchidopexy testicular tissue. Similar results were also found for miR-217, miR-206 etc. Li et al. also found that miR-217 could regulate apoptosis by targeting TNFSF11 in human podocyte cells [29]. This

study also identified a significant downregulation of miR-217 in post-cryptorchidopexy testicular tissue. Similarly, miR-206 was significantly upregulated in post-cryptorchidopexy testicular tissue and was shown to promoted cell apoptosis in Legg–Calvé–Perthes disease [30].

Conclusions

In summary, miRNA expression in post-cryptorchidopexy testicular tissue was profiled using NGS and compared with that of OA men with normal spermatogenesis. Several signalling pathways that are likely to be involved in spermatogenesis arrest in these patients were addressed. The results provide an important platform for future investigations into the roles of miRNAs in the progression of cryptorchidism as well as therapeutic

Table 4 A collection of the top 30 most upregulated known miRNAs detected by deep sequencing in cryptorchid tissues

MiRNA name	baseMean	log2FoldChange	lfcSE	stat	p	Adjust p
hsa-miR-7151-3p	6.026	2.634	0.892	2.953	0.0031	0.014
hsa-miR-376a-2-5p	10.918	2.202	0.724	3.042	0.0023	0.011
hsa-miR-1224-5p	17.708	2.193	0.615	3.565	0.00036	0.0024
hsa-miR-1299	187.854	1.958	0.426	4.600	4.22E-06	5.73E-05
hsa-miR-142-5p	697.547	1.898	0.583	3.255	0.0011	0.0060
hsa-miR-543	1281.559	1.869	0.450	4.152	3.29E-05	0.00036
hsa-miR-487a-3p	80.564	1.865	0.591	3.155	0.0016	0.0079
hsa-miR-584-3p	19.666	1.829	0.562	3.254	0.0011	0.0060
hsa-miR-665	18.416	1.798	0.710	2.534	0.011	0.036
hsa-miR-134-3p	29.541	1.778	0.598	2.975	0.0029	0.013
hsa-miR-369-3p	500.851	1.692	0.432	3.916	8.99E-05	0.00082
hsa-miR-377-3p	96.245	1.665	0.551	3.023	0.0025	0.011
hsa-miR-33a-5p	28.103	1.664	0.550	3.025	0.0025	0.011
hsa-miR-376a-3p	112.0733	1.602	0.436	3.704	0.00021	0.0015
hsa-miR-758-3p	520.1303	1.589	0.439	3.620	0.00029	0.0020
hsa-miR-654-3p	4175.568	1.587	0.388	4.095	4.22E-05	0.00044
hsa-miR-134-5p	2747.859	1.558	0.424	3.675	0.00024	0.0017
hsa-miR-889-3p	740.3619	1.552	0.468	3.312	0.00093	0.0052
hsa-miR-127-3p	40,871.646	1.548	0.392	3.955	7.65E-05	0.00071
hsa-miR-1185-1-3p	161.457	1.539	0.506	3.039	0.0024	0.011
hsa-miR-1185-2-3p	38.541	1.534	0.587	2.614	0.0089	0.030
hsa-miR-154-5p	267.267	1.516	0.346	4.385	1.16E-05	0.00014
hsa-miR-381-3p	7512.422	1.511	0.382	3.957	7.57E-05	0.00070
hsa-miR-127-5p	768.176	1.511	0.401	3.765	0.00017	0.0013
hsa-miR-337-5p	44.570	1.510	0.439	3.437	0.00059	0.0036
hsa-miR-379-3p	262.022	1.508	0.401	3.756	0.00017	0.0013
hsa-miR-136-3p	937.135	1.506	0.389	3.868	0.00011	0.00096
hsa-miR-376c-3p	327.216	1.492	0.402	3.713	0.00020	0.0015
hsa-miR-495-3p	884.797	1.443	0.390	3.696	0.00022	0.0016
hsa-miR-376b-5p	24.828	1.442	0.590	2.445	0.014	0.045

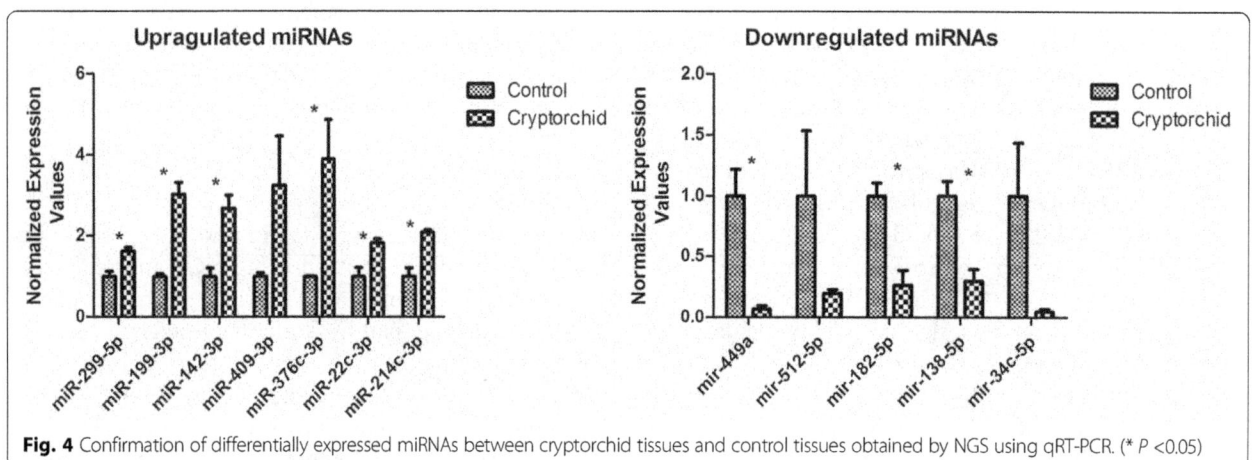

Fig. 4 Confirmation of differentially expressed miRNAs between cryptorchid tissues and control tissues obtained by NGS using qRT-PCR. (* $P < 0.05$)

Table 5 Top 30 most enriched GO terms for predicted targets of differentially expressed miRNAs between cryptorchid and normal tissues

GO number	Term*	GO process	Ratio in study	Ratio in pop	p
GO:0007165	BP	signal transduction	19.68%	23.63%	1.04E-05
GO:0002250	BP	adaptive immune response	0.70%	1.83%	1.56E-05
GO:0050789	BP	regulation of biological process	47.95%	52.34%	4.14E-05
GO:0050794	BP	regulation of cellular process	45.10%	49.34%	7.66E-05
GO:0008150	BP	biological_process	78.42%	81.73%	8.25E-05
GO:0065007	BP	biological regulation	51.05%	55.25%	8.51E-05
GO:0006956	BP	complement activation	0.25%	0.98%	0.000114
GO:0006958	BP	complement activation, classical pathway	0.20%	0.88%	0.000134
GO:0048518	BP	positive regulation of biological process	21.53%	25.03%	0.00014
GO:0050776	BP	regulation of immune response	3.95%	5.72%	0.000229
GO:0044425	CC	membrane part	28.37%	34.86%	1.03E-10
GO:0005886	CC	plasma membrane	17.68%	23.38%	1.11E-10
GO:0031224	CC	intrinsic component of membrane	23.23%	29.30%	2.06E-10
GO:0016021	CC	integral component of membrane	22.68%	28.69%	2.24E-10
GO:0005575	CC	cellular_component	84.22%	88.01%	1.38E-07
GO:0005794	CC	Golgi apparatus	3.35%	5.84%	1.42E-07
GO:0005840	CC	ribosome	2.20%	1.09%	7.38E-06
GO:0000139	CC	Golgi membrane	1.85%	3.41%	1.92E-05
GO:0044459	CC	plasma membrane part	9.84%	12.81%	1.93E-05
GO:0004872	MF	receptor activity	5.39%	8.48%	5.53E-08
GO:0060089	MF	molecular transducer activity	5.39%	8.48%	5.53E-08
GO:0005179	MF	hormone activity	1.55%	0.54%	6.49E-08
GO:0004871	MF	signal transducer activity	5.79%	8.78%	2.25E-07
GO:0038023	MF	signaling receptor activity	4.45%	7.13%	3.21E-07
GO:0099600	MF	transmembrane receptor activity	4.25%	6.85%	4.09E-07
GO:0003823	MF	antigen binding	0.50%	1.75%	4.18E-07
GO:0004888	MF	transmembrane signaling receptor activity	4.15%	6.63%	9.33E-07
GO:0032553	MF	ribonucleotide binding	6.34%	8.94%	1.10E-05
GO:0003674	MF	molecular_function	77.82%	81.17%	7.79E-05

*BP Biological process; CC Cellular component; MF Molecular function

Table 6 KEGG pathway analysis for predicted target genes of differentially expressed miRNAs between cryptorchid and normal tissues

Pathway ID	Description	GeneRatio	BgRatio	p	Adjust p	GeneName
hsa00190	Oxidative phosphorylation	28/664	133/7297	1.80E-05	0.0053	ATP5G2;COX6C;SDHD;COX7A2L; COX8C;ATP6V1D
hsa05012	Parkinson's disease	28/664	142/7297	6.29E-05	0.0093	ATP5G2;COX6C;SDHD;UBB;UBE2L6; COX7A2L;GNAL;COX8C
hsa03010	Ribosome	29/664	154/7297	0.0001112	0.0110	MRPL16;RPL38;RPS4X;MRPL35; RPS6;MRPS18C;RPL26;RPS27L
hsa05016	Huntington's disease	33/664	193/7297	0.0002633	0.0187	ATP5G2;COX6C;UCP1;SDHD; POLR2J3;COX7A2L;COX8C;POLR2K
hsa05010	Alzheimer's disease	30/664	171/7297	0.0003147	0.0187	ATP5G2;COX6C;CASP12;SDHD; PPP3CC;COX7A2L;LPL;COX8C

targets to help these patients recover fertility. However, the comprehensive modulating behaviours of genes remain unclear, therefore determining the target genes and regulatory networks of these differentially-expressed miRNAs is essential in future investigations.

Additional files

Additional file 1: Primers used for the quantification of representative deregulated miRNAs. (XLS 23 kb)

Additional file 2: Length distribution of clean reads from smRNA next-generation deep sequencing. (TIF 2836 kb)

Additional file 3: Number of smRNA sequencing tags that locate on each chromosome. (TIF 3575 kb)

Additional file 4: A collection of all the downregulated known miRNAs detected by deep sequencing in cryptorchid tissues. (XLS 45 kb)

Additional file 5: A collection of all the upregulated known miRNAs detected by deep sequencing in cryptorchid tissues. (XLS 35 kb)

Abbreviations

HE: Hematoxylin-eosin; miRNAs: MicroRNAs; NGS: Next-generation sequencing; NOA: Non-obstructive azoospermia; OA: Obstructive azoospermia; qRT-PCR: Quantitative real-time reverse transcription-polymerase chain reaction

Acknowledgements

We thank all subjects who provided the tissues for this study.

Funding

This study was funded by the the National Natural Science Foundation of China (No. 81370749).

Authors' contributions

DT, XH and XZ designed the study.ZH and HW performed the experiments.LZ and DP analyzed the data.DT and ZH wrote the paper. All authors read and approved the final manuscript.

Competing interests

The authors declare that they have no competing interests.

Author details

[1]Reproductive Medicine Center, Department of Obstetrics and Gynecology, The First Affiliated Hospital of Anhui Medical University, Hefei, Anhui, People's Republic of China. [2]Anhui Province Key Laboratory of Reproductive Health and Genetics, Anhui Medical University, Hefei, Anhui, People's Republic of China. [3]Anhui Provincial Engineering Technology Research Center for Biopreservation and Artificial Organs, Hefei, Anhui, People's Republic of China. [4]Department of Urology, The First Affiliated Hospital of Anhui Medical University, Hefei, Anhui, People's Republic of China.

References

1. Matzuk MM, Lamb DJ. Genetic dissection of mammalian fertility pathways. Nat Cell Biol. 2002;4(Suppl):s41–9.
2. Practice Committee of the American Society for Reproductive Medicine. Diagnostic evaluation of the infertile male: a committee opinion. Fertil Steril. 2015;103:e18–25.
3. Kolon TF, Herndon CD, Baker LA, Baskin LS, Baxter CG, Cheng EY, et al. Evaluation and treatment of cryptorchidism: AUA guideline. J Urol. 2014;192: 337–45.
4. Barthold JS, Gonzalez R. The epidemiology of congenital cryptorchidism, testicular ascent and orchiopexy. J Urol. 2003;170:2396–401.
5. Bao J, Li D, Wang L, Wu J, Hu Y, Wang Z, et al. MicroRNA-449 and microRNA-34b/c function redundantly in murine testes by targeting E2F transcription factor-retinoblastoma protein (E2F-pRb) pathway. J Biol Chem. 2012;287:21686–98.
6. Bouhallier F, Allioli N, Lavial F, Chalmel F, Perrard MH, Durand P, et al. Role of miR-34c microRNA in the late steps of spermatogenesis. RNA. 2010;16: 720–31.
7. Bartel DP. MicroRNAs: genomics, biogenesis, mechanism, and function. Cell. 2004;116:281–97.
8. Tang D, Huang Y, Liu W, Zhang X. Up-regulation of microRNA-210 is associated with spermatogenesis by targeting IGF2 in male infertility. Med Sci Monit. 2016;22:2905–10.
9. Hilz S, Modzelewski AJ, Cohen PE, Grimson A. The roles of microRNAs and siRNAs in mammalian spermatogenesis. Development. 2016;143:3061–73.
10. Lian J, Zhang X, Tian H, Liang N, Wang Y, Liang C, et al. Altered microRNA expression in patients with non-obstructive azoospermia. Reprod Biol Endocrinol. 2009;7:13.
11. Comazzetto S, Di Giacomo M, Rasmussen KD, Much C, Azzi C, Perlas E, et al. Oligoasthenoteratozoospermia and infertility in mice deficient for miR-34b/c and miR-449 loci. PLoS Genet. 2014;10:e1004597.
12. Duan Z, Huang H, Sun F. The functional and predictive roles of miR-210 in cryptorchidism. Sci Rep. 2016;6:32265.
13. Moritoki Y, Hayashi Y, Mizuno K, Kamisawa H, Nishio H, Kurokawa S, et al. Expression profiling of microRNA in cryptorchid testes: miR-135a contributes to the maintenance of spermatogonial stem cells by regulating FoxO1. J Urol. 2014;191:1174–80.
14. Ensembl database. http://asia.ensembl.org/index.html. Accessed 28 Sept 2017.
15. MiRDeep2 http://www.mdc-berlin.de/8551903/en/research/research_teams/ systems_biology_of_gene_regulatory_elements/projects/miRDeep. Accessed 29 Sept 2017.
16. Zhang L, Wei P, Shen X, Zhang Y, Xu B, Zhou J, et al. MicroRNA expression profile in penile Cancer revealed by next-generation small RNA sequencing. PLoS One. 2015;10:e0131336.
17. TargetScan. http://www.targetscan.org/vert_71. Accessed 2 Oct 2017.
18. John B, Enright AJ, Aravin A, Tuschl T, Sander C, Marks DS. Human MicroRNA targets. PLoS Biol. 2004;2:e363.
19. Zhou Y, Wang X, Zhang Y, Zhao T, Shan Z, Teng W. Circulating microrna profile as a potential predictive biomarker for early diagnosis of spontaneous abortion in patients with subclinical hypothyroidism. Front Endocrinol (Lausanne). 2018;9:128.
20. Agoulnik AI, Huang Z, Ferguson L. Spermatogenesis in cryptorchidism. Methods Mol Biol. 2012;825:127–47.
21. Taran I, Elder JS. Results of orchiopexy for the undescended testis. World J Urol. 2006;24:231–9.
22. Hadziselimovic F, Thommen L, Girard J, Herzog B. The significance of postnatal gonadotropin surge for testicular development in normal and cryptorchid testes. J Urol. 1986;136:274–6.
23. Yin Y, DeWolf WC, Morgentaler A. Experimental cryptorchidism induces testicular germ cell apoptosis by p53-dependent and -independent pathways in mice. Biol Reprod. 1998;58:492–6.
24. Yin Y, Stahl BC, DeWolf WC, Morgentaler A. P53 and Fas are sequential mechanisms of testicular germ cell apoptosis. J Androl. 2002;23:64–70.
25. Mu X, Liu Y, Collins LL, Kim E, Chang C. The p53/retinoblastoma-mediated repression of testicular orphan receptor-2 in the rhesus monkey with cryptorchidism. J Biol Chem. 2000;275:23877–83.
26. Li W, Bao W, Ma J, Liu X, Xu R, Wang RA, et al. Metastasis tumor antigen 1 is involved in the resistance to heat stress-induced testicular apoptosis. FEBS Lett. 2008;582:869–73.

## 8

Effects of Levonorgestrel and progesterone on Oviductal physiology in mammals

Cheng Li[1,2,3†], Hui-Yu Zhang[1†], Yan Liang[1], Wei Xia[1], Qian Zhu[1], Duo Zhang[1], Zhen Huang[1,2], Gui-Lin Liang[1], Rui-Hong Xue[2,3], Hang Qi[1], Xiao-Qing He[1], Jiang-Jing Yuan[1], Ya-Jing Tan[2,3], He-Feng Huang[2,3*] and Jian Zhang[1,2*] (ID)

Abstract

Background: Our previous study indicated that emergency contraception, including levonorgestrel and progesterone, could lead to ectopic pregnancy following contraception failure. However, our understanding of the effects of levonorgestrel and progesterone on oviductal physiology is limited.

Methods: The receptivity of the fallopian tubal epithelium after levonorgestrel and progesterone treatment was examined through western blots for receptivity markers and JAr-spheroid-fallopian tubal epithelial cell attachment assays. The ciliary beat frequency was analyzed using an inverted bright-field microscope. Furthermore, an in vivo animal model of embryo-tubal transplantation was also studied to determine the effects of levonorgestrel- and progesterone-induced ciliary beat reduction.

Results: Our results showed that levonorgestrel and progesterone did not change the levels of fallopian tubal epithelial cell receptive markers, including LIF, STAT3, IGFBP1, ITGB3, MUC1, and ACVR1B, or affect JAr-spheroid implantation. However, levonorgestrel and progesterone reduced the ciliary beat frequency in fallopian tubes in a dose-dependent manner. An in vivo model also showed that levonorgestrel and progesterone could lead to embryo retention in the oviducts.

Conclusions: These findings show that levonorgestrel and progesterone can reduce the ciliary beat frequency without altering receptivity, indicating a possible mechanism for progesterone- or levonorgestrel-induced tubal pregnancy.

Keywords: Progesterone, Levonorgestrel, Oviduct, Receptivity, Ciliary beat frequency

Background

Progesterone (P4) plays a crucial role in the regulation of female reproductive physiology [1]. It has been reported that a high level of P4 can interrupt follicular development and thus delay or inhibit ovulation [2]. For this reason, progesterone and its synthetic analogue, levonorgestrel (LNG), are used as contraceptive methods by women of reproductive age.

Levonorgestrel-only pills for emergency contraception (LNG-EC) are available in an over-the-counter form in many countries and can prevent unwanted pregnancies with an efficacy of 52–94% when used within 120 h of unprotected intercourse [3]. Similar to other contraceptive methods, LNG-EC reduces the chance of pregnancy, including both intrauterine pregnancy and occasional ectopic pregnancy (EP); however, cases of EP following LNG-EC failure have been reported in various countries [4, 5]. To confirm the association between EP and LNG-EC, we previously conducted a multi-center case-control study and found that the risk of EP after LNG contraceptive failure was approximately 5-fold higher than that of intrauterine pregnancy [6].

Tubal inflammation, which is typically secondary to genital infection, was generally regarded an important

* Correspondence: Huanghefg@sjtu.edu.cn; zhangjian_ipmch@sjtu.edu.cn
†Cheng Li and Hui-Yu Zhang contributed equally to this work.
²Institute of Embryo-Fetal Original Adult Disease Affiliated to Shanghai Jiao Tong University School of Medicine, Shanghai Jiao Tong University, Shanghai, China
¹Department of Gynecology, International Peace Maternity and Child Health Hospital, School of Medicine, Shanghai Jiao Tong University, Shanghai, China
Full list of author information is available at the end of the article

risk factor for EP, but we previously confirmed that tubal pregnancy following LNG-EC failure is associated with lower rates of Chlamydia trachomatis infection, fallopian tubal inflammation, and/or fibrosis compared with general tubal pregnancy [7]. Thus, we hypothesize that LNG, combined with a high progesterone level, might influence fallopian tube physiology rather than tubal morphology or salpingitis.

The transport of embryos in the fallopian tubes is believed to be facilitated through the fallopian tube physiology, which involves ciliary activity and muscular contractions. Previous studies have reported that progesterone can suppress the epithelial ciliary beat frequency in human fallopian tubes by 40–50% [8]. In addition, the administration of progesterone also decreases the contractions of the longitudinal muscular layer of human fallopian tubes compared with the baseline value [9]. Although previous studies have investigated the physiological effects of progesterone on tubal ciliary beats and smooth muscle contractions [8, 9], the effects of the super-physiological P4 levels induced by LNG-EC remain unclear. Although LNG-EC is a synthetic analogue of progesterone, its structure and pharmacological properties, including its effective dose, metabolism, pharmacokinetics, bioavailability and binding to serum binding proteins, differs from those of progesterone. Furthermore, there is no reliable information regarding the influence of LNG on fallopian tubal receptivity, embryo-tubal transportation or implantation. For these reasons, we explored whether LNG, combined with a super-physiological progesterone level, would affect oviduct function, which is involved in the occurrence of EP.

Methods
Collection and incubation of human fallopian tubes
After obtaining written consent and approval from the local ethical committee, we collected samples of fallopian tubes at the mid-luteal phase from patients undergoing hysterectomies for benign conditions (uterine leiomyoma). All patients had regular menstrual cycles and had not used any hormonal medication within 3 months. The collected tissues were rinsed several times to remove all visible blood, and the muscularis and serosa were then removed. Pieces of tissue (1–2 mm^2) were dissected from the ampulla portions of the fallopian tubes and treated with different doses of LNG (Sigma-Aldrich, St Louis, MO, USA) and P4 (Sigma-Aldrich, St Louis, MO, USA) for 24 h in an incubator at 37 °C.

Cell culture
A human fallopian tubal epithelial cell line (OE-E6/E7) was obtained from Dr. Kai-Fai Lee, University of Hong Kong. The OE-E6/E7 cell line is an immortalized human fallopian tubal epithelium cell line established by the University of Hong Kong, and these cells are characterized by human oviduct-specific glycoproteins, estrogen receptors, and cytokeratin [10]. The OE-E6/E7 cells were cultured at 37 °C in DMEM/F12 culture media (Invitrogen, Paisley, UK) supplemented with 1% penicillin and streptomycin (Invitrogen), 10% fetal bovine serum (Invitrogen) and L-glutamine (Invitrogen) in a 5% CO_2 atmosphere.

JAr spheroid-fallopian tubal epithelial cell attachment assays
JAr cells (JAr, HTB-144, ATCC, Manassas, VA, USA) are a trophoblastic tumor cell line of placental origin that express the placental hormone and differentiate into syncytiotrophoblasts. We used multicellular spheroids of human choriocarcinoma JAr cells as an in vitro attachment model as previously described [11]. We treated OE-E6/E7 cells at 40–50% confluency with 10 nmol/L 17β-estradiol (Sigma-Aldrich, St Louis, MO, USA) and 1 nmol/L P4 (Sigma-Aldrich, St Louis, MO, USA) to mimic the hormonal environment under normal physiological conditions. The cells were treated with LNG and P4 at various concentrations until full confluency was reached. At 80–90% confluency, the OE-E6/E7 cells were treated with various concentrations of LNG and P4 for 24 h, and JAr spheroids were transferred onto the surface of a confluent monolayer of OE-E6/E7 cells. The cultures were maintained in the culture medium for 6 h. Non-adherent spheroids were removed by centrifugation of the cell culture plates with the cell surface facing down at 15 g for 10 min. We counted the attached spheroids under a light microscope, and the results are expressed as percentages of the total number of seeded spheroids (% adhesion).

Measurement of the ciliary beat frequency
The ciliary beat frequency (CBF) was measured at 37 °C under an inverted bright-field microscope (Nikon TE2000, Nikon Instruments, Inc., Melville, NY, USA). Video sequences of the moving cilia were acquired with a 12-bit high-speed camera (Prosilica EC1020, Prosilica Inc., Burnaby, Canada) at a rate of 30 frames per s for 10 s. The CBF was calculated using ciliaFA software, a plugin for ImageJ (software version 1.49 t; NIH, USA) that extracts pixel intensities and performs fast Fourier transformation using Microsoft Excel (2016 professional edition; Microsoft Corporation, WA, USA) [12].

Quantitative real time-PCR (qRT-PCR) analyses
The total RNA from scraped cells was extracted using the RNAiso reagent (TAKARA, Dalian, China) and then reverse-transcribed according the manufacturer's instructions (TAKARA, Dalian, China). qRT-PCR was performed with a QuantStudio™ 7 flex system (Applied Biosystems,

Table 1 Primer sequences of PCR

Gene	Forward primer	Reverse primer
18 s	GTAACCCGTTGAACCCCATT	CCATCCAATCGGTAGTAGCG
STAT3	CAGTGACAGCTTCCCAATGG	ACTGCTGGTCAATCTCTCCC
IGFBP1	TGATGGCCCCTTCTGAAGAG	TCTCCTGTGCCTTGGCTAAA
ITGB3	TGACGAAAATACCTGCAACCG	GCATCCTTGCCAGTGTCCTTAA
MUC1	GAAAGAACTACGGGCAGCTG	GCCACCATTACCTGCAGAAA
LIF	TGAACCAGATCAGGAGCCAA	GACTATGCGGTACAGCTCCA
ACVR1B	AAAGACAAGACGCTCCAGGA	ATACTTCCCCAAACCGACCC

Foster City, CA, USA) using the primer sequences listed in Table 1. The threshold cycles were determined, and relative gene expression levels were calculated using the $2^{-\Delta\Delta CT}$ method with glyceraldehyde-3-phosphate dehydrogenase as the endogenous control.

Western blotting
OE-E6/E7 cells were lysed in RIPA buffer supplemented with a protease inhibitor cocktail (Millipore, Darmstadt, Germany). Protein loading was normalized using the total protein concentrations determined through Bradford assays. Samples (30 μg/lane) were separated on a 12% sodium dodecyl sulfate-polyacrylamide gel and transferred onto Protran Immun-Blot nitrocellulose transfer membranes (Schleicher & Schuell Bioscience GmbH, Dassel, Germany). Antibodies against β-actin (1:5000, Proteintech, IL, USA), IGFBP1 (1:1000, Proteintech, IL, USA), ITGB3 (1:1000, Proteintech, IL, USA), MUC1 (1:1000, Proteintech, IL, USA), ACVR1B (1:1000, Proteintech, IL, USA) and STAT3 (1:1000, Cell Signaling Technology, Danvers, MA, USA) were used as primary antibodies, and horseradish peroxidase-conjugated goat anti-rabbit IgG (1:5000, Cell Signaling Technology, Danvers, MA, USA) and goat anti-mouse IgG (1:5000, Cell Signaling Technology, Danvers, MA, USA) were used as secondary antibodies. Specific signals were visualized by the enhanced chemiluminescence method as previously described [13].

Animal experiments and embryo-tube transportation assays
Eight-week-old C57BL/6 J mice were used in this study (Shanghai Research Center for Model Organisms). All animal experiments were approved by the Medical Ethics Committee of Shanghai Research Center for Model Organisms. The mice were housed in a room at 25 °C with a 12-h light:12-hdark cycle and 50–60% humidity and were given a standard diet (containing 10% fat) and water. Female mice (6–8 weeks of age) were mated randomly, and vaginal plug-positive mice were immediately injected intraperitoneally with saline, LNG (8 mg/kg), or P4 (8 mg/kg). Twelve hours after observation of the vaginal plug,

the mice were sacrificed via cervical dislocation to measure the CBF. Embryo-tube transportation assays were conducted as described by Ning et al. [14]. Seventy-four hours after observation of the vaginal plug, the oviducts and uterus were ligated. The embryos were flushed from the oviducts or uteri with PBS. We counted the embryos remaining in the oviducts, and the results are expressed as percentages of the total number of embryos.

Statistical analysis
All the results are expressed as the means ± standard deviation. To determine the statistical significance of the differences among the treatments, one-way analysis of variance and Tukey-Kramer multiple comparisons tests were performed to compare the relative efficacy of each treatment (PRISM software version 6.0; GraphPad). A probability of $p < 0.05$ was considered to indicate a significant difference.

Results
Effect of LNG on fallopian tube epithelium receptivity
To determine whether LNG affects the receptivity of the fallopian tubal epithelium, we subjected the tubal epithelial cell line OE-E6/E7 to different doses of LNG and P4 and detected the expression of various receptive markers, including LIF, STAT3, IGFBP1, ITGB3, MUC1, and ACVR1B, through qRT-PCR and western blot analyses. However, the expression of these receptive markers did not show any significant changes following the administration of LNG or P4, regardless of the dose (Fig. 1). Furthermore, we performed JAr spheroid-fallopian tubal epithelial cell attachment assays. Spheroids of approximately 60–150 μm were produced from JAr cells and allowed to attach to a monolayer of OE-E6/E7 cells (Fig. 2a) that had been previously treated with different doses of LNG and P4, and the percentages of attached JAr spheroids did not show any significant differences among the groups (Fig. 2c-d).

Effect of different concentrations of LNG on the CBF
To determine whether LNG, together with altered P4 levels, had a dose-dependent effect on the tubal CBF, we cultured tubal epithelial explants with LNG and P4 at doses ranging from 10^{-8} to 10^{-5} mol/L. The CBF decreased with increases in the LNG concentration (Fig. 3a-b). The CBF of the explants incubated with LNG at a concentration of 10^{-6} mol/L (6.92 ± 0.36 Hz) and 10^{-5} mol/L (6.89 ± 0.30 Hz) was decreased significantly compared with that of explants in the control medium (8.23 ± 0.32 Hz). Similar results were obtained with the P4 treatments. Treatment with P4 at 10^{-6} mol/L and 10^{-5} mol/L decreased the CBF to 6.89 ± 0.38 Hz and 6.69 ± 0.33 Hz, respectively, from 8.26 ± 0.32 Hz, which was

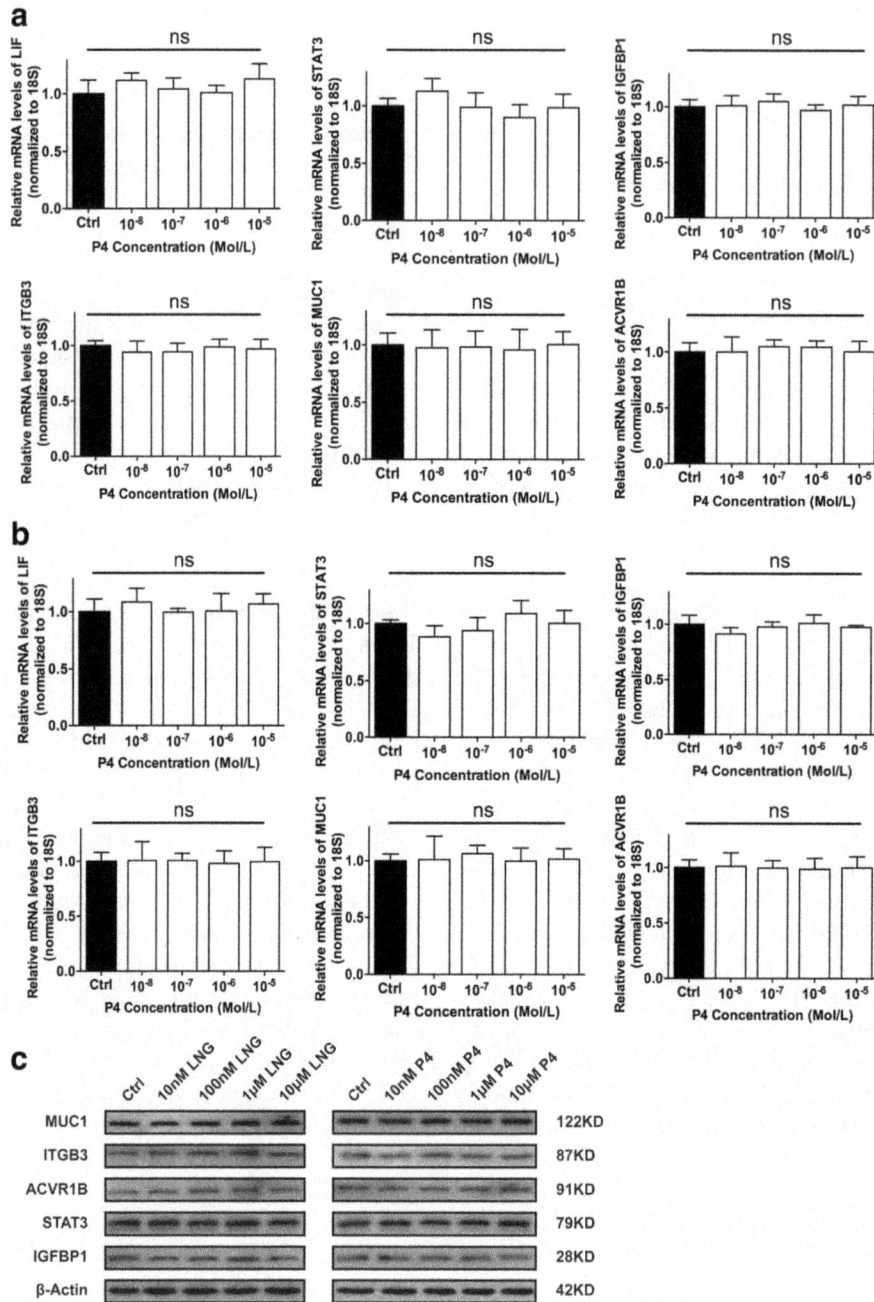

Fig. 1 Effects of different concentrations of LNG and P4 on the expression of receptivity markers in the fallopian tubes. **a-b** mRNA expression levels of LIF, STAT3, IGFBP1, ITGB3, MUC1, and ACVR1B in OE-E6/E7 cells following treatment with different concentrations of LNG and P4 ($n = 3$ in each group; ns, not significant); **c** protein expression levels of MUC1, ITGB3, ACVR1B, STAT3, and IGFBP1 in OE-E6/E7 cells following treatment with different concentrations of LNG and P4

the value obtained for the explants in the control medium (Fig. 3c-d).

To further confirm these findings in vivo, we analyzed the CBF of C57BL6/J mice after an intraperitoneal injection of saline, LNG (8 mg/kg), or P4 (8 mg/kg). The in vivo CBF of mice was significantly decreased after treatment with LNG (9.39 ± 0.45 Hz vs. 11.69 ± 0.60 Hz, $p = 0.012$) or P4 (8.80 ± 0.56 Hz vs. 11.69 ± 0.60 Hz, $p = 0.006$) compared with that of the saline-treated control mice (Fig. 4).

Effect of LNG on embryo-tube transportation in mice

Because the ciliary beat in the fallopian tubes plays a critical role in embryo transport, we further observed

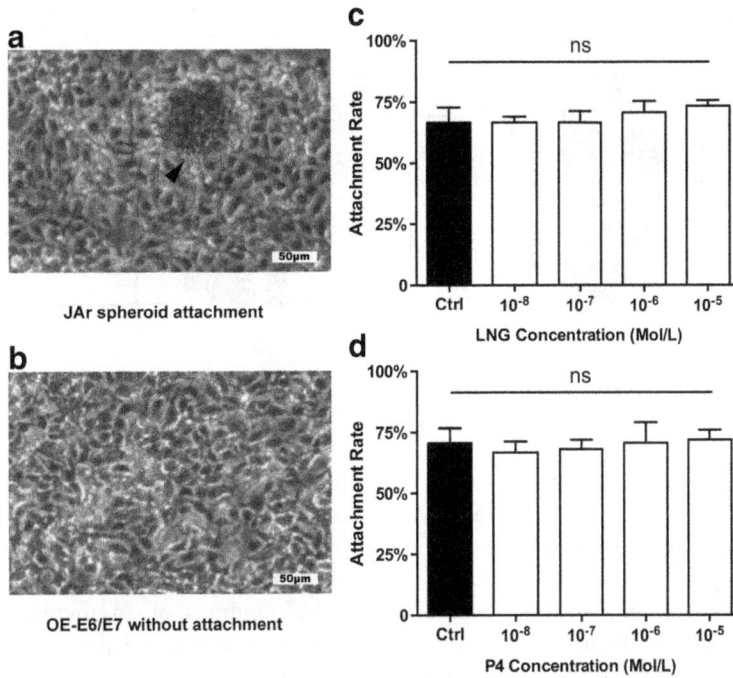

Fig. 2 Effects of different concentrations of LNG and P4 on JAr spheroid- fallopian tubal attachment rates. **a** JAr spheroids were selected (arrow) and attached to OE-E6/E7 monolayers; **b** OE-E6/E7 monolayer without attached JAr spheroids; **c-d** rates of the attachment of JAr spheroids to OE-E6/E7 cells treated with different concentrations of LNG and P4 ($n = 3$ in each group; ns, not significant)

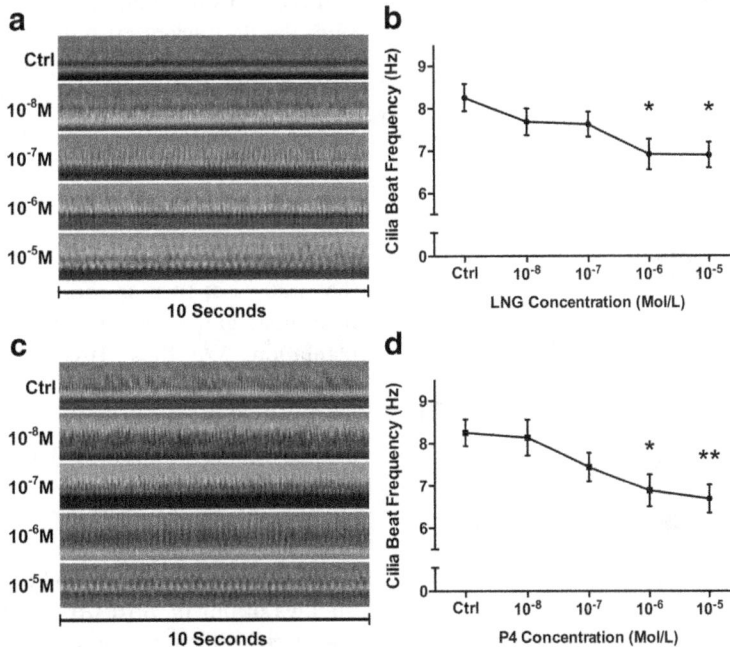

Fig. 3 Effects of different concentrations of LNG and P4 on the tubal CBF in vitro. **a** Orthographic views of the ciliary beat frequency following treatment with different concentrations of LNG (one ciliary beat represents one shift from bright to dark on the timeline); **b** LNG decreased the CBF in vitro in a dose-dependent manner ($n = 8$ in each group; *, $p < 0.05$); **c** orthographic views of the ciliary beat frequency following treatment with different concentrations of P4; **d** P4 decreased the CBF in vitro in a dose-dependent manner ($n = 8$ in each group; *, $p < 0.05$; **, $p < 0.01$)

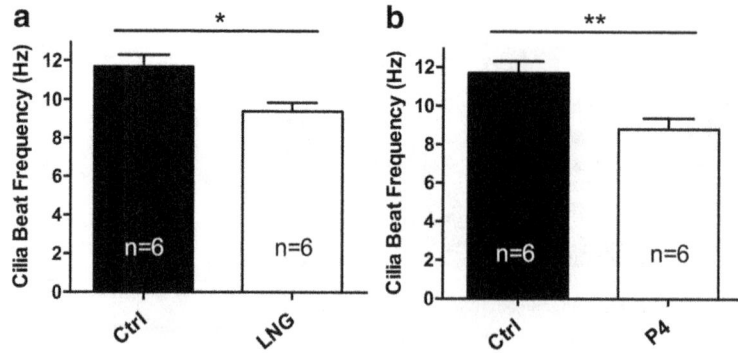

Fig. 4 Effects of LNG and P4 on the tubal CBF in mice. **a** LNG decreased the tubal CBF in mice ($n = 6$ in each group; 9.39 ± 0.45 Hz vs. 11.69 ± 0.60 Hz, $p = 0.012$); **b** P4 decreased the tubal CBF in mice ($n = 6$ in each group; 8.80 ± 0.56 Hz vs. 11.69 ± 0.60 Hz, $p = 0.006$)

the effects of LNG and the super-physiological level of P4 on embryo transport through the fallopian tube. We counted the percentages of embryos retained in the fallopian tubes in each group and found that all the mice in the LNG group experienced embryo-tube retention, with an average percentage of embryo retention of 18.27%, whereas none of the mice in the saline-treated group experienced embryo-tube retention (Fig. 5a). Consistently, the same effect was also observed in the P4 group, which had an average percentage of embryo retention of 15.37%, compared with the control group, which had an average percentage of 0% (Fig. 5b).

Discussion

Our findings show that LNG had no effect on fallopian tubal receptivity but revealed a dose-dependent effect on

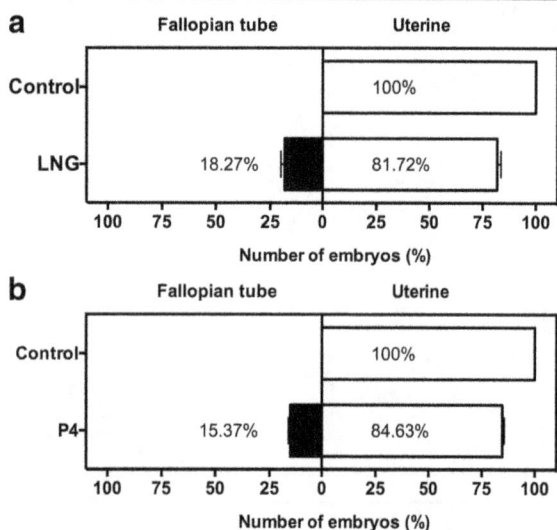

Fig. 5 Effects of LNG and P4 on embryo-tubal transportation in mice. **a** An embryo recovery of 18.27% was obtained from the oviducts following the administration of LNG ($n = 5$ in each group); **b** 15.37% of embryos were recovered from the oviducts following the administration of P4 ($n = 5$ in each group)

ciliary motility: increases in the concentration of LNG resulted in decreases in the tubal ciliary beat frequency, which ultimately led to embryo retention in the fallopian tubes of mice. This phenomenon might account for the clinical findings of an increased risk of EP following LNG contraceptive failure observed in our previous study [6].

With regard to the mechanism of EP, it is believed that an altered tubal environment and impaired embryo-tubal transportation allow implantation of an embryo in the fallopian tube [15]. Thus, we further explored the effects of LNG, together with a super-physiological P4 level, on both of these physiological functions.

Successful implantation requires a receptive endometrium that is appropriately primed with estrogen and progesterone. In an EP, alterations to the fallopian tubal receptivity might be a response to the sequence of factors or cytokines that alter various physiological functions, including the promotion of embryo implantation [15]. However, no previous studies have that indicated whether LNG, together with a super-physiological P4 level, can change the secretion of implantation factors that induce apposition, adhesion and invasion in fallopian tubal epithelium cells to promote embryo-tubal implantation. We thus detected the expression of LIF, MUC1, ITGB3, ACVR1B, STAT3, and IGFBP1, which are known implantation factors, in the human fallopian tubal cell line OE-E6/E7 after treatment with different does of LNG and P4. The results suggest that LNG and P4 have no effects on the receptivity of fallopian tubal cells by stimulating secretion or altering the expression levels of receptive factors. The results also confirm the findings of our in vitro JAr spheroid-fallopian tubal epithelial cell attachment assays, which showed that LNG, together with a super-physiological P4 level, do not affect fallopian tubal receptivity. However, an in vivo model for tubal pregnancy in rodents has not been established because the abdominal cavity is the most frequent extra-uterine implantation site and only a few cases of tubal pregnancy in primates have been reported to date [16]. Therefore, the in vivo evaluation of tubal implantation is difficult.

Embryo transport through the fallopian tube is managed mainly by the ciliary beat frequency and muscular contractions. Almost 80% of EPs occur in the ampulla, which is characterized by a thin smooth muscle layer and long longitudinal mucosal folds with a high percentage of ciliated cells in the epithelium. However, the isthmus has a thick smooth muscle layer and only one-fourth the number of ciliated cells found in the ampulla [17]. Halbert et al. confirmed that the rate of ovum transport remains unchanged after smooth muscle activity is blocked with isoproterenol, which indicated that ciliary motility was capable of transporting embryos in the absence of muscle contraction [18]. Thus, this study focused on the effect of LNG on the tubal CBF and showed that LNG and P4 decreased the tubal CBF in a dose-dependent manner. Furthermore, our in vivo experiment revealed embryo retention in the fallopian tubes of mice following LNG and P4 administration. However, LNG cannot prevent pregnancies if it is taken after the luteinizing hormone level has begun to increase and ovulation has occurred [2]. At this point, the fertilized ovum would be transported slowly due to the LNG-induced decrease in the CBF. This slow transport will increase the risk of tubal implantation, as reported in our previous study [6]. Because of these findings, we believe that high levels of LNG or P4 decrease the tubal CBF and might contribute to the occurrence of tubal pregnancy following LNG-EC failure.

In addition to the clinical findings of a correlation between EP and contraceptive doses of LNG, the association between high levels of P4 and EP might also provide insight into the reason for the increased EP rates found among women using assisted reproductive technology. Our previous epidemiology study revealed that the risk of EP is significantly increased among women who underwent assisted reproductive technology treatment [19]. Several studies have also indicated that the risk of EP is closely related to fresh embryo transfer [20] and controlled ovarian stimulation (COH) [21]. Notably, transferred embryos are more likely to move from their original transfer position to the fallopian tubes due to the cervix-to-fundus direction of uterine peristalsis following COH [22, 23]. Moreover, the supraphysiological hormone levels induced by COH, particularly elevated P4 levels, might reduce ciliary motility and lead to subsequent embryo retention in the fallopian tube. This finding could also help explain the lower rate of EP in embryo transfer cycles without ovarian hyperstimulation, such as frozen embryo transfer, compared with that observed with fresh embryo transfer. Extension of the clinical implications of the present findings indicates that an increased P4 level in the tubal-uterine environment contributes to ectopic implantation after embryo transfer.

Conclusion
In summary, our data show that LNG, combined with a super-physiological level of progesterone, can decrease the tubal ciliary beat frequency and thus lead to embryo retention in the fallopian tube without changing tubal receptivity. A better understanding of the role of LNG in modulating the physiology of the human fallopian tube might help delineate the underlying mechanism leading to tubal pregnancies and better prevent tubal pregnancies in the future.

Abbreviations
ACVR1B: Activin A receptor type 1B; CBF: Ciliary beat frequency; IGFBP1: Insulin-like growth factor binding protein 1; ITGB3: Integrin subunit beta 3; LIF: Leukemia inhibitory factor; LNG: Levonorgestrel; LNG-EC: Levonorgestrel emergency contraception; MUC1: Mucin 1; P4: Progesterone; qRT-PCR: Quantitative real-time polymerase chain reaction; STAT3: Signal transducer and activator of transcription 3

Funding
This study was supported by the National Natural Science Foundation of China [grant numbers 81671482 and 31401226].

Authors' contributions
HFH and JZ conceived the study, participated in its design, supervised the study and critically revised the manuscript. CL and HYZ were responsible for the animal study and for writing the manuscript. YL critically revised the manuscript. WX and QZ participated in the cell culture experiments. ZH, GLL, RHX, HQ, and XQH participated in the sample collection and in the writing and revision of the manuscript. JJY and YJT contributed to the statistical analysis. All the authors substantially contributed to the revision of the manuscript. All authors read and approved the final manuscript.

Competing interests
The authors declare that they have no competing interests.

Author details
[1]Department of Gynecology, International Peace Maternity and Child Health Hospital, School of Medicine, Shanghai Jiao Tong University, Shanghai, China. [2]Institute of Embryo-Fetal Original Adult Disease Affiliated to Shanghai Jiao Tong University School of Medicine, Shanghai Jiao Tong University, Shanghai, China. [3]Center of Reproductive Medicine, International Peace Maternity and Child Health Hospital, School of Medicine, Shanghai Jiao Tong University, No. 910, Hengshan Rd, Shanghai 200030, China.

References
1. Graham JD, Clarke CL. Physiological action of progesterone in target tissues. Endocr Rev. 1997;18(4):502–19.
2. Gemzell-Danielsson K. Mechanism of action of emergency contraception. Contraception. 2010;82(5):404–9.
3. von Hertzen H, Piaggio G, Ding J, et al. Low dose mifepristone and two regimens of levonorgestrel for emergency contraception: a WHO

multicentre randomised trial. Lancet. 2002;360(9348):1803–10.

4. Ghosh B, Dadhwal V, Deka D, Ramesan CK, Mittal S. Ectopic pregnancy following levonorgestrel emergency contraception: a case report. Contraception. 2009;79(2):155–7.

5. Kozinszky Z, Bakken RT, Lieng M. Ectopic pregnancy after levonorgestrel emergency contraception. Contraception. 2011;83(3):281–3.

6. Zhang J, Li C, Zhao WH, et al. Association between levonorgestrel emergency contraception and the risk of ectopic pregnancy: a multicenter case-control study. Sci Rep. 2015;5:8487.

7. Li C, Meng CX, Sun LL, et al. Reduced prevalence of chronic tubal inflammation in tubal pregnancies after levonorgestrel emergency contraception failure. Pharmacoepidemiol Drug Saf. 2015;24(5):548–54.

8. Mahmood T, Saridogan E, Smutna S, Habib AM, Djahanbakhch O. The effect of ovarian steroids on epithelial ciliary beat frequency in the humaallopian tube. Hum Reprod. 1998;13(11):2991–4.

9. Wanggren K, Stavreus-Evers A, Olsson C, Andersson E, Gemzell-Danielsson K. Regulation of muscular contractions in the human fallopian tube through prostaglandins and progestagens. Hum Reprod. 2008;23(10):2359–68.

10. Lee YL, Lee KF, Xu JS, Wang YL, Tsao SW, Yeung WS. Establishment and characterization of an immortalized human oviductal cell line. Mol Reprod Dev. 2001;59(4):400–9.

11. Kodithuwakku SP, Pang RT, Ng EH, et al. Wnt activation downregulates olfactomedin-1 in fallopian tubal epithelial cells: a microenvironment predisposed to tubal ectopic pregnancy. Lab Investig. 2012;92(2):256–64.

12. Smith CM, Djakow J, Free RC, et al. ciliaFA: a research tool for automated, high-throughput measurement of ciliary beat frequency using freely available software. Cilia. 2012;1:14.

13. Liu XM, Ding GL, Jiang Y, et al. Down-regulation of S100A11, a calcium-binding protein, in human endometrium may cause reproductive failure. J Clin Endocrinol Metab. 2012;97(10):3672–83.

14. Ning N, Zhu J, Du Y, Gao X, Liu C, Li J. Dysregulation of hydrogen sulphide metabolism impairs oviductal transport of embryos. Nat Commun. 2014; 5:4107.

15. Shaw JL, Dey SK, Critchley HO, Horne AW. Current knowledge of the aetiology of human tubal ectopic pregnancy. Hum Reprod Update. 2010; 16(4):432–44.

16. Corpa JM. Ectopic pregnancy in animals and humans. Reproduction. 2006; 131(4):631–40.

17. Noreikat K, Wolff M, Kummer W, Kolle S. Ciliary activity in the oviduct of cycling, pregnant, and muscarinic receptor knockout mice. Biol Reprod. 2012;86(4):120.

18. Halbert SA, Becker DR, Szal SE. Ovum transport in the rat oviductal ampulla in the absence of muscle contractility. Biol Reprod. 1989;40(6):1131–6.

19. Li C, Zhao WH, Zhu Q, et al. Risk factors for ectopic pregnancy: a multi-center case-control study. BMC Pregnancy Childbirth. 2015;15:187.

20. Shapiro BS, Daneshmand ST, De Leon L, Garner FC, Aguirre M, Hudson C. Frozen-thawed embryo transfer is associated with a significantly reduced incidence of ectopic pregnancy. Fertil Steril. 2012;98(6):1490–4.

21. Weiss A, Beck-Fruchter R, Golan J, Lavee M, Geslevich Y, Shalev E. Ectopic pregnancy risk factors for ART patients undergoing the GnRH antagonist protocol: a retrospective study. Reprod Biol Endocrinol. 2016;14:12.

22. Rombauts L, McMaster R, Motteram C, Fernando S. Risk of ectopic pregnancy is linked to endometrial thickness in a retrospective cohort study of 8120 assisted reproduction technology cycles. Hum Reprod. 2015;30(12): 2846–52.

23. van Gestel I, Ijland MM, Hoogland HJ, Evers JL. Endometrial waves in in vitro fertilization cycles: a validation study. Fertil Steril. 2005;83(2):491–3.

## 9

Using appropriate pre-pregnancy body mass index cut points for obesity in the Chinese population

Yanxin Wu, Wai-Kit Ming, Dongyu Wang, Haitian Chen, Zhuyu Li and Zilian Wang[*] ⓘ

Abstract

Background: Appropriate classification of obesity is vital for risk assessment and complication prevention during pregnancy. We aimed to explore which pre-pregnancy BMI cut-offs of obesity, either BMI ≥ 25 kg/m^2 as recommended by the WHO for Asians or BMI ≥ 28 kg/m^2 as suggested by the Working Group on Obesity in China (WGOC), best predicts the risk of adverse maternal and perinatal outcomes.

Methods: We retrospectively reviewed 11,494 medical records for live singleton deliveries in a tertiary center in Guangzhou, China, between January 2013 and December 2016. The primary outcomes included maternal obesity prevalence, adverse maternal and perinatal outcomes. Data were analyzed using the Chi-square test, logistic regression, and diagnostics tests.

Results: Among the study population, 824 (7.2%) were obese according to the WHO criteria for Asian populations, and this would be reduced to 198 (1.7%) based on the criteria of WGOC. Obesity-related adverse maternal and perinatal outcomes were gestational diabetes mellitus, preeclampsia, cesarean section, and large for gestational age ($P < 0.05$). Compared to the WGOC criterion, the WHO for Asians criterion had a higher Youden index in our assessment of its predictive value in identifying risk of obesity-related adverse outcomes for Chinese pregnant women. Women in the BMI range of 25 to 28 kg/m^2 are at high risks for adverse maternal and perinatal outcomes, which were similar to women with BMI ≥ 28 kg/m^2.

Conclusions: A lower pre-pregnancy BMI cutoff at 25 kg/m^2 for defining obesity may be appropriate for pregnant women in South China. If WGOC standards are applied to pregnant Chinese populations, a significant proportion of at-risk patients may be missed.

Keywords: Obesity, Pregnancy, Body mass index, Outcome

Background

The prevalence of obesity is on the rise throughout China and the rest of the world in recent decades, including women of childbearing age [1, 2]. Greater adiposity in pregnancy is associated with increased risk of gestational diabetes, hypertensive disorders of pregnancy, higher birth weight, preterm delivery, large for gestational age, and cesarean section (C/S) [3–6]. Therefore, to ensure these women can receive medical advice and closer monitoring, many national and international antenatal guidelines recommend an early diagnosis of overweight and obesity in women of childbearing age [7, 8].

According to the World Health Organization (WHO), the cut-offs of BMI for defining overweight and obesity for Caucasian populations are 25 and 30 kg/m^2 [9]. Previous studies have shown that the Chinese, as well as other Asian populations, have a lower BMI but a higher percentage of body fat than Caucasians of similar age and gender [10, 11]. As such, the BMI criterion for Asian populations should be lowered so as to better suit the characteristics of this racial group. For Asian populations, the expert

* Correspondence: wangzilian2016@aliyun.com
Department of Obstetrics and Gynecology, The First Affiliated Hospital of Sun Yat-sen University, No. 58 Zhongshan Road 2, Guangzhou 510000, P. R. China

group of the WHO defines BMIs of 23.0–24.9 kg/m^2 as overweight and ≥ 25.0 kg/m^2 as obesity [12]. This expert group has labeled these recommendations as temporary and stated that these need to be further validated by additional epidemiological research, owing to limited information available about Asian populations [13]. BMI cut-off points of 24.1–27.9 kg/m^2 for overweight and ≥ 28.0 kg/m^2 for obesity have been proposed by the Working Group on Obesity in China (WGOC) and the International Life Sciences Institute Focal Point in China [14, 15]. The proposal was primarily based on a large, national population (20- to 70-years-old), cross-sectional study of anthropometric indices and cardiovascular risk factors. Optimal classification of obesity is vital for risk assessment and weight management, for both the individual and health professionals. However, it is unclear whether these recommendations can also adequately reflect the risk of adverse maternal and perinatal outcomes among pregnant women.

The objective of this study was to investigate the application of obesity criterion of BMI recommended by the WHO for Asians and WGOC in pregnant Chinese women to identify which recommendation best identifies those at risk of adverse maternal and perinatal outcomes.

Methods

Study population and clinical data

This study is a retrospective cohort study. We reviewed the medical records of ethnically Chinese women with singleton pregnancy and a live delivery at the First Affiliated Hospital of Sun Yat-sen University, Guangzhou, China, between January 2013 and December 2016. Inclusion criteria were as follows: gave birth at 28 or more completed weeks of gestation; and complete antenatal and birth data. Exclusion criteria were as follows: preexisting diabetes and hypertension. A total of 11,494 women were included, among which 9,178 (79.9%) were nulliparous. The study was approved by an ethics committee of The First Affiliated Hospital of Sun Yat-sen University.

Demographic data were collected for each participant and included maternal age (years), clinical history, pre-pregnancy weight (self-reported or any measured weights during the 1 year before pregnancy), height, and prenatal care (date of prenatal visit and complications of pregnancy). Pre-pregnancy BMI was calculated as weight in kilograms (kg) before pregnancy, divided by height in meters squared (m^2). Maternal obesity was defined using the WHO classification for Asian populations (BMI ≥ 25kg/m^2) and WGOC (BMI ≥ 28kg/m^2). All possible thresholds were defined for BMIs between 19 and 28kg/m^2 in three unit increments. Adverse obstetrics outcomes were compared in the classification among the study population.

Maternal and perianaloutcomes included prevalence of C/S,operative vaginal delivery (OVD), preeclampsia (gestational systolic BP ≥ 140mmHg ordiastolic BP ≥

90mmHg [at least two readings, 4h apart], with 1+ of proteinuria or more on dipstick), gestational diabetes (according to the criteria established by the American Diabetes Association) [16], and postpartum hemorrhage. Outcomes among neonates included preterm birth (delivered <37^{+0} weeks gestation), shoulder dystocia, large for gestational age (LGA), small for gestational age (SGA), a low Apgar score (1 or 5-min Apgar score less than 7), and admission to the neonatal intensive care unit (NICU). LGA and SGAwere defined as birth weight above or below the 90th and 10th centiles of the local scale, respectively, after adjusting for gender and gestational age [17].

Statistical analysis

All statistical analyses were performed using the Statistical Package for Social Science version 21.0 (SPSS, Inc., Chicago, IL, USA) and R 3.3.1 (R Project for Statistical Computing., Vienna, Austria). Data are expressed as mean ±standard deviations (SD) for normally distributed variables, median with interquartile range for skewed data, and as frequencies for categorical variables. Differences between groups were assessed using the Mann-Whitney U-test, Kruskal-Wallis test or Chi-squared test, as appropriate. The BMI group of 19~22 kg/m^2 was used as the reference or comparison group. Maternal age and previous C/S were considered as confounding factors in the determination of all adjusted odds ratios in relation to BMI level. The risks of maternal and perinatal complications were presented as adjusted odds ratio with 95% confidence interval (95% CI) after adjusting for the confounding factors. We adopted the Chi-square test for trend to investigate whether the prevalence of adverse obstetric outcomes in different BMI groups manifested a linear trend. Moreover, bootstrap resampling was performed 1000 times to calculate the 95%CI of the Youden indexes criteria and the 95%CI of the difference of Youden indexes between the two criteria, thereby revealing their predictive effect on adverse maternal and perinatal outcomes. P-value less than 0.05 was defined as of statistical significance. If the 95%CI of the difference of Youden indexes between the two criteria did not cover a zero value, it was indicated that the Youden indexes of the two criteria were at statistically different levels.

Results

Obesity prevalence

The prevalence of obesity was 7.2% (95% CI, 6.7~7.7) according to the WHO criteria for Asian populations (BMI ≥ 25kg/m^2); this proportion decreased to 1.7% (95% CI, 1.5~2.0) when using the Chinese-specific threshold (BMI ≥ 28kg/m^2) (Fig. 1). The characteristics of the women are listed in Table 1. Mothers with obesity were more likely to be older, have a previous cesarean

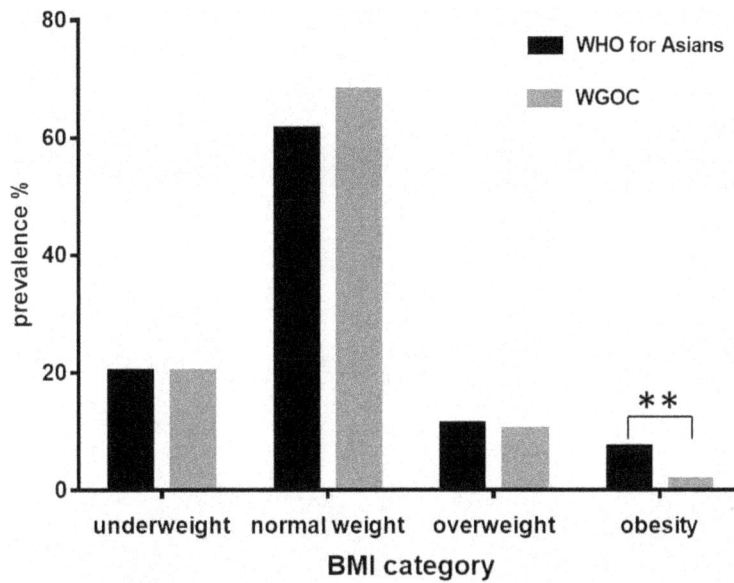

Fig. 1 Obesity defined by WHO for Asian population and WGOC specific BMI cut-offs among women from the First Affiliated Hospital of Sun Yat-sen University, Guangzhou, China. BMI (kg/m²) < 18.5 = Underweight. BMI for Asian population (kg/m²): 18.5-22.9 = normal weight, 23.0-24.9 = overweight, ≥ 25 = obesity. BMI for WGOC (kg/m²): 18.5-23.9 = normal weight, 24.0-27.9 = overweight, ≥ 28 = obesity. ** P<0.001

delivery, shorter gestational week, and higher birth weight of their offspring ($p < 0.001$).

Trends in maternal obesity and associated risks of adverse maternal and perinatal outcomes

As presented in Table 2, with increasing BMI, the risk of GDM, preeclampsia, LGA, and C/S increased, indicating that women with obesity are at increased risks of the above complications. The prevalence of GDM, pre-eclampsia, C/S, and LGA manifested a positive linear trend with increasing BMI (P for trend < 0.001). In contrast, risks for SGA and OVD decreased with increasing BMI. Increasing BMI was not associated with an increased risk of PPH, preterm birth, shoulder dystocia, low Apgar's score or admission to the NICU. Thus, we considered GDM, preeclampsia, C/S, and LGA as obesity-related adverse maternal and perinatal outcomes (Fig. 2).

Variable BMI group and obesity related adverse perinatal complications.

Table 3 showed the odds ratios associated with obesity-related adverse maternal and perinatal outcomes in the group of BMI ≥ 28kg/m² in comparison with the group of 25 ≤ BMI < 28kg/m². The risks of preeclampsia, C/S, and LGA were similar between the two groups, except that the risk of GDM was a little higher in the group of BMI ≥ 28kg/m² (AOR was 1.47[95% CI: 1.05~2.07]).

Effectiveness of the two obesity criteria to predict adverse outcomes

The sensitivities, specificities and Youden indexes of BMI ≥ 25 kg/m² and BMI ≥ 28 kg/m² in predicting adverse outcomes were shown in Table 4. Compare to BMI ≥ 28 kg/m², the sensitivity of BMI ≥ 25 kg/m² rose by 3-4 folds, while the decrease in specificity was minor. The Youden index of BMI ≥ 25 kg/m² predicting the risk of GDM was higher than that of BMI ≥ 28kg/m². Similar

Table 1 Baseline characteristics of this study's population[a]

	Prepregnancy BMI category (kg/m²)					
	BMI<19 (n= 3135)	19≤BMI<22 (n= 5113)	22≤BMI<25 (n= 2422)	25≤BMI<28 (n= 626)	BMI≥28 (n= 198)	P
Maternal age (years)	29.7 ± 4.0	31.4 ± 4.2	32.5 ± 4.3	33.0 ± 4.2	32.5 ± 4.4	<0.001
Nulliparity	2482 (79.2)	4093 (80.1)	1943 (80.2)	504 (80.5)	156 (78.8)	0.82
Previous C/S	276 (8.8)	711 (13.9)	448 (18.5)	147 (23.5)	41 (20.7)	<0.001
Gestational week	38.9 ± 1.56	38.9 ± 1.5	38.7 ± 1.6	38.6 ± 1.7	38.4 ± 1.9	<0.001
Birth weight (grams)	3060.7 ± 425.6	3159.9 ± 437.2	3210.6 ± 477.7	3263.4 ± 486.1	3272.5 ± 545.3	<0.001

BMI body mass index; *C/S* caesarean section.
[a]Continuous variables were presented as mean ± SD; qualitative variables were presented as N (%)

Table 2 Maternal and neonatal complications of singleton pregnancies among women by pre-pregnancy obesity

Outcomes	BMI<19(kg/m²)		19≤BMI<22(kg/m²)		22≤BMI<25(kg/m²)		25≤BMI<28(kg/m²)		BMI≥28(kg/m²)		P for trend
	N (%)	OR (95% CI)[a]	N (%)		N (%)	OR (95% CI)[a]	N (%)	OR (95% CI)[a]	N (%)	OR (95% CI)[a]	
Maternal complications											
GDM	424 (13.5)	0.87 (0.77-0.99)	896 (17.5)	Reference group 1	584 (24.1)	1.34 (1.20-1.52)	193 (30.8)	1.82 (1.51-2.19)	76 (38.4)	2.73 (2.02-3.69)	<0.001
Preeclampsia	62 (2.0)	0.85 (0.62-1.56)	119 (2.3)	1	85 (3.5)	1.53 (1.15-2.03)	37 (5.9)	2.64 (1.81-3.85)	12 (6.1)	2.71 (1.47-4.99)	<0.001
PPH	163 (5.2)	0.73 (0.60-0.88)	355 (6.9)	1	161 (6.6)	0.97 (0.80-1.17)	52 (8.3)	1.25 (0.92-1.69)	12 (6.1)	0.88 (0.49-1.60)	0.008
Delivery mode											
OVD	293 (9.3)	1.28 (1.08-1.50)	350 (6.8)	1	152 (6.3)	0.99 (0.81-1.20)	24 (3.8)	0.63 (0.41-0.96)	2(1.0)	0.15 (0.04-0.62)	<0.001
C/S	1235 (39.4)	0.77 (0.70-0.85)	2543 (49.7)	1	1403 (57.9)	1.24 (1.12-1.38)	409 (65.3)	1.56 (1.29-1.88)	133 (67.2)	1.88 (1.36-2.59)	<0.001
Neonatal complications											
Preterm birth	222 (7.1)	1.02 (0.86-1.22)	366 (7.2)	1	216 (8.9)	1.24 (1.04-1.47)	58 (9.3)	1.25 (0.93-1.67)	22 (11.1)	1.56 (0.99-2.46)	0.001
LGA	220 (7.0)	057 (0.48-0.67)	605 (11.8)	1	416 (17.2)	1.53 (1.34-1.75)	142 (22.7)	2.14 (1.74-2.63)	49 (24.7)	2.42 (1.73-3.38)	<0.001
SGA	260 (8.3)	1.47 (1.23-1.75)	291 (5.7)	1	104 (4.3)	0.76 (0.60-0.95)	18 (2.9)	0.51 (0.32-0.83)	6 (3.0)	0.53 (0.23-1.21)	<0.001
Shoulder dystocia	1 (0.0)	0.06 (0.01-0.42)	27 (0.5)	1	7 (0.3)	0.58 (0.25-1.33)	2 (0.3)	0.68 (0.16-2.87)	1 (0.5)	1.04 (0.14-7.69)	0.102
Low Apgar's score	106 (3.4)	1.09 (0.85-1.41)	152 (3.0)	1	82 (3.4)	1.18 (0.90-1.55)	16 (2.6)	0.90 (0.53-1.51)	12 (6.1)	2.17 (1.18-3.98)	0.656
Admission to NICU	665 (21.2)	0.99 (0.89-1.11)	1056 (20.7)	1	520 (21.5)	1.08 (0.96-1.22)	146 (23.3)	1.23 (1.01-1.50)	50 (25.3)	1.34 (0.97-1.86)	0.159

BMI body mass index; *GDM* gestational diabetes mellitus; *PPH* Postpartum hemorrhage; *OVD* Operative vaginal delivery; *C/S* caesarean section; *LGA* large for gestational age; *SGA* small for gestational age; *NICU* neonatal intensive care unit; *OR* Odds ratio; *CI* confidence interval
[a]Data adjusted for maternal age and previous caesarean section.

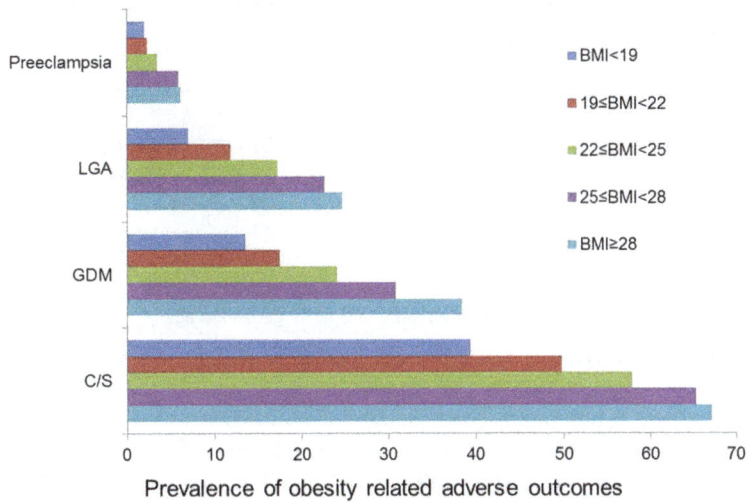

Fig. 2 Prevalence of adverse pregnancy and birth outcomes by cumulative BMI. BMI: body mass index; GDM: gestational diabetes mellitus; C/S: caesarean section; LGA: large for gestational age

patterns were also detected for preeclampsia, C/S, and LGA. Finally, to predict the risk of the obesity-related adverse maternal and perinatal outcomes, we analyzed the Youden indexes of BMI ≥ 25 kg/m² and BMI ≥ 28 kg/m². The Youden index of BMI ≥ 25 kg/m² was higher than BMI ≥ 28 kg/m² (the difference of the Youden indexes was 0.065 [95% CI:0.051~0.079]), indicating that the former better identifies women at risk of obesity-related adverse maternal and perinatal outcomes.

Discussion

In our study, women with obesity were at significantly increased risk of maternal and perianal complications. Although women whose BMI ≥ 28 kg/m² were at high risk of complications, it was similar to those whose BMIs were between 25 and 28kg/m². We found that BMI ≥ 25kg/m² is better at predicting the risk of maternal and perianal complications than BMI ≥ 28kg/m². Therefore, we suggested that BMI ≥ 25 kg/m² is more appropriate than BMI ≥ 28 kg/m² for defining obesity for pregnant women in South China.

Table 3 Variable BMI group and obesity related adverse perinatal complications[a]

	25≤BMI<28 (kg/m²)	BMI≥28(kg/m²)	
	Reference group	OR (95% CI)	AOR (95% CI) [a]
GDM	1	1.40 (1.00-1.95)	1.47 (1.05-2.07)
Preeclampsia	1	1.03 (0.53-2.01)	1.03 (0.53-2.01)
C/S	1	1.09 (0.77-1.52)	1.20 (0.83-1.72)
LGA	1	1.12 (0.77-1.63)	1.12 (0.77-1.63)

BMI body mass index; GDM gestational diabetes mellitus; C/S caesarean section; LGA large for gestational age; OR Odds ratio; CI confidence interval.
[a]Data adjusted for maternal age and previous caesarean section.

BMI is a single acceptable predictor of adverse outcomes [18]. Our results show that increasing BMI is associated with increased risks of GDM, preeclampsia, C/S, and LGA, supporting results of previous studies [3–5, 19, 20]. SGA and operative vaginal delivery were negatively associated with increasing BMI, indicating that obesity was not associated with increased risk of SGA and operative vaginal delivery. Therefore, we considered GDM, preeclampsia, C/S, and LGA as obesity-related maternal and perinatal outcomes. Chui and colleagues concluded that a BMI of 25kg/m² in Chinese adults was equivalent to a BMI of 30 kg/m² in Caucasian subjects in terms of identifying those at risk of diabetes; [21] this finding indicates that the criterion of BMI should be race-specific. Leung et al. found that, compared with Caucasians, the impact of high BMI on gestational diabetes and preeclampsia in Chinese women was stronger [19]. However, the effect of different obesity criteria on predicting the risk of maternal and perinatal outcomes has not been addressed.

Youden's index (also known as Youden's J statistic) is a single statistic that captures the performance of a dichotomous diagnostic test. A higher value of the Youden's index indicates better test authenticity. Aye M et al. used Youden's index to identify the optimal cut-off point of BMI to predict the metabolic risk factors for metabolic syndrome among people aged 13–91 years [22]. Oliveira et al. used sensitivity, specificity, and overall accuracy (area under the curve) to describe the predictive performance of different diagnostic criteria of obesity as predictors of metabolic syndrome in adolescents [23]. In the research, we aimed to compare the WHO for Asians and WGOC obesity criteria's effectiveness in predicting adverse maternal and perinatal outcomes, rather than

Table 4 Sensitivities, specificities and Youden indexes of the two obesity criteria in predicting the risk of adverse outcomes

	Sensitivity (%)		Specificity (%)		Youden index (95% CI)		Difference of Youden index (95% CI)
	BMI_{25}	BMI_{28}	BMI_{25}	BMI_{28}	BMI_{25}	BMI_{28}	
GDM	12.4	3.5	94.0	98.7	0.06 (0.05~0.08)	0.02 (0.01~0.03)	0.04 (0.03~0.06)[b]
Preeclampsia	15.6	3.81	93.1	98.3	0.09 (0.05~0.13)	0.02 (0.01~0.04)	0.07 (0.03~0.10)[b]
C/S	9.47	2.32	95.1	98.9	0.05 (0.04~0.06)	0.01 (0.01~0.02)	0.03 (0.03~0.04)[b]
LGA	13.3	3.42	93.7	98.5	0.07 (0.05~0.09)	0.02 (0.01~0.03)	0.05 (0.04~0.07)[b]
Obesity related outcomes[a]	14.5	3.82	94.6	98.8	0.09 (0.08~0.11)	0.03 (0.02~0.03)	0.07 (0.05~0.08)[b]

BMI body mass index; *GDM* gestational diabetes mellitus; *C/S* caesarean section; *LGA* large for gestational age; *CI* confidence interval.
[a]Obesity related outcomes required at least one in the following items: GDM, preeclampsia, C/S, and LGA
[b]The difference of Youden index between the two groups was statistically significant

finding the cut-point of the maximum predictive ability. Therefore, we use sensitivity, specificity and Youden index to evaluate the two cut-points' predictive abilities. The sensitivity of BMI $\geq$ 25 kg/m^2 was 3-4 folds higher than BMI $\geq$ 28 kg/m^2, while the decrease in specificity was minor. The Youden index of BMI $\geq$ 25 kg/m^2 was higher than that for BMI $\geq$ 28 kg/m^2, indicating that BMI $\geq$ 25 kg/m^2 has a better predictive value on the risk of obesity-related maternal and perinatal outcomes.

The association between the BMI and adverse maternal and perinatal outcome is likely to be driven by body fat. Although body fat was not measured in our study, many researchers have shown that BMI is an accurate assessment of the amount of adiposity. Chang et al. have revealed that Taiwan people with a BMI $\geq$ 25 kg/m^2 had a similar body fat rate as Caucasians with BMI $\geq$ 30 kg/m^2 [24]. Chen et al. have shown that, compared with the percent body fat obesity cut-off ($\geq$ 40%), the BMI-obesity (BMI $\geq$ 25 kg/m^2) criteria resulted in a better Youden index than the WGOC BMI criteria among middle-aged Chinese women [25]. In our study, the prevalence of obesity was 7.2% according to the WHO for the Asian BMI-obesity criterion; but was just 1.7% based on the WGOC criterion. This is because most of our subjects were from South China, which is a relatively slim population. However, if the WGOC standards (defining BMI $\geq$ 28 kg/m^2 as obesity) are applied, a significant proportion of at-risk patients might be missed (about 5.5%). A lower BMI cut-off at 25 kg/m^2 for defining obesity would better predict those at risk of adverse obstetric and perinatal outcomes and, therefore, enable the development of adequate support to reduce the incidence of adverse maternal and perinatal outcomes.

To our knowledge, this study is the first to compare the different obesity criteria's effectiveness in predicting adverse maternal and perinatal outcomes. However, some limitations of our study should also be noted. Pre-pregnancy BMI was calculated using weight and height, and most of these data were likely to be self-reported. Nevertheless, self-reported BMI has been shown to have high specificity (96–98%) and sensitivity (86–92%) in women of childbearing age (20–49 years) [26]. Also, pre-pregnancy self-reported weight seems to be highly correlated with early pregnancy measured weight (r = 0.95) [27]. Also, this single-center study might not be representative of the general population. However, the center is the national key clinical department in South China with about 4000-delivery per year. Relevant guidelines were strictly followed in the management and care of pregnant women in this hospital, thereby avoiding the occurrence of adverse outcomes owing to the subjective factors of medical staff, which makes the outcomes more objective and reliable. In addition, the Youden indexes of BMI cut-offs for obesity were not high, because the sensitivities of them were low, which implicated that we couldn't identify diseased and non-diseased individuals respectively only by BMI in clinical practice. We need to set up a model to predict a specific complication of pregnancy, in which more indicators should be included. These results could provide some evidence for further study. Lastly, lower BMI cut-off for obesity would cause a larger number of Chinese pregnant women to be treated as high-risk pregnancies. Therefore, a large, multi-center trial and further research addressing cost-effectiveness are warranted.

Conclusions

Our results support the notion that obesity is associated with adverse perinatal outcomes. A lower BMI cut-off of 25 kg/m^2 for defining obesity might be appropriate for Chinese pregnant women and help to identify those at risk of adverse maternal and perinatal outcomes. These results are important for women who are pregnant or are planning to become pregnant, as well as for clinicians who guide or provide prenatal counseling for women.

Acknowledgments
The authors thank associated Professor Jinxin Zhang from the Department of

Medical Statistics and Epidemiology, School of Public Health, Sun Yat-sen University for a critical review of the study design and the sponsor of Danone Nutricia Early Life Nutrition.

Funding
The study was supported by Clinical Medical Project 5010 of Sun Yat-sen University, China (Grant No: 2012004 (Zilian Wang, PI)).

Authors' contributions
YW and ZW were responsible for the design of the study, interpretation of data, and the manuscript draft. WM and DW reviewed and commented on the manuscript. HC and ZL were involved in data cleaning and verification. All authors revised the manuscript, had full access to all of the data in the study and can take responsibility for the integrity of the data and the accuracy of the data analysis, and had authority over approval of final manuscript version and the decision to submit for publication.

Authors' information
Zilian Wang is a clinical professor in the division of Maternal-fetalMedicine, Department of Obstetrics and Gynecology, the First Affiliated Hospital of Sun Yat-sen University of China. Yanxin Wu, Dongyu Wang and Zhuyu Li are senior attending physicians of the same institution. Wai-kit Ming and Haitian Chen are associate professors of the same institution.

Competing interests
The authors declare that they have no competing interests.

References
1. Collaborators GBDO, Afshin A, Forouzanfar MH, Reitsma MB, Sur P, Estep K, Lee A, Marczak L, Mokdad AH, Moradi-Lakeh M, et al. Health Effects of Overweight and Obesity in 195 Countries over 25 Years. N Engl J Med. 2017;377:13–27.
2. Wang Z, Hao G, Wang X, Chen Z, Zhang L, Guo M, Tian Y, Shao L, Zhu M. Current prevalence rates of overweight, obesity, central obesity, and related cardiovascular risk factors that clustered among middle-aged population of China. Zhonghua Liu Xing Bing Xue Za Zhi. 2014;35:354–8.
3. Xiong C, Zhou A, Cao Z, Zhang Y, Qiu L, Yao C, Wang Y, Zhang B. Association of pre-pregnancy body mass index, gestational weight gain with cesarean section in term deliveries of China. Sci Rep. 2016;6:37168.
4. Kim SS, Zhu Y, Grantz KL, Hinkle SN, Chen Z, Wallace ME, Smarr MM, Epps NM, Mendola P. Obstetric and neonatal risks among obese women without chronic disease. Obstetrics and gynecology. 2016;128:104.
5. Schummers L, Hutcheon JA, Bodnar LM, Lieberman E, Himes KP. Risk of adverse pregnancy outcomes by prepregnancy body mass index: a population-based study to inform prepregnancy weight loss counseling. Obstet Gynecol. 2015;125:133–43.
6. Liu Y, Dai W, Dai X, Li Z. Prepregnancy body mass index and gestational weight gain with the outcome of pregnancy: a 13-year study of 292,568 cases in China. Arch Gynecol Obstet. 2012;286:905–11.
7. Overcash RT, Lacoursiere DY. The clinical approach to obesity in pregnancy. Clin Obstet Gynecol. 2014;57:485–500.
8. Kominiarek MA, Gay F, Peacock N. Obesity in Pregnancy: A Qualitative Approach to Inform an Intervention for Patients and Providers. Matern Child Health J. 2015;19:1698–712.
9. WHO. Obesity: preventing and managing the global epidemic. Report of a WHO Consultation. WHO Technical Report Series 894. Geneva: World Health Organization; 2000.
10. Carpenter CL, Yan E, Chen S, Hong K, Arechiga A, Kim WS, Deng M, Li Z, Heber D. Body fat and body-mass index among a multiethnic sample of college-age men and women. J Obesity. 2013;2013.
11. Shaikh S, Jones-Smith J, Schulze K, Ali H, Christian P, Shamim AA, Mehra S, Labrique A, Klemm R, Wu L. Excessive adiposity at low BMI levels among women in rural Bangladesh. J Nutr Sci. 2016;5.
12. Choo V. WHO reassesses appropriate body-mass index for Asian populations. Lancet. 2002;360:235.
13. WHO EC. Appropriate body-mass index for Asian populations and its implications for policy and intervention strategies. Lancet. 2004;363:157.
14. Zhou B. Coorperative Meta-Analysis Group Of China Obesity Task F: [Predictive values of body mass index and waist circumference to risk factors of related diseases in Chinese adult population]. Zhonghua Liu Xing Bing Xue Za Zhi. 2002;23:5–10.
15. Zhou BF. Cooperative Meta-Analysis Group of the Working Group on Obesity in C: Predictive values of body mass index and waist circumference for risk factors of certain related diseases in Chinese adults--study on optimal cut-off points of body mass index and waist circumference in Chinese adults. Biomed Environ Sci. 2002;15:83–96.
16. American Diabetes A. Standards of medical care in diabetes--2011. Diabetes Care. 2011;34(Suppl 1):S11–61.
17. Gong XM, Li ZH, Yu RJ: Maternal and fetal general parameters. In: W.Y. Zhang, eds. Chinese Perinatology. Beijing: People's Medical Publishing House; 2012. pp. 1592–1593.
18. Bryant M, Santorelli G, Lawlor DA, Farrar D, Tuffnell D, Bhopal R, Wright J. A comparison of South Asian specific and established BMI thresholds for determining obesity prevalence in pregnancy and predicting pregnancy complications: findings from the Born in Bradford cohort. Int J Obes (Lond). 2014;38:444–50.
19. Leung TY, Leung TN, Sahota DS, Chan OK, Chan LW, Fung TY, Lau TK. Trends in maternal obesity and associated risks of adverse pregnancy outcomes in a population of Chinese women. Bjog. 2008;115:1529–37.
20. Scott-Pillai R, Spence D, Cardwell CR, Hunter A, Holmes VA. The impact of body mass index on maternal and neonatal outcomes: a retrospective study in a UK obstetric population, 2004-2011. Bjog. 2013;120:932–9.
21. Chiu M, Austin PC, Manuel DG, Shah BR, Tu JV. Deriving ethnic-specific BMI cutoff points for assessing diabetes risk. Diabetes Care. 2011;34:1741–8.
22. Mra A, Malek S. Waist circumference and BMI cut-off points to predict risk factors for metabolic syndrome among outpatients in a district hospital. Singapore Med J. 2012, Aug;53(8):545–50.
23. Oliveira RG, Guedes DP. Performance of different diagnostic criteria of overweight and obesity as predictors of metabolic syndrome in adolescents. J Pediatr (Rio J). 2017;93:525–31.
24. Chang CJ, Wu CH, Chang CS, Yao WJ, Yang YC, Wu JS, Lu FH. Low body mass index but high percent body fat in Taiwanese subjects: implications of obesity cutoffs. Int J Obes Relat Metab Disord. 2003;27:253–9.
25. Chen YM, Ho SC, Lam SS, Chan SS. Validity of body mass index and waist circumference in the classification of obesity as compared to percent body fat in Chinese middle-aged women. Int J Obes (Lond). 2006;30:918–25.
26. Kuczmarski MF, Kuczmarski RJ, Najjar M. Effects of age on validity of self-reported height, weight, and body mass index: findings from the Third National Health and Nutrition Examination Survey, 1988-1994. J Am Diet Assoc. 2001;101:28–34. quiz 35-26
27. Park S, Sappenfield WM, Bish C, Bensyl DM, Goodman D, Menges J. Reliability and validity of birth certificate prepregnancy weight and height among women enrolled in prenatal WIC program: Florida, 2005. Matern Child Health J. 2011;15:851–9.

## 10

Follicle-stimulating hormone (FSH) promotes retinol uptake and metabolism in the mouse ovary

Zhuo Liu[1†], Yongfeng Sun[2†], Yanwen Jiang[1†], Yuqiang Qian[1], Shuxiong Chen[1], Shan Gao[1], Lu Chen[1], Chunjin Li[1*] and Xu Zhou[1*]

Abstract

Background: Retinoids (retinol and its derivatives) are required for the development and maintenance of normal physiological functions of the ovary. However, the mechanisms underlying the regulation of ovarian retinoid homeostasis during follicular development remain unclear.

Methods: The present study determined retinoid levels and the expression levels of genes involved in the retinol uptake and its metabolic pathway in the ovaries of follicle-stimulating hormone (FSH)-treated mice and in granulosa cells treated with FSH using ultra performance liquid chromatography (UPLC) combined with quadrupole time-of-flight high-sensitivity mass spectrometry (Q-TOF/HSMS) and real-time PCR analysis.

Results: The levels of total retinoids and retinoic acid (RA) and expressions of retinol-oxidizing enzyme genes alcohol dehydrogenase 1 (*Adh1*) and aldehyde dehydrogenase (*Aldh1a1*) are increased in the ovaries of mice treated with FSH; in contrast, the retinyl ester levels and retinol-esterifying enzyme gene lecithin: retinol acyltransferase (*Lrat*) expression are diminished. In FSH-treated granulosa cells, the levels of retinyl esters, retinaldehyde, and total retinoids are augmented; and this is coupled with an increase in the expressions of stimulated by retinoic acid 6 (*Stra6*) and cellular retinol-binding protein 1 (*Crbp1*), genes in the retinol uptake pathway, and *Adh1*, *Adh7*, and *Aldh1a1* as well as a diminution in *Lrat* expression.

Conclusions: These data suggest that FSH promotes retinol uptake and its conversion to RA through modulating the pathways of retinol uptake and metabolism in the mouse ovary. The present study provides a possible mechanism for the regulation of endogenous RA signaling in the developing follicles.

Keywords: Follicle-stimulating hormone, Retinol, Ovary, Granulosa cells

Background

Follicles are the functional units of the ovary, with primary functions being oocyte maturation and steroid hormone biosynthesis and secretion. After entering puberty, some follicles begin to grow under the indirect stimulation of gonadotropin-releasing hormone (GnRH) and ultimately culminate in either atresia or ovulation. The processes of follicular development and ovulation are primarily controlled by neuroendocrine activities in the hypothalamus–pituitary–ovary (HPO) axis, although early stages appear to occur independently of the HPO axis. Follicle-stimulating hormone (FSH) and luteinizing hormone (LH), which are released by the pituitary gland, principally control follicular development and ovulation by regulating estradiol (E₂) secretion and the functions of granulosa and theca cells [1]. In addition to neuroendocrine mechanisms, cell-cell communications between oocyte and somatic (granulosa and theca) cells play critical roles in the initiation and coordination of somatic cell and oocyte differentiation [2–5]. Paracrine interactions between oocyte and their surrounding granulosa cells during oocyte and follicular development ensure proper coordination of oocyte and somatic cell functions

* Correspondence: llcjj158@163.com; xzhou65@vip.sina.com
†Zhuo Liu, Yongfeng Sun and Yanwen Jiang contributed equally to this work.
1College of Animal Science, Jilin University, 5333 Xian Road, Changchun 130062, Jilin, China
Full list of author information is available at the end of the article

[2, 4, 5]. It has been well established that the retinoid pathway plays a fundamental role in maintaining the normal ovarian function [6]. Kawai et al. [7] reported that retinoic acid (RA) in antral follicles was required for FSH-regulated granulosa cell differentiation and ovarian reproductive competence, and that retinoid deficiency prevented the development of oocytes and reduced the number of ovulated oocytes in mice. RA is also required for both nuclear and cytoplasmic maturation of mouse and bovine oocytes [8, 9], and can stimulate steroidogenesis, such as for testosterone synthesis in human theca cells and estradiol synthesis in mouse granulosa cells [6, 10]. In addition, ovarian retinoid levels vary with the estrous cycle [11], and the concentration of retinol is greater in the fluid of dominant follicles relative to that of small follicles [12, 13]. However, the regulatory mechanisms underlying ovarian retinoid homeostasis are not currently fully understood.

Retinol (vitamin A) and its derivatives (retinyl esters, retinal, and RA) are collectively known as retinoids. It is generally understood that most retinoids are taken up by extrahepatic tissues from retinol-binding protein 4 (RBP4)-bound retinol in the circulation through transmembrane-spanning protein stimulated by RA 6 (STRA6), which acts as the cell surface receptor for RBP4 and can facilitate the transport of retinol from RBP4-retinol complexes into cells [14]. To be biologically active, intracellular retinol must first be oxidized to retinaldehyde and then to RA and a large number of enzymes and binding proteins are involved in these processes. Upon entering cells, retinol is bound by free cellular retinol-binding protein 1 (CRBP1). STRA6, as a bidirectional transporter of retinol, is potentially involved in maintaining intracellular retinoid homeostasis along with RBP4 and CRBP1 [14–17]. Within cells, retinol can either be converted to retinaldehyde and RA via 2 enzymatic steps or be stored in cells as retinyl esters catalyzed by lecithin: retinol acyltransferase (LRAT). First, retinol can be oxidized to retinaldehyde by alcohol dehydrogenases (ADHs, such as ADH1 and ADH7), and then retinal can be oxidized to RA by aldehyde dehydrogenases (ALDHs, such as ALDH1A1) [18]. Most of the cellular actions of retinoids are thus realized due to the transcriptional regulatory activity of RA, which binds nuclear RA receptors (RARs: RARα, RARβ, and RARγ) as well as the peroxisome proliferator activated receptor β/δ (PPARβ/δ); RARs and PPARβ/δ then associate with retinoid X receptors (RXRs: RXRα, RXRβ, and RXRγ) to form heterodimers and combine with RA response elements (RAREs) or peroxisome proliferator response elements (PPREs) within the promoters of retinoid-responsive genes [6, 19]. It was reported that the partition of RA between the two signaling pathways exerts opposing action on cell growth and apoptosis and that the

alternative pathways are coordinated by cellular RA-binding protein 2 (CRABP2) and fatty acid–binding protein 5 (FABP5), which bind and transport RA to RARs and PPARβ/δ, respectively [19, 20]. In addition to the classical direct nuclear receptor signaling pathways, RA stimulates rapid, nongenomic signaling events by inducing kinase phosphorylation and activation via binding to extra-nuclear RARs, which subsequently leads to downstream nuclear effects on transcription [21].

The present study was aimed to investigate the regulatory mechanisms underlying ovarian retinoid accumulation and metabolism. To this end, we examined retinoid levels using ultra performance liquid chromatography (UPLC) combined with quadrupole time-of-flight high-sensitivity mass spectrometry (Q-TOF/HSMS) in ovaries of FSH-treated mice and in follicular granulosa cells treated with FSH. We also determined the expressions of genes of enzymes and binding proteins involved in retinol uptake and metabolism. Our data showed that FSH promoted retinol uptake and its conversion to RA in both mouse ovaries in vivo and in granulosa cells cultured in vitro.

Material and methods
Animals
Three-week-old immature female BALB/c mice were obtained from the Medical Department of Jilin University (Changchun, China), raised in an environment with controlled temperature (22–24 °C) and humidity (60–70%) in a 12-h light/dark cycle, and provided with food and water ad libitum. They were injected intraperitoneally with a single dose of FSH (10 IU/mouse; Ningbo Second Hormone Factory, Ningbo, China) [22–24] and sacrificed via cervical dislocation 24 or 48 h after injection. Ovary tissues were rapidly collected and stored at − 80 °C. All animal studies were conducted in strict accordance with the protocol approved by the Animal Care and Use Committee of Jilin University.

Isolation of follicular granulosa cells and culture in vitro
Primary granulosa cells were isolated from immature female mouse ovaries, as described previously [25, 26]. In brief, mice were sacrificed via cervical dislocation after being anesthetized, and the follicles were isolated with no. 5 fine needles. The follicles were then treated with trypsin (Hyclone, USA) for 1 h and filtered using a 100-μm filter (Life Technologies, USA). The isolated granulosa cells were cultured in Dulbecco's Modified Eagle Medium/F12 1:1 (Hyclone, USA) supplemented with 10% fetal bovine serum (Hyclone, USA), 1% insulin–transferrin–selenium (Sigma, USA), and 1% antibiotics (Hyclone, USA) at 37 °C in an atmosphere of 5% CO_2 in compressed air at high humidity. Twenty-four hours later, non-adherent cells were removed and

adherent cells were treated with FSH (100 IU/L) in the presence of all-*trans*-retinol (1 μM, approximately to the concentration of retinol in 100% serum; Sigma, USA).

Sample preparation and liquid chromatography–mass spectrometry (LC-MS) analysis

Ovary tissues (50 mg) and granulosa cells (5×10^6) were each homogenized in 800 μL of methanol with an internal standard (5 μg/ml, DL-o-chlorophenylalanine), the homogenates were centrifuged at 13,000 rpm for 15 min, and the supernatants (200 μl) were collected. LC-MS was carried out on a Waters Acquity™ UPLC system (Waters, USA) coupled with a Waters XevoTM G2 QTOF-MS (Waters, UK). Chromatography was performed on an Acquity UPLC high strength silica (HSS) T3 column (2. 1 mm × 100 mm, 1. 8 μm, UK) at 40 °C. The mobile phases were water (A) and acetonitrile (B) containing 0.1% formic acid. The optimized elution conditions for LC are shown in Table 1. 6-μL sample solution was injected for each run, and MS analysis was performed on a mass spectrometer XevoTM G2 QTof (Waters, UK). For the positive electrospray mode, the capillary and cone voltage were set at 1.4 kV and 40 V, respectively. The desolvation gas flow was set to 600 L/h at 350 °C, the cone gas flow was set to 50 L/h and the source temperature was set to 120 °C. The collision and ion energies were 10–40 V and 1 V, respectively. The data acquisition rate was set to 0.1 s, with a 0.1 s interscan delay; the scan range was from 50 to 1500 m/z. Rutin solution was used as the lockmass to ensure accuracy and reproducibility. All the acquisition and analysis of data were performed using Waters MassLynx v4.1 software.

Total RNA extraction and real-time quantitative PCR assay

Total RNA from ovarian tissues and granulosa cells cultured in vitro was extracted using an RNAprep pure Micro Kit (Tiangen, Beijing, China) and reverse transcribed into cDNA using a PrimeScript RT reagent kit (Takara, Japan) according to the manufacturer's instructions. Real-time PCR was performed on a sequence-detection system (Agilent Technologies, USA) using the SYBR Premix Ex TaqII kit (Takara, Japan), with *β-Actin* used as an internal reference. The relative mRNA expression

Table 1 UPLC elution conditions

Time (min)	Flow rate (ml/min)	Pressure limit (bar)	Solv Ratio B (%)
0	0.35	800	5
1	0.35	800	5
6	0.35	800	20
9	0.35	800	50
13	0.35	800	95
15	0.35	800	95

levels were calculated using the $2^{-\Delta\Delta Ct}$ method. All primers were obtained from Sangon Biotech (Shanghai, China), and information for the primers is shown in Table 2. All experiments were repeated at least three times.

Statistical analyses

Statistical analyses of the data were conducted via independent sample t-tests or one-way ANOVA (Fig. 2a), followed by Tukey's test. Differences were considered to be significant at $P < 0.05$. All the statistical analyses were performed using SPSS 22.0 for Windows (StatSoft, USA).

Results

Retinoid levels in ovaries of mice treated with FSH

The retinoid levels in ovaries of mice left untreated or treated with FSH were examined using semi-quantitative LC-MS analysis. Representative LC-MS total-ion chromatograms (TICs) of the samples are displayed in Fig. 1. The retinoid metabolites were identified by searching against the METLIN Metabolite Database (http:// metlin.scripps.edu/) and Human Metabolome Database (HMDB, http://www.hmdb.ca/) and comparing the accurate masses or mass-to-charge ratios (m/z). The retinoid levels were calculated using the formula $C_x = S_x/S_s{}^*\rho_s{}^*V/m/M_x$ (μmol/mg) for tissue samples or $= S_x/S_s{}^*\rho_s/M_x$ (umol/ml) for cell samples, where S_x and S_s indicate integral areas of the peaks of metabolite X and internal standard, respectively; ρ_s indicates the concentrations of internal standard (ug/ml); V indicates the volume of extraction solvent (ml); M_x indicats the molar mass of metabolite X; and m indicates the weight of tissue samples (mg). The results showed that the levels of RA and total retinoids increased in the ovaries of mice treated with FSH for 48 h; in contrast, retinyl esters diminished (Fig. 2a).

Expression of genes in retinol uptake and metabolism pathways in ovaries of mice treated with FSH

We further determined the expression of the genes involved in retinol uptake and metabolism. The data showed that the expression of the alcohol dehydrogenase gene *Adh1* and aldehyde dehydrogenase gene *Aldh1a1* increased with FSH, but that the expression of the lecithin: retinol acyltransferase gene *Lrat* decreased (Fig. 2b).

Retinoid levels in follicular granulosa cells treated with FSH

Since granulosa cells are the main cell types regulated by FSH in the ovary, we further evaluated the effects of FSH on retinoid levels in granulosa cells. The TICs of the samples are displayed in Fig. 3. The results showed that the levels of retinyl esters, retinaldehyde, and total retinoids increased significantly in cells treated with FSH

Table 2 Primer list

Gene	Forward	Reverse	Size (bp)	Annealing temperature
β-Actin	5′-TCTGGCACCACACCTTCTA-3′	5′-AGGCATACAGGGACAGCAC-3′	180	60
Stra6	5′-AGGGCCCTGGAAGCTACTG-3′	5′-AGGCCAGCAAGGAGTAGTC-3′	197	60
Crbp1	5′-GCCTTACGCAAAATCGCCAA-3′	5′-ACAGTGGTCATGCACTTGCG-3′	176	60
Adh1	5′-TTGGCTGTAAAGCAGCAGGA-3′	5′-CATGGGGTTCATGGAGAGGT-3′	293	60
Adh7	5′-CTGGTGCCTCCAGGATCATT-3′	5′-CCCAGTGAAGAGCAGCATTG-3′	293	60
Aldh1a1	5′-CCCGGATTTTTGTTGAGGAG-3′	5′-GAGAACACTGTGGGCTGCAC-3′	244	60
Lrat	5′-AGGTGACACGGACCCATTTT-3′	5′-CTGCTCCGTAGGCAAAGTCC-3′	205	60

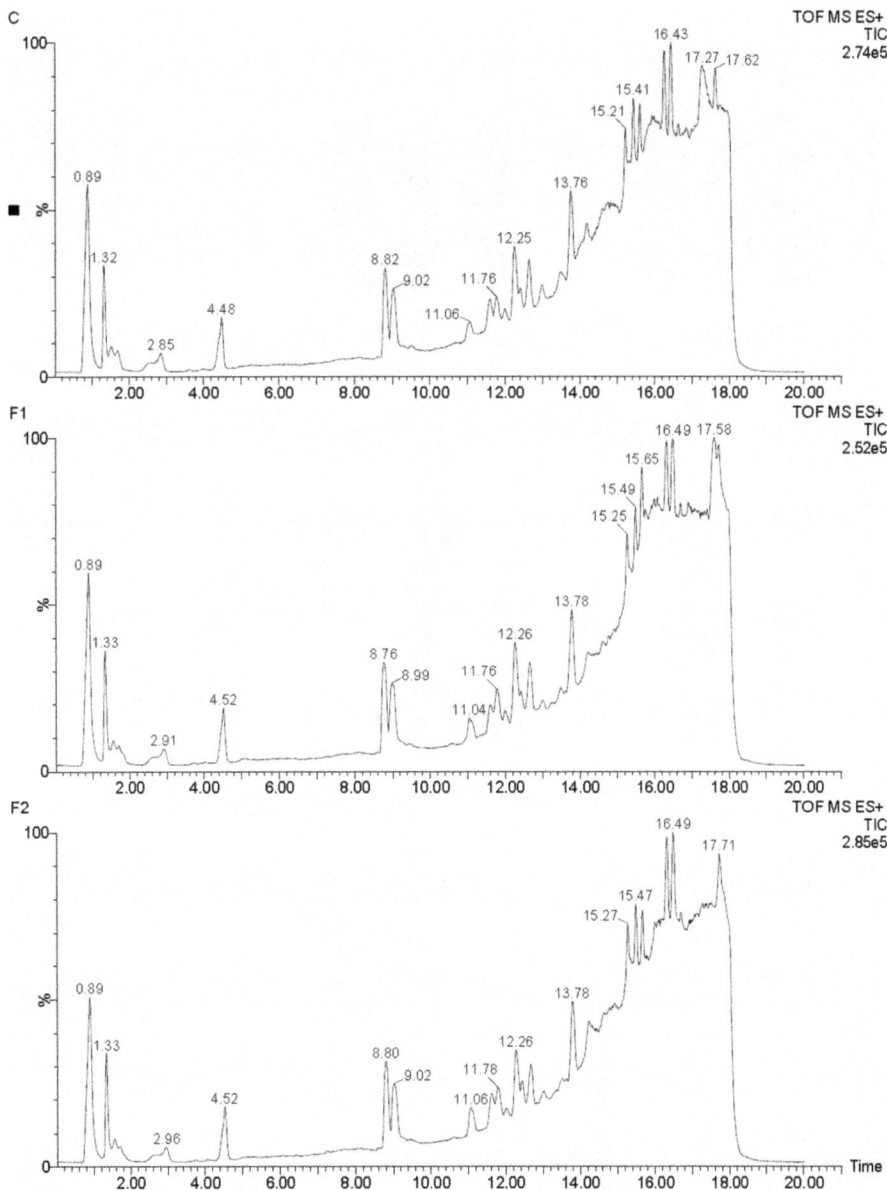

Fig. 1 Representative LC-MS TICs of samples from the ovaries of mice treated with (C) or without FSH for 24 (F1) or 48 h (F2)

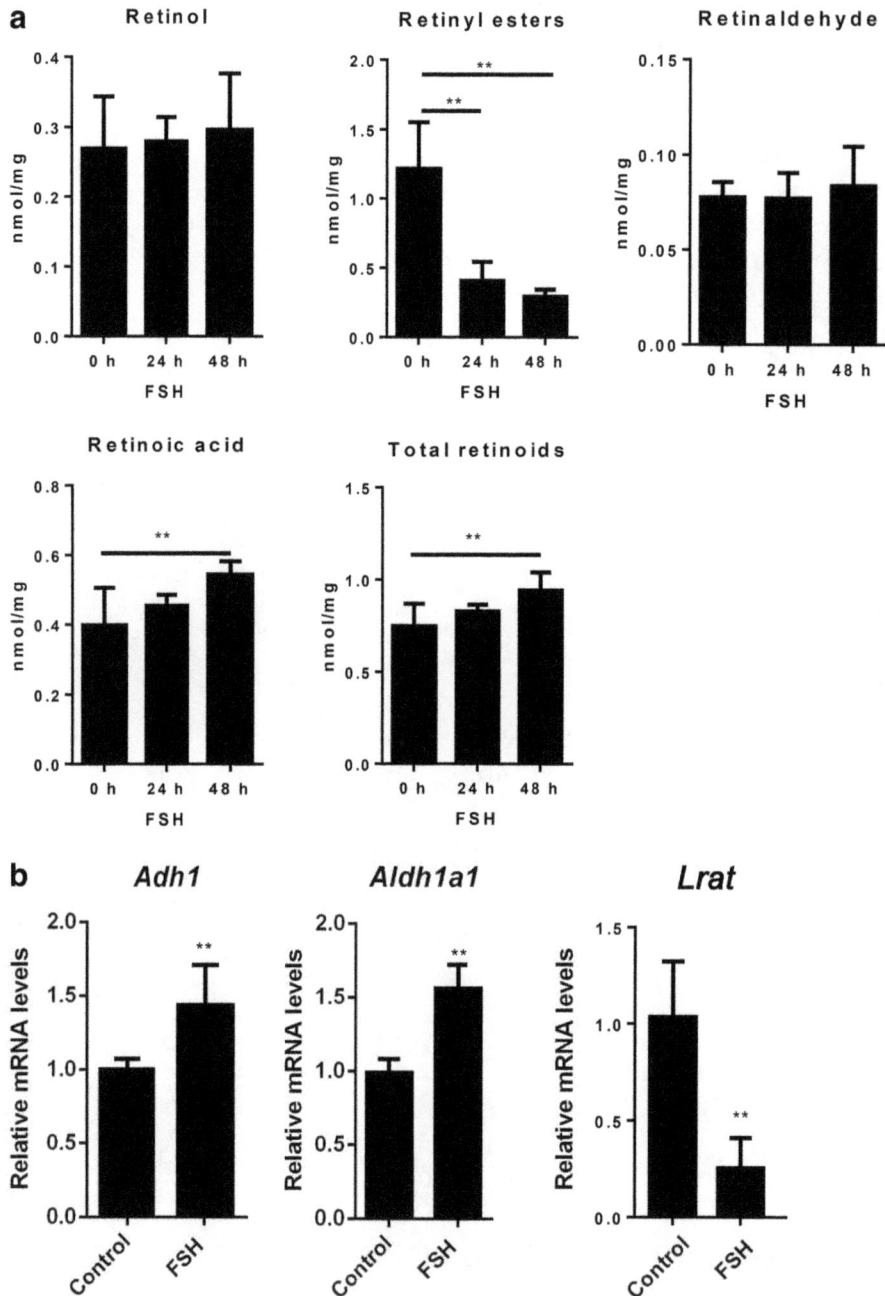

Fig. 2 Effects of FSH on retinol uptake and metabolism in the mouse ovaries. **a** Semi-quantitative LC-MS analysis of retinoid levels in ovaries from untreated mice or mice treated with FSH for 24 or 48 h. **b** Real-time PCR analyses of the expression of genes in retinol uptake and metabolism pathways in ovaries from untreated mice or mice treated with FSH for 48 h. Data are presented as means ± SEM, $n = 5$. $*p < 0.05$, $**p < 0.01$

for 24 h compared with untreated controls (Fig. 4a). The levels of retinol and RA also tended to show an increase (though not significant) (Fig. 4a).

Expression of genes in retinol uptake and metabolism pathways in ovarian follicular cells treated with FSH
We also determined the expression of genes involved in retinol uptake and metabolism in granulosa cells.

The results showed that the mRNA levels for *Stra6*, *Crbp1*, *Adh1*, *Adh7*, and *Aldh1a1* were increased when treated with FSH; however, that of *Lrat* decreased (Fig. 4b).

Discussion
Results from previous studies have shown that de novo synthesized RA, a potent, bioactive member of the

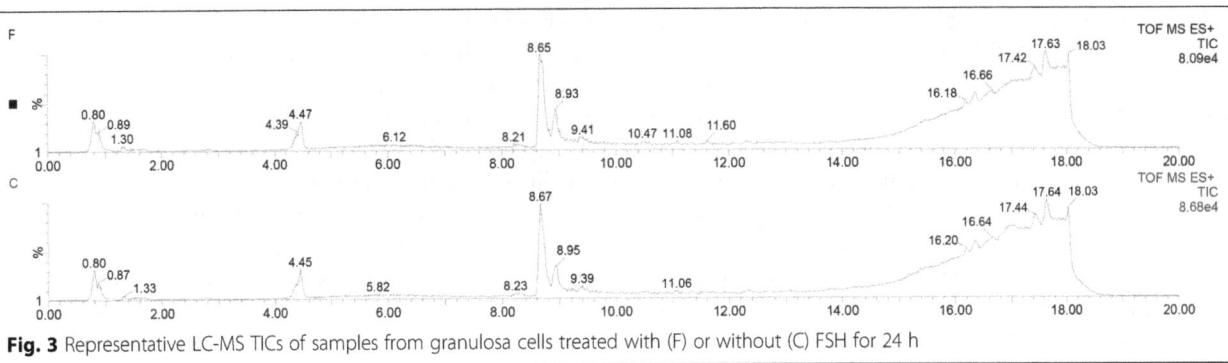

Fig. 3 Representative LC-MS TICs of samples from granulosa cells treated with (F) or without (C) FSH for 24 h

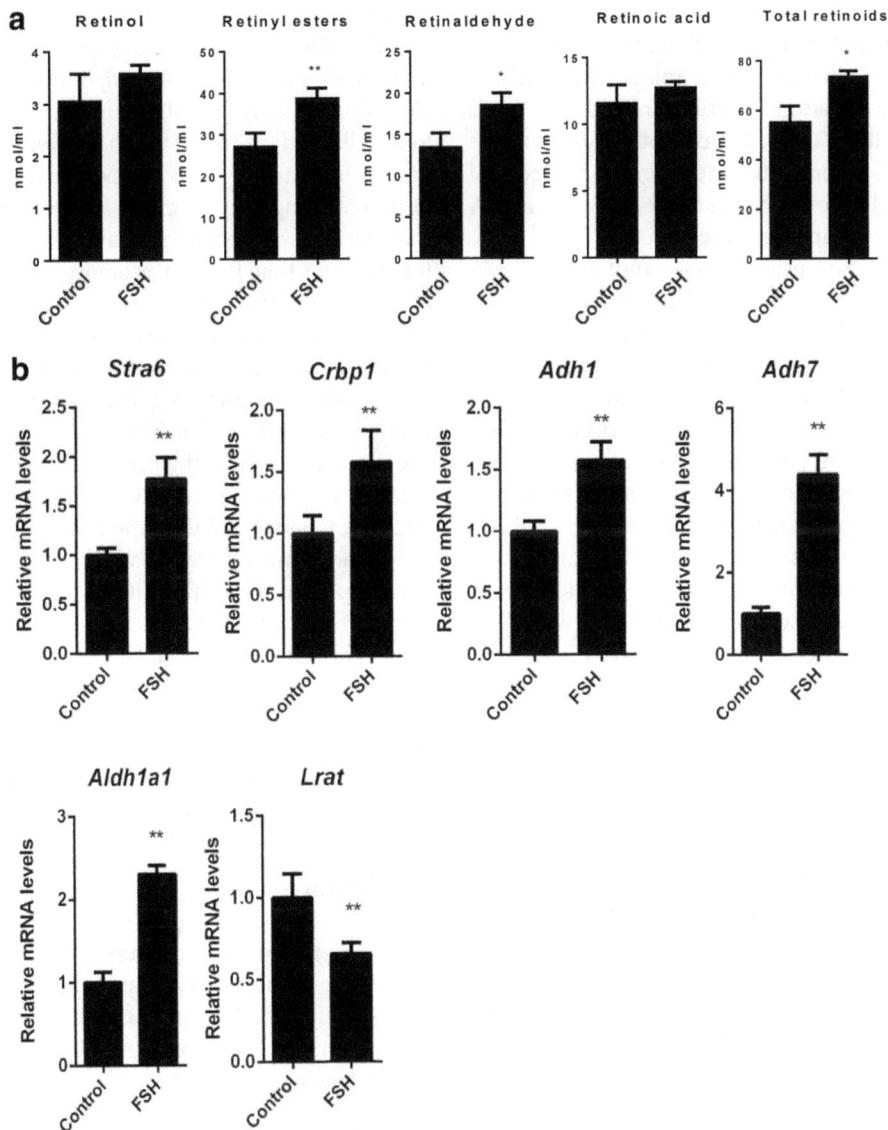

Fig. 4 Effects of FSH on retinol uptake and metabolism in granulosa cells. **a** Semi-quantitative LC-MS analysis of retinoid levels in mouse follicular granulosa cells in the presence or absence of FSH for 24 h. **b** Real-time PCR analyses of the expression of genes in retinol uptake and metabolism pathways in mouse follicular granulosa cells in the presence or absence of FSH for 24 h. Data are presented as means ± SEM, $n = 4$. *$p < 0.05$, **$p < 0.01$

retinoid signaling family, plays crucial roles in ovarian functions [7–10, 27]. RA can enhance LHR expression, stimulate steroidogenesis in granulosa cells and promote oocyte mutation. In addition, the levels of retinoids vary during the estrous cycle and follicular growth, with higher levels in the follicular fluids of large antral follicles [11–13]. However, the mechanisms underlying the regulation of ovarian retinoid accumulation and RA biosynthesis during follicular development remain unclear.

FSH, the primary reproductive hormones that control follicular development and ovarian functions, may be involved in the regulation of ovarian retinoid accumulation and metabolism. Our previous data showed that FSH can stimulate RBP4 expression in developing follicles [23]. RBP4, which acts as the mediator for the systemic and intercellular transport of retinol, plays an important role in the cellular retinol influx, efflux, and exchange of retinol [28]; and seems to play a role in intercellular transport and accumulation of retinol in follicular fluids of dominant follicles [12, 23]. Besides, other studies have also shown that FSH stimulated the expression of several enzymes and binding proteins that are involved in RA synthesis in granulosa and Sertoli cells [7, 23, 29].

In the present study, using semi-quantitative LC-MS analyses, we demonstrated that FSH increased the levels of total retinoids and RA in mouse ovaries in vivo. The results from real-time PCR analyses showed correspondingly that FSH stimulated the expression of ADH1 and ALDH1 genes, which catalyze the conversion of retinol to retinal and retinal to RA, respectively [6]. In contrast, FSH decreased the levels of retinyl esters and inhibited the expression of LRAT, which catalyzes the esterification of retinol [6]. Retinyl esters, such as retinyl palmitate, are thought to be a storage form of retinol [15]; under certain conditions, these retinyl esters are hydrolyzed by cells to produce retinol and bioactive retinoids such as RA. Thus, FSH likely promotes retinol uptake and the conversion of retinol to retinal and RA, and inhibits the esterification of retinol in the mouse ovary in vivo.

As follicular granulosa cells constitute the primary FSH-responsive cell types in the ovary, we employed mouse granulosa cells in primary culture as an in vitro cell model to further confirm the effect of FSH on retinol uptake and metabolism in the mouse ovary. The results showed that FSH increased the levels of total retinoids and retinal; and that FSH also stimulated the gene expression of STRA6 and CRBP1 (which are thought to play important roles in retinol uptake by cells [14–17]), ADH1 and ADH7 (which catalyze the conversion of retinol to retinal [6]), and ALDH1A1 (which catalyzes the conversion of retinal to RA [6]). Therefore, FSH also enhances the uptake and metabolism of retinol in granulosa cells, though the increase in RA levels was not significant. The increase in retinyl ester levels may

be caused by the quick uptake of retinol into cells under the stimulation of FSH, which may then result in the accumulation of retinyl esters. Another study showed that FSH can also increase retinyl ester levels in the presence of physiological concentration of retinol (i.e. 1 μM) in Sertoli cells cultured in vitro [29].

Kawai et al. [7] reported that STRA6, the transmembrane-spanning bidirectional transporter of retinol, was primarily distributed in granulosa cells of large antral follicles. Besides, CRBP1, which also plays an important role in the transportation of retinol into cells, was also reported to be expressed in granulosa cells [12]. ADH1 and ALDH1A1 were also expressed in granulosa cells, though higher expression levels were observed in the theca cell layer [7]. Thus, it is likely that granulosa cells could take up retinol and transform it into retinal and RA. RA synthesized from retinol exerts fundamental actions in granulosa cell differentiation and functions [6]; meanwhile, it may then be secreted from the granulosa cells and delivered to the developing oocytes as a paracrine factor to assist oocyte development and maturation through its receptor RARs. It has been proved that RARs are expressed in all cell types in developing follicles and that RA can promote the nuclear and cytoplasmic maturation of oocytes cultured in vitro [6].

In this study, the increase in RA levels in FSH-stimulated granulosa cells cultured in vitro was not significant but the RA levels increased significantly in the ovaries of FSH-injected mice. This inconsistency may be caused by two possibilities. First, the cells were treated for 24 h in the presence of physiological concentrations of retinol; the time might be too long and the increased RA might be degraded. In another similar study, in which Sertoli cells (one major FSH-responsive cell type in testis) were pre-cultured with FSH for 24 h, followed by incubation with retinol, Guo et al. [29] showed that total RA increased significantly within 2 h and by 12 h no difference was seen from the control. Besides, the cell culture condition may be not very mimic to in vivo environment; in the physical condition, there are many other factors (for example testosterone) existing in the surroundings of granulosa cells.

Conclusion

In conclusion, in the present study, we demonstrated that FSH promoted retinol uptake and its conversion to RA in the mouse ovary. This information is significant when elucidating the mechanisms by which production of endogenous RA-signaling molecules are regulated in the developing follicles.

Abbreviations
ADH: Alcohol dehydrogenase; ALDH: Aldehyde dehydrogenases; CRBP: Cellular retinol-binding protein; FSH: Follicle-stimulating hormone; HPLC: Ultra performance liquid chromatography; LRAT: Lecithin:retinol acyltransferase; MS: Mass spectrometry; RA: Retinoic acid; RAR: Receptor;

RBP4: Retinol-binding protein 4; RXR: Retinoid X receptor; STRA6: Stimulated by RA 6

Acknowledgements
We would like to thank LetPub (www.letpub.com) for providing linguistic assistance during the preparation of this manuscript.
Summary sentence: FSH stimulates retinol uptake and its conversion to retinoic acid in the mouse ovaries and follicular granulosa cells.

Funding
This work was supported by the National Natural Science Foundation of China (grants numbers 31372308, 31672417 and 31301969).

Authors' contributions
YJ, CL and XZ conceived and designed the study; ZL, YS, and YJ performed the experiments and analyzed the data; YJ wrote the manuscript. All authors read and approved the final manuscript.

Competing interests
The authors declare that they have no competing interests.

Author details
¹College of Animal Science, Jilin University, 5333 Xian Road, Changchun 130062, Jilin, China. ²College of Animal Science and Technology, Jilin Agricultural University, 2888 Xincheng Street, Changchun 130118, Jilin, China.

References
1. Walker DM, Gore AC. Transgenerational neuroendocrine disruption of reproduction. Nat Rev Endocrinol. 2011;7:197–207.
2. Thomas FH, Vanderhyden BC. Oocyte-granulosa cell interactions during mouse follicular development: regulation of kit ligand expression and its role in oocyte growth. Reprod Biol Endocrinol. 2006;4:19.
3. Eppig JJ. Reproduction: oocytes call, Granulosa Cells Connect. Curr Biol. 2018;28:R354–R6.
4. Canipari R. Oocyte–granulosa cell interactions. Hum Reprod Update. 2000;6:279–89.
5. Orisaka M, Tajima K, Tsang BK, Kotsuji F. Oocyte-granulosa-theca cell interactions during preantral follicular development. J Ovarian Res. 2009;2:9.
6. Jiang YW, Li CJ, Chen L, Wang FG, Zhou X. Potential role of retinoids in ovarian physiology and pathogenesis of polycystic ovary syndrome. Clin Chim Acta. 2017;469:87–93.
7. Kawai T, Yanaka N, Richards JS, Shimada M. De novo-synthesized retinoic acid in ovarian antral follicles enhances FSH-mediated ovarian follicular cell differentiation and female fertility. Endocrinology. 2016;157:2160–72.
8. Ikeda S, Kitagawa M, Imai H, Yamada M. The roles of vitamin A for cytoplasmic maturation of bovine oocytes. J Reprod Dev. 2005;51:23–35.
9. Tahaei LS, Eimani H, Yazdi PE, Ebrahimi B, Fathi R. Effects of retinoic acid on maturation of immature mouse oocytes in the presence and absence of a granulosa cell co-culture system. J Assist Reprod Genet. 2011;28:553–8.
10. Wickenheisser JK, Nelson-DeGrave VL, Hendricks KL, Legro RS, Strauss JF, McAllister JM. Retinoids and retinol differentially regulate steroid biosynthesis in ovarian theca cells isolated from normal cycling women and women with polycystic ovary syndrome. J Clin Endocrinol Metab. 2005;90:4858–65.
11. Haliloglu S, Baspinar N, Serpek B, Erdem H, Bulut Z. Vitamin A and beta-carotene levels in plasma, corpus luteum and follicular fluid of cyclic and pregnant cattle. Reprod Domest Anim. 2002;37:96–9.
12. Brown JA, Eberhardt DM, Schrick FN, Roberts MP, Godkin JD. Expression of retinol-binding protein and cellular retinol-binding protein in the bovine ovary. Mol Reprod Dev. 2003;64:261–9.
13. Schweigert FJ, Zucker H. Concentrations of vitamin A, beta-carotene and vitamin E in individual bovine follicles of different quality. J Reprod Fertil. 1988;82:575–9.
14. Kawaguchi R, Yu J, Honda J, Hu J, Whitelegge J, Ping P, et al. A membrane receptor for retinol binding protein mediates cellular uptake of vitamin A. Science. 2007;315:820–5.
15. D'Ambrosio DN, Clugston RD, Blaner WS. Vitamin A metabolism: an update. Nutrients. 2011;3:63–103.
16. Isken A, Golczak M, Oberhauser V, Hunzelmann S, Driever W, Imanishi Y, et al. RBP4 disrupts vitamin A uptake homeostasis in a STRA6-deficient animal model for Matthew-wood syndrome. Cell Metab. 2008;7:258–68.
17. Kim YK, Wassef L, Hamberger L, Piantedosi R, Palczewski K, Blaner WS, et al. Retinyl ester formation by lecithin: retinol acyltransferase is a key regulator of retinoid homeostasis in mouse embryogenesis. J Biol Chem. 2008;283:5611–21.
18. Conaway HH, Henning P, Lerner UH. Vitamin A metabolism, action, and role in skeletal homeostasis. Endocr Rev. 2013;34:766–97.
19. Jiang Y, Chen L, Taylor RN, Li C, Zhou X. Physiological and pathological implications of retinoid action in the endometrium. J Endocrinol. 2018;236:R169–R88.
20. Delva L, Bastie JN, Rochette-Egly C, Kraiba R, Balitrand N, Despouy G, et al. Physical and functional interactions between cellular retinoic acid binding protein II and the retinoic acid-dependent nuclear complex. Mol Cell Biol. 1999;19:7158–67.
21. Rochette-Egly C. Retinoic acid signaling and mouse embryonic stem cell differentiation: cross talk between genomic and non-genomic effects of RA. Biochimica Et Biophysica Acta-Molecular And Cell Biology Of Lipids. 2015;1851:66–75.
22. Zhou J, Li C, Yao W, AA M, Huo L, Liu H, et al. Hypoxia-inducible factor-1alpha-dependent autophagy plays a role in glycolysis switch in mouse granulosa cells. Biol Reprod. 2018; https://doi.org/10.1093/biolre/ioy061.
23. Jiang Y, Zhao Y, Chen S, Chen L, Li C, Zhou X. Regulation by FSH of the dynamic expression of retinol-binding protein 4 in the mouse ovary. Reprod Biol Endocrinol. 2018;16:25.
24. Gong S, Sun GY, Zhang M, Yuan HJ, Zhu S, Jiao GZ, et al. Mechanisms for the species difference between mouse and pig oocytes in their sensitivity to glucocorticoids. Biol Reprod. 2017;96:1019–30.
25. Liang N, Xu YL, Yin YM, Yao GD, Tian H, Wang GS, et al. Steroidogenic Factor-1 is required for TGF-beta 3-mediated 17 beta-estradiol synthesis in mouse ovarian granulosa cells. Endocrinology. 2011;152:3213–25.
26. Yao GD, Yin MM, Lian J, Tian H, Liu L, Li X, et al. MicroRNA-224 is involved in transforming growth factor-beta-mediated mouse granulosa cell proliferation and granulosa cell function by targeting Smad4. Mol Endocrinol. 2010;24:540–51.
27. Kipp JL, Golebiowski A, Rodriguez G, Demczuk M, Kilen SM, Mayo KE. Gene expression profiling reveals Cyp26b1 to be an activin regulated gene involved in ovarian granulosa cell proliferation. Endocrinology. 2011;152:303–12.
28. Kawaguchi R, Zhong M, Kassai M, Ter-Stepanian M, Sun H. Vitamin a transport mechanism of the multitransmembrane cell-surface receptor STRA6. Membranes (Basel). 2015;5:425–53.
29. Guo X, Morris P, Gudas L. Follicle-stimulating hormone and leukemia inhibitory factor regulate Sertoli cell retinol metabolism. Endocrinology. 2001;142:1024–32.

## 11

GnRH dysregulation in polycystic ovarian syndrome (PCOS) is a manifestation of an altered neurotransmitter profile

Nirja Chaudhari, Mitali Dawalbhakta and Laxmipriya Nampoothiri[*] ⓘ

Abstract

Background: GnRH is the master molecule of reproduction that is influenced by several intrinsic and extrinsic factors such as neurotransmitters and neuropeptides. Any alteration in these regulatory loops may result in reproductive-endocrine dysfunction such as the polycystic ovarian syndrome (PCOS). Although low dopaminergic tone has been associated with PCOS, the role of neurotransmitters in PCOS remains unknown. The present study was therefore aimed at understanding the status of GnRH regulatory neurotransmitters to decipher the neuroendocrine pathology in PCOS.

Methods: PCOS was induced in rats by oral administration of letrozole (aromatase inhibitor). Following PCOS validation, animals were assessed for gonadotropin levels and their mRNA expression. Neurotrasnmitter status was evaluated by estimating their levels, their metabolism and their receptor expression in hypothalamus, pituitary, hippocampus and frontal cortex of PCOS rat model.

Results: We demonstrate that GnRH and LH inhibitory neurotransmitters – serotonin, dopamine, GABA and acetylcholine – are reduced while glutamate, a major stimulator of GnRH and LH release, is increased in the PCOS condition. Concomitant changes were observed for neurotransmitter metabolising enzymes and their receptors as well.

Conclusion: Our results reveal that increased GnRH and LH pulsatility in PCOS condition likely result from the cumulative effect of altered GnRH stimulatory and inhibitory neurotransmitters in hypothalamic-pituitary centre. This, we hypothesise, is responsible for the depression and anxiety-like mood disorders commonly seen in PCOS women.

Keywords: PCOS, GnRH, LH, FSH, Neurotransmitters

Background

The reproductive system is governed by the hypothalamic-pituitary-gonadal axis (HPG), wherein a pulsatile release of GnRH from the hypothalamus stimulates anterior pituitary gonadotropes to release LH and FSH, leading to steroid production from the ovaries. The regulation of HPG axis is quite complex, involving several intrinsic factors (estrogens, progesterone, inhibin, activin, etc) [1] as well as extrinsic factors (neurotransmitters, neuropeptides, stress, etc) [2]. However, any abnormality that prevents or interferes with the function of these factors may culminate into reproductive endocrine anomalies. One of the most prevalent reproductive endocrinopathies is polycystic ovarian syndrome

(PCOS), affecting 6–10% of women worldwide [3]. The key features of PCOS include hyperandrogenemia, oligo-/ano-vulation and peripheral cyst formation in ovaries [4]. In addition, PCOS is a disorder underpinning neuroendocrine abnormalities, characterized by increased GnRH and LH:FSH ratio [5]. However, in spite of its widespread occurrence and profound implications, the etiology of this disease remains poorly understood.

While reduced norepinephrine, dopamine and serotonin has been reported in the serum of PCOS women [6], their levels in GnRH regulatory regions of the brain are unknown due to the obvious difficulties in obtaining these tissues from patients. A tissue-specific understanding of the neurotransmitters would help us gain an insight into the pathogenesis of PCOS. Thereby, the objective of the current study was to evaluate the status of GnRH-regulatory neurotransmitters in a PCOS rat model.

* Correspondence: lpnmsubaroda@gmail.com
Reproductive-Neuro-Endocrinology Lab, Department of Biochemistry, Faculty of Science, The Maharaja Sayajirao University of Baroda, Vadodara, Gujarat, India

To address the above objective, Letrozole, an aromatase inhibitor, was used to induce PCOS in rats [7]. Evaluation of the neurotransmitter levels was performed from hypothalamus, pituitary as well as from hippocampus and frontal cortex. The reasons for selecting these areas of brain mainly include i) presence of GnRHR in the described tissues, which contributes to regulation of reproduction and reproductive behaviour [8, 9]; ii) active steroidogenesis occurring in these regions [10, 11] and iii) them being important sites of neurotransmitter synthesis [12]. The rates of neurotransmitter synthesis and clearance were monitored by estimating the activities of neurotransmitter metabolizing enzymes. Gene expression analysis of specific neurotransmitter receptors that profoundly influence pulsatile release of GnRH/LH and other reproductive processes was performed in PCOS and normal rats.

Methods
Animals
Charles Foster female rats (2–3 months old) were housed in controlled conditions of temperature, humidity and light with ad libitum availability of food and water. Animals were allowed to acclimatize for one week before treatment. All experimental protocols listed herein were approved by the Institutional animal ethical committee (IAEC), Department of Biochemistry, The M. S. University of Baroda, India and they are in accordance with the ethical standards of the Committee For the Purpose of Control and Supervision of Experiments on Animals (CPCSEA), India.

Induction of PCOS in rats
PCOS was induced in rats by oral administration of letrozole, a non-steroidal aromatase inhibitor [7]. For PCOS induction, 100 rats were randomly assigned to two different groups ($n = 50$ per group). A daily treatment regime of 21 days included oral administration through gavage of 0.5 ml of 1% carboxymethyl cellulose (CMC) for control group and 0.5 mg/kg body weight of letrozole dissolved in CMC for PCOS group. After 21 days of treatment, body weight, oral glucose tolerance, estrus cyclicity, serum estrogen, progesterone and testosterone levels and ovarian histology profile were analysed to check for development of PCOS.

Estrus cyclicity
Estrus cyclicity was monitored daily before (for 14 days) and also during (for 21 days) the course of treatment by microscopic examination of the predominant cell type in vaginal smears [13]. Animals showing regular cycles of 4–5 days complete with the proestrus, estrus, metestrus and diestrus stages were defined as normal cyclic rats, whereas animals in which the estrus cycle was found arrested in any one of the stages for 4 consecutive days were termed as acyclic rats.

Oral glucose tolerance test (OGTT)
OGTT was performed according to the method of Buchanan et al. [14], wherein 12 h fasting blood plasma was collected from orbital sinus into vials containing sodium fluoride and EDTA, followed by oral administration of glucose at 1 g/kg body weight. The blood was then collected every 30 min for 2 h and plasma glucose levels were estimated using Glucose oxidase-peroxidase (GOD-POD) kit (Reckon diagnostics, Vadodara, India).

Blood and tissue collection
Blood and tissue collection was performed during diestrus stage of estrus cycle and between 8 and 9 AM in the morning. Blood was withdrawn through orbital sinus in a tube and centrifuged at 5000 g for 15 min at room temperature. Supernatant containing serum was separated and immediately stored at -80 °C. Following blood collection, animals were euthanized by cervical dislocation. Pituitary, hypothalamus, hippocampus and frontal cortex were dissected out and stored at -80 °C.

Hormone profile
For estimation of hormones, commercially available ELISA kits were used (17β Estradiol ELISA kit-DKO003; Testosterone ELISA kit-DKO002 and Insulin ELISA kit-DKO076; Diametra. Italy). Progesterone was measured through ELISA kit (CAN-P-35) from Diagnostics Biochem Canada Inc., Canada. FSH and LH were estimated in serum using ELISA kits (rat FSH ELISA kit-E-EL-R0391; rat LH ELISA kit-E-EL-R0026) from Elabscience Biotechnology Co., Ltd., USA. Assays were performed according to manufacturers' protocols. Sensitivity of methods are 8.68 pg/ml (17β Estradiol), 0.01 ng/ml (Testosterone), 0.1 ng/ml (Progesterone), 0.025 μIU/ml (Insulin), 0.38 ng/ml (FSH) and 0.19 ng/ml (LH) at 95% confidence limit.

Histology
Ovaries of 6 different animals from each group were removed and fixed in Bouin's fixative. For histological examination, 5 μm thick sections were prepared and stained with Hematoxylin-Eosin and histo-anatomical changes were observed under light microscope [15].

Neurotransmitter estimation
Neurotransmitters were estimated using reverse phase HPLC coupled with electrochemical detector (Waters 2465; Waters corporation, Milford, USA) [16]. Tissues were homogenized in 0.17 M perchloric acid, centrifuged at 12000 g for 20 min at 4 °C and supernatant was immediately used for neurotransmitter estimation or kept at -80 °C until use. For HPLC analysis, tissue samples as well as neurotransmitter standards were mixed with derivatization reagent (37 mM orthopthalaldehyde, 50 mM sodium sulfite, 90 mM tetraborate buffer-pH 10.4 and

5% methanol) for 10 min and 20 µl of sample was injected in HPLC. Glutamate and GABA were separated using a Sunfire® C18 column containing 0.1 M monosodium phosphate, 0.5 mM EDTA and 25% (v/v) methanol (pH 4.5) as mobile phase. For separation of norepinephrine, dopamine and serotonin, mobile phase containing a solution (pH 4.2) of 32 mM citric acid, 12.5 mM disodium hydrogen orthophosphate, 0.5 mM octyl sodium sulfate, 0.5 mM EDTA, 2 mM KCl and 15% (v/v) methanol was used. Standard curves were used to quantify the amount of neurotransmitter in each sample by calculating area under the curve (AUC).

Epinephrine estimation

For epinephrine estimation, a colorimetric method was used [17]. Tissues were homogenized in 10% trichloroacetic acid followed by centrifugation at 10000 g for 10 min at 4 °C. Supernatant (0.2 ml) was added to a tube containing 0.25 ml of 10% (w/v) sodium carbonate and incubated for 30 min at room temperature followed by addition of 0.125 ml of Folin's reagent and 0.375 ml of 5% (w/v) NaOH. Absorbance of epinephrine was recorded at 486 nm within 90 s of incubation.

5-Hydroxy tryptophan decarboxylase (TDC)

TDC was measured spectroflourimetrically as described by Sangwan and group [18]. Tissue homogenates were prepared in 0.1 M sodium phosphate buffer (pH 7.5) containing 5 mM thiourea, 1 mM EDTA and 5 mM β-mercaptoethanol. Tubes containing homogenates were centrifuged at 10000 g for 10 min at 4 °C, supernatant was separated and used as an enzyme source. For TDC assay, 0.1 ml of homogenate was added to a tube containing 0.7 ml of assay buffer (0.1 M sodium phosphate buffer-pH 8.5, 10% glycerol and 5 mM β-mercaptoethanol), 0.1 ml of 10 mM 5-hydroxytryptophan and 0.1 ml of 10 mM pyridoxal phosphate (PLP). The solutions were mixed properly and incubated at 37 °C for 40 min, followed by termination of enzyme reaction by adding 2 ml of 4 N NaOH. Serotonin formed was extracted by adding 3.5 ml of ethyl acetate followed by centrifugation at 1000 g for 10 min. Fluorescence measurement of upper organic layer was taken at 350 nm with prior excitation at 280 nm using a Hitachi F-7000 fluorescence spectrophotometer.

GABA-transaminase (GABAT)

GABAT was estimated by kinetic method using spectrophotometer [19]. Tissues were homogenized in phosphate buffer (50 mM NaH$_2$PO$_4$, 5 mM KCl, 120 mM NaCl, pH 7.4) and centrifuged at 12,000 g for 15 min at 4 °C. The pellet was resuspended in phosphate buffer and was used for enzyme assay. Tissue homogenates (50 µl) were incubated with 1 ml of 100 mM potassium pyrophosphate buffer (pH 8.6) containing 5 mM α-ketoglutarate, 4 mM NAD, 3.5 mM β-mercaptoethanol and 10 µM pyridoxal

phosphate for 15 min at 37 °C. The absorbance of blank was measured at 340 nm followed by addition of 0.1 ml of 100 mM GABA. The absorbance was immediately monitored at 340 nm for every 10 s for 2 min.

Glutamic acid decarboxylase (GAD)

GABA formed by the enzyme GAD was estimated using spectroflourimetry method [20]. Tissues were homogenized in 0.15 M KCl containing 5 mM EDTA and 0.5% triton-X, incubated for 30 min on ice and centrifuged at 3000 g for 10 min. Supernatant (0.1 ml) was incubated with a solution containing 80 mM potassium phosphate buffer (pH 6.2), 25 mM sodium glutamate and 0.5 mM pyridoxal phosphate for 30 min at 37 °C.The reaction of GAD was terminated by addition of 0.5 ml of 15% TCA followed by centrifugation at 5000 g for 10 min. GABA containing supernatant was mixed with 0.5 ml of 14 mM ninhydrin solution and the tubes were kept in a water-bath set at 60 °C for 30 min. The samples were incubated with 5 ml of copper tartarate reagent (160 mg sodium bicarbonate, 30 mg copper sulphate and 33 mg tartaric acid dissolved in 100 ml of distilled water) for 15 min. The fluorescence emission was measured at 451 nm with prior excitation at 377 nm using a Hitachi F-7000 fluorescence spectrophotometer.

Monoamine oxidase (MAOA & MAOB)

Spectrophotometric method was employed for estimation of MAOA and MAOB activity [21]. Tissue homogenates were prepared in homogenate buffer (0.25 M sucrose, 20 mM EDTA and 0.1 M tris- pH 7.4) and cell debris was removed by centrifugation at 800 g for 10 min at 4 °C. The supernatant was centrifuged at 12000 g for 20 min at 4 °C and resultant pellet was dissolved in 0.01 M sodium phosphate buffer (pH 7.4) containing 320 mM sucrose by keeping in ice for 20 min. The tubes were again centrifuged at 3000 g for 10 min at 4 °C and supernatant obtained was used as enzyme source. The assay mixture for MAOA included 0.1 M sodium phosphate buffer (pH 7.4) containing 0.4 mM 5-hydroxytryptamine whereas for MAOB 10 mM of benzylamine was used as a substrate. The reaction was terminated by addition of 0.2 ml of 1 M HCl after 20 min of incubation at 37 °C. Product formed was extracted by vortexing for 5 min with 2 ml of butyl acetate for MAOA or cyclohexane for MAOB. Tubes were centrifuged at 3000g for 5 min and upper organic layer was measured at wavelength of 280 nm for MAO-A activity and 242 nm for MAO-B activity with spectrophotometer, respectively.

Glutamate dehydrogenase (GDH)

GDH activity was measured in the direction of oxidative deamination of glutamate into α-ketoglutarate [22]. Tissues were homogenized in 10 volume of 0.25 M sucrose-10 mM HEPES, pH -7.4 and centrifuged at 1000 g for

10 min at 4 °C. The supernatant was collected in a fresh vial and centrifuged at 12000 g for 30 min at 4 °C to yield mitochondrial pellet which was dissolved in homogenate buffer and used as enzyme source. The enzyme (0.05 ml) was added to assay mixture (50 mM tris buffer-pH 9.5, 1 M glutamate, 0.1 M EDTA, 56 mM NAD and 40 mM ADP) and absorbance was monitored immediately at 340 nm for every 10 s for 1 min.

Acetylcholine esterase (AChE)

Acetylcholine is degraded by enzyme AChE, which was estimated by kinetic method [23]. Tissue homogenates were prepared in 0.1 M sodium phosphate buffer (pH 8.0), centrifuged at 12000 g for 5 min at 4 °C and resulting supernatant was used as enzyme source. Tubes containing 1.5 ml of 0.1 M phosphate buffer (pH 8.0), 0.01 ml of freshly prepared substrate (75 mM acetylcholine iodide in distilled water) and 0.05 ml of freshly made Ellman's reagent (10 mM DTNB and 17.85 mM $NaHCO_3$ dissolved in 0.1 M sodium phosphate buffer – pH 7.0) were incubated at 25 °C. Absorbance of blank was measured at 405 nm followed by addition of 0.2 ml of enzyme. The change in absorbance was monitored thereafter for 10 min at every 2 min-interval.

RNA isolation and PCR

Total RNA was extracted using TRIsoln reagent (GeNei, India) and 2 μg of RNA was reverse-transcribed using Verso cDNA synthesis kit with Oligo-dT primers (ThermoScientific, USA). Real-time quantitative polymerase chain reaction (qPCR) was performed using Quantstudio Real Time PCR system (Life Technologies, USA). Primers were procured from IDT (CA, USA) and their sequences are given in Table 1. All the samples were run in triplicate and accompanied by a non-template control. PCR was performed with SYBR select PCR Master Mix (Applied Biosystems, USA) according to manufacturer's protocol. Thermal cycling conditions included initial denaturation in one cycle of 15 min at 95 °C, followed by 45 cycles of 15 s at 94 °C, 30 s at 60 °C and 30 s at 72 °C. The fold changes in the mRNA were calculated for each sample group using the $2^{-\Delta\Delta CT}$ method [24]. Fold changes in expression of less than 0.5 and greater than 2 were considered biologically significant.

Statistical analysis

Statistical analysis was performed using Student's t-test and Two-way ANOVA, followed by Bonferroni *post-hoc* test using GraphPad Prism 5 software. P values of < 0.05 were deemed to be statistically significant.

Table 1 Primer sequences of rat targeted genes

Targeted Genes	Primer sequence	Accession number
GnRH1	F: 5′ CCGCTGTTGTTCTGTTGACTG 3′ R: 5′ TCACACTCGGATGTTGTGGA 3′	NM_012767
GnRHR	F: 5′ TCTGCAATGCCAAAATCATC 3′ R: 5′ GTAGGGAGTCCAGCAGATGAC 3′	NM_031038.3
FSHβ	F: 5′ AGGAAGAGTGCCGTTTCTGC 3′ R: 5′ GCTGTCACTATCACACTTGC 3′	NM_001007597.2
LHβ	F: 5′ CTGTCCTAGCATGGTTCGAGT 3′ R: 5′ AGTTAGTGGGTGGGCATCAG 3′	NM_012858.2
TH	F: 5′ CATTGGACTTGCATCTCTGG 3′ R: 5′ GTTCCTGAGCTTGTCCTTGG 3′	NM_012740.3
COMT	F: 5′ GACGCGAAAGGCCAAATCAT 3′ R: 5′ ACGTTGTCAGCTAGGAGCA 3′	NM_012531.2
5HT1A	F:5′CCCCCCAAGAAGAGCCTGAA3′ R:5′GGCAGCCAGCAGAGGATGAA3′	NM_012585.1
α1AR	F: 5′ ACCAGCTCCGGTGAACATTT 3′ R: 5′ GCCGCCCAGATATTGCAGAA 3′	NM_017191.2
D2R	F:5′ TGAACCTGTGTGCCATCAGCA 3′ R:5′ TTGGCTCTGAAAGCTCGACTG 3′	NM_012547.1
GABAB1	F:5′CGCTACCATCCAACAGACCA3′ R:5′TGTCAGCATACCACCCGATG3′	NM_031028.3
M2-AchR	F:5′CACAGTTTCCACTTCGCTGG 3′ R:5′ CACCTTTTTGGGCCTTGGTG 3′	NM_031016.1
NMDAR	F:5′ ACACCGACCAAGAAGCCATC 3′ R:5′ GGACTCATCCTTATCCGCCA 3	NM_012574.1
β-Actin	F: 5′ AGGCCCCTCTGAACCCTAAG 3′ R: 5′ GGAGCGCGTAACCCTCATAG 3′	NM_031144.3

Results

Induction of PCOS in rats

Testosterone levels were significantly elevated in serum of letrozole treated animals ($P < 0.001$) with a decrease in progesterone levels ($P < 0.05$) and no change in serum estradiol levels (Table 2). Figure 1 demonstrates the ovarian histology. Control sections showed follicles in various stages of development (Fig. 1a) whereas treatment group sections had numerous peripheral cysts along with low number of corpus lutea (Fig. 1b, c and d). Treatment group also had a high percentage of acyclic rats (disturbed estrus cycle) (Fig. 1e); mainly arrested in diestrus stage. Further, there was a significant increase in the body weight (Fig. 1f) ($P < 0.01$), glucose intolerance (Fig. 1g), area under the curve for glucose (Fig. 1h), serum insulin level ($P < .001$) and HOMA-IR index (Table 2) of letrozole treated group as compared to the CMC control group. All the animals of letrozole-treated group exhibited hormonal and structural alterations and were considered as PCOS positive rats for further experiments.

Gonadotropin status in PCOS

GnRH1 plays a pivotal role in stimulating pituitary release of FSH and LH. When analysed for gene expression (Fig. 2a) , PCOS rats demonstrated significantly increased transcripts of hypothalamic *GnRH1* ($P < 0.01$) and pituitary *GnRHR* ($P < 0.01$), while hypothalamic *GnRHR* expression was reduced ($P < 0.001$) as compared to control rats. GnRH released from the hypothalamus stimulates gonadotropin secretion from anterior pituitary. Gonadotropin estimations revealed no change in FSH levels among both the groups while a significant increase was observed in LH levels of PCOS rats ($P < 0.001$), leading to an elevated LH:FSH ratio (Table 3). To examine whether the origin of this alteration lies at the genetic level, transcript analysis was carried out. In present study, both the *FSHβ* ($P < 0.05$) as well as *LHβ* ($P < 0.01$) mRNA were found significantly increased in the pituitary of PCOS rats as compared to control (Fig. 2b).

Neurotransmitter levels in PCOS rats

GnRH and LH release are mainly influenced by various neurotransmitters secreted by discrete brain regions. When estimated, serotonin levels (Fig. 3a) were significantly reduced in all the tissues analysed with greatest decrease in hypothalamus ($P < 0.001$) and pituitary ($P < 0.001$) of PCOS group rats as compared to control. A similar trend was observed for norepinephrine (Fig. 3b) content. Epinephrine

levels (Fig. 3c) were also decreased in hypothalamus ($P < 0.01$) and pituitary ($P < 0.01$) of PCOS animals; however no difference was observed in hippocampus and frontal cortex. Furthermore, notably low levels of dopamine (Fig. 3d) and GABA (Fig. 3e) were also seen in all tested brain tissues of PCOS animals as compared to control rats. In contrast to all these neurotransmitters, the amount of glutamate was significantly elevated (Fig. 3f) in hypothalamus ($P < 0.001$), pituitary ($P < 0.001$), hippocampus ($P < 0.01$) and frontal cortex ($P < 0.01$) of PCOS rats as compared to control.

Neurotransmitter synthesizing enzymes in PCOS rats

The turnover of neurotransmitters is tightly regulated by the activities of their metabolising enzymes. Serotonin synthesizing enzyme Tryptophan decarboxylase (TDC) was reduced in all analysed brain tissues of PCOS animals ($P < 0.01$), except in the hippocampus (Fig. 4a). GABA-T, which acts as a synthesizing enzyme for glutamate and degrading enzyme for GABA, showed heightened activity in hypothalamus ($P < 0.01$), pituitary ($P < 0.01$), hippocampus ($P < 0.05$) and frontal cortex ($P < 0.05$) of PCOS rats as compared to control animals (Fig. 4b). Glutamic acid decarboxylase (GAD) enzyme catalyses the conversion of glutamate into GABA. GAD activity exhibited notable decrease in hypothalamus ($P < 0.01$) and pituitary ($P < 0.01$) of PCOS rats but no change was observed in other tissues (Fig. 4c). Furthermore, gene expression of tyrosine hydroxylase *(TH)*, a rate limiting enzyme for all catecholamine synthesis, was reduced in hypothalamus ($P < 0.01$) and pituitary ($P < 0.05$) of PCOS rats as compared to control (Fig. 4d).

Neurotransmitter degrading enzymes in PCOS rats

Neurotransmitters are quickly metabolized through degrading enzymes secreted into the synaptic cleft. Serotonin, norepinephrine, dopamine and epinephrine are metabolized by monoamine oxidase (MAO). When analysed for activity, a significant increase in MAO-A was observed in hypothalamus ($P < 0.001$), pituitary ($P < 0.001$), hippocampus ($P < 0.01$) and frontal cortex ($P < 0.01$) of PCOS rats as compared to control animals (Fig. 5a). MAO-B also followed a similar trend in all the tissues but it was less obvious as compared to MAO-A activity (Fig. 5b). Another major enzyme which degrades catecholamines dopamine, norepinephrine and epinephrine is Catechol-O-methyl transferase (COMT). The transcript level of *COMT* was markedly elevated in hypothalamus ($P < 0.01$) and pituitary ($P < 0.05$) of PCOS rats while no change was observed in

Table 2 Serum hormone profile after 21 days of letrozole treatment

	Estradiol (pg/ml)	Testosterone (ng/ml)	Progesterone (ng/ml)	Insulin(μIU/ml)	HOMA-IR
Control	132.3 ± 17.37	0.315 ± 0.05	12.25 ± 0.54	7.42 ± 1.04	1.56 ± 0.14
Let-treated	139.3 ± 19.10	1.177 ± 0.07***	9.95 ± 0.39*	15.54 ± 1.27***	4.40 ± 0.21***

All values are presented as Mean ± SEM; $n = 6$ per group; *$P < 0.05$; ***$P < 0.001$ as compared to control

$$\text{HOMA - IR} = \frac{\text{Glucose (mg/dl)} \times \text{Insulin (μIU/ml)}}{405}$$

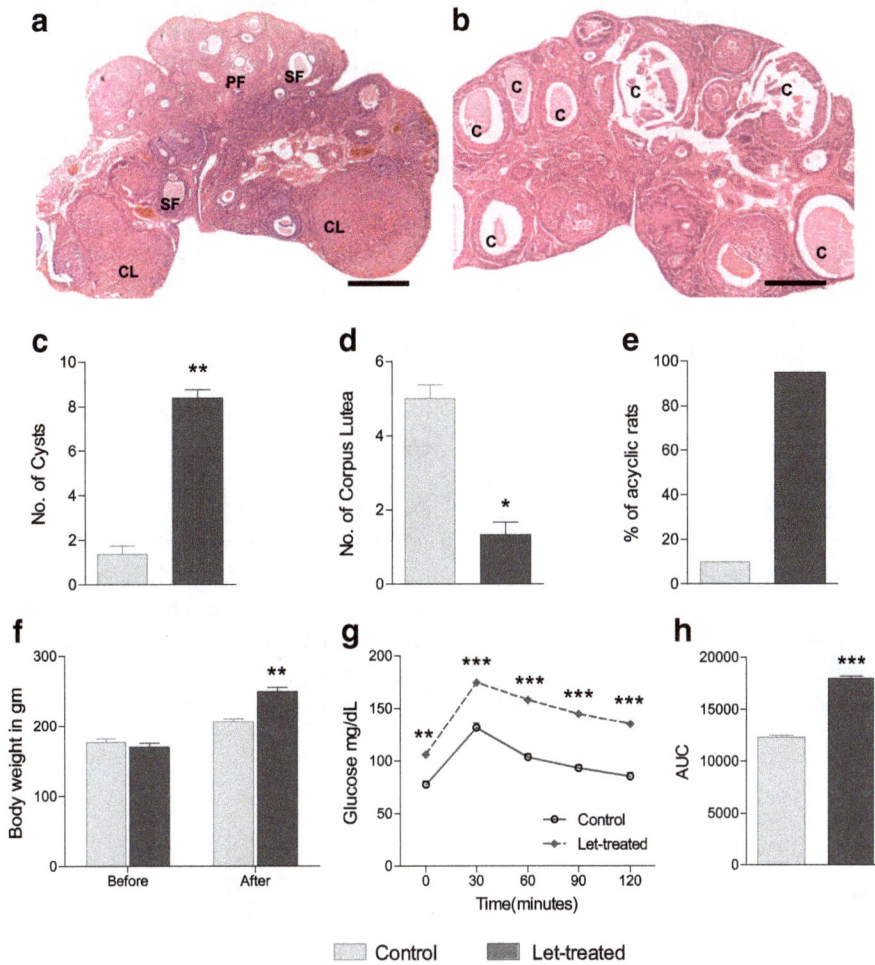

Fig. 1 Validation of PCOS rat model after 21 days of letrozole treatment. Hematoxylin-Eosin stained ovarian sections of Control group (**a**) and letrozole treatment group (**b**) under 4X magnification (Scale bar = 500μm). PF: Primary follicle; SF: secondary follicle; CL: Corpus luteum; C: Cyst. **c** Number of cystic follicles, **d** number of CL, and **e** percent of females that were acyclic after letrozole treatment. Change in body weight (**f**); Oral glucose tolerance test profile (**g**) and area under the curve (AUC) for glucose tolerance (**h**) in control and treated rats. Error bars represent SEM; $n = 6$–10 per group; **$P < 0.01$; ***$P < 0.001$ as compared to control group

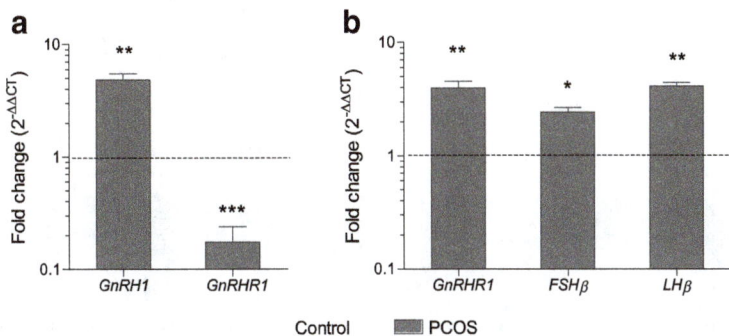

Fig. 2 Gonadotropin status in letrozole-induced PCOS animals. **a** Expression profile of hypothalamic *GnRH1*, *GnRHR1*, and **b** pituitary *GnRHR1*, *FSHβ* and *LHβ*. *β-Actin* was used as internal control and fold change in expression was calculated by $2^{-\Delta\Delta CT}$ method. Values are mean fold change in gene expression of PCOS group samples as compared to control samples (represented by black dashed line). Error bars represent SEM; $n = 6$ per group; **$P < 0.01$; ***$P < 0.001$ as compared to control group

Table 3 Serum Gonadotropin levels in letrozole induced PCOS rat model

	FSH (ng/ml)	LH (ng/ml)	LH: FSH
Control	2.20 ± 0.099	2.40 ± 0.138	1.08: 1
PCOS	2.29 ± 0.180	6.76 ± 0.132 ***	2.97: 1***

All values are presented as Mean ± SEM; $n = 6$ per group; ***$P < 0.001$ as compared to control values

other tissues (Fig. 5c). In addition, metabolizing enzymes glutamate dehydrogenase (GDH) and acetylcholine esterase (AChE), which degrade glutamate and acetylcholine respectively, were also assessed. Acetylcholine esterase activity (Fig. 5d) was also higher in PCOS animals as evident in hypothalamus ($P < 0.01$), pituitary ($P < 0.01$) and hippocampus ($P < 0.05$). In contrast to other metabolizing enzymes activity, that is increased in PCOS animals, GDH activity (Fig. 5e) was significantly low in hypothalamus ($P < 0.01$), pituitary ($P < 0.01$), hippocampus ($P < 0.05$) and frontal cortex as compared to control tissues.

Neurotransmitter receptor profile in PCOS rats

Neurotransmitter receptors expressed on pre- or postsynaptic neurons relay their biological action. An mRNA expression profile of various neurotransmitter receptors was thus generated using quantitative real-time PCR. Transcript levels for serotonin receptor *5HT1A*, adrenergic alpha1 receptor *(α1AR)*, dopamine D2 receptor (*D2R*) and *GABAB1* receptor declined significantly in all tissues tested in PCOS rats as compared to control (Fig. 6a-d). Transcriptional down-regulation of muscarinic acetylcholine 2 receptor (*M2AchR*) receptor (Fig. 6e) was also observed in hypothalamus (P < 0.05) and pituitary ($P < 0.05$) of PCOS animals. Contrary to all these and in line with glutamate content, *NMDA* receptor expression (Fig. 6f) was found markedly high in hypothalamus ($P < 0.01$), pituitary ($P < 0.001$), hippocampus ($P < 0.05$) and frontal cortex ($P < 0.05$) of PCOS animals when compared with control tissues.

Discussion

PCOS is a very common endocrine disorder in women of reproductive age and is characterized by increased androgen production and abnormal gonadotropin secretion, resulting in chronic anovulation. To understand the etiopathology of PCOS, the present study employed a letrozole-treated rat model, which exhibits hormonal,

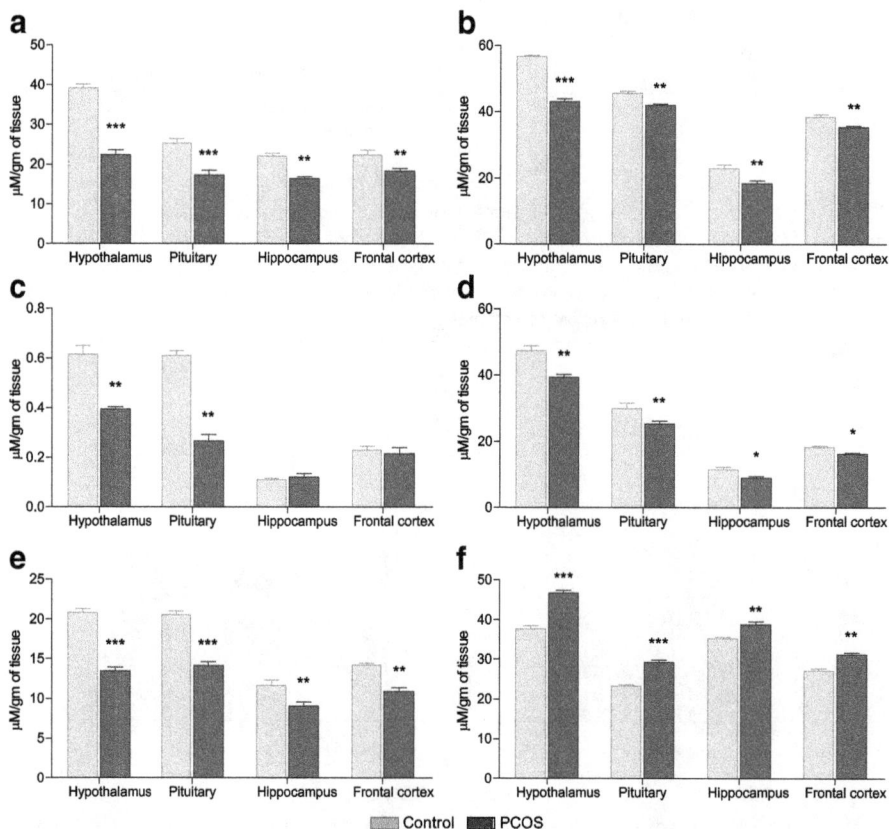

Fig. 3 Neurotransmitter levels in control and PCOS animals. **a** Serotonin, **b** norepinephrine, **c** epinephrine, **d** dopamine, **e** GABA and **f** glutamate levels in different tissues of control and PCOS rats. All values are represented as Mean ± SEM; $n = 6$ per group; *$P < 0.05$; **$P < 0.01$; ***$P < 0.001$ as compared to control group

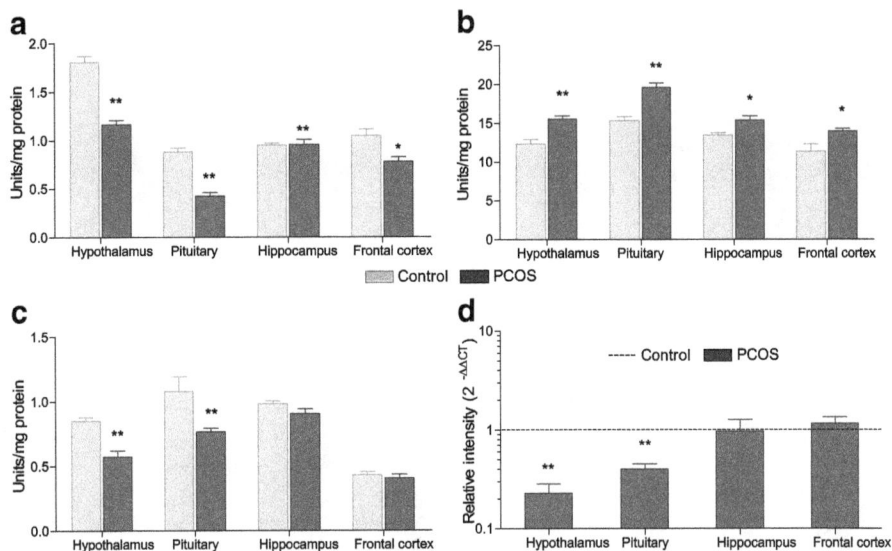

Fig. 4 Status of neurotransmitter synthesizing enzymes. Activity of **a** tryptophan decarboxylase (TDC), **b** GABA transaminase (GABA-T), and **c** glutamic acid decarboxylase (GAD) in different tissues of control and PCOS rats. **d** Values are mean fold change in tyrosine hydroxylase (TH) mRNA expression of PCOS group samples as compared to control samples (represented by black dashed line). β-Actin was used as internal control for mRNA studies and fold change in expression was calculated by $2^{-\Delta\Delta CT}$ method. Error bars represent SEM; $n = 6$ per group; $*P < 0.05$; $**P < 0.01$; $***P < 0.001$ as compared to control group

reproductive and metabolic signs similar to the human PCOS condition [7, 25, 26]. Furthermore, it was observed currently that the PCOS rats had a high serum LH:FSH ratio, a characteristic feature of PCOS. This, we believe, must stem from increased transcription of the *GnRH* in the hypothalamus and *GnRHR* in the pituitary, as also observed by Kauffman and group [26]. Thus, letrozole-induced PCOS rat model possesses similar neuroendocrine traits as seen in PCOS women, making it a favourable model for use in PCOS research.

A number of studies using dual-label immunohisto-chemistry and in situ hybridization have shown that several neurotransmitter and neuropeptide receptors are expressed in GnRH neurons and they directly regulate GnRH, LH and FSH release [2]. The effect of serotonin on GnRH neurons is biphasic in nature wherein activation of 5-HT2A receptor increases GnRH neuronal activity via PKC (Protein kinase C) pathway, while activation of 5-HT1A receptor suppresses GnRH neuronal firing through adenylate cyclase [27, 28]. Serotonin content was found significantly reduced in all brain tissues of PCOS animals as compared to control, which can be well correlated with the observed decrease in TDC activity (serotonin synthesis) and heightened MAO activity. Also, the expression of 5HT1A receptor was decreased in PCOS animals. Based on this, and the above-cited references, increased GnRH and LH release in PCOS may result, at least partially, from reduced inhibition of GnRH by serotonin.

In addition to serotonin, the role of catecholamines is also known in GnRH regulation. Norepinephrine has been shown to rapidly increase GnRH mRNA levels in

ovariectomised rats [29]. It is also responsible for the pre-ovulatory LH surge through the α- and β-adrenergic receptors. Propranolol, an α-adrenergic receptor blocker stimulates NE-induced LH release, while treatment of β-antagonist blocked the release of pre-ovulatory LH surge [30, 31]. This indicates that the stimulatory effect of norepinephrine on LH release is mediated by β-adrenergic receptors while α-adrenergic receptor inhibits LH release. Moreover, α-adrenergic receptor is also involved in steroid mediated feedback regulation of GnRH [32]. In the case of epinephrine, although reports on GnRH regulation are rare, a positive relation is implied, where the former stimulates release of GnRH and LH, also through the α-adrenergic receptor [33, 34]. Whereas both epinephrine and norepinephrine were reduced in the brain of PCOS rats, the GnRH and LH were still elevated, pointing towards the involvement of other regulatory factors in this outcome.

Unlike norepinephrine and epinephrine, dopamine is a major suppressor for GnRH release [35]. It also inhibited the firing and anteroventral paraventricular (AVPV)-evoked GABA/glutamate postsynaptic currents in the GnRH neu-rons in vitro mediated by D1 and D2-like receptors in male and female mice [35]. Recent study in ewes also suggests that D2 dopamine receptor not only affects the GnRH release but also GnRH and GnRHR gene expression in hypothalamus. Also, LH pulse frequency increases upon local injection of Sulpride (D2R antagonist) in ewes, reflect-ing the potency of D2R in inhibiting GnRH and LH pulsati-lity [36]. In addition to its influence on GnRH/LH, it has an inhibitory effect on prolactin release. A positive association between PCOS, low dopamine and hyperprolactinemia has

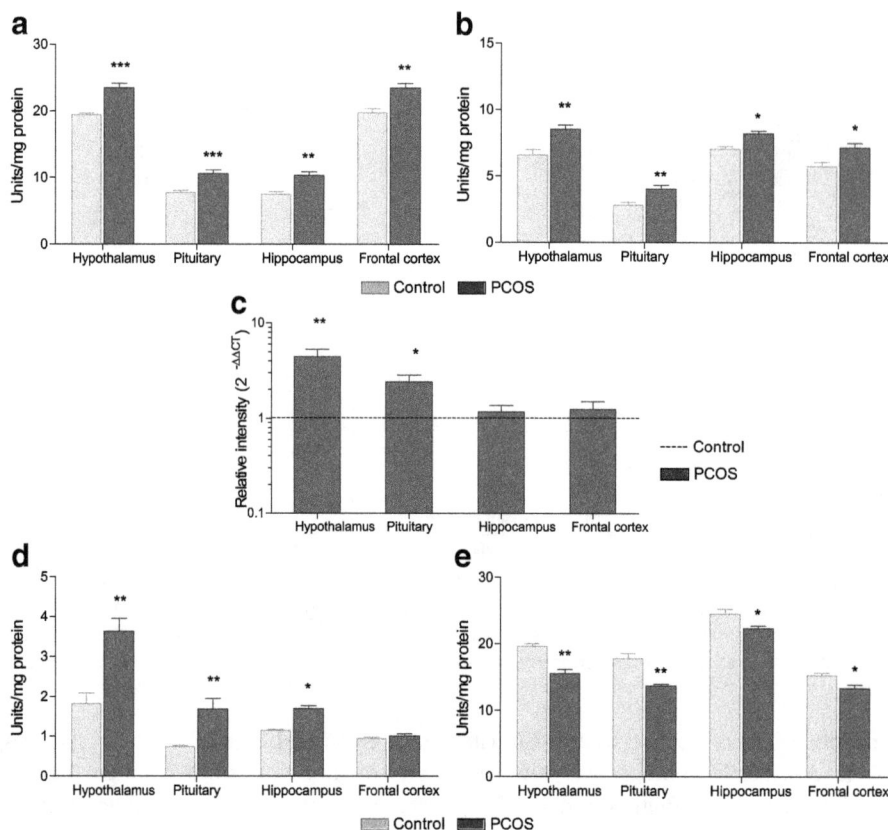

Fig. 5 Status of neurotransmitter degrading enzymes in PCOS rats. Enzyme activity of **a** monoamine oxidase A (MAOA) and **b** MAOB in various tissues of control and PCOS rats. **c** Bar graph represents values of mean fold change in gene expression of Catechol-O-methyl transferase (COMT) in PCOS animals as compared to control rats (represented by black dashed line). β-Actin was used as internal control for mRNA studies and fold change in expression was calculated by $2^{-\Delta\Delta CT}$ method. Activity of **d** acetylcholine esterase (AChE) and **e** glutamate dehydrogenase (GDH) in tissues of control and PCOS animals. Error bars represent SEM; $n = 6$ per group; *$P < 0.05$; **$P < 0.01$; ***$P < 0.001$ as compared to control group

been suggested [37]. Further, hyperprolactinemia exerts an inhibitory effect on the gonadotrophs [38]. In the present case, dopamine content in brain of PCOS rats was significantly decreased along with reduced expression of D2R, which may result into hypersecretion of prolactin in PCOS condition. Supporting our data, many studies suggest the role of reduced dopaminergic tone in increased LH release in PCOS [39, 40]. Additionally, treatment with bromocriptine, a D2 receptor agonist, can restore normal menstrual cycle and ovulation in PCOS women [39].

GABA is the major inhibitory neuron of the central nervous system. GABAB1 knockout mice demonstrated abnormal estrus cyclicity and reduced fecundity with significantly increased GnRH release as well as GnRH pulse frequency [41], whereas GABAA knockdown mice had normal estrus cycle and puberty onset [42]. In addition, treatment of GABA or muscimol, a GABAA/C receptor agonist, to cultured anterior pituitary cells results into increased secretion of LH through Ca2+ release [43]. However, when cultured pituitary cells were incubated with baclofen, a GABAB agonist, GnRH-induced LH

release was inhibited while basal LH secretion did not change [43, 44]. This suggests that GABAA/C stimulate basal LH secretion whereas GABAB suppresses GnRH-induced LH release. Reduced signalling of GABA through GABAB1 observed in our system may have contributed to an increased GnRH/LH pulse. Interestingly, a study in prenatally androgenised mouse model of PCOS demonstrated increased GABA innervations to GnRH neurons [45]. This disparity in the result is likely due to the fact that Moore and group have used arcuate nucleus for their study while we have used whole hypothalamus, which includes many such nuclei. Also, this group has used prenatally androgenised mouse model of PCOS [45] and in utero androgen exposure can lead to epigenetic changes, which could result in developmental alterations in neural circuits.

In contrast to GABA, Glutamate is the major excitatory neurotransmitter for GnRH release. GnRH neurons express both ionotropic glutamate receptors (AMPA, Kainate and NMDA) and metabotropic glutamate receptors. However, reports describing the role of metabotropic

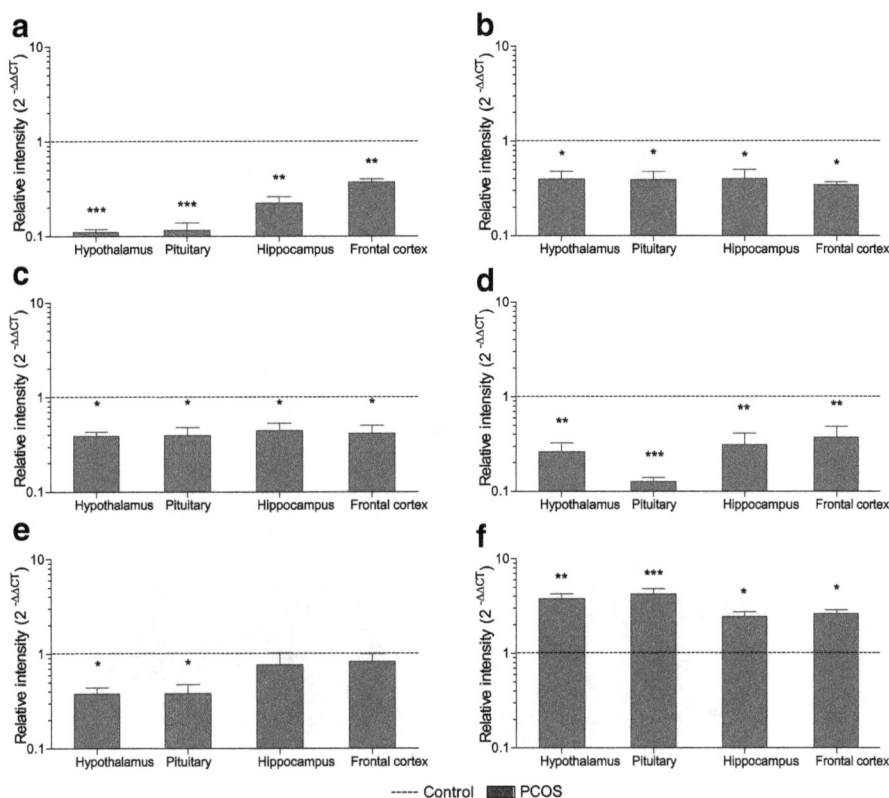

Fig. 6 Transcript analysis of neurotransmitter receptor in PCOS rats. mRNA expression profile of **a** serotonin 5HT1A receptor (5HT$_{1A}$); **b** alpha1-adrenergic receptor (α$_1$AR); **c** dopamine D$_2$ receptor (D$_2$R); **d** GABA B1 receptor (GABA$_{B1}$); **e** muscarinic acetylcholine 2 receptor (M$_2$AchR) and **f** NMDA glutamate receptor (NMDA) in control and PCOS brain tissues. Bar graph represents values of mean fold change in gene expression of PCOS animals as compared to control rats (represented by black dashed line). β-Actin was used as internal control for mRNA studies and fold change in expression was calculated by 2$^{-\Delta\Delta CT}$ method. Error bars represent SEM; n = 6 per group; *P < 0.05; **P < 0.01; ***P < 0.001 as compared to control group

glutamate receptors in GnRH regulation are scanty [46]. NMDA receptor antagonist-MK801 abolished endogenous pulses of GnRH secretion whereas pulsatile release of GnRH was not affected in the presence of 6,7-dinitroquinoxaline-2,3-dione (kainate receptor blocker) [47]. In addition, mRNA and protein expression study has revealed the presence of vesicular glutamate transporter in gonadotrophs of anterior pituitary and a stimulatory role for glutamate in LH release was also documented [48, 49]. In PNA-induced PCOS mouse model, no effect of glutamate was observed in GnRH pulsatility [45]. However, significantly high glutamate levels and NMDA receptor expression in PCOS animals were observed in the current study, suggesting direct overstimulation of GnRH and LH release. Further, the activities of GAD and GDH were significantly decreased in PCOS rats while that of GABA-T was markedly elevated suggesting that in PCOS condition the flux of reaction is towards the glutamate and not towards GABA.

Along with all the above-stated neurotransmitters, the role of acetylcholine in GnRH regulation is also emerging. In cultured GT1–7 cell line, acetylcholine stimulates GnRH

release through activation of nicotinic receptor whilst an inhibitory effect of acetylcholine on GnRH activity was mediated by muscarinic receptor activation [50]. Also, in GT1–7 cells, acetylcholine treatment activates M2 muscarinic receptor that further reduces forskolin-induced cAMP production followed by suppression of GnRH release [51]. Similarly, treatment of exogenous acetylcholine to cultured anterior pituitary cells resulted in decreased response of GnRH-induced LH release. This response was counteracted by muscarinic receptor antagonist atropine [52]. Currently, activity of acetylcholine esterase (AChE), a hydrolytic enzyme of acetylcholine, was found elevated in the hypothalamus and pituitary of PCOS rats along with decreased expression of M2 muscarinic acetylcholine receptor (M2AChR), thus, suggesting reduced levels of acetylcholine in PCOS condition which may contribute to increased GnRH and LH pulse frequency in PCOS women.

It should be noted that along with neurotransmitters, HPG axis is governed by several neuropeptides of the like of kisspeptin, a major factor which directly or through its interaction with steroids and neurotransmitters, stimulates the release and expression of GnRH/LH [53, 54]. Various

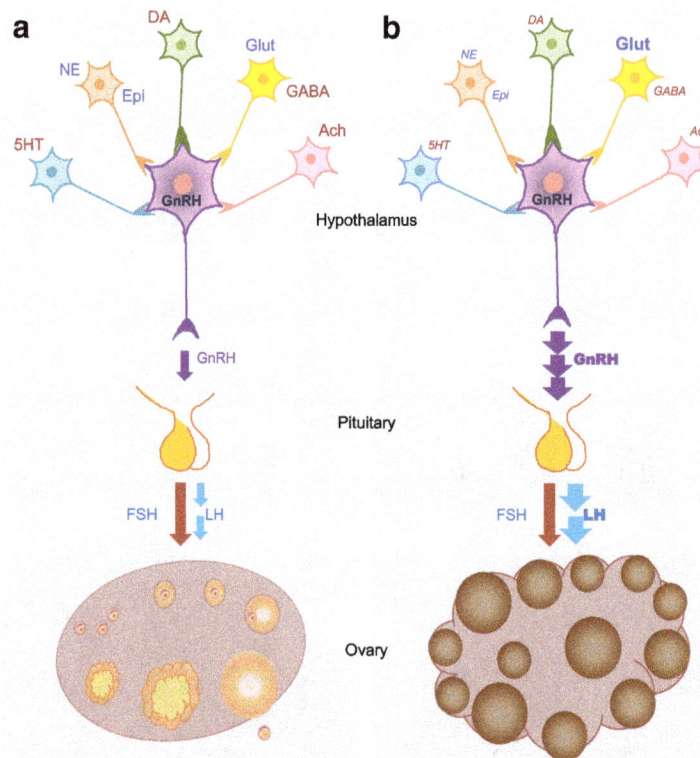

Fig. 7 Diagrammatic summary of results. Hypothalamic-pituitary-ovarian axis in normal (**a**) and in PCOS (**b**) conditions. Blue font: Stimulatory molecules; Red font: Inhibitory molecules; Bold font: Increased in PCOS condition; *Italic font*: Decreased in PCOS condition. Thick arrow: increased in PCOS condition as compared to control. 5HT: Serotonin; DA: Dopamine; NE: Norepinephrine; Epi: Epinephrine; Glut: Glutamate; Ach: Acetylcholine

immnohistochemical studies have demonstrated co-localization of GABAB, NMDAR glutamate receptor and D2 dopamine receptor in kisspeptin neurons. Furthermore, antagonists of GABAB and D2R dopamine receptors increase Kisspeptin-mediated GnRH and LH release [55, 56], whereas treatment with MK801-NMDA receptor antagonist blocks kisspeptin-dependent reinstatement of LH surge [57]. Data from our lab has revealed significant increases in expression of both *Kiss1* and its receptor *Gpr-54* in the hypothalamus of PCOS rats (manuscript under preparation) that also falls in line with a previous study [26]. Thus, alteration of neurotransmitters and neuropeptide together are likely to be responsible for the increased GnRH and LH pulsatility in PCOS condition.

Besides the regulation of endocrine axis, neurotransmitters are also implicated in several psychiatric manifestations. The vast majority of anti-depressants include inhibitors of monoamine oxidase and serotonin reuptake transporters (SSRI), indicating the role of serotonin, dopamine and norepinephrine in mood regulation [58–61]. Glutamate and GABA are also emerging candidates for depression and anxiety disorders [62, 63]. Alterations in acetylcholine signalling have also been shown to lead to symptoms of depression and anxiety wherein overactive or hyper-responsive muscarinic cholinergic system has

been documented [58]. All these references suggest that alteration in neurotransmitter profile seen in letrozole-induced PCOS model may result into development of depression and anxiety-like symptoms (manuscript communicated). In light of these references and our data, the occurrence of depression, anxiety and other mood disorders, which affect upto 40% of PCOS women [64, 65], can be linked to an altered neurotransmitter profile. We have indeed observed symptoms of depression and anxiety in behavioural experiments on letrozole-induced PCOS rat model (manuscript communicated).

Current study clearly demonstrated severe neurotransmitter modulation in letrozole-induced PCOS rat model. Likewise, in a study, rat treated with letrozole demonstrated decreased norepinephrine and dopamine content in hippocampus and frontal cortex [66]. However, the concentration and duration of letrozole treatment in that study was much higher as compared to our study. Furthermore, the possibility that the currently observed changes in neurotransmitters are due to other interactions of letrozole can be ruled out by our previous study wherein testosterone propionate-induced PCOS rat model also demonstrated similar neurotransmitter profile [67]. This thereby strengthens the result of present study indicating that neurotransmitter modulation is a pivotal attribute of PCOS condition.

Conclusion

Results from our study thus suggest the presence of heightened excitatory signal (glutamate) and decreased inhibitory currents (serotonin, dopamine, GABA and acetylcholine), which may be responsible for the increased pulsatility of GnRH and LH, leading to increased LH/FSH ratio as observed in PCOS (Fig. 7). It is also evident that the observed changes in neurotransmitter levels of the brain are mainly due to altered rates of their catabolism. Further, the dysregulated neurotransmitter profile in PCOS could also be the reason for low self-esteem, anxiety, frequent mood swings and depression, features closely associated with PCOS women. This is the first study which explicitly demonstrates that neurotransmitter modulation may act as a key feature in the development of PCOS pathology with increasing risk of other co-morbidities such as stress and mood.

Abbreviations

$5HT_{1A}$: Serotonin $5HT_{1A}$ receptor; AChE: Acetyl cholinesterase; COMT: Catecholamine-O-methyl transferase; D_2R: Dopamine D_2 receptor; FSH: Follicle stimulating hormone; GABA: γ-amino butyric acid; $GABA_{B1}$: $GABA_{B1}$ receptor; GABA-T: GABA transaminase; GAD: Glutamic acid decarboxylase; GDH: Glutamate dehydrogenase; GnRH: Gonadotropin-releasing hormone; HOMA-IR: Homeostatic Model Assessment of Insulin Resistance; HPG axis: Hypothalamic-pituitary-gonadal axis; LH: Luteinizing hormone; M_2AchR: Muscarinic acetylcholine 2 receptor; MAO: Monoamine oxidase; NMDA: N-methyl-D-aspartate glutamate receptor; OGTT: Oral glucose tolerance test; TDC: Tryptophan decarboxylase; TH: Tyrosine hydroxylase; $α_1AR$: $α_1$-adrenergic receptor

Acknowledgements

Dr. B. Suresh, Department of Zoology, The M. S. University of Baroda, Vadodara, India for photomicrographs of ovarian sections. DBT-MSUB-ILSPARE program and Dr. T. Bagchi, Department of Microbiology, The M. S. University of Baroda, Vadodara, India for real-time PCR instrumentation.

Funding

This research did not receive any specific grant from any funding agency in the public, commercial or not-for-profit sector.

Authors' contributions

NC and LN designed and conceptualized this study. All experiments were performed by NC and MD. Data analysis, interpretation and manuscript writing was carried out by NC. LN critically reviewed the manuscript. All authors read and approved the final manuscript.

Competing interests

The authors declare that they have no competing interests.

References

1. Levine JE. An introduction to neuroendocrine systems. Handbook of Neuroendocrinology. Academic press; 2011. p. 3.
2. Smith MJ, Jennes L. Neural signals that regulate GnRH neurones directly during the oestrous cycle. Reproduction. 2001;122:1–10.
3. Joshi B, Mukherjee S, Patil A, Purandare A, Chauhan S, Vaidya R. A cross-sectional study of polycystic ovarian syndrome among adolescent and young girls in Mumbai, India. Indian J Endocrinol Metab. 2014;18:317.
4. Diamanti-Kandarakis E. Polycystic ovarian syndrome: pathophysiology, molecular aspects and clinical implications. Expert Rev Mol Med. 2008;10:e3. https://doi.org/10.1017/S1462399408000598.
5. Azziz R, Carmina E, Chen Z, Dunaif A, Laven JS, Legro RS, Lizneva D, Natterson-Horowtiz B, Teede HJ, Yildiz BO. Polycystic ovary syndrome. Nat Rev Dis Primers. 2016;2:16057.
6. Shi X, Zhang L, Fu S, Li N. Co-involvement of psychological and neurological abnormalities in infertility with polycystic ovarian syndrome. Arch Gynecol Obstet. 2011;284:773–8.
7. Kafali H, Iriadam M, Ozardalı I, Demir N. Letrozole-induced polycystic ovaries in the rat: a new model for cystic ovarian disease. Arch Med Res. 2004;35: 103–8.
8. Badr M, Pelletier G. Characterization and autoradiographic localization of LHRH receptors in the rat brain. Synapse. 1987;1:567–71.
9. Maggi R. Physiology of gonadotropin-releasing hormone (GnRH): beyond the control of reproductive functions. MOJ Anat Physiol. 2016;2:1–5.
10. Furukawa A, Miyatake A, Ohnishi T, Ichikawa Y. Steroidogenic acute regulatory protein (StAR) transcripts constitutively expressed in the adult rat central nervous system: Colocalization of StAR, cytochrome P-450SCC (CYP XIA1), and 3β-Hydroxysteroid dehydrogenase in the rat brain. J Neurochem. 1998;71:2231–8.
11. Zwain IH, Yen SS. Neurosteroidogenesis in astrocytes, oligodendrocytes, and neurons of cerebral cortex of rat brain. Endocrinology. 1999;140:3843–52.
12. Hrabovszky E, Liposits Z. Afferent neuronal control of type-I gonadotropin releasing hormone neurons in the human. Front Endocrinol. 2013;4:130.
13. Marcondes FK, Bianchi FJ, Tanno AP. Determination of the estrous cycle phases of rats: some helpful considerations. Braz J Biol. 2002;62:609–14.
14. Buchanan TA, Sipos GF, Gadalah S, Yip KP, Marsh DJ, Hsueh W, Bergman RN. Glucose tolerance and insulin action in rats with renovascular hypertension. Hypertension. 1991;18:341–7.
15. Lillie RD. Histopathologic technic and practical histochemistry. New York: Blakiston; 1947.
16. Bhattacharyya S, Khanna S, Chakrabarty K, Mahadevan A, Christopher R, Shankar SK. Anti-brain autoantibodies and altered excitatory neurotransmitters in obsessive–compulsive disorder. Neuropsychopharmacology. 2009;34:2489–96.
17. Ghosh NC, Deb C, Banerjee S. Colorimetric determination of epinephrine in blood and adrenal gland. J Biol Chem. 1951;192:867–74.
18. Sangwan RS, Mishra S, Kumar S. Direct Fluorometry of phase-extracted tryptamine-based fast quantitative assay ofl-tryptophan decarboxylase fromCatharanthus roseusLeaf. Anal Biochem. 1998;255:39–46.
19. Basu N, Scheuhammer AM, Rouvinen-Watt K, Evans RD, Trudeau VL, Chan LH. In vitro and whole animal evidence that methylmercury disrupts GABAergic systems in discrete brain regions in captive mink. Comp Biochem Physiol C Toxicol Pharmacol. 2010;151:379–85.
20. MacDonnell P, Greengard O. The distribution of glutamate decarboxylase in rat tissues; isotopic vs fluorimetric assays. J Neurochem. 1975;24:615–8.
21. Yu ZF, Kong LD, Chen Y. Antidepressant activity of aqueous extracts of Curcuma longa in mice. J Ethnopharmacol. 2002;83:161–5.
22. Lee WK, Shin S, Cho SS, Park JS. Purification and characterization of glutamate dehydrogenase as another isoprotein binding to the membrane of rough endoplasmic reticulum. J Cell Biochem. 2000;76:244–53.
23. Ellman P. Pulmonary manifestations in the systemic collagen diseases. Postgrad Med J. 1956;32:370.
24. Livak KJ, Schmittgen TD. Analysis of relative gene expression data using real-time quantitative PCR and the 2− ΔΔCT method. Methods. 2001;25: 402–8.
25. Maharjan R, Nagar PS, Nampoothiri L. Effect of aloe barbadensis mill. Formulation on Letrozole induced polycystic ovarian syndrome rat model. J Ayurveda Integr Med. 2010;1:273.
26. Kauffman AS, Thackray VG, Ryan GE, Tolson KP, Glidewell-Kenney CA, Semaan SJ, Poling MC, Iwata N, Breen KM, Duleba AJ, Stener-Victorin EA. Novel letrozole model recapitulates both the reproductive and metabolic phenotypes of polycystic ovary syndrome in female mice. Biol Reprod. 2015;93:69–1.
27. De Vivo M, Maayani S. Characterization of the 5-hydroxytryptamine1a receptor-mediated inhibition of forskolin-stimulated adenylate cyclase activity in Guinea pig and rat hippocampal membranes. J Pharmacol Exp Ther. 1986;238:248–53.
28. Bhattarai JP, Roa J, Herbison AE, Han SK. Serotonin acts through 5-HT1 and 5-HT2 receptors to exert biphasic actions on GnRH neuron excitability in the mouse. Endocrinology. 2014;155:513–24.

29. He JR, Molnar J, Barraclough CA. Morphine amplifies norepinephrine (NE)-induced LH release but blocks NE-stimulated increases in LHRH mRNA levels: comparison of responses obtained in ovariectomized, estrogen-treated normal and androgen-sterilized rats. Mol Brain Res. 1993;20:71–8.

30. Krieg RJ, Sawyer CH. Effects of intraventricular catecholamines on luteinizing hormone release in ovariectomized-steroid-primed rats. Endocrinology. 1976;99:411–9.

31. Leung PC, Arendash GW, Whitmoyer DI, Gorski RA, Sawyer CH. Differential effects of central adrenoceptor agonists on luteinizing hormone release. Neuroendocrinology. 1982;34:207–14.

32. Jacobi JS, Martin C, Nava G, Jeziorski MC, Clapp C, De La Escalera GM. 17-Beta-estradiol directly regulates the expression of adrenergic receptors and kisspeptin/GPR54 system in GT1-7 GnRH neurons. Neuroendocrinology. 2007;86:260–9.

33. Rubinstein L, Sawyer CH. Role of catecholamines in stimulating the release of pituitary ovulating hormone (s) in rats. Endocrinology. 1970;86:988–95.

34. Plant TM, Zeleznik AJ, editors. Knobil and Neill's physiology of reproduction. Academic Press; 2014.

35. Liu X, Herbison AE. Dopamine regulation of gonadotropin-releasing hormone neuron excitability in male and female mice. Endocrinology. 2013;154:340–50.

36. Ciechanowska M, Lapot M, Mateusiak K, Przekop F. Neuroendocrine regulation of GnRH release and expression of GnRH and GnRH receptor genes in the hypothalamus-pituitary unit in different physiological states. Reprod Biol. 2010;10:85–124.

37. Hernández I, Parra A, Méndez I, Cabrera V, del Carmen Cravioto M, Mercado M, Díaz-Sánchez V, Larrea F. Hypothalamic dopaminergic tone and prolactin bioactivity in women with polycystic ovary syndrome. Arch Med Res. 2000;31:216–22.

38. Henderson HL, Townsend J, Tortonese DJ. Direct effects of prolactin and dopamine on the gonadotroph response to GnRH. J Endocrinol. 2008;197:343–50.

39. Kalro BN, Loucks TL, Berga SL. Neuromodulation in polycystic ovary syndrome. Obstet Gynecol Clin N Am. 2001;28:35–62.

40. Gómez R, Ferrero H, Delgado-Rosas F, Gaytan M, Morales C, Zimmermann RC, Simón C, Gaytan F, Pellicer A. Evidences for the existence of a low dopaminergic tone in polycystic ovarian syndrome: implications for OHSS development and treatment. J Clin Endocrinol Metab. 2011;96:2484–92.

41. Catalano PN, Di Giorgio N, Bonaventura MM, Bettler B, Libertun C, Lux-Lantos VA. Lack of functional GABA B receptors alters GnRH physiology and sexual dimorphic expression of GnRH and GAD-67 in the brain. Am J Physiol Endocrinol Metab. 2010;298:E683–96.

42. Lee K, Porteous R, Campbell RE, Lüscher B, Herbison AE. Knockdown of GABAA receptor signaling in GnRH neurons has minimal effects upon fertility. Endocrinology. 2010;151:4428–36.

43. Virmani MA, Stojilković SS, Catt KJ. Stimulation of luteinizing hormone release by gamma-aminobutyric acid (GABA) agonists: mediation by GABAA-type receptors and activation of chloride and voltage-sensitive calcium channels. Endocrinology. 1990;126:2499–505.

44. Anderson RA, Mitchell R. Effects of β-aminobutyric acid receptor agonists on the secretion of growth hormone, luteinizing hormone, adrenocorticotrophic hormone and thyroid-stimulating hormone from the rat pituitary gland in vitro. J Endocrinol. 1986;108:1–8.

45. Moore AM, Prescott M, Marshall CJ, Yip SH, Campbell RE. Enhancement of a robust arcuate GABAergic input to gonadotropin-releasing hormone neurons in a model of polycystic ovarian syndrome. Proc Nat Acad Sci USA. 2015;112:596–601.

46. Iremonger KJ, Constantin S, Liu X, Herbison AE. Glutamate regulation of GnRH neuron excitability. Brain Res. 2010;1364:35–43.

47. Bourguignon JP, Gerard A, Mathieu J, Simons J, Franchimont P. Pulsatile release of gonadotropin-releasing hormone from hypothalamic explants is restrained by blockade of N-methyl-D, L-aspartate receptors. Endocrinology. 1989;125:1090–6.

48. Hrabovszky E, Csapo AK, Kallo I, Wilheim T, Turi GF, Liposits ZS. Localization and osmotic regulation of vesicular glutamate transporter-2 in magnocellular neurons of the rat hypothalamus. Neurochem Int. 2006;48:753–61.

49. Zanisi M, Galbiati M, Messi E, Martini L. The anterior pituitary gland as a possible site of action of kainic acid. Proc Soc Exp Biol Med. 1994;206:431–7.

50. Krsmanovic LZ, Mores N, Navarro CE, Saeed SA, Arora KK, Catt KJ. Muscarinic regulation of intracellular signaling and neurosecretion in gonadotropin-releasing hormone neurons. Endocrinology. 1998;139:4037–43.

51. Arai Y, Ishii H, Kobayashi M, Ozawa H. Subunit profiling and functional characteristics of acetylcholine receptors in GT1-7 cells. J Physiol Sci. 2017;67:313–23.

52. Zemkova H, Kucka M, Bjelobaba I, Tomić M, Stojilkovic SS. Multiple cholinergic signaling pathways in pituitary gonadotrophs. Endocrinology. 2013;154:421–33.

53. Ansel L, Bolborea M, Bentsen AH, Klosen P, Mikkelsen JD, Simonneaux V. Differential regulation of kiss1 expression by melatonin and gonadal hormones in male and female Syrian hamsters. J Biol Rhythm. 2010;25:81–91.

54. García-Galiano D, van Ingen Schenau D, Leon S, Krajnc-Franken MA, Manfredi-Lozano M, Romero-Ruiz A, Navarro VM, Gaytan F, van Noort PI, Pinilla L, Blomenröhr M. Kisspeptin signaling is indispensable for neurokinin B, but not glutamate, stimulation of gonadotropin secretion in mice. Endocrinology. 2012;153:316–28.

55. Zhang C, Bosch MA, Rønnekleiv OK, Kelly MJ. γ-aminobutyric acid B receptor mediated inhibition of gonadotropin-releasing hormone neurons is suppressed by kisspeptin-G protein-coupled receptor 54 signaling. Endocrinology. 2009;150:2388–94.

56. Goodman RL, Maltby MJ, Millar RP, Hileman SM, Nestor CC, Whited B, Tseng AS, Coolen LM, Lehman MN. Evidence that dopamine acts via kisspeptin to hold GnRH pulse frequency in check in anestrous ewes. Endocrinology. 2012;153:5918–27.

57. Neal-Perry G, Lebesgue D, Lederman M, Shu J, Zeevalk GD, Etgen AM. The excitatory peptide kisspeptin restores the luteinizing hormone surge and modulates amino acid neurotransmission in the medial preoptic area of middle-aged rats. Endocrinology. 2009;150:3699–708.

58. Drevets WC, Price JL, Furey ML. Brain structural and functional abnormalities in mood disorders: implications for neurocircuitry models of depression. Brain Struct Func. 2008;213:93–118.

59. Darlington CL, Goddard M, Zheng Y, Smith PF. Anxiety-related behavior and biogenic amine pathways in the rat following bilateral vestibular lesions. Ann N Y Acad Sci. 2009;1164:134–9.

60. Hasler G. Pathophysiology of depression: do we have any solid evidence of interest to clinicians? World Psychiatry. 2010;1(9):155–61.

61. Garcia-Garcia AL, Newman-Tanaredi A, Leonardo ED. P5-HT1 a receptors in mood and anxiety: recent insights into autoreceptor versus heteroreceptor function. Psychopharmacology. 2013;15:112–8.

62. Brambilla P, Perez J, Barale F, Schettini G, Soares JC. GABAergic dysfunction in mood disorders. Mol Psychiatry. 2003;8:721–37.

63. Sanacora G, Treccani G, Popoli M. Towards a glutamate hypothesis of depression: an emerging frontier of neuropsychopharmacology for mood disorders. Neuropharmacology. 2012;62:63–77.

64. Kerchner A, Lester W, Stuart SP, Dokras A. Risk of depression and other mental health disorders in women with polycystic ovary syndrome: a longitudinal study. Fertil Steril. 2009;91:207–12.

65. Goodarzi MO, Dumesic DA, Chazenbalk G, Azziz R. Polycystic ovary syndrome: etiology, pathogenesis and diagnosis. Nat Rev Endocrinol. 2011;7:219–31.

66. Aydin M, Yilmaz B, Alcin E, Nedzvetsky VS, Sahin Z, Tuzcu M. Effects of letrozole on hippocampal and cortical catecholaminergic neurotransmitter levels, neural cell adhesion molecule expression and spatial learning and memory in female rats. Neuroscience. 2008;151:186–94.

67. Chaudhari NK, Nampoothiri LP. Neurotransmitter alteration in a testosterone propionate-induced polycystic ovarian syndrome rat model. Horm Mol Biol Clin Investig. 2017;29:71–7.

## 12

The relationship between gonadotropin releasing hormone and ovulation inducing factor/nerve growth factor receptors in the hypothalamus of the llama

Rodrigo A. Carrasco, Jaswant Singh and Gregg P. Adams*ⓘ

Abstract

Background: A molecule identical to nerve growth factor, with ovulation-inducing properties has been discovered in the seminal plasma of South American camelids (ovulation-inducing factor/nerve growth factor; OIF/NGF). We hypothesize that the ovulatory effect of OIF/NGF is initiated at the level of the hypothalamus, presumably by GnRH neurons. The objective of the present study was to determine the structural relationship between GnRH neurons and neurons expressing high- and low-affinity receptors for NGF (i.e., TrkA and p75, respectively) in the hypothalamus.

Methods: Mature llamas ($n = 4$) were euthanized and their hypothalamic tissue was fixed, sectioned, and processed for immunohistochemistry on free-floating sections. Ten equidistant sections per brain were double stained for immunofluorescence detection of TrkA and GnRH, or p75 and GnRH.

Results: Cells immunoreactive to TrkA were detected in most hypothalamic areas, but the majority of cells were detected in the diagonal band of Broca (part of the ventral forebrain) and the supraoptic nuclei and periventricular area. The number of cells immunoreactive to p75 was highest in the diagonal band of Broca and lateral preoptic areas and least in more caudal areas of the hypothalamus ($p < 0.05$) in a pattern similar to that of TrkA. A low proportion of GnRH neurons were immunoreactive to TrkA (2.5% of total GnRH cells), and no co-localization between GnRH and p75 was detected. GnRH neuron fibers were detected only occasionally in proximity to TrkA immunopositive neurons.

Conclusions: Results do not support the hypothesis that the effect of OIF/NGF is driven by a direct interaction with GnRH neurons, but rather provide rationale for the hypothesis that interneurons exist in the hypothalamus that mediate OIF/NGF-induced ovulation.

Keywords: GnRH, TrkA, p75, Llamas, Hypothalamus, Ovulation-induction factor, Nerve growth factor

Background

As induced ovulators, llamas and alpacas ovulate in response to copulation [1, 2]. The physical stimulation of coitus, however, is not the primary trigger for ovulation, as initially proposed, but rather ovulation occurs in response to a factor present in seminal plasma that induces a preovulatory LH surge [3–6]. The seminal ovulation-inducing factor (OIF) is a potent stimulator of LH release [4, 7], and is capable of inducing ovulation in

* Correspondence: gregg.adams@usask.ca
Department of Veterinary Biomedical Sciences, Western College of Veterinary Medicine, University of Saskatchewan, 52 campus drive, Saskatoon, Saskatchewan S7N5B4, Canada

llamas and alpacas at dose 1/100th of that present in a normal ejaculate [8]. Mass spectrometry and protein crystallography allowed the identification of OIF as ß-nerve growth factor [6] and will be herein-after referred to as OIF/NGF (seminal plasma derived NGF). In a study designed to determine the mechanism by which OIF/NGF elicits LH release from the pituitary gland [9], llamas pretreated with a GnRH receptor antagonist and subsequently treated with OIF/NGF failed to have a preovulatory LH surge. While the main site of action of OIF/NGF in vivo appears to be at the level of the hypothalamus, treatment of primary cell cultures of alpaca, cattle and rat pituitaries with OIF/NGF or seminal plasma also induced LH release [10, 11].

Ovarian follicular development in llamas and alpacas occurs in a wave-like pattern [12], as described in other farm animals [13, 14]. As a monotocous species, each follicular wave involves development of a single dominant follicle which, in llamas and alpacas, is capable of ovulating when it is ≥7 mm in diameter [12, 15]. In the absence of mating, ovulation does not occur, a corpus luteum does not develop, and successive follicular waves emerge at periodic intervals. In contrast, spontaneous ovulators ovulate irrespective of mating, a corpus luteum is present during the majority of the estrous cycle, and progesterone plays a role in follicle maturation and oocyte competence [16]. Ovarian estradiol is not associated with positive feedback on the hypothalamic-pituitary axis to elicit the LH surge in induced ovulators, as it is in spontaneous ovulators, but it does modulate pituitary LH secretion in OIF/NGF-treated llamas [17].

Nerve growth factor is a molecule that has the effect of maintaining and enhancing neuron survival [18], and is present in restricted areas of the central nervous system in rodents, such as the cerebral cortex, the hippocampus, cholinergic pathways in the septal area and the dorsal root ganglia [19, 20]. As well, NGF receptors have been detected by autoradiography in the diagonal band of Broca, caudal putamen, lateral preoptic area and globus palidus in rats [21]. The effect of NGF is mediated through interaction with two different receptors, TrkA and p75. TrkA (also known as NTRK1) is a specific high-affinity receptor that mediates most of the classical actions of NGF, whereas p75 (also known as NGFR) is a less specific low-affinity receptor that has been associated with NGF-activated cell death in oligodendrocytes [22, 23]. Despite the apparent opposing effects mediated by the two receptors, a large proportion of cells in the septal/diagonal band of Broca region [24, 25] and the nucleus basalis [25] bear both p75 and TrkA (mRNA or protein). Pharmacological blockade of TrkA eliminated most of the effects of NGF [26], and p75 is capable of binding to neurotrophins other than NGF (Reviewed by [27]); hence, it is likely that the ovulation-inducing effect of OIF/NGF is driven by interaction with the high-affinity receptor, TrkA.

GnRH secretion is a fundamental signal for the preovulatory LH surge [28]. In an initial effort to address the hypothesis that OIF/NGF induces ovulation through direct interaction with GnRH neurons in llamas, the objective of the present study was to determine if the high- and low-affinity receptors of OIF/NGF are expressed in GnRH neurons of llamas.

Methods
Animals and tissue collection
Non-pregnant, non-lactating adult female llamas ($n = 4$) weighting 100 to 140 kg were euthanized using an overdose of pentobarbital during summer (Euthanyl Forte, Bimeda MTC Animal health Inc., Cambridge, Ontario, Canada). The head was separated and immediately perfused via the carotid arteries with 2 l of cold heparinized (10,000 IU Na heparin/L) saline (0.9% NaCl) solution, followed by 2 l of a solution of 4% formaldehyde in phosphate buffered saline (PBS; 0.1 M, pH = 7.4). After the brain was extracted from the cranium, a piece of tissue containing part of the septum and the hypothalamus was dissected out and immersed in the same fixative overnight at 4 °C. The next day, tissues were washed 3 times in PBS and stored in PBS with 0.1% sodium azide at 4 °C until cryoprotection. Samples were immersed in cryoprotectant solution (30% sucrose in PBS) until the tissues sank, and then frozen at – 80 °C until sectioning. Tissues were sectioned transversely (coronal plane) at a thickness of 50 um using a cryostat, and each section was stored in a mixture of 30% sucrose and 30% ethylene glycol in PBS at – 20 °C until immunostaining. Single and double immunohistochemistry was carried out on free-floating sections to optimize staining of thick (50 μm) sections (see below). Animal procedures were approved by the University of Saskatchewan Committee on Animal Care in accordance with guidelines of the Canadian Council on Animal Care.

Single immunohistochemistry
Anatomical detail and TrkA immunoreactivity were assessed by light microscopy, using adjacent sections stained with Cresyl violet or by immunohistochemistry against TrkA [29]. Briefly, sections were rinsed in PBS and incubated in 3% hydrogen peroxide to block endogenous peroxidases. Sections were heated to 90 °C in sodium citrate buffer for 30 mins (0.1 M; pH = 6.0; Sigma) and incubated in blocking buffer for 1 h. TrkA antibody was applied at 1:500 dilution in blocking buffer for 24 h, sections were rinsed three times in PBS, and goat anti-rabbit antibody conjugated to horseradish peroxidase was used to detect the antigen-antibody complex [29]. Sections were washed three times in PBS, immersed in a solution of DAB for 10 min, rinsed in PBS, mounted on glass slides, air dried and cover-slipped until examination. Anatomical organization was determined using the aid of the *Lama glama* brain atlas of the University of Wisconsin, Madison (http://brainmuseum.org/) and stereotaxic atlases of other mammals [30–32].

Double immunofluorescence
Two sets of ten equidistant sections per brain (approximately one every 1500 um) were selected for double immunofluorescence labelling for either GnRH with TrkA or GnRH with p75. After removing the cryoprotectant solution, sections were rinsed 4 times in PBS for 10 min each. To expose epitopes to antibodies in tissue sections

(Antigen retrieval), samples were heated at 80 °C for 35 min in sodium citrate solution (0.1 M; pH = 6.0; Sigma). After cooling to room temperature, section non-specific binding was blocked with 0.5% BSA 0.5% triton X-100 in PBS for 3 h. Sections were incubated for 48 h at 4 °C in a cocktail consisting of two primary antibodies diluted in 0.5% BSA (Sigma), 0.5% triton x-100, and 0.1% sodium azide in PBS. For both sets of sections (TrkA and p75), anti-GnRH antibody (mouse anti-GnRH SMI 41; Sternberger Monoclonals; Cedarlane, Burlington, Ontario, Canada) was used at a dilution of 1:10,000 in blocking buffer. Anti-TrkA (rabbit anti-TrkA, Santa Cruz biotechnologies; Dallas, Texas, USA) was used at a dilution of 1:500, and rabbit anti-p75 (gift from Dr. Louis F Reichardt, University of California San Francisco, USA) was used at a 1:5000 dilution. Sections were washed 3 times with PBS and incubated in a mixture of secondary antibodies consisting of goat anti-rabbit antibody conjugated to biotin (1:500 for TrkA, 1:1000 for p75; Life Technologies;

Burlington, Ontario, Canada) and goat anti-mouse antibody conjugated to Alexa 546 (1:500; Life Technologies; Burlington, Ontario, Canada) for 2 to 3 h at 37 °C in blocking buffer. After washing the secondary antibodies, samples were incubated with streptavidin conjugated to Alexa 488 diluted in blocking buffer (1:200 for TrkA, and 1:5000 for p75; Life Technologies; Burlington, Ontario, Canada) for 1 to 2 h [29]. Finally, sections were washed and mounted on poly-L-lysine coated slides, air dried, incubated for 10 min in a solution of 0.3% sudan black in 70% ethanol (to reduce autofluorescence), air dried again, covered with Vectashield mounting medium (Vectorlabs, Burlington, Ontario, Canada) containing DAPI, and a coverslip was applied. Coverslipped sections were stored at 4 °C in the dark until examination.

Cell numbers were counted manually by a single observer using a wide-field fluorescent microscope at 20× magnification (Zeiss Axioskop 40; Thornwood, New York, USA). To avoid double counting and overestimation, only those cells that displayed a single distinguishable nucleus

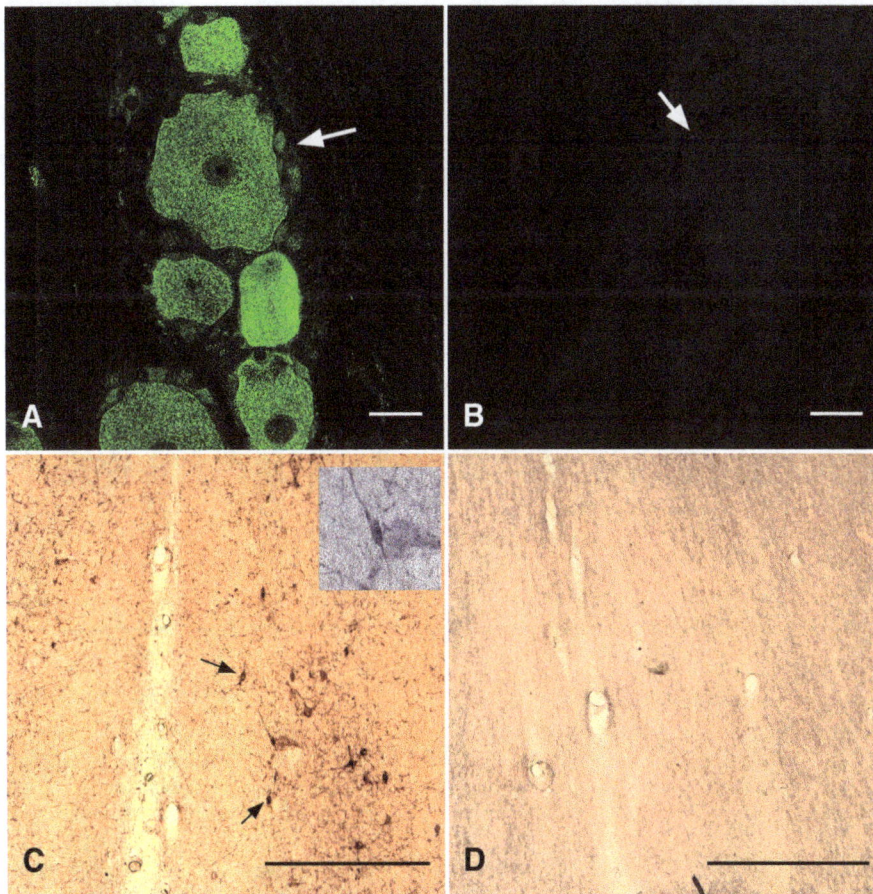

Fig. 1 Validation of antibodies against TrkA (**a** positive control; **b** negative control) and p75 (**c** positive control; **d** negative controls) using sections of a dorsal root ganglium (for TrkA) or medial septum (for p75) of a llama. For the negative control sections, primary antibodies were pre-absorbed with the corresponding immunogen. **a**, **b**. Scale bar = 30 um; **c**, **d** 50 um

were counted. Confocal microscopy was performed on a Leica LSM confocal microscope (Leica Microsystems, Concord, Ontario, Canada) with lasers for excitation of Alexa 488, Alexa 546, and DAPI. Stacks were obtained by using a 63× oil immersion objective lens, with a numerical aperture of 1.4. Optical section thickness was 0.7 μm.

Antibody controls

The TrkA antibody was raised in rabbit against a fragment of the C terminus of human TrkA receptor. Preadsorption of the primary anti-TrkA antibody with TrkA immunogen (Santa Cruz Biotechnologies; Dallas, Texas, USA) was performed in a 1 to 5 ratio (protein content) with no resultant immunodetection. Llama dorsal root ganglia were used as a positive control (Fig. 1). GnRH is highly conserved among species [33] and use of the anti-GnRH antibody has been validated previously with different species (rat, [34]; sheep, [35]. We have tested the specificity of the GnRH antibody by pre-adsorption with the GnRH peptide (ab 120184; Abcam, Cambridge, MA, USA) and by replacing the primary antibody with a mouse isotype (IgG 1), both procedures resulted in no immunoreaction. The p75 antibody was raised against the extracellular domain of rat p75 receptor. Anti-p75 antibody specificity was tested by omission of the primary antibody and by preincubating with 5 μg of a fragment containing the extracellular domain of the recombinant human protein (ab157276, Abcam, Cambridge, MA, USA), with no resultant immunoreaction [36].

Data analysis

Data are expressed as mean ± SEM or as a percentage of the total number of cells displaying double immunoreactivity. The number of GnRH (from both set of double-stained sections), TrkA, and p75 immunopositive cells was compared among anatomical areas by analysis of variance for repeated measures. The total number of cells per brain (GnRH vs TrkA, and GnRH vs p75) were compared by t tests. Differences were considered significant with a p-value ≤0.05.

Results
Distribution of TrkA immunoreactive cells

Llama dorsal root ganglia stained against TrkA receptor showed a strong immunoreaction (Fig. 1a). The signal was restricted to sensory neurons; no reaction was detected in satellite cells of the dorsal root ganglia. When the antibody was pre-incubated with TrkA peptide, no signal was detected (Fig. 1b), documenting the specificity of the antibody signal. The immunoreactivity was restricted primarily to the cytoplasm surrounding the neuronal nuclei, whereas no identifiable neuronal projections (fibers) were detected.

TrkA immunoreactivity was present in all hypothalamic areas and nuclei examined, except in the median eminence, dorsal hypothalamus, and the optic chiasma. The variation in the number of TrkA positive cells was sufficiently high that no significant difference was detected among the immunoreactive areas, but was numerically greatest in the area of the diagonal band of Broca and medial septum, and least in the medio-basal hypothalamus (Fig. 2a). Importantly, relative accumulations of TrkA immunopositive cells were found in the diagonal band of Broca (part of the ventral forebrain), and the supraoptic and periventricular areas (part of the anterior hypothalamus and mediobasal hypothalamus; Fig. 3). TrkA immunoreactive neurons were only occasionally detected in the arcuate nucleus and retrochiasmatic area (data not shown).

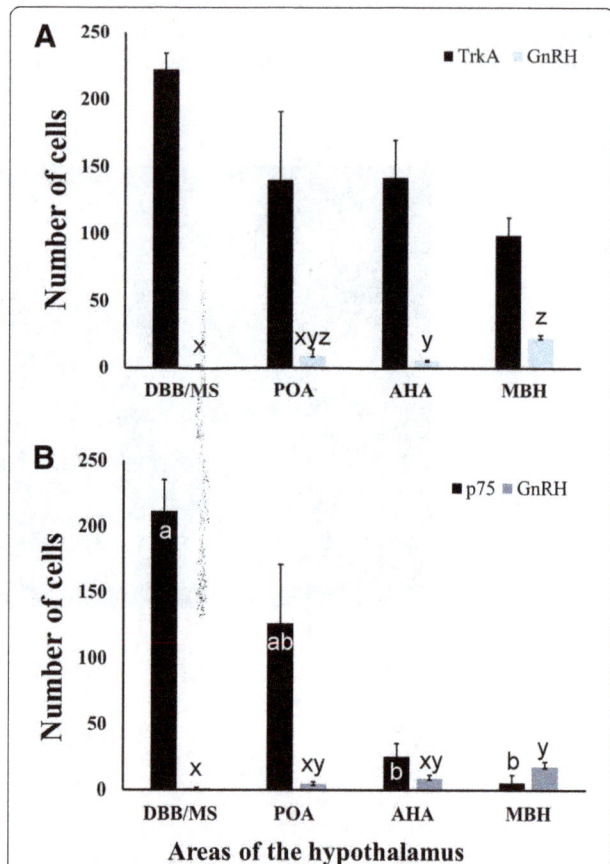

Fig. 2 Distribution of cells expressing immunoreactivity to GnRH, TrkA, and p75 (mean ± SEM number of cells) in the hypothalamus and preoptic areas of llama brains ($n = 4$). Double staining was done on separate sets of sections; hence, cell numbers for TrkA and GnRH are presented in (**a**), and cell numbers for P75 and GnRH are presented in (**b**). DBB/MS: diagonal band of Broca/medial septum, POA: preoptic area, AHA: anterior hypothalamic area, MBH: medio-basal hypothalamus. [ab] For TrkA and p75 neurons, values with no common superscript among regions are different ($p < 0.05$). [xyz] For GnRH neurons, values with no common superscript among regions are different ($p < 0.05$)

Distribution of p75 immunoreactive neurons

A dense network of p75 immunoreactive fibers and cells was detected in the ventral forebrain (i.e., diagonal band of Broca and medial septum), decreasing caudally ($p < 0.05$) in a pattern similar to that of TrkA (Fig. 2b). Low immunoreactivity was found in the medio-basal hypothalamus and none in the mammillary hypothalamus. An abundance of immunoreactive cells was found in the bed nucleus of the stria terminalis, surrounding the anterior commissure in the preoptic area. Strong immunoreactivity was detected in the ependymal cells of the lateral and third ventricles. Individual fibers were detected in proximity to the lateral ventricle and a dense network of fibers appeared in the organum vasculosum and the ventral aspect of the third ventricle at the level of the arcuate nucleus and median eminence. Representative images of P75 neurons are shown in Fig. 3c-d.

Morphological relationship between NGF receptors and GnRH

Overall, TrkA and p75 immunoreactive cells were found in abundance in the llama hypothalamus (2390.2 ± 131 and 1097.5 ± 209.7 cells, respectively), and GnRH cell counts did not differ between slides co-stained with TrkA vs p75 (40.5 ± 7.3 vs 33.7 ± 10.5 cells, respectively; $p = 0.68$). Of the total number of cells (among 4 animals) in the hypothalamus displaying immunoreactivity to GnRH, 156/160 (97.5%) stained for GnRH alone, and 4/160 (2.5%) stained for both GnRH and TrkA. Of the number of cells displaying immunoreactivity to TrkA in the hypothalamus of 4 animals, 9477/9481 (> 99%) stained for TrkA alone; i.e., only 4/9481 (0.042%) stained for both TrkA and GnRH. Aside from the low degree of co-localization, TrkA and GnRH neurons were not commonly visualized in the same anatomical plane, and on only three occasions appeared closely related (i.e., within the same microscopic field; Fig. 4a-d). In the three

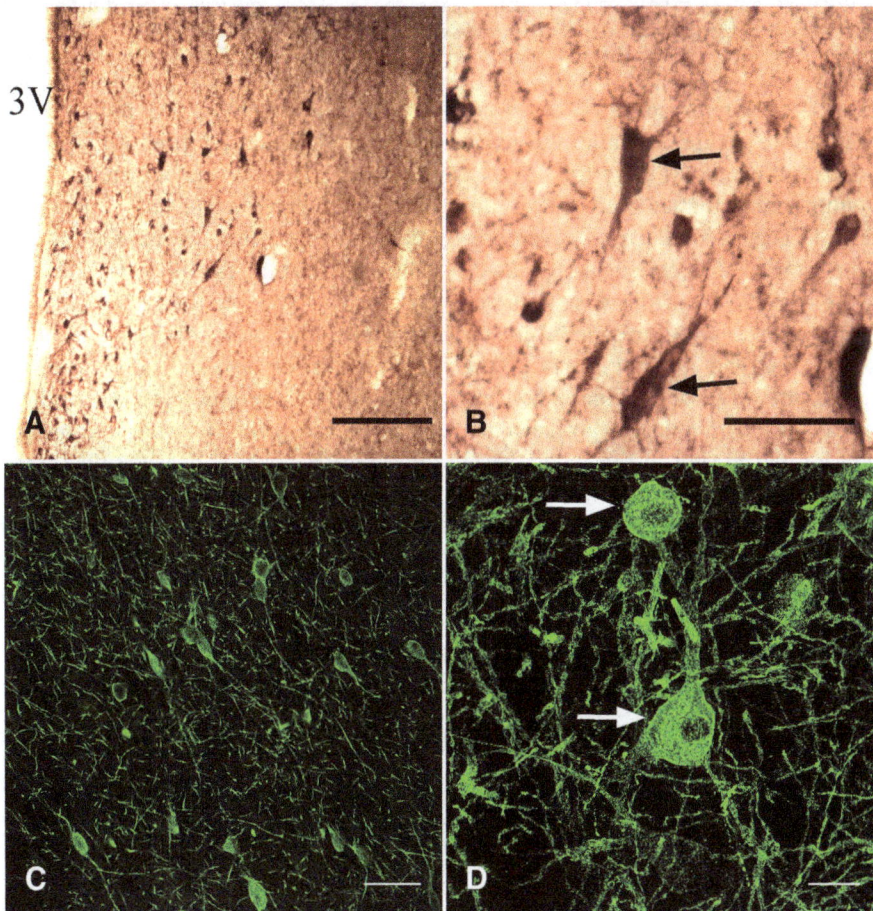

Fig. 3 Immunoreactivity to TrkA and p75 receptor in the hypothalamus of llamas. Low (**a**) and high (**b**) magnification of TrkA immunoreactive neurons (arrows) in the periventricular area, as detected by light microscopy. Note that B is a magnification of A. P75 immunoreactive neurons (arrows) in the septal area at low (**c**) and high magnification (**d**), as detected by immunofluorescence. 3 V: third ventricle. Scale bars: **a** 200 μm., **b** 50 μm., **c** 100 μm., **d** 30 μm

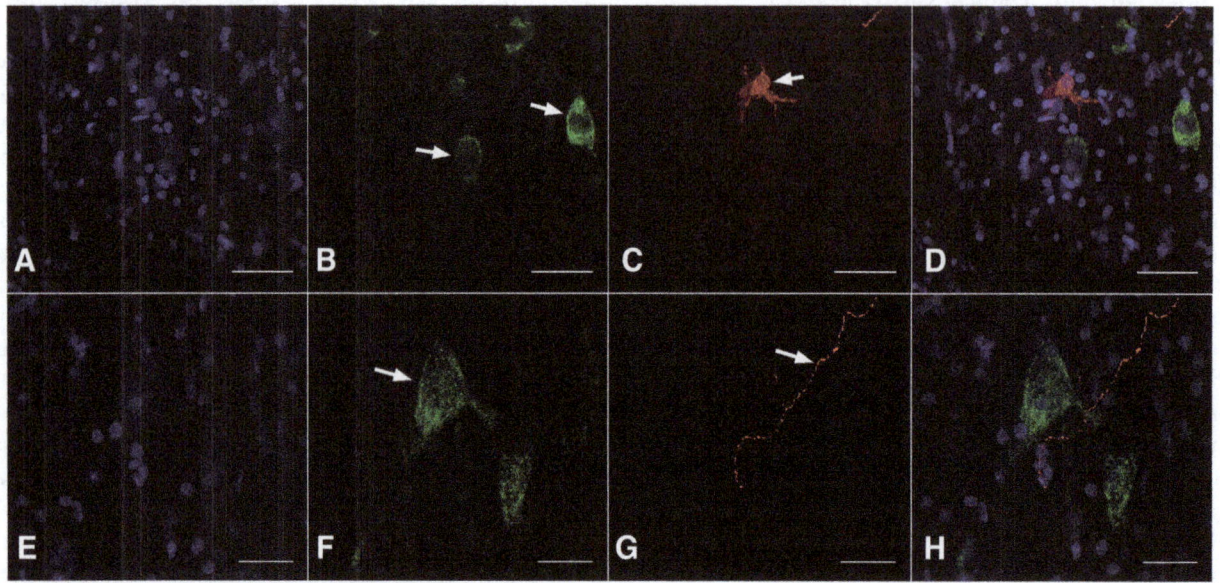

Fig. 4 Immunoreactivity to GnRH and TrkA in the llama hypothalamus, detected by double immunofluorescence. The upper panel (**a-d**; maximum intensity projections) shows the relationship between TrkA neurons (**b**; arrows; green) and GnRH neurons (**c**; arrow; red). The lower panel (maximum intensity projections) illustrates the relationship between TrkA neurons (**f**; arrow) and GnRH fibers (**g**; arrow). Images **d** and **h** depict the overlay of the corresponding panels (**a-d** and **e-h**) including the nuclear counter-stain (**a**, **e**). Scale bars: **a-d** 30, E-H 50 μm

instances where GnRH immunoreactive fibers were found in close relationship to TrkA immunoreactive cells, there was no apparent contact (Fig. 4e-h).

GnRH and p75 immunoreactivities were never detected in the same cell. The two cell types were occasionally located in the same microscopic field (Fig. 5a-c), but the majority of the respective neurons were detected in different areas. P75 neurons were present in greater numbers in the septal area and anterior areas of the hypothalamus (i.e., preoptic area), and virtually non-existent in posterior areas (i.e., mammillary hypothalamus). GnRH neurons were located mostly in the medio-basal hypothalamus and were generally sparse. GnRH cell counts did not differ between slides co-stained with TrkA vs p75 ($p = 0.68$). P75 immunoreactive fibers were occasionally located in proximity to GnRH neurons (Fig. 5d). A scheme of the relationship between GnRH, TrkA and p75 among examined sections is shown in Fig. 6.

Discussion

Ovulation-inducing factor has been shown to induce ovulation in a high proportion of llamas and alpacas after parenteral administration. The effect appears to be mediated via GnRH neurons (directly or indirectly) resulting in preovulatory LH secretion from the gonadotropes in the anterior pituitary [9]. Results of the present study do not support the hypothesis that OIF/NGF effects a response through direct interaction with GnRH neurons in llamas since the high- and low-affinity receptors for OIF/NGF were detected in 2% and 0% of GnRH

neurons, respectively. It is unlikely that such a low proportion of GnRH neurons would drive the preovulatory LH surge. In mice and sheep, for instance, detection of the c-FOS proto-oncogene (a marker of neuronal activation) revealed that about 40% of GnRH neurons are activated during the LH surge [37–39]. Similar to the triggering factor for the LH surge in spontaneous ovulators (estradiol), the triggering factor in camelids (OIF/NGF) must involve an intermediate cell type to interact with GnRH neurons (e.g., kisspeptin neurons, norepinephrine neurons). This view is consistent with the notion that GnRH neurons act as a final output for a complex interplay between neurons [40].

In the present study, TrkA immunoreactive cells were present in most areas examined but were accumulated in three major structures: 1) the diagonal band of Broca in the ventral forebrain, 2) the supraoptic nucleus, and 3) the periventricular area of the third ventricle. These findings are similar to those of studies in rats and macaques [25, 41]. The presence of TrkA immunoreactive cells in the periventricular area offers interesting insight into the route of action of the OIF/NGF system. This area is in close contact with the third ventricle and if OIF/NGF crosses the blood-brain barrier into the cerebrospinal fluid, it would be available to interact with the TrkA receptors in regions of the brain that influence GnRH neurons. In an autoradiographic study of rats, radiolabelled NGF injected into the cerebral ventricle was detected in a layer of the parenchyma surrounding the lateral, third and fourth ventricles [42], consistent with the idea that the ependymal epithelium lining the third ventricle is permeable to such molecules.

Whether NGF crosses the blood-brain barrier in llamas remains unknown. In mice, both the high molecular weight form (7 s NGF) and the low molecular weight form (2.5 s NGF or β-NGF) were detected in the central nervous system after radiolabelling and intravenous administration [43]. With a molecular weight of 26 kDa [6], it seems unlikely that OIF/NGF can simply diffuse through the blood brain barrier [44]. Thus, we hypothesize two routes of NGF entry into the brain: 1) by interacting with the choroid plexus with subsequent active secretion into the cerebrospinal fluid, or 2) by interacting with neurons or their projections in the vicinity of the organum vasculosum and the median eminence (reviewed by [45, 46]). If OIF/NGF crosses the blood-brain barrier by interacting with the epithelium of the choroid plexus, the expression of a specific receptor is required. Such a mechanism has been theorized as one of the pathways for leptin, a 16 kDa hormone produced by adipocytes, which exerts a suppressive effect on appetite possibly via the choroid plexus to act in the arcuate nucleus [47, 48]. Although the low-affinity receptor, p75, has been identified in the rat choroid plexus [49], as well as mRNA of NGF and other neurotrophins, the high affinity receptor, TrkA, has not been detected at high levels in the choroid plexus [50]. Hence, the expression of NGF receptors and their association with a transport system in the choroid plexus of llamas remain unknown.

Circumventricular organs, including the organum vasculosum and the median eminence in the hypothalamus, are areas of the brain where the blood-brain barrier is modified, allowing the secretion of peptides/proteins or sensing the internal milieu by neurons [45]. Thus, the presence of receptors in these structures would allow interaction with neurotrophins circulating in the vascular system. Consistent with studies of other species [51], we found abundant expression of the low-affinity receptor in the diagonal band of Broca/medial septum, lateral

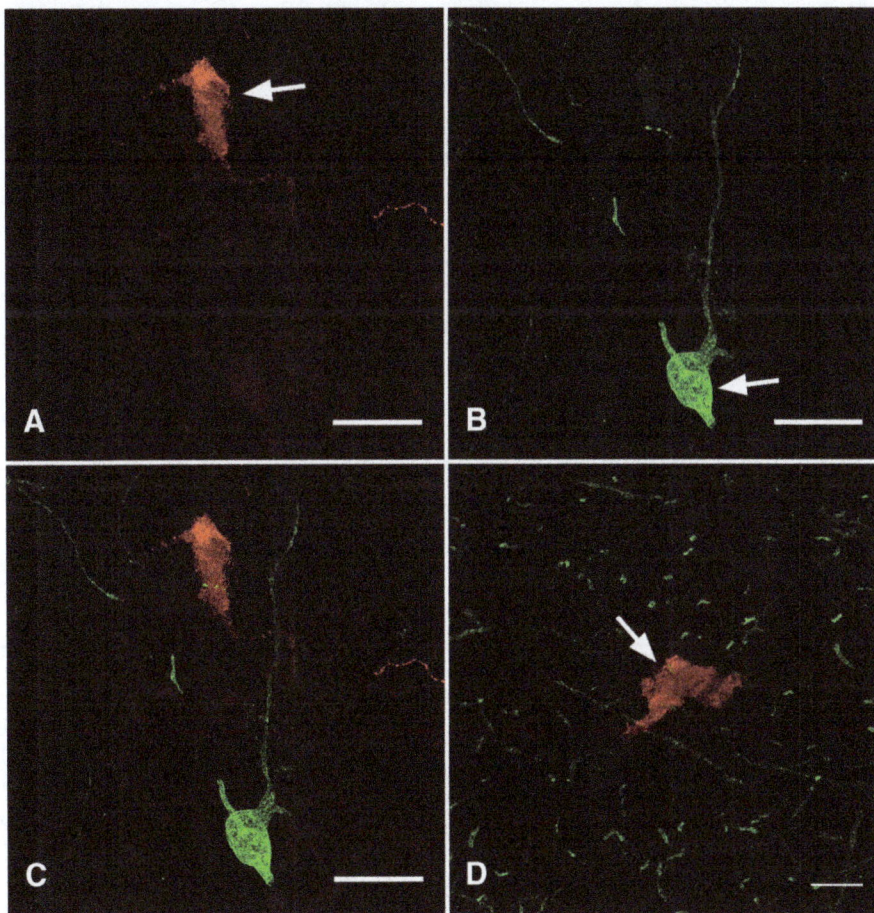

Fig. 5 Immunoreactivity to GnRH and p75 in the llama hypothalamus, detected by double immunofluorescence. A single microscopic field (**a-c**; maximum intensity projection displaying cells immunoreactive for GnRH (red), p75 (green), and both channels (merged). A GnRH immunoreactive neuron (**d**, red) in proximity to p75 immunoreactive fibers (D, green). Arrows indicate nerve cell bodies. Scale bars: **a-c**, 50 μm. **d** 30 μm

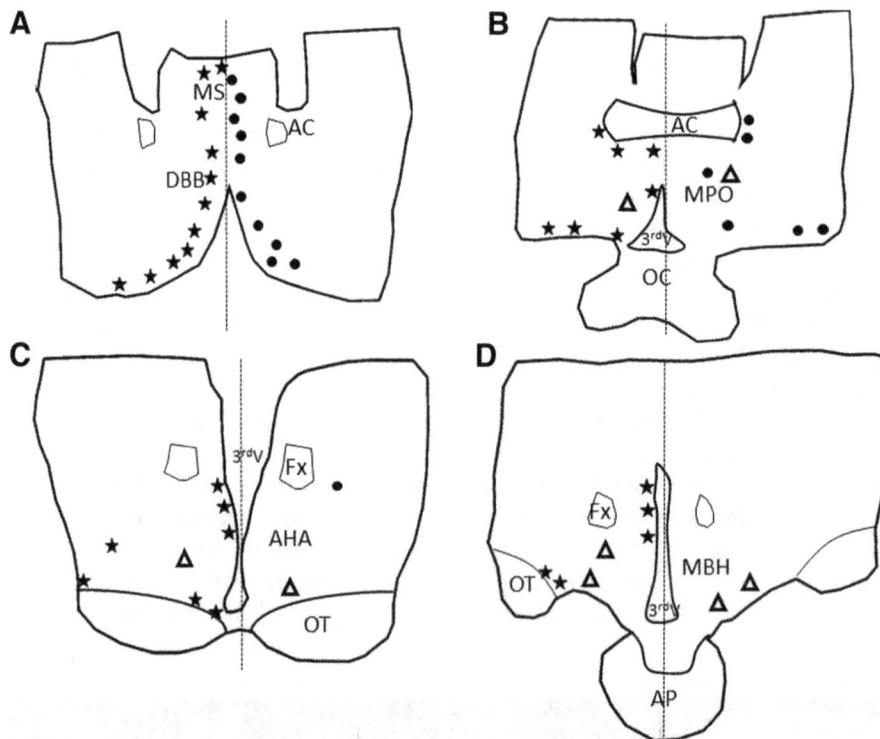

Fig. 6 A representation of the distribution of TrkA (stars), p75 (dots), and GnRH (triangles) neurons in the hypothalamus of llamas. Tracings were made from transverse (coronal) sections, progressing from cranial to caudal, of the diagonal band of Broca/medial septum (**a**), preoptic area (**b**), anterior hypothalamus (**c**), and medio-basal hypothalamus (**d**). For a given histological section, each symbol represents approximately 10 neurons for TrkA and p75, and 5 neurons for GnRH. Each diagram is divided at the midline (dashed line) to permit representation of TrkA on the left and p75 on the right. MS: medial septum, DBB: diagonal band of Broca, MPOA: medial preoptic area, AC: anterior commissure, OC: optic chiasma, Fx: fornix, AHA: anterior hypothalamic area, OT: optic tract, MBH: medio-basal hypothalamus, 3rdV: third ventricle, AP: anterior pituitary

preoptic area and circumventricular organs (organum vasculosum and median eminence). The expression of the low affinity receptor in the median eminence and ependymal layer could be the reflex of important physiological functions. It has been shown that the administration of fluorescent leptin labels the ependymal/tanycyte layer as soon as 15 min after treatment, and the mechanism is associated to the leptin receptor [52]. Given the ability of p75 to bind to several neurotrophins besides NGF (reviewed in [53]), the presence of p75 in circumventricular organs may be attributed a role in mediating neurotrophin entry into the brain or activating signaling pathways. Based on results of PC$_{12}$ neuronal culture experiments, the p75 receptor is capable of internalizing NGF independent of TrkA [54]. However, it remains to be determined if p75 receptor-expressing cells are involved in OIF/NGF-induced ovulation in South American camelids.

Kisspeptin has been documented as an important mediator of GnRH neuron function in several species, such as laboratory rodents [55], sheep [56], and monkeys [57]. In the musk shrew, an induced ovulator, mating activated kisspeptin neurons in the preoptic area, and administration of kisspeptin mimicked mating-induced ovulation [58]. Although no data were reported, authors of a recent review on camelids speculated that kisspeptin may be a mediator of OIF/NGF-induced ovulation [59]. Concentrations of kisspeptin neurons have been identified in the preoptic area and in the arcuate nucleus, and these two populations display different functions in mediating tonic or surge secretion of GnRH [60]. The role of kisspeptin neurons in the ovulatory mechanism in camelids remains to be elucidated.

Conclusion

Results of the present study do not support the hypothesis that OIF/NGF interacts directly with GnRH neurons through receptors to elicit ovulation in llamas. The presence of both high- and low-affinity receptors in the hypothalamus of llamas provides rationale for the hypothesis that OIF/NGF interacts with an interneuron or a group of interneurons that provide inputs to GnRH neurons. The neurochemical identity of the TrkA and p75 immunoreactive cells in the hypothalamus of llamas, however, remains to be established.

Abbreviations
BSA: Bovine serum albumin; GnRH: Gonadotrophin-releasing hormone; LH: Luteinizing hormone; OIF: Ovulation-inducing factor; OIF/NGF: Ovulation-inducing factor/nerve growth factor; PBS: Phosphate buffer saline

Acknowledgements
Authors would like to acknowledge to Carlos Leonardi for help with animal handling and tissue collection, and Dr. Louis F Reichardt (University of California, San Francisco, USA) for kindly providing the p75 antisera used in the present study.

Funding
Research supported by the Natural Sciences and Engineering Research Council of Canada (NSERC).

Authors' contributions
RC participated in study design, data collection, data analysis, data interpretation and manuscript preparation. JS participated in data analysis and manuscript preparation. GPA (principal investigator) participated in the study design, data collection, and manuscript preparation. All authors read and approved the final manuscript.

Consent for publication
Not applicable.

Competing interests
The authors declare that they have no competing interests.

References

1. England BG, Foot WC, Matthews DH, Cardozo AG, Riera S. Ovulation and corpus luteum function in the llama (Lama glama). J Endocrinol. 1969;45:505–13.
2. Fernandez-Baca S, Madden DHL, Novoa C. Effect of different mating stimuli on induction of ovulation in the alpaca. J Reprod Fert. 1970;22:261–7.
3. Adams GP, Ratto MH, Silva ME, Carrasco RA. Ovulation-inducing factor (OIF/NGF) in seminal plasma: a review and update. Reprod Domest Anim. 2016; 51(Suppl. 2):4–17.
4. Adams GP, Ratto MH, Huanca W, Singh J. Ovulation - inducting factor in the seminal plasma of llamas and alpacas. Biol Reprod. 2005;73:452–7.
5. Berland MA, Ulloa-Leal C, Barria M, Wright H, Dissen GA, Silva ME, Ojeda SR, Ratto MH. Seminal plasma induces ovulation in llamas in the absence of a copulatory stimulus: role of nerve growth factor as an ovulation-inducing factor. Endocrinology. 2016;157:3224–32.
6. Ratto MH, Leduc YA, Valderrama XP, Van Straten KE, Delbaere LT, Pierson RA, Adams GP. The nerve of ovulation-inducing factor in semen. Proc Natl Acad Sci U S A. 2012;109:15042–7.
7. Ratto MH, Delbaere LT, Leduc YA, Pierson RA, Adams GP. Biochemical isolation and purification of ovulation-inducing factor (OIF) in seminal plasma of llamas. Reprod Biol Endocrinol. 2011;10:9–24.
8. Tanco VM, Ratto MH, Lazzarotto M, Adams GP. Dose response of female llamas to ovulation-inducing factor (OIF) from seminal plasma. Biol Reprod. 2011;85:452–6.
9. Silva ME, Smulders JP, Guerra M, Valderrama XP, Letelier C, Adams GP, Ratto MH. Cetrorelix suppresses the preovulatory LH surge and ovulation induced by ovulation-inducing factor (OIF) present in llama seminal plasma. Reprod Biol Endocrinol. 2011;9:74.
10. Bogle OA, Ratto MH, Adams GP. Ovulation-inducing factor induces LH secretion from pituitary cells. Anim Reprod Sci. 2012;133:117–22.
11. Paolicchi F, Urquieta B, Del Valle L, Bustos-Obregon E. Biological activity of the seminal plasma of alpacas: stimulus for the production of LH by pituitary cells. Anim Reprod Sci. 1999;54:203–10.
12. Adams GP, Sumar J, Ginther OJ. Effects of lactational status and reproductive status on ovarian follicular waves in llamas (Lama glama). J Reprod Fert. 1990;90:535–45.
13. Adams GP. Comparative patterns of follicle development and selection in ruminants. J Reprod Fert. 1999;54:17–32.
14. Draincourt MA. Regulation of ovarian follicular dynamics in farm animals: implications for manipulation of reproduction. Theriogenology. 2001;55:1211–39.
15. Bravo PW, Stabenfeldt GH, Lasley BL, Fowler ME. The effect of ovarian follicle size on pituitary and ovarian responses to copulation in domesticated South American camelids. Biol Reprod. 1991;45:553–9.
16. Fair T, Lonergan P. The role of progesterone in oocyte acquisition of developmental competence. Reprod Domest Anim. 2012;47:142–7.
17. Silva ME, Recabarren MP, Recabarren SE, Adams GP, Ratto MH. Ovarian estradiol modulates the stimulatory effect of ovulation-inducing factor (OIF) on pituitary LH secretion in llamas. Theriogenology. 2012;77:1873–82.
18. Levi-Montalcini R. The nerve growth factor: thirty years after. EMBO J. 1987;6:1145–54.
19. Conner JM, Muir D, Varon S, Hagg T, Manthorpe M. The localization of nerve growth factor-like immunoreactivity in the adult basal forebrain and hippocampal formation. J Comp Neurol. 1992;319:454–62.
20. Whitemore SR, Ebendal T, Larkfors L, Olson L, Seiger A, Stromberg I, Persson H. Developmental and regional expression of β nerve growth factor messenger RNA and protein in the rat central nervous system. Proc Natl Acad Sci U S A. 1986;83:817–21.
21. Richardson PM, Verge Issa VMK, Riopelle RJ. Distribution of neuronal receptors for nerve growth factor in the rat. J Neurosci. 1986;6:2312–21.
22. Casaccia-Bonnefil P, Carter BD, Dobrowski RT, Chao MV. Death of oligodendrocites mediated by the interaction of nerve growth factor with its receptor p75. Nature. 1996;383:716–9.
23. Yoon SO, Casaccia-Bonnefil P, Carter B, Chao MV. Competitive signaling between TrkA and p75 nerve growth factor receptors determines cell survival. Neuroscience. 1998;18:3273–81.
24. Gibbs RB, Pfaff DW. In situ hybridization detection of trka mRNA in brain: distribution, colocalization with p75NGFR and up-regulation by nerve growth factor. J Comp Neurol. 1994;341:324–39.
25. Sobreviela T, Clary DO, Reichardt LF, Brandabur MM, Kordower JH, Mufson EJ. TrkA-immunoreactive profiles in the central nervous system: Colocalization with neurons containing p75 nerve growth factor receptor, choline acetyltransferase, and serotonin. J Comp Neurol. 1994; 350:587–611.
26. Ohmichi M, Decker SJ, Pang L, Saltiel AR. Inhibition of the cellular actions of nerve growth factor by staurosporine and k252a from the attenuation of the activity of the trk tyrosine kinase. Biochemistry. 1992;31:4034–9.
27. Chao MV. Neurotrophins and their receptors: a convergent point for many signaling pathways. Nat Rev Neurosci. 2003;4:299–309.
28. Clarke IJ, Cummins JT. The relationship between gonadotropin releasing hormone (GnRH) and luteinizing hormone (LH) secretion in ovariectomized ewes. Endocrinology. 1982;111:1737–9.
29. Hoffman GE, Le WW, Sita LV. The importance of titrating antibodies for immunocytochemical methods. Curr Protoc Neurosci. 2008;2:12.
30. Felix B, Léger ME, Fessard DA. Stereotaxic atlas of the pig brain. 1st ed. New York: Elsevier; 1999.
31. Girgis M, Shih-Cjang W. A new stereotaxic atlas of the rabbit brain. 1st ed. St. Louis: W.H. Green; 1981.
32. Urban I, Richard P. A stereotaxic atlas of the New Zealand's rabbit brain. 1st ed. Springfield: Charles C Thomas; 1972.
33. Fernald RD, White RB. Gonadotropin-releasing hormone genes: phylogeny, structure, and functions. Front Neuroendocrinol. 1999;20:224–40.
34. Egginger J, Parmentier C, Garrel G, Cohen-Tannougji J, Camus A, Calas A, Hardin-Prouzet H, Grange-Messent V. Direct evidence for the co-expression of URP and GnRH in a sub-population of rat hypothalamic neurons: anatomical and functional correlation. PLoS One. 2011;6:e26611.
35. Tillet Y, Tourlet S, Picard S, Sizaret P, Caraty A. Morphofunctional interactions between galanin and GnRH-containing neurones in the diencephalon of the ewe. The effect of oestradiol. J Chem Neuroanat. 2012;43:14–9.
36. Weskamp G, Reichardt LF. Evidence that biological activity of NGF is mediated through a novel subclass of high affinity receptors. Neuron. 1991;6:649–63.

37. Lee WS, Smith MS, Hoffman GE. Luteinizing hormone-releasing hormone neurons express fos protein during the proestrus surge of luteinizing hormone. Proc Natl Acad Sci U S A. 1990;87:5163–7.

38. Moenter SM, Karsch FJ, Lehman MN. Fos expression during the estradiol-induced gonadotrophin-releasing hormone (GnRH) surge of the ewe: induction in GnRH and other neurons. Endocrinology. 1993;133:896–903.

39. Wu TJ, Segal AZ, Miller GM, Gibson MJ, Silverman AJ. FOS expression in gonadotropin-releasing hormone neurons: enhancement by steroid treatment and mating. Endocrinology. 1992;131:2045–50.

40. Herbison A. Physiology of the gonadotropin-releasing hormone neuron network. In: Neil J, editor. Knobil and Neil's physiology of reproduction. St Louis: Elsevier; 2005. p. 1415–82.

41. Holtzman DM, Kilbridge J, Li Y, Cunningham ETJ, Lenn NJ, Clary DO, Reichardt LF, Mobley WC. TrkA expression in the CNS: evidence for the existence of several novel NGF-responsive CNS neurons. J Neurosci. 1995;15:1567–76.

42. Ferguson IA, Schweitzer JB, Bartlett PF, Johnson EM Jr. Receptor mediated retrograde transport in CNS neurons after intraventricular administration or NGF and growth factors. J Comp Neurol. 1991;313:680–92.

43. Pan W, Banks WA, Kastin AJ. Permeability of the blood–brain barrier to neurotrophins. Brain Res. 1998;788:87–94.

44. Banks WA. Characteristics of compounds that cross the blood brain barrier. BMC Neurol. 2009;9:S3.

45. Rodriguez EM, Blazquez JL, Guerra M. The design of barriers in the hypothalamus allows the median eminence and the arcuate nucleus to enjoy private milieus: the former opens to the portal blood and the latter to the cerebrospinal fluid. Peptides. 2010;31:757–76.

46. Herde MK, Geist K, Campbell RE, Herbison AE. Gonadotrophin-releasing hormone neurons extend complex highly branched dendritic trees outside the blood brain barrier. Endocrinology. 2012;152:3832–41.

47. Cowley MA, Smart JL, Rubinstein M, Gerdán MG, Diano S, Horvath TL, Cone RD, Low MJ. Leptin activates anorexigenic POMC neurons through a neural network in the arcuate nucleus. Nature. 2001;411:480–4.

48. Zlokovic BV, Jovanovic S, Miao W, Samara S, Verma S, Farrel CL. Differential regulation of leptin transport by the choroid plexus and blood-brain barrier and high affinity transport systems for entry into the hypothalamus and across the blood-cerebrospinal fluid barrier. Endocrinology. 2001;141:1434–41.

49. Spuch C, Carro E. The p75 neurotrophin receptor localization in blood-CSF barrier: expression in choroid plexus epithelium. BMC Neurosci. 2011;12:39.

50. Timmusk T, Mudó G, Metis M, Belluardo N. Expression of mRNAs for neurotrophin and their receptors in the rat choroid plexus and dura mater. Neuroreport. 1995;15:1997–2000.

51. Ferreira G, Meurisse M, Tillet Y, Lévy F. Distribution and co-localization of choline acetyltransferase and p75 neurotrophin receptors in the sheep basal forebrain: implications for the use of a specific cholinergic immunotoxin. Neuroscience. 2001;104:419–39.

52. Balland E, Dam J, Langlet F, Caron E, Steculorum S, Messina A, Rasika S, Falluel-morel A, Anouar Y, Dehouck B, Trinquet E, Jockers R, Bouret S, Prevot V. Hypothalamic tanycytes area an ERK- gated conduit for leptin into the brain. Cell Metab. 2014;19:293–301.

53. Roux PP, Barker PA. Neurotrophin signaling through the p75 neurotrophin receptor. Prog Neurobiol. 2002;67:203–33.

54. Bronfman FC, Tcherpakov M, Jovin TM, Fainzilber M. Ligand-induced internalization of the p75 neurotrophic receptor: a slow route to the signaling endosome. J Neurosci. 2003;23:3209–20.

55. Gottsch ML, Cunningham MJ, Smith JT, Popa SM, Acohido BV, Crowley WF, Seminara S, Clifton DK, Steiner RA. A role for Kisspeptins in the regulation of gonadotropin secretion in the mouse. Endocrinology. 2004;145:4073–7.

56. Messager S, Chatzidaki EE, Ma D, Hendrick AG, Zahn D, Dixon J, Thresher RR, Malinge I, Lomet D, Carlton MB, Colledge WH, Caraty A, Aparicio SA. Kisspeptin directly stimulates gonadotropin-releasing hormone release via G protein-coupled receptor 54. Proc Natl Acad Sci U S A. 2005;102:1761–6.

57. Plant TM, Ramaswamy S, Dipietro MJ. Repetitive activation of hypothalamic G protein-coupled receptor 54 with intravenous pulses of kisspeptin in the juvenile monkey (Macaca mulatta) elicits a sustained train of gonadotropin-releasing hormone discharges. Endocrinology. 2006;147:1007–13.

58. Inoue N, Sasaqawa K, Ikai K, Sasaki Y, Tomikawa J, Oishi S, Fuji N, Uenoyama Y, Ohmori Y, Yamamoto N, Hondo E, Maeda K, Tsukamura H. Kisspeptin neurons mediate reflex ovulation in the musk shrew (Suncus murinus). Proc Natl Acad Sci U S A. 2011;108:17527–32.

59. El Allali K, El Bousmaki N, Ainani H, Simonneaux V. Effect of Camelid's seminal plasma ovulation-inducing factor/ β-NGF: a kisspeptin target hypothesis. Front Vet Sci. 2017;4:99.

60. Goodman RL, Lehman MN. Kisspeptin neurons from mice to men: similarities and differences. Endocrinology. 2012;153:5105–18.

## 13

The thermo-sensitive gene expression signatures of spermatogenesis

Santosh K. Yadav[1†], Aastha Pandey[1†], Lokesh Kumar[1], Archana Devi[1,2], Bhavana Kushwaha[1,2], Rahul Vishvkarma[1], Jagdamba P. Maikhuri[1], Singh Rajender[1,2] and Gopal Gupta[1,2*]

Abstract

Background: Spermatogenesis in most mammals (including human and rat) occurs at ~ 3 °C lower than body temperature in a scrotum and fails rapidly at 37 °C inside the abdomen. The present study investigates the heat-sensitive transcriptome and miRNAs in the most vulnerable germ cells (spermatocytes and round spermatids) that are primarily targeted at elevated temperature in a bid to identify novel targets for contraception and/or infertility treatment.

Methods: Testes of adult male rats subjected to surgical cryptorchidism were obtained at 0, 24, 72 and 120 h post-surgery, followed by isolation of primary spermatocytes and round spermatids and purification to > 90% purity using a combination of trypsin digestion, centrifugal elutriation and density gradient centrifugation techniques. RNA isolated from these cells was sequenced by massive parallel sequencing technique to identify the most-heat sensitive mRNAs and miRNAs.

Results: Heat stress altered the expression of a large number of genes by ≥2.0 fold, out of which 594 genes (286↑; 308↓) showed alterations in spermatocytes and 154 genes (105↑; 49↓) showed alterations in spermatids throughout the duration of experiment. 62 heat-sensitive genes were common to both cell types. Similarly, 66 and 60 heat-sensitive miRNAs in spermatocytes and spermatids, respectively, were affected by ≥1.5 fold, out of which 6 were common to both the cell types.

Conclusion: The study has identified *Acly, selV, SLC16A7*(MCT-2), *Txnrd1* and *Prkar2B* as potential heat sensitive targets in germ cells, which may be tightly regulated by heat sensitive miRNAs rno-miR-22-3P, rno-miR-22-5P, rno-miR-129-5P, rno-miR-3560, rno-miR-3560 and rno-miR-466c-5P.

Background

In most mammals, normal spermatogenesis occurs in a scrotum at a temperature lower than body (~ 3 °C), but fails rapidly inside the abdomen at body temperature. In contrast to other developmental and biological processes, which occur normally at body temperature (~ 37 °C), spermatogenesis completely ceases at this temperature. The scrotum is nature's uniquely designed organ to maintain testes at ~ 3 °C lower than the body-temperature. Limited clinical studies have reported that transient testicular heating of adult human males results in reversible spermatogenic arrest, and hence could be used as a method of contraception [1]. However, the practical-feasibility of physically heating the testis by thermal insulators and/or electrical devices [2] has limited its wide-scale potential clinical application as a method of contraception.

Cryptorchidism (undescended testes) is a condition in which the testes fail to descend into the scrotum and remain in abdomen due to developmental defects. It is one of the most common congenital abnormalities observed in 1–5% of full-term male births and is a risk factor for infertility [3]. It has been well documented that meiotic (pachytene/diplotene spermatocytes) and post-meiotic (round spermatids) are the most heat sensitive germ cell types that undergo quick apoptosis under heat-stress/cryptorchidism in men [4] and rats [5, 6]. The higher sensitivity of germ cells to mild heat stress in comparison to the somatic cells (e.g. Sertoli and Leydig cells) could apparently be due to their high proliferative activity [7], making it an attractive target for contraceptive intervention.

The spermatogenesis is regulated at transcriptional, post-transcriptional and epigenetic levels by integrated expressions of an array of testicular genes in a precise temporal fashion [8, 9]. In recent years, several high

* Correspondence: g_gupta@cdri.res.in
†Santosh K. Yadav and Aastha Pandey contributed equally to this work.
[1]Division of Endocrinology, CSIR-Central Drug Research Institute, BS-10/1, Sector-10, Jankipuram Extension, Sitapur Road, Lucknow 226031, India
[2]Academy of Scientific and Innovative Research (AcSIR), New Delhi 110001, India

throughput differential gene expression studies on spermatogenesis have been performed in rodents, mostly using microarray technology, either in whole testes of prepubertal animals [10–12] or elutriation/Staput-enriched primary spermatocytes and round spermatids [13–15]. Though microarray technique has been employed as a potential tool to identify candidate genes playing important roles in fertility [16, 17], it is limited by its application to known transcripts, and does not contemplate testicular peculiarities such as the remarkable number of splice variants that are differentially expressed in spermatogenic cells [18, 19]. Recently, massive parallel sequencing has been applied successfully to undertake gene expression analysis because of its better sensitivity and capability to identify and quantify novel transcribed regions and splice variants [20–22]. Most recently, da Cruz et al. [23] employed this technology to analyze meiotic and post-meiotic gene expression signatures of mouse transcriptome. However, the thermo-sensitive transcriptome of germ cells reflecting early degenerative changes in these cells have not been explored. In addition to improving our understanding of molecular regulation of spermatogenesis, identification of thermo-sensitive genes could be exploited to achieve contraception by 'molecular heating' in testis instead of actual physical heating. The present study investigates the changes in transcriptome profile of spermatocytes and spermatids from rat testes subjected to surgical cryptorchidism to identify the most heat-sensitive genes in testes.

Methods
Animals
The Institutional Animal Ethics Committee of CDRI, Lucknow, approved the study. Adult male Sprague-Dawley (SD) rats, aged 14 to 16 weeks and weighing 220–250 g, maintained in institute's air conditioned (24 ± 1 °C) quarters with constant photoperiod of 12 h light and 12 h dark and free access to the standard pellet diet and water ad libitum, were used in these investigations.

Surgical cryptorchidism
Rats were anesthetized with ketamine (50 mg/kg) and xylazine (10 mg/kg), and bilateral cryptorchidism was induced surgically through the abdominal route by anchoring both the testes to the inner lateral abdominal wall using a suture passing through the connective tissue of the cauda epididymis. The animals were autopsied 24, 72 and 120 h after the surgery and the testes were removed. One testis from each animal of every group was fixed in 10% formalin for histological studies while the other testis was used for isolation of germ cells. Each group consisted of 5 animals and sham-operated rats served as controls.

Hematoxylin and eosin (H&E) and TUNEL assay
Testes tissues fixed in 10% buffered formalin were embedded in paraffin and 5 μ sections were cut using a microtome (Leica Biosystems, Nussloch, Germany). Sections were processed for H&E staining and thereafter analyzed under a light microscope (Nikon) and their images were captured using NIS elements software, at suitable magnification. Tunel assay was performed using paraffin embedded tissue sections by following the instructions provided with Promega Tunel assay kit (cat no. G3250). Briefly, the paraffin embedded tissue sections were deparaffinised, rehydrated in a series of ethanol, fixed with 4% paraformaldehyde, treated with proteinase-K solution followed by treatment with equilibrating buffer and rTDT incubation buffer for 1 h. Finally the tissues were washed counterstained with DAPI and stored at 4 °C. Thereafter tissue sections were analysed under flourescence microscope (Nikon) and the images were captured using NIS elements software, at suitable magnification. For statistical analysis of the number of primary spermatocytes and round spermatids present in sham (control), 24, 72 and 120 h of cryptorchid testes, the same were counted in three different areas of three different sections from each group, and the data has been analysed by one-way analysis of variance (ANOVA). P values less than 0.05 were considered as significant.

Isolation and purification of spermatocytes and round spermatids from rat testis
Primary spermatocytes and round spermatids were isolated by trypsin digestion and purified by centrifugal elutriation and density gradient centrifugation by the method of Meistrich et al. [24]. Briefly, the testes were decapsulated and minced with scissors in Basal Medium Eagle (BME). Subsequently, the minced suspension was incubated for 15 min with shaking in a water bath at 34 °C in Basal Medium Eagle (BME) supplemented with 0.1% trypsin (w/v), 0.1% glucose and 17 μg/ml DNase. After incubation, the enzyme reaction was stopped by addition of Soybean trypsin inhibitor (0.04% w/v), and the cell-suspension was filtered through a nylon mesh (36 μm) and passed through a column of glass wool to remove sperm. The ensued cell suspension was centrifuged at 400 g for 5 min at 4 °C and the cell pellet obtained was washed twice with BME. The mixed germ cell population was suspended in BME containing DNase (2 μg/ml) and FBS (8% V/V) and kept on ice. Later, the cell suspension was elutriated with a Beckman Elutriator Rotor (JE-5) fitted with a standard chamber and mounted on a Beckman High Speed Centrifuge (Avanti J-26S–XP). Two fractions (I and II) were collected at 3000 rpm at flow rates of 18.0 and 31.5 ml/min, and then the rotor speed was reduced to 2000 rpm and another two fractions (III and IV) were collected at

flow rates of 23.0 and 40.0 ml/min, respectively. Fractions II and IV contained pachytene spermatocytes and round spermatids at purities of ~ 80% and ~ 75%, respectively. The fractions II and IV were layered separately over linear Percoll gradients of 25–37% and 23–33% Percoll, respectively, and centrifuged at 4025 g for 60 min in a swinging bucket rotor fitted on to a Sigma 3-30 K refrigerated centrifuge. The major band was recovered through a puncture in the side of the tube, washed and diluted with BME. Further, the purity of isolated cells was checked visually under a microscope and through DNA quantitation using flow cytometry.

RNA isolation and sequencing

A Qiagen RNeasy Micro Kit (74,004, Qiagen) was used to extract RNA from the sorted cells. The extraction was performed according to Quick-Start Protocol suggested by the manufacturers. miRNA was isolated from the total RNA population by the ligation of a 3' RNA adapter using t4 RNA ligase and ligation buffer. The 3'adapter ligated small RNA was again 5' ligated with 5'RNA adapter and then the corresponding small RNA was reverse transcribed and amplified to generate cDNA constructs. These cDNA constructs were purified using 6% PAGE and the corresponding small RNA bands were excised between 140 and 160 bp lengths. The cDNA construct from the gel was recovered by filtration and subsequently precipitated with ethanol. These were quantified and subjected to sequencing and data analysis. The integrity and quality of the extracted RNAs were checked by Agilent 2100 bioanalyzer and the qualified RNA samples were used for sequencing. A total of 3 pools were prepared for each type of cells to have three biological replicates. Dynabeads mRNA DIRECTTM kit (610.12, Life Technologies) was used to enrich RNAs with polyA tail. mRNA-seq library was prepared using TruSeq RNA kit (RS-122-2001, Illumina). Sequencing was performed on Illumina Hiseq 2500 next generation sequencing platform. Sequencing-v3 (634,848, Clontech Laboratories) was used to amplify the cDNA derived from these cells before sequencing was performed.

Raw data production and preprocessing

TopHat (v2.0.8b, http://tophat.cbcb.umd.edu/) was used to map the RNA-seq reads to rat genome build hg19 (UCSC). The reads with low quality were removed from the raw sequencing reads. Read mapping were performed using Tophat (R software), reads count were obtained using HTSeq (http://www-huber.embl.de/users/anders/HTSeq/doc/overview.html). Differentially expressed genes were analysed using DESeq R software pack. Benjamini-Hochberg multiple testing corrections were employed to reveal the differentially expressed genes.

Validation of mRNA expression by real time RT-PCR

Total RNA was isolated using Trizol reagent (Invitrogen Life Technologies, Carlsbad, CA) and 3 μg of RNA was converted to cDNA using the RevertAid H Minus First Strand cDNA Synthesis Kit (Fermentas, Waltham, MA) following the manufacturer's instructions. Real time PCR was performed on a Light Cycler 480 (Roche, Basel, Switzerland) detection system using SYBR Green I Master mix (Roche, Basel, Switzerland) in 96-well plates. All reactions were run in triplicates and relative gene expression was normalized to steady state expression of GAPDH, calculations made by using the 2-ΔΔCt method.

Results

Histology of control and cryptorchid testes

The H & E stained testes sections of control and cryptorchid rat suggest that at 24 h there was negligible visible change in any stage of spermatogenesis and most of the stages were present (Fig. 1b), as in control (Fig. 1a). However, at 72 h there was a marked increase in the incidence of germ cell apoptosis predominantly at stages I–V and the late stages XI–XIV, while stages V–X were comparatively less affected (Fig. 1c). On the other hand, at 120 h stages I–VI were badly distorted while stages X–XIV were not distinguishable at all. However, stages VII and VIII were visible but cell apoptosis was quite significant (Fig. 1d). There was a significant reduction in number of spermatocytes at 72 ($P < 0.05$) and 120 ($P < 0.01$) h of cryptochidism (Fig. 1e). In case of spermatids, a significant reduction in their number was evident at 24 ($P < 0.05$), 72 and 120 ($P < 0.001$) h (Fig. 1f).

Tunnel assay of paraffin embedded testis tissues

Tunnel assay was performed to check whether the loss of cells in cryptorchid testes was due to heat-induced apoptosis (Fig. 2). Results indicated that apoptosis was induced in testicular germ cells at body temperature and the number of apoptotic cells gradually increased with the duration of heat exposure (Fig. 2a, d, g, j). Though very few yet significant number of apoptotic cells were observed at 24 h ($P < 0.05$) of heat-stress, the number increased significantly thereafter at 72 h ($P < 0.001$) and 120 h ($P < 0.001$) (Fig. 2m), which was in agreement with H&E data.

Isolation, purification and characterization of primary spermatocytes and round spermatids

The enzymatic digestion of testicular parenchyma resulted in complete dispersion of testicular cells (Fig. 3a). The two cell types i.e. spermatocytes and round spermatids were isolated up to the purity of ~ 75% and ~ 80%, respectively, by using centrifugal elutriation method. The homogeneity of spermatocytes and round spermatids was

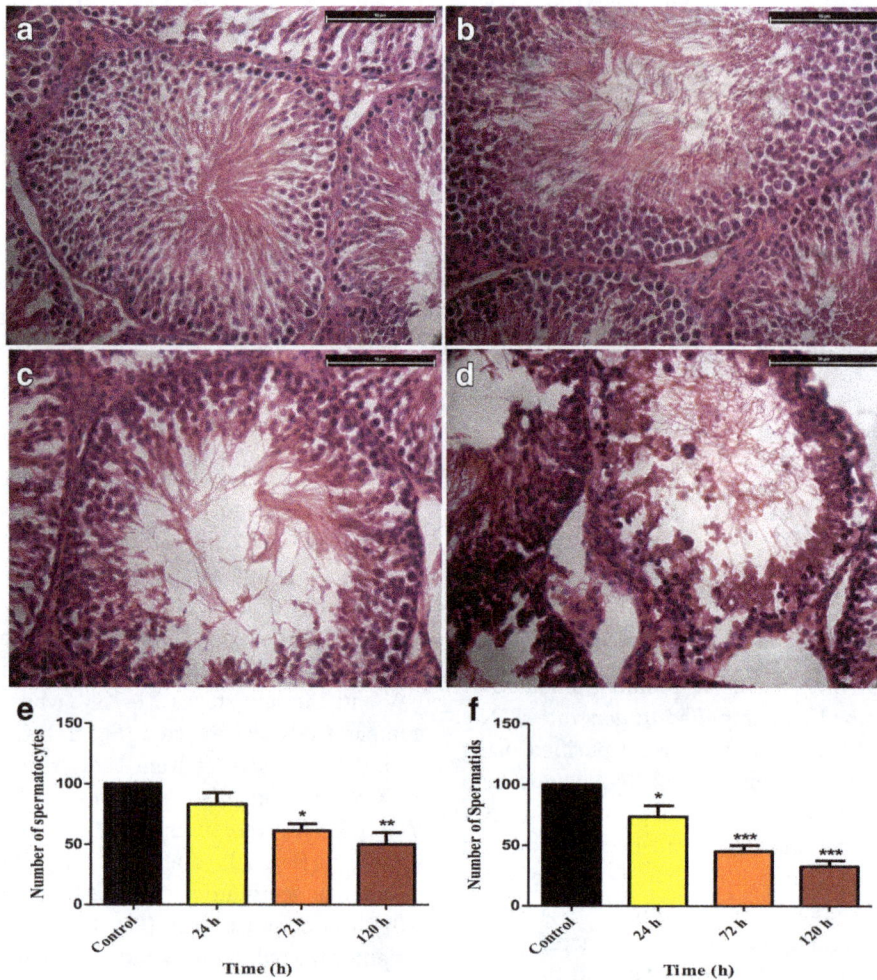

Fig. 1 Representative picture of testes histology at 0 h [sham, **a**], 24 h [**b**], 72 h [**c**] and 120 h [**d**] of cryptorchidism (Bar = 10 µm). Average number of spermatocytes (**e**) and spermatids (**f**) after 0, 24, 72 and 120 h of cryptorchidism. (Mean ± SE; *$P < 0.05$; **$P < 0.01$; ***$P < 0.001$)

further increased to ~ 90 and > 92%, respectively, by Percoll density gradient centrifugation method (Fig. 3b and c). The purity of the two cell types was confirmed by FACS, which exhibited a single peak in both the cell preparations with negligible number of contaminating cells (Fig. 3d and e). The trypan blue exclusion test showed > 95% viability of the purified cells in the two fractions (data not shown).

Transcriptome profiling and differential gene expression analysis

Total RNA was extracted from highly purified primary spermatocytes and round spermatids, isolated from the testicular tissues of all the experimental groups, and subjected to sequencing using Illumina NextSeq 2500. We performed pairwise differential gene expression (DGE) comparisons between samples to detect the genes exhibiting differences in expression by at least 2-fold. The transcriptome from spermatocytes of control testis (0-Cr-Sc) was compared with that of 24 h crypt (24-Cr-Sc) and 72 h crypt (72-Cr-Sc) testes. Similarly, the transcriptome from control spermatids (0-Cr-Sd) was compared with 24, 72 and 120 h crypt spermatids (24-Cr-Sd; 72-Cr-Sd; 120-Cr-Sd). In spermatocytes, the expression of total 1602 genes was altered (897 up regulated and 705 down regulated) after 24 h of cryptorchidism, and the expression of 1807 genes was altered (987 up regulated and 820 down regulated) after 72 h of cryptorchidism. Similarly in spermatids, after 24, 72, 120 h of cryptorchidism altered expression of 1210 (505 up regulated and 705 down regulated), 1718 (990 up regulated and 728 down regulated) and 3559 (2180 up regulated and 1379 down regulated) transcripts, respectively, was seen. The genes showing change in the expression within 24 h could be categorized as early response genes while those showing alteration after 24 h could be termed as mid and late

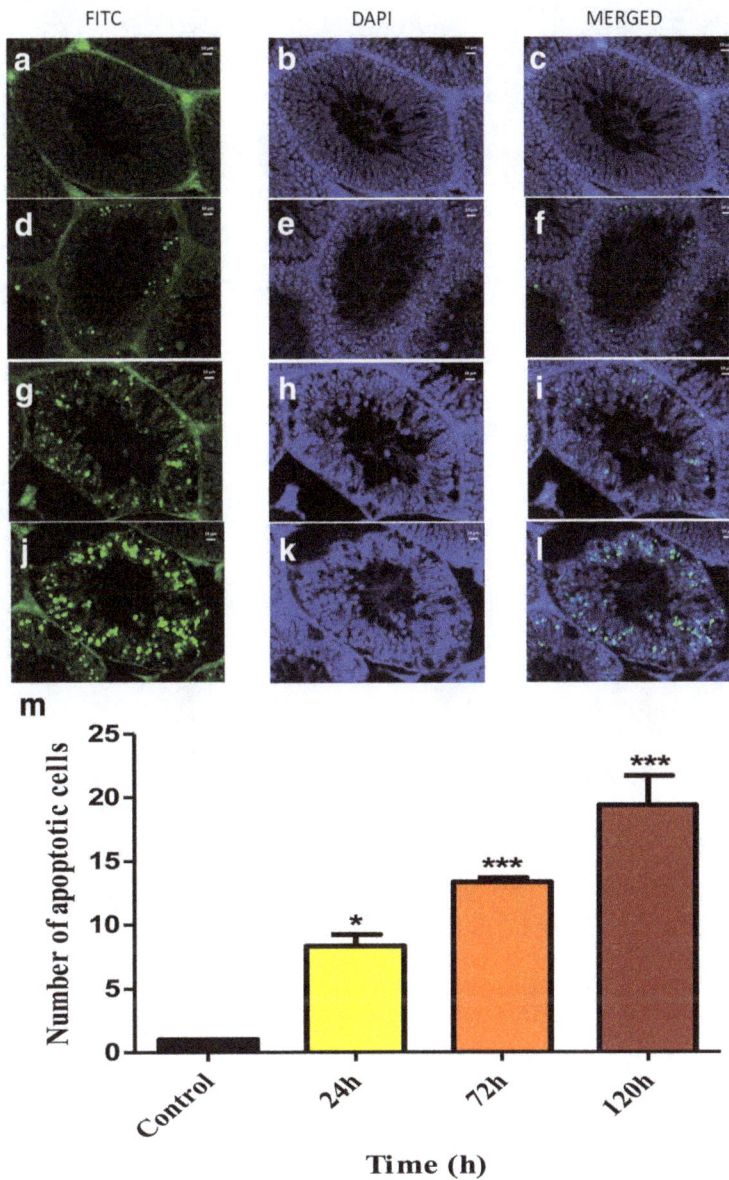

Fig. 2 Apoptosis of germ cells by Tunel Assay in rat testis at 0 h [1**a**, **b**, **c**]; 24 h [1**d**, **e**, **f**]; 72 h [1**g**, **h**, **i**] and 120 h [1 **j**, **k**, **l**] of cryptorchidism. (**a**, **d**, **g**, **j** – FITC staining for DNA fragmentation; **b**, **e**, **h**, **k** – DAPI staining of DNA; **c**, **f**, **i**, **l** – merged images) (Bar = 10 μm). Average number of TUNEL positive cells (M; Mean ± SE; *$P < 0.05$; ***$P < 0.001$)

response genes. Overall observations clearly indicate that the number of genes with altered expression increased with an increase in the time period of heat exposure.

Venn analysis indicated that all through 24–72 h of cryptorchidism, a total of 286 genes were up-regulated and 308 genes were down-regulated in spermatocytes. Similarly, in spermatids 105 genes were up-regulated and 49 genes were down-regulated during 24–120 h of cryptorchidism. Further, Venn analysis suggested that 62 genes were altered in both the cell types during the entire period of hyperthermia (Fig. 4). A heat map of the

expression profile of temperature-sensitive genes in the two cell types has been prepared (Fig. 5). A number of genes showed more than one transcript variant, which exhibited different expression patterns in spermatocytes and spermatids.

Gene ontology

With the aim of finding the pathways/biological processes prominently affected by heat stress, gene ontology of 62 crucial genes was performed. The PANTHER online analysis tool indicated that the

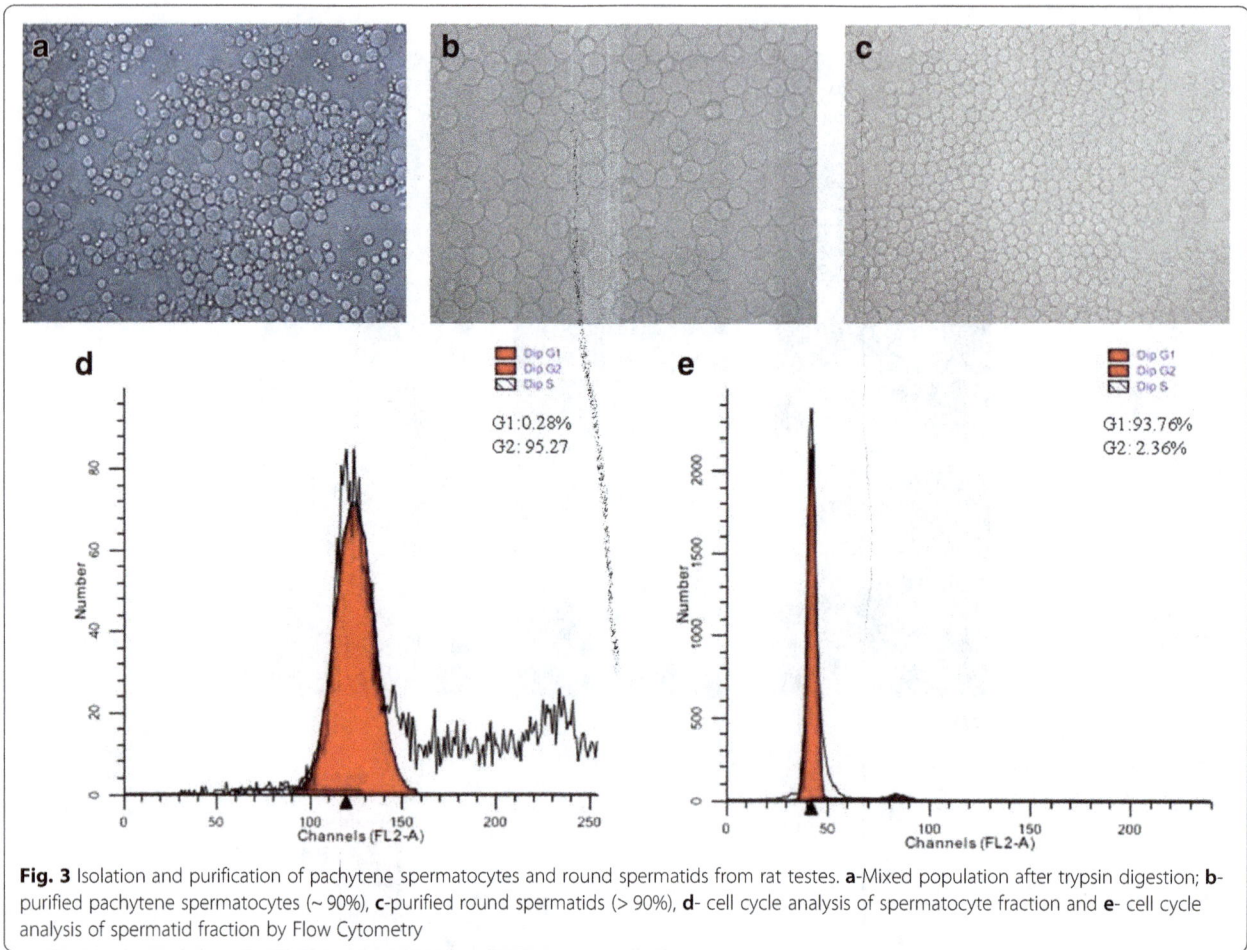

Fig. 3 Isolation and purification of pachytene spermatocytes and round spermatids from rat testes. **a**-Mixed population after trypsin digestion; **b**-purified pachytene spermatocytes (~ 90%), **c**-purified round spermatids (> 90%), **d**- cell cycle analysis of spermatocyte fraction and **e**- cell cycle analysis of spermatid fraction by Flow Cytometry

affected transcripts had catalytic (26), binding (21), structural (7), and transporter (6) functions (Table 1). These transcripts were mostly related to cellular (29) and metabolic processes (26), or to biological regulation (6), localization (9), reproduction (1), developmental process (6), or to cellular component organization and biogenesis (8). A single gene may be involved in more than one process. According to the PANTHER tool, the shortlisted genes encoded proteins belonging to the class of nucleic acid binding (9), enzyme modulators (5), hydrolases (8), transferases (5), transcription factors (4), and signaling molecules (3).

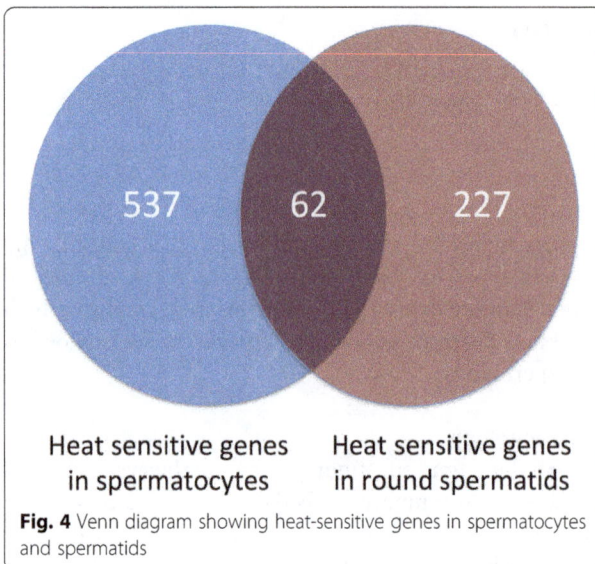

Fig. 4 Venn diagram showing heat-sensitive genes in spermatocytes and spermatids

Validation of deep sequencing data by qPCR

For validation of deep sequencing data, we selected 15 heat-sensitive genes related to important biological processes i.e. metabolism (Mct1, Mct2, Mct4, Glut3, Ldhc), lipid biogenesis (Acly), ROS and Ca^{++} mediated signaling pathway (Daxx, Camk2d), apoptotic signaling pathway (p53, Daxx), gene expression

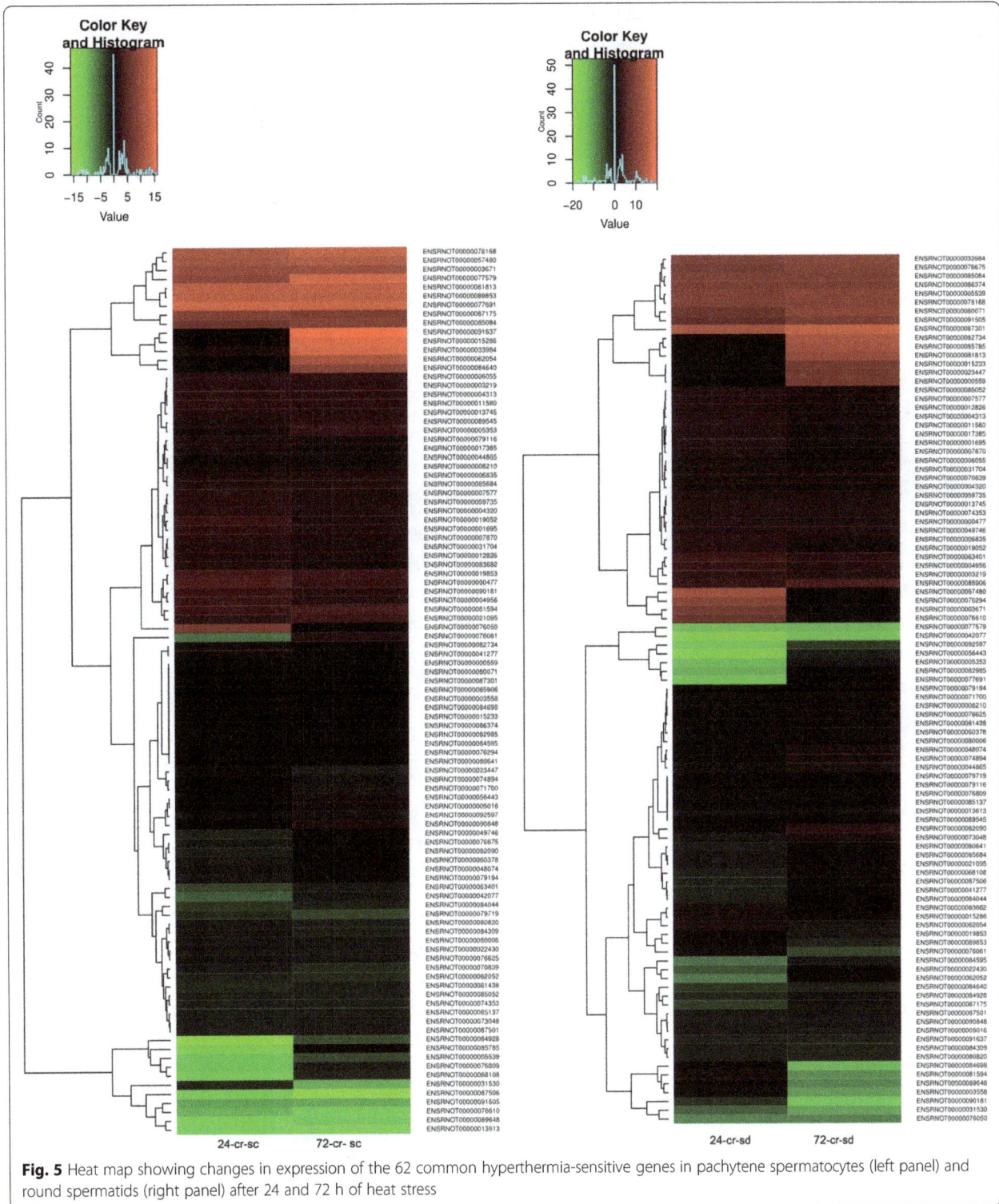

Fig. 5 Heat map showing changes in expression of the 62 common hyperthermia-sensitive genes in pachytene spermatocytes (left panel) and round spermatids (right panel) after 24 and 72 h of heat stress

regulation (Taf9, Gtf2b, Cnot8), spermatogenesis (spata22), redox pathway (Txnrd1) and mitochondria related pathway (Mrps14) for validation by RT-PCR. For all the 15 genes, the qPCR data followed almost the same pattern as depicted by sequencing data for both the cell types (Fig. 6).

miRNA profiling of heat stressed spermatocytes and spermatids by deep sequencing

Similar to mRNA sequencing data analysis, we also performed miRNA sequencing data analysis for spermatocytes and round spermatids from normal and cryptorchid rat testes. A change of ≥1.5 fold in

Table 1 Gene ontology of genes affected by heat in both spermatocytes and spermatids

	No. of genes	Name of genes
Molecular functions		
Binding (GO:0005488)	21	Taf9, Cast, Apbb1, Crip1, Zfp202, Timp1, Lilrb3l, AC120291 (Mbd3), Sptbn1, Cast, Sept4, AC120291 (Mex3d), Prpf8, Rabgap1l, Gtf2b, Tdrd5, Micu1, Upf1, Prelp, Micu2, Camk2d
Catalytic activity (GO:0003824)	26	Cst, Clk3, Hsd11b1, Mink1, Timp1, Abcc12, AC120291 (Atp8b3), Scpep1, Cast, Sept4, Grip1, AC120291 (Mex3d), Acly, Serpinf1, Prpf8, Ptpru, Rabgap1l, Tdrd5, Txnrd1, Upf1, Nt5c3b, Idhc, Mipep, Scamp1, LOC316124, Camk2d
Receptor activity (GO:0004872)	2	Lilrb3l, Ptpru
Signal transducer activity (GO:0004871)	1	Mink1
Structural molecule activity (GO:0005198)	7	Emp1, Crip1, Mgp, C1qa, Sptbn1, Sept4, Mrps14
Transporter activity (GO:0005215)	6	Abcc12, AC120291 (Atp8b3), Mct4, LOC316124, Mct2,Mct1
Biological process		
Biological adhesion (GO:0022610)	7	Cfb, Col6a2, Ccdc80, C1qa, Cfb, Rabgap1l, Prelp
Biological regulation (GO:0065007)	6	Crip1, Mink1, Timp1, AC120291 (Atp8b3), AC120291 (Mbd3), Serpinf1
Cellular component organization or biogenesis (GO:0071840)	8	Col6a2, Crip1, Mink1, AC120291 (Atp8b3), C1qa, AC120291 (Mbd3)
Cellular process (GO:0009987)	29	Emp1, Cfb, Col6a2, Apbb1, Ccdc80, AC120291 (Plk5), Zfp202, Mink1, Timp1, AC120291 (Atp8b3), C1qa, Lilrb3l, AC120291 (Mbd3), Wdr36, Scpep1, Sptbn1, Cfb, Sept4, Grip1, Prpf8, Rabgap1l, Prkar2b, Upf1, Prelp, Mipep, Mct4, Mrps14, Mct2, Camk2d
Developmental process (GO:0032502)	6	Crip1, Mink1, C1qa, Sptbn1, Prelp, Camk2d
Immune system process (GO:0002376)	9	Cfb, Col6a2, Crip1, Ccdc80, Abcc12, C1qa, Col3a1, Cfb, LOC316124
Localization (GO:0051179)	9	Abcc12, AC120291, Cast, Rabgap1l, Scamp1, Mct4, LOC316124, Mct2, Mct1
Metabolic process (GO:0008152)	26	Taf9, Cast, Apbb1, Crip1, Zfp202, Hsd11b1, Mink1, Timp1, AC120291 (Atp8b3), AC120291 (Mbd3), Wdr36, Scpep1, AC120291 (Mex3d), Acly, Prpf8, Ptpru, Sdhaf3, Gtf2b, Tdrd5, Txnrd1, Upf1, Idhc, Prelp, Mipep, LOC316124, Mrps14
Multicellular organismal process (GO:0032501)	4	Mink1, Col3a1, Grip1, Prelp
Reproduction (GO:0000003)	1	Crip1
Response to stimulus (GO:0050896)	8	Taf9, Cfb, Lilrb3, Crip1, Mink1, Timp1, Abcc12, Cfb
Cellular Component		
Cell junction (GO:0030054)	1	Grip1
Cell part (GO:0044464)	15	Emp1, Apbb1, Crip1, Zfp202, Mink1, AC120291 (Atp8b3), AC120291 (Mbd3), Wdr36, Sptbn1, Sept4, Prpf8, Ptpru, Mipep, Mrps14, Camk2d
Extracellular matrix (GO:0031012)	4	Col6a2, Timp1, C1qa, Prelp
Extracellular region (GO:0005576)	4	Timp1, C1qa, Serpinf1, Prelp
Macromolecular complex (GO:0032991)	3	Wdr36, Prpf8, Mrps14
Membrane (GO:0016020)	4	AC120291 (Atp8b3), Grip1, Mct4, Mct1
Organelle (GO:0043226)	9	Apbb1, Zfp202, AC120291 (Atp8b3), AC120291 (Mbd3), AC120291, Sept4, Prpf8, Prelp, Mipep
Protein class		
Calcium-binding protein (PC00060)	3	Mgp, Micu1, Micu2
Cell adhesion molecule (PC00069)	1	C1qa
Cell junction protein (PC00070)	1	Grip1
Cytoskeletal protein (PC00085)	5	Emp1, Crip1, Ivns1abp, Sptbn1, Sept4
Defense/immunity protein (PC00090)	1	Lilrb3l
Enzyme modulator (PC00095)	5	Cast, Cast (Erc2), Sept4, Serpinf1, Rabgap1l
Extracellular matrix protein (PC00102)	3	Mgp, C1qa, Prelp
Hydrolase (PC00121)	8	Ivns1abp, AC120291 (Atp8b3), Scpep1, Ptpru, Rabgap1l, Upf1, Nt5c3b, Mipep
Ligase (PC00142)	3	AC120291 (Mex3d), Acly, LOC316124

Table 1 Gene ontology of genes affected by heat in both spermatocytes and spermatids *(Continued)*

	Nō. of genes	Name of genes
lyase (PC00144)	1	*Acly*
Membrane traffic protein (PC00150)	1	*Cast*
Nucleic acid binding (PC00171)	9	*Taf9, Crip1, AC120291 (Mbd3), Wdr36, AC120291 (Mex3d), Prpf8, Tdrd5, Upf1, Mrps14*
Oxidoreductase (PC00176)	3	*Hsd11b1, Txnrd1, ldhc*
Signaling molecule (PC00207)	3	*Apbb1, Mgp, Lilrb3l*
Structural protein (PC00211)	1	*Mgp*
Transcription factor (PC00218)	4	*Taf9, Crip1, Ivns1abp, Gtf2b*
Transferase (PC00220)	5	*Clk3, Grip1, Acly, Scamp1, Camk2d*
Transporter (PC00227)	5	*Abcc12, AC120291 (Atp8b3), Mct4, Mct2, Mct1*
Transfer carrier protein	1	*Scamp1*
Receptors	2	*Ptpru, Prelp*
Pathways		
Alzheimer disease-amyloid secretase pathway (P00003)	1	*Apbb1*
Alzheimer disease-presenilin pathway (P00004)	1	*Apbb1*
Angiogenesis (P00005)	1	*AC120291 (Apc2)*
Cytoskeletal regulation by Rho GTPase (P00016)	2	*Arpc2, Gtf2b*
General transcription regulation (P00023)	2	*Taf9, Gtf2b*
Inflammation mediated by chemokine and cytokine signaling pathway (P00031)	3	*Col6a2, Arpc2, camk2d*
Integrin signalling pathway (P00034)	3	*Col6a2, Arpc2, Col3a1*
Parkinson disease (P00049)	1	*Sept4*
Pyruvate metabolism (P02772)	1	*Acly*
Transcription regulation by bZIP transcription factor (P00055)	3	*Taf9, Gtf2b, Prkar2b*
Wnt signaling pathway (P00057)	1	*AC120291 (Apc2)*
5HT receptor Mediated signaling	1	*Prkar2b*
Apoptosis signalling pathway	1	*daxx*
b 1 adrenergic signaaling	1	*Prkar2b*
b2 adrenegenic signalling	1	*Prkar2b*
dopamine receptor mediated signaling	1	*Prkar2b*
fas signalling pathway	1	*daxx*
endothilin signalling pathway	1	*Prkar2b*
muscarinie acetylcholine receptor 2 and 4 signalling	1	*Prkar2b*
metabotropic glutamate receptor III pathway	1	*Prkar2b*
metabotropic glutamate receptor II pathway	1	*Prkar2b*
ionotropic glutamate receptor pathway	1	*Camk2d*
GABA b receptor signaling	1	*Prkar2b*

expression of miRNAs under heat stress was considered as significant. In spermatocytes, after 24, 72 and 120 h of cryptorchidism, 175 (93 upregulated and 82 down regulated), 185 (71 upregulated and 114 down regulated) and 280 (126 upregulated and 154 down regulated) miRNAs exhibited altered expression, respectively. Venn analysis (Fig. 7) indicated that 66 miRNAs remained affected throughout 24–120 h of heat stress in spermatocytes, which included 3 novel miRNAs (Table 2). On the other hand, in spermatids after 24, 72 and 120 h of cryptorchidism, 265 (147 upregulated and 118 down

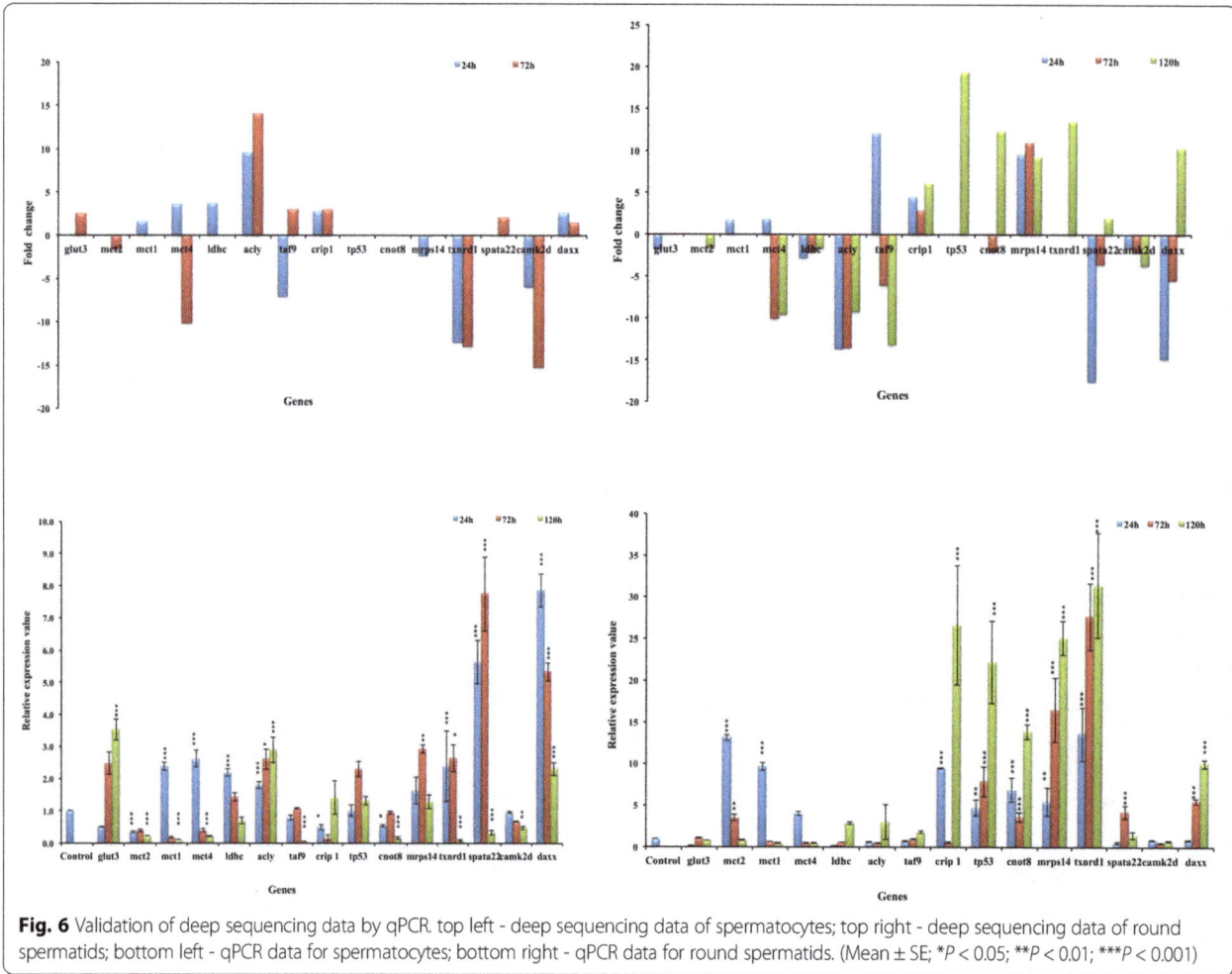

Fig. 6 Validation of deep sequencing data by qPCR. top left - deep sequencing data of spermatocytes; top right - deep sequencing data of round spermatids; bottom left - qPCR data for spermatocytes; bottom right - qPCR data for round spermatids. (Mean ± SE; *P < 0.05; **P < 0.01; ***P < 0.001)

regulated), 301 (160 upregulated and 141 down regulated), and 328 (162 upregulated and 166 down regulated) genes exhibited altered expression, respectively. Venn analysis (Fig. 7) showed that 60 miRNAs (including 6 novel) (Table 2) remained significantly affected throughout 24–120 h of cryptorchidism. The heat map of the expression profile of

common miRNAs in both the cell types is presented in Fig. 8.

Prediction of novel miRNAs
Among novel miRNAs, we identified 3 and 6 miRNAs that were most heat-sensitive in spermatocytes and round spermatids, respectively (Table 3).

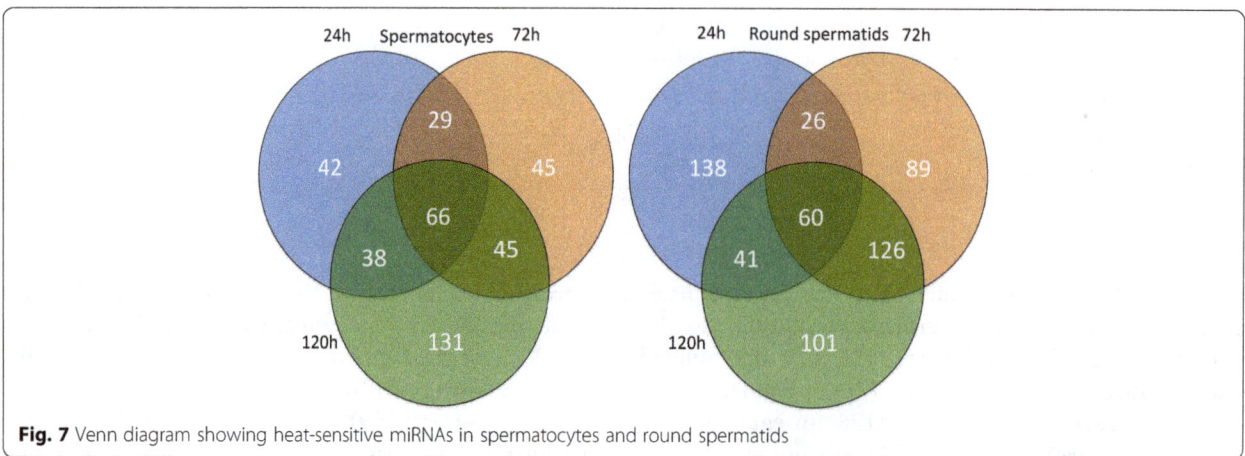

Fig. 7 Venn diagram showing heat-sensitive miRNAs in spermatocytes and round spermatids

Table 2 miRNAs with altered expression in spermatocytes and round spermatid under heat stress

Major miRNAs altered by heat in spermatocytes	Major miRNAs altered by heat in round spermatids
bta-miR-339a; bta-miR-339b; bta-miR-423-3p; bta-miR-99a-5p; cfa-miR-101; cfa-miR-1306; cgr-miR-28-5p; cgr-miR-298-5p; chi-miR-15a-5p; efu-miR-29a; efu-miR-34a; efu-miR-381; ggo-miR-146a; ggo-miR-148a; ggo-miR-151a; ggo-miR-381; hsa-let-7c-5p; hsa-miR-100-5p; hsa-miR-101-3p; hsa-miR-10a-5p; hsa-miR-1306-5p; hsa-miR-148a-3p; hsa-miR-202-5p; hsa-miR-28-5p; hsa-miR-381-3p; hsa-miR-423-3p; hsa-miR-99a-5p; mdo-miR-100-5p; mdo-miR-10b-5p; mdo-miR-199b-2-5p; mmu-let-7i-5p; mmu-miR-101c; mmu-miR-146a-5p; mmu-miR-151-5p; mmu-miR-201-5p; mmu-miR-202-5p; mmu-miR-296-5p; mmu-miR-298-5p; mmu-miR-300-3p; mmu-miR-3074-5p; mmu-miR-3470b; mmu-miR-501-3p; mmu-miR-674-3p; Novel_1015; Novel_3011; Novel_66; oan-miR-1386; oar-miR-10a; oar-miR-374b; oar-miR-99a; ppy-miR-378d; rno-miR-148a-5p; rno-miR-25-5p; rno-miR-339-5p; rno-miR-3560; rno-miR-3585-5p; rno-miR-3586-3p; rno-miR-466c-5p; rno-miR-483-3p; rno-miR-501-3p; rno-miR-547-3p; rno-miR-676; sha-miR-202; ssc-let-7i; ssc-miR-186; ssc-miR-339	bta-miR-22-3p; bta-miR-3600; bta-miR-363; cgr-miR-222-3p; cgr-miR-24-5p; cgr-miR-28-5p; cgr-miR-664-3p; cgr-miR-7b; chi-miR-361-3p; chi-miR-363-3p; efu-miR-30a; efu-miR-34a; efu-miR-7a; efu-miR-7b; ggo-miR-151a; ggo-miR-328; ggo-miR-423; hsa-miR-100-5p; hsa-miR-151b; hsa-miR-22-3p; hsa-miR-22-5p; hsa-miR-3184-3p; hsa-miR-32-3p; hsa-miR-361-3p; hsa-miR-423-5p; hsa-miR-449b-5p; mdo-miR-100-5p; mdo-miR-106-5p; mdo-miR-15a-5p; mdo-miR-22-3p; mml-miR-32-3p; mml-miR-411-3p; mml-miR-99b-3p; mmu-miR-129-5p; mmu-miR-151-5p; mmu-miR-204-3p; mmu-miR-24-2-5p; mmu-miR-28c; mmu-miR-301a-5p; mmu-miR-3074-2-3p; mmu-miR-32-3p; mmu-miR-7b-5p; mmu-miR-99b-3p; mmu-miR-99b-5p; Novel_1113; Novel_1204; Novel_2956; Novel_3356; Novel_4066; Novel_4398; rno-miR-298-3p; rno-miR-301a-5p; rno-miR-32-3p; rno-miR-328a-3p; rno-miR-3586-3p; rno-miR-411-3p; rno-miR-423-5p; rno-miR-664-3p; ssc-miR-20a; ssc-miR-411

Target prediction of heat-sensitive miRNAs in round spermatids and gene ontology of predicted targets

The heat-sensitive miRNAs, among known miRNAs in rat species, were selected for target prediction. The gene ontologies of predicted targets have been detailed for spermatocytes (Table 4) and spermatids (Table 5).

The crucial thermo-sensitive genes regulated tightly by miRNAs have been selected with the help of online miRDB tool. The table below lists the most heat sensitive miRNAs and their probable target proteins in temperature vulnerable meiotic and post-meiotic germ cells of rat testis at 24/72/120 h of heat stress, during which their numbers decrease to significantly low numbers. Capturing molecular changes early in heat exposure could identify the core thermo-regulators, while longer exposure may result in a host of secondary molecular changes, which may not be the key thermo-regulators.

Thermo-sensitive miRNAs	Fold change in miRNA	Fold change in target mRNA	Predicted gene targets	Cell Type
rno-miR-22-3P	+ 3.4	−13.5	Acly	Spermatid
rno-miR-22-5P	+ 1.8	−13.5	Acly	Spermatid
rno-miR-129-5P	−1.9	+ 8.5	selV	Spermatocyte
rno-miR-3560	+ 2.1	−1.6	MCT2	Spermatocyte
rno-miR-3560	+ 2.1	−12.3	Txnrd1	Spermatocyte
rno-miR-466c-5P	+ 1.5	−1.8	Prkar2B	Spermatid

Discussion

Crytorchidism is a state wherein the loss of germ cells takes place by apoptosis leading to infertility, and transient testicular heating has been shown to provide reversible contraception in men [25] and temporary sterility in rats [26]. Therefore, determining the dynamics

of gene expression during spermatogenesis under heat stress could be advantageous in identifying key heat-sensitive genes regulating gamete production for the development of male contraceptives. While a few studies have investigated the differential gene expression (DGE) in mouse during normal spermatogenesis [20–22], none has tried to study the regulation of transcriptome in the vulnerable germ cell types (spermatocytes and spermatids) during cryptorchidism. A careful analysis of transcriptome data suggested that though there is a general disturbance in metabolic/biological processes and pathways under heat stress in both spermatocytes and spermatids, the most strongly affected genes were related to solute carrier family (transporters), energy metabolism, ROS, ribosomal, ring/zinc finger, proteasomal, ubiquitination, HSPs, transcription factors, apoptotsis and transmembrane proteins. However, the expression profile in the two cell populations was distinct for several genes.

The site of spermatogenesis i.e. seminiferous tubules is one of the most heterogenic niches of the body where about 30 types of cells coexist. These cells not only vary in their size, morphology, and function, but also in their DNA content; e.g. 2C (spermatogonia, Sertoli cells, Leydig cells etc), 4C (G2 phase spermaocytes), and 1C or C (round and elongating spermatids, and spermatozoa). The heterogeneity of testicular cells and the lack of in vitro systems for spermatogenic cell culture [27] are the major hurdles in gene expression studies at different stages of spermatogenesis [23]. To overcome this, enrichment of stage-specific germ-cell populations is mandatory. The gravimetric decantation in BSA gradients (staput) [28–30] and the centrifugal elutriation [31] are amongst the most widely used techniques of germ cell enrichment. Using the centrifugal elutriation technique coupled with Percoll® density gradient centrifugation, successful enrichment of pachytene spermatocytes and round spermatids to purity

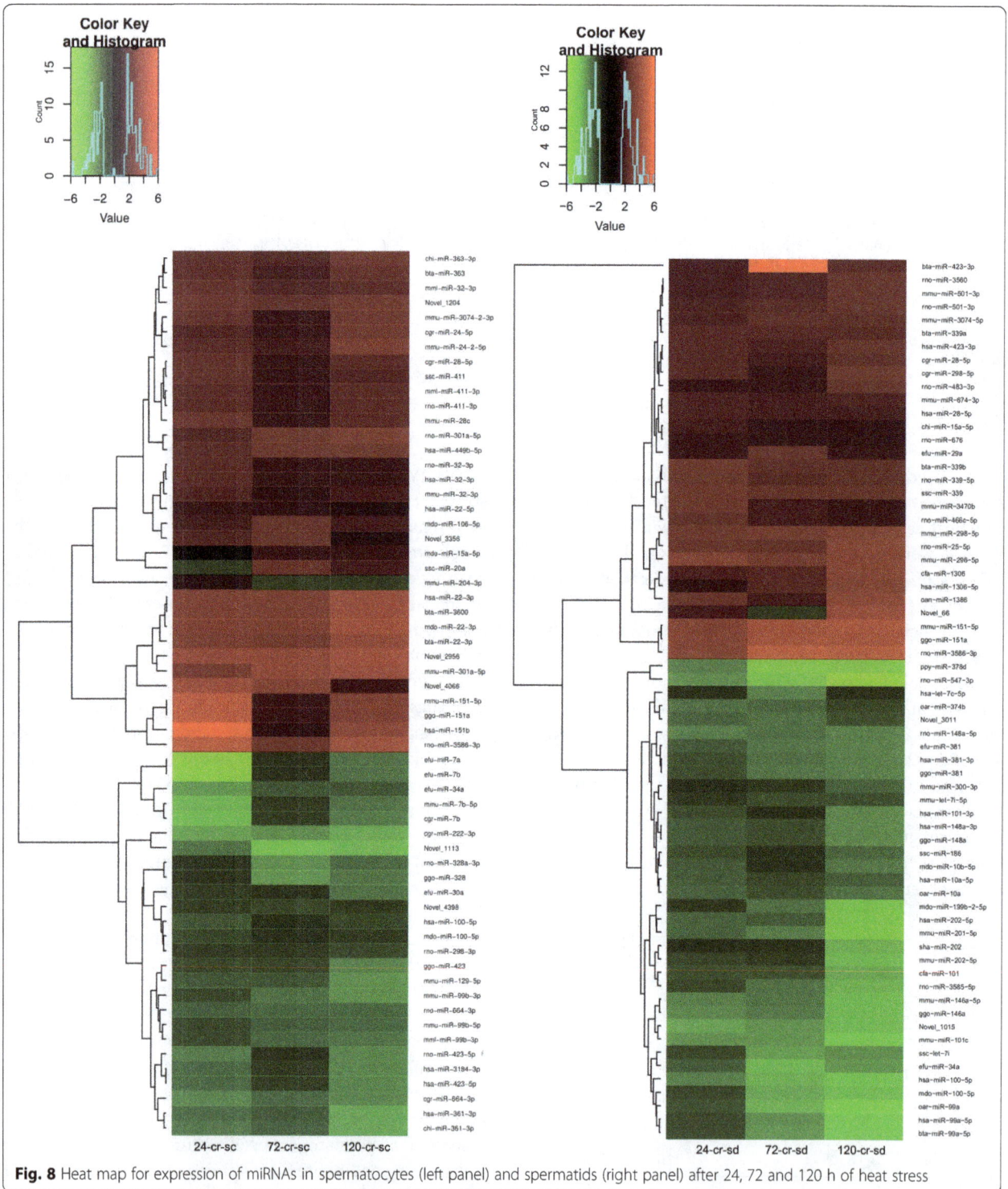

Fig. 8 Heat map for expression of miRNAs in spermatocytes (left panel) and spermatids (right panel) after 24, 72 and 120 h of heat stress

levels of > 90% was achieved. To our understanding, this is the best method of achieving germ cell purification to a high level. Nevertheless, less than 10% cross-contamination would not affect the findings of the study except screening out genes with minor differences between the two cell types.

We observed altered expression of HSP members belonging to *Hspa*, *Hsp90*, *Hspe*, *Hspd* and *Hspb*. *Hspe1* is a mitochondrial co-chaperonin, necessary for the folding of newly imported and stress-denatured mitochondrial proteins and works in association with *Hsp60* (Hspd) in the presence of ATP [32]. Hspe1 showed > 3.0 fold up-regulation in heat

Table 3 Details of novel miRNAs common in spermatocytes and round spermatids

S. no	Name	Sequence	Nucleotide length (bases)
Common in spermatids			
1	Novel_1204	CAAGAGGTGCATGCTGACAG	20
2	Novel_2956	GATTTAGCTCAGTGGTAGAG	20
3	Novel_3356	GGCTATTCTCGGCTGTCAGC	20
4	Novel_4066	TACCTCACTGTAGTCTAGGG	20
5	Novel_4398	TCCAGGTCCACTCTGCTGAGCACT	24
6	Novel_1113	ATTCTGGCTGTGTCTCTCAGGAGC	24
Common in round spermatocytes			
7	Novel_1015	ATGGGCTGTAGAATTTCTCT	20
8	Novel_3011	GCAGTGGAACATGTATTTAA	20
9	Novel_66	AACTGGAGGGCAACATGTATTA	22

stressed round spermatids and its companion protein Hspd1 was up-regulated (3.2 fold) after 120 h of cryptorchidism. However, in case of pachytene spermatocytes the Hspd1 exhibited higher expression after 24 h of cryptorchidism but expression of Hspe1 remained unchanged. Thus, it can be assumed that round spermatids could delay the apoptotic response due to heat stress with the help of these HSPs. On the other hand, *Hspa13* was continuously down-regulated from 24 h of heat stressed in both the cell types and maximum down expression (– 9.9 fold) was observed in spermatocytes at 72 h of heat stress. According to Yunoki et al. [33] Hspa13 is non-inducible to heat stress in human fibroblast cells. *Hspa13* is over expressed under UVB treatment and inhibits apoptosis [34] in the presence of alkannin. Thus higher under expression of *Hspa13* in spermatocytes suggest higher susceptibility to apoptosis. When we observed expression of *Hsf2*, an important heat stress transcription factor, we didn't find any change in round spermatids while a slight down regulation in spermatocytes was reported.

It is well known that the more mature germ cells, specifically spermatocytes and spermatids, rely on lactate as their energy source [35, 36], which is provided by the Sertoli cells. This lactate is further converted into pyruvate with the help of *LDHc* and is accompanied by the generation of reduced NAD$^+$. *LDHc* is testis specific isozyme of LDH expressed in male germ cells [37]. Moreover the fertility of *Ldhc* null males was severely compromised, which further confirmed the importance of this isozyme in fertility [38]. Due to this fact, *LDHc* attracted the attention of researchers as a fertility target for developing contraceptive vaccine [39, 40]. Significant changes in the expression levels of *LDHc*, lactate transporters (MCT1, MCT2, MCT4) and GLUT3 genes in germ cells was observed under heat stress, which were further validated by real time PCR. The lactate formed in the Sertoli cells is transferred to the germ cells with help of monocarboxylate transporters i.e., MCT1, MCT2, MCT4 which are present on germ cells. MCT1 is present on spermatogonia, spermatocytes and spermatids, while MCT2 is reported to be present on the tails of elongated spermatids and sperm [41]. This indicated that the metabolism of heat stressed germ cells is disturbed which may lead to apoptosis of the spermatids and spermatocytes. Furthermore, lactate taken up by germ cells is metabolized to pyruvate with the resultant increase in NADH, which is a substrate for NOX4. Reactive Oxygen Species (ROS) produced by NOX4 activity may act as second messengers in regulating the signal transduction pathways and gene expression. This indicates that besides energy metabolism, lactate also has a paracrine role and may also play a decisive role as a cell-signalling molecule in the seminiferous tubules after being secreted by the Sertoli cells [42].

The other targets include ATP-citrate lyase (*ACLY*), which is known to be the primary enzyme responsible for the synthesis of cytosolic acetyl-CoA in many tissues for the synthesis of lipids to meet the great demand for membrane expansion of rapidly proliferating cells [43]. Inhibition of ATP citrate lyase (*ACLY*), leads to growth suppression and apoptosis in a subset of human cancer cells [44]. In heat stressed testis, the level of *Acly* was found to be decreased in spermatids which could also be a reason for apoptosis of the germ cells. *Acly* is target of the miRNAs rno-miR-22-3p and rno-miR-22-5p. Acetyl-CoA is the requisite building block for the endogenous synthesis of fatty acids, cholesterol, and isoprenoids as well as acetylation reactions that modify proteins. ACL-generated oxaloacetate is reduced to malate, which can return to the mitochondria, recycling carbon and shuttling reducing equivalents into the mitochondria. The conversion of cytosolic oxaloacetate to malate is driven by the high cytosolic NADH/NAD+ ratio present in glycolytic cells. Malate can enter the mitochondrial matrix and be converted there to oxaloacetate to complete the substrate cycle. The coupled conversion of NAD+ to NADH provides a continuing mechanism to preserve the mitochondrial membrane potential (MMP) and sustain a high

Table 4 Gene ontology of predicted targets for heat-sensitive miRNAs found in pachytene spermatocytes

	No of genes	Predicted targets
Molecular functions		
Binding	15	Taf9b, Syt4, Cpeb1, Upf2, Arhgef2, Plch1, Net1, Arid3b, Enc1, Pole4, Impad1, Rfx7, Camk1d, Aph1a, Nfyb
Catalytic activity	22	Atp11c, Upf2, Dusp10, Arhgef2, Plch1, Mtor, Net1, Tmtc3, Casp9, Cnot8, Kbtbd8, Pole4, Impad1, Tesk2, Camk1d, Mapk8, Map3k14, Aph1a, Map4k3, Acly, Map3k3, Nfyb
Receptor activity	1	Net1
Signal transducer activity	2	Dusp10, Map4k3
Structural molecule activity	1	Enc1
Translation regulator activity	1	Cpeb1
Transporter activity	3	Atp11c, Cacna1a, Slc30a4
Biological processes		
Biological adhesion	3	Arhgef2, Net1, Net1
Biological regulation	9	Atp11c, Syt4, Cacna1a, Dusp10, Casp9, Slc30a4, Map3k14, Map4k3, Map3k3
Cellular component organization or biogenesis	3	Atp11c, Syt4, Tesk2
Cellular process	28	Atp11c, Syt4, Cpeb1, Cacna1a, Dusp10, Arhgef2, Plch1,Mtor, Net1, Tmtc3, Net1, Cltc, Casp9, Cnot8, Enc1, Slc30a4, Kbtbd8, Smurf1, Impad1, Rfx7, Tesk2, Camk1d, Gphn, Mapk8, Map3k14, Map4k3, Map3k3, Nfyb
Developmental process	11	Lmtk2, Arhgef2, Epha4, Net1, Net1, Casp9, Enc1, Tesk2, Map3k14, Map4k3, Map3k3
Immune system process	2	Tesk2, Mapk8
Localization	2	Atp11c, Cltc
Metabolic process	23	Taf9b, Atp11c, Cpeb1, Upf2, Dusp10, Plch1, Mtor, Tmtc3, Arid3b, Cnot8, Kbtbd8, Smurf1, Pole4, Impad1, Rfx7, Tesk2, Gphn, Map3k14, Aph1a, Map4k3, Acly, Map3k3, Nfyb
Multicellular organismal process	3	Syt4, Net1, Cltc
Reproduction	1	Tesk2
Response to stimulus	11	Taf9b, Dusp10, Mtor, Casp9, Slc30a4, Smurf1, Tesk2, Mapk8, Map3k14, Map4k3, Map3k3
Cellular components		
Cell part	16	Atp11c, Cpeb1, Cltc, Casp9, Cnot8, Enc1, Kbtbd8, Smurf1, Pole4, Impad1, Rfx7, Camk1d, Gphn, Map3k14, Map4k3, Map3k3
Extracellular matrix	1	Net1
Extracellular region	1	Net1
Macromolecular complex	4	Cpeb1, Cltc, Cnot8, Kbtbd8
Membrane	3	Atp11c, Syt4, Cacna1a
Organelle	4	Atp11c, Cpeb1, Pole4, Rfx7
Protein classes		
Calcium binding protein	1	Plch1
Cytoskeletal protein	1	Enc1

Table 4 Gene ontology of predicted targets for heat-sensitive miRNAs found in pachytene spermatocytes (Continued)

	No of genes	Predicted targets
Enzyme modulator	5	Arhgef2,Plch1,Net1,Casp9,Aph1a
Extracellular matrix protein	1	Net1
Hydrolase	4	Atp11c,Plch1,Casp9,Impad1
Ligase	2	Smurf1,Acly
Lyase	1	Acly
Membrane traffic protein	2	Syt4,Cltc
Nucleic acid binding	8	Taf9b,Cpeb1,Upf2,Mtor,Arid3b, Pole4, Rfx7, Nfyb
Receptor	1	Net1
Signalling molecule	1	Plch1
Transcription factor	6	Taf9b,Arid3b, Cnot8, Pole4, Rfx7, Nfyb
Transferase	6	Mtor, Tmtc3, Tesk2, Camk1d, Mapk8, Acly
Transporter	3	Atp11c, Cacna1a, Slc30a4
Pathways		
5HT2 type receptor mediated signaling pathway	1	Plch1
Alzheimer disease-amyloid secretase pathway	2	Mapk8, Aph1a
Alzheimer disease-presenilin pathway	1	Aph1a
Angiogenesis	2	Casp9, Mapk8
Apoptosis signaling pathway	4	Casp9, Mapk8, Map3k14, Map4k3
Axon guidance mediated by Slit/Robo	1	Net1
Axon guidance mediated by netrin	1	Net1
B cell activation	2	Mapk8, Map3k3
CCKR signaling map	2	Mapk8, Map3k14
EGF receptor signaling pathway	2	Mapk8, Map3k3
Endogenous cannabinoid signaling	1	Cacna1a
FAS signaling pathway	2	Casp9, Mapk8
FGF signaling pathway	2	Mapk8, Map3k3
GABA-B receptor II signaling General transcription regulation	1	Cacna1a
Gonadotropin-releasing hormone receptor pathway	6	Syt4, Mapk8, Map3k3, Map3k14, Map4k3, Nfyb
Heterotrimeric G-protein signaling pathway-Gi alpha and Gs alpha mediated pathway	1	Cltc
Heterotrimeric G-protein signaling pathway-Gq alpha and Go alpha mediated pathway	2	Cacna1a, Cltc
Histamine H1 receptor mediated signaling pathway	1	Plch1

Table 4 Gene ontology of predicted targets for heat-sensitive miRNAs found in pachytene spermatocytes (*Continued*)

	No of genes	Predicted targets
Hypoxia response via HIF activation	1	*Mtor*
Inflammation mediated by chemokine and cytokine signaling pathway	1	*Plch1*
Integrin signalling pathway	2	*Mapk8, Map3k3*
Interferon-gamma signaling pathway	1	*Mapk8*
Interleukin signaling pathway	1	*Mtor*
Ionotropic glutamate receptor pathway	1	*Cacna1a*
Metabotropic glutamate receptor group II pathway	1	*Cacna1a*
Metabotropic glutamate receptor group III pathway	1	*Cacna1a*
Notch signaling pathway	1	*Aph1a*
Oxidative stress response	2	*Dusp10, Mapk8*
Oxytocin receptor mediated signaling pathway	1	*Plch1*
PDGF signaling pathway	2	*Mtor, Mapk8*
PI3 kinase pathway	1	*Casp9*
Parkinson disease	1	*Mapk8*
Pyruvate metabolism	1	*Acly*
Ras Pathway	1	*Mapk8*
T cell activation	1	*Mapk8*
TGF-beta signaling pathway	2	*Smurf1, Mapk8*
Thyrotropin-releasing hormone receptor signaling pathway	2	*Cacna1a* *Plch1*
Toll receptor signaling pathway	1	*Mapk8*
Transcription regulation by bZIP transcription factor	1	*Taf9b*
Ubiquitin proteasome pathway	1	*Smurf1*
VEGF signaling pathway	1	*Casp9*
p38 MAPK pathway	1	*Dusp10*
p53 pathway by glucose deprivation	1	*Mtor*

Table 5 Gene ontology of predicted targets for heat-sensitive miRNAs found in round spermatids

	No. of genes gene	Name of genes
Molecular functions		
Binding	7	Pak7, Arhgef2, Cast, Tp63, Cast, Dazl, Wnt5b
Catalytic activity	18	Grip1, Ddx4, Mapk8, Rictor, Pak7, Arhgef2, Ddx6, Cast, Txnrd1, Mapk6, Cnot7, Dhx57, Arhgap1, Cybrd1, Map2k1, RragB, Cdk14 Gsk3a
Receptor activity	1	Calcr
Structural molecule activity	1	Slc25a43
Translation regulator activity	1	Eif4e2,Eif4g2
Transporter activity	17	Slc6a6, Slc38a11, Cacna1d, Slc38a2, Slc6a8, Slc13a5, Slc16a7, Slc30a7, Slc5a9, Slc35a2, Slc44a1, Slc17a5, Slc6a1, Slc23a2, Slc4a10, Slc20a2, Slc1a3
Biological functions		
Biological adhesion	1	Arhgef2
Biological regulation	13	Ddx4, Rictor, Pak7, Cacna1d, Ddx6, Tp63, Slc30a7, Cnot7, Wnt5b, Arhgap1, Map2k1, Slc4a10, RragB
Cellular component organisation or biogenesis	3	Rictor, Pak7, Ddx6
Cellular process	36	Calcr, Slc6a6, Slc25a43, Grip1, Slc38a11, Ddx4, Slc12a6, Mapk8, Rictor, Pak7, Cacna1d, Slc38a2, Slc6a8, Arhgef2, Slc13a5, Ddx6, Slc16a7, Tp63, Slc8a3, Mapk6, Slc30a7, Slc5a9, Cnot7, Prkar2b, Dhx57, Wnt5b, Slc17a5, Arhgap1, Slc6a1, Map2k1 Slc4a10, RragB, Slc20a2, Cdk14, Slc1a3, Gsk3a
Developmental process	8	Calcr,Pak7, Notch4, Arhgef2, Tp63, Wnt5b Map2k1, Cdk14, Gsk3a,Eif4g2
Immune system process	2	Mapk8, Mapk6
Localization	17	Calcr, Slc6a6, Slc38a11, Pak7, Slc38a2, Slc6a8, Slc13a5, Slc16a7, Cast, Slc5a9, Slc35a2, Slc17a5, Slc6a1, Slc23a2, Slc4a10, Slc20a2, Slc1a3
Locomotion	1	Pak7
Metabolic process	15	Slc25a43, Ddx4, Ddx6, Cast, Tp63, Txnrd1, Slc35a2, Cnot7, Dhx57, Arhgap1, Slc23a2, RragB, Cdk14, Slc1a3, Gsk3a
Multicellular organismal process	8	Calcr, Grip1, Slc12a6, Wnt5b, Slc6a1, Cdk14, Slc1a3, Gsk3a
Reproduction	2	Calcr, Dazl
Response to stimulus	10	Calcr, Mapk8, Rictor, Pak7, Tp63, Mapk6, Slc30a7, Wnt5b, Map2k1, RragB
Cellular components		
cell junction	1	Grip1
cell part	23	Slc6a6, Grip1, Ddx4, Rictor, Pak7, Cacna1d, Slc38a2,Slc6a8, Slc13a5, Ddx6,Slc16a7,Tp63, Slc30a7, Slc5a9, Cnot7, Dhx, Arhgap1,Slc6a1, Cybrd1, Map2k1,Slc4a10,RragB,Slc20a2
extracellular region	1	Wnt5b
macromolecular complex	6	Ddx4, Rictor, Ddx6, Tp63, Cnot7, RragB
membrane transporter	12	Slc6a6, Slc38a2, Slc6a8, Slc13a5, Slc16a7, Slc5a9, Slc17a5, Slc6a1, Cybrd1, Slc4a10, RragB, Slc20a2
Organelle	9	Ddx4, Slc38a2, Ddx6, Tp63, Slc30a7, Cnot7, Dhx57, Cybrd1, RragB

Table 5 Gene ontology of predicted targets for heat-sensitive miRNAs found in round spermatids (*Continued*)

	No. of genes gene	Name of genes
Protein classes		
calcium-binding protein	1	Slc25a43
cell junction protein	1	Grip1
defense/immunity protein	1	Calcr
enzyme modulator	4	Arhgef2, Cast,Arhgap1,RragB
membrane traffic protein	1	Cast
nucleic acid binding	7	Slc25a43, Ddx4, Ddx6, Eif4e2, Dazl, Dhx57, Eif4g2
Oxidoreductase	2	Txnrd1, Cybrd1
receptor	1	Calcr
signaling molecule	1	Wnt5b
transcription factor	2	Tp63, Cnot7
transfer/carrier protein	1	Slc25a43
transferase	5	Grip1, Mapk8, Mapk6, Cdk14, Gsk3a
transporter	17	Slc6a6, Slc25a43, Slc38a11, Cacna1d,Slc38a2 Slc6a8, Slc13a5,Slc16a7, Slc30a7, Slc5a9, Slc35a2, Slc44a1, Slc17a5, Slc6a1, Slc23a2, Slc4a10, Slc1a3
Pathways		
5HT1 type receptor mediated signaling pathway	1	Prkar2b
5HT2 type receptor mediated signaling pathway	1	Cacna1d
Alzheimer disease-amyloid secretase pathway	3	Mapk8, Cacna1d, Mapk6
Alzheimer disease-presenilin pathway	2	Notch4, Wnt5b
Angiogenesis	6	Mapk8, Notch4, Mapk6, Wnt5b, Arhgap1,Map2k1
Angiotensin II-stimulated signaling through G proteins and beta-arrestin	1	Map2k1
Apoptosis signaling pathway	1	Mapk8
B cell activation	2	Mapk8, Map2k1
Beta1 adrenergic receptor signaling pathway	2	Cacna1d, Prkar2b
Beta2 adrenergic receptor signaling pathway	2	Cacna1d, Prkar2b
CCKR signaling map	2	Mapk8, Map2k1
Cadherin signaling pathway	1	Wnt5b
Cytoskeletal regulation by Rho GTPase	2	Pak7, Arhgap1
Dopamine receptor mediated signaling pathway	1	Prkar2b
EGF receptor signaling pathway	2	Mapk8, Map2k1
Endothelin signaling pathway	2	Prkar2b, Map2k1

Table 5 Gene ontology of predicted targets for heat-sensitive miRNAs found in round spermatids (Continued)

	No. of genes gene	Name of genes
Enkephalin release	1	Prkar2b
FAS signaling pathway	1	Mapk8
FGF signaling pathway	2	Mapk8,Map2k1
GABA-B receptor II signaling	1	Prkar2b
Gonadotropin-releasing hormone receptor pathway	4	Mapk8,Cacna1d, Map3k7,Map2k1
Hedgehog signaling pathway	1	Prkar2b
Heterotrimeric G-protein signaling pathway-Gi alpha and Gs alpha mediated pathway	2	Prkar2b, Gsk3a
Histamine H2 receptor mediated signaling pathway	1	Prkar2b
Huntington disease	1	Tp63
Inflammation mediated by chemokine and cytokine signaling pathway	2	Pak7, Map3k7
Insulin/IGF pathway-mitogen activated protein kinase kinase/MAP kinase cascade	1	Map2k1
Ionotropic glutamate receptor pathway	1	Slc1a3
Insulin/IGF pathway-protein kinase B signaling cascade	1	Gsk3a
Integrin signalling pathway	3	Mapk8, Mapk6, Map2k1
Interferon-gamma signaling Pathway	1	Mapk8
Interleukin signaling pathway	2	Map3k7, Mapk6
Muscarinic acetylcholine receptor 2 and 4 signaling pathway	2	Slc6a8, Prkar2b
Metabotropic glutamate receptor group III pathway	2	Prkar2b, Slc1a3
Metabotropic glutamate receptor group II pathway	1	Prkar2b
Nicotinic acetylcholine receptor signaling pathway	2	Cacna1d, Slc6a8
Notch signaling pathway	2	Notch4, Gsk3a
Oxidative stress response	1	Mapk8
Oxytocin receptor mediated signaling pathway	1	Cacna1d
P53 pathway feedback loops 1	1	Tp63
PDGF signaling pathway	4	Mapk8, Mapk6,Arhgap1,Map2k1
Parkinson disease	1	Mapk8
Ras Pathway	3	Mapk8,Map2k1,Gsk3a
T cell activation	2	Mapk8,Map2k1
TGF-beta signaling pathway	2	Mapk8, Map3k7
Toll receptor signaling pathway	3	Mapk8, Map3k7, Map2k1
Transcription regulation by bZIP transcription factor	1	Prkar2b

Table 5 Gene ontology of predicted targets for heat-sensitive miRNAs found in round spermatids (*Continued*)

	No. of gene	Name of genes
VEGF signaling pathway		*Mapk6, Arhgap1, Map2k1*
Wnt signaling pathway		*Map3k7,Wnt5b*
p38 MAPK pathway		*Map3k7*
p53 pathway by glucose deprivation		*Tp63*
p53 pathway feedback loops 2		*Tp63*
p53 pathway		*Tp63*

mitochondrial NADH/NAD+ ratio that maintains the TCA cycle in a repressed state. Thus, ACL enzymatic activity is poised to affect both glucose-dependent lipogenesis and cellular bioenergetics [45].

Conclusions

In conclusion, transcriptome analysis on the most heat sensitive germ cells in the testis identified a large number of genes that were altered by ≥2.0 fold, out of which 594 genes (286↑; 308↓) showed alterations in spermatocytes and 154 genes (105↑; 49↓) showed alterations in spermatids throughout the duration of experiment. 62 heat-sensitive genes were common to both cell types. Similarly, 66 and 60 heat-sensitive miRNAs in spermatocytes and spermatids, respectively, were affected by ≥1.5 fold, out of which 6 were common to both the cell types. Among various pathways affected significantly by heat stress, the study has identified *Acly, selV, SLC16A7*(MCT-2), *Txnrd1* and *Prkar2B* as potential heat sensitive targets in germ cells, which may be under tight regulation of heat sensitive miRNAs, rno-miR-22-3P, rno-miR-22-5P, rno-miR-129-5P, rno-miR-3560, rno-miR-3560 and rno-miR-466c-5P, as predicted by miRDB tool. The regulatory targets of these miRNAs, particularly their effect on the top genes altered by heat stress, remain to be worked out. This study has not only advanced our understanding of molecular cues in spermatogenesis but also identified the potential targets for fertility regulation.

Acknowledgments

The authors gratefully acknowledge the grant of research fellowships by the Council of Scientific and Industrial Research, New Delhi, India (SKY and RV), the Indian Council of Medical Research New Delhi, India (AP) and the Department of Biotechnology New Delhi, India (AD). Thanks are due to the SAIF division for their help in obtaining FACS data.

Funding

This study was supported by the CSIR-network project BSC0101.

Authors' contributions

SKY, AP, LK, AD, BK and RV performed the animal surgeries, cell purification, histology and FACS, gene-expression analysis and all other bench experiments, analysed the data and drafted the manuscript. GG, JPM and SR supervised the experiments, data analysis and bioinformatics. GG and SR conceived the study, designed the experiments and finalized the manuscript. All authors read, edited and approved the final manuscript.

Competing interests

The authors declare that they have no competing interests.

References

1. Mieusset R, Bujan L. The potential of mild testicular heating as a safe, effective and reversible contraceptive method for men. Int J Androl. 1994; 17(4):186–91.

2. Fahim MS, Fahim Z, Der R, Hall DG, Harman J. Heat in male contraception (hot water 60 °C, infrared, microwave, and ultrasound). Contraception. 1975; 11(5):549–62.

3. Toppari J, Larsen JC, Christiansen P, Giwercman A, Grandjean P, Guillette LJ, Jégou B, Jensen TK, Jouannet P, Keiding N, Leffers H, McLachlan JA, Meyer O, Müller J, Rajpert-De Meyts E, Scheike T, Sharpe R, Sumpter J, Skakkebaek NE. Male reproductive health and environmental xenoestrogens. Environ Health Perspect. 1996;104:741–803.

4. Carlsen E, Andersson AM, Petersen JH, Skakkebaek NE. History of febrile illness and variation in semen quality. Hum Reprod. 2003;18:2089–92.

5. Chowdhury AK, Steinberger E. Early changes in the germinal epithelium of rat testes following exposure to heat. J Reprod Fertil. 1970;22:205–12.

6. Lue YH, Hikim AP, Swerdloff RS, Im P, Taing KS, Bui T, Leung A, Wang C. Single exposure to heat induces stage-specific germ cell apoptosis in rats: role of intratesticular testosterone on stage specificity. Endocrinology. 1999; 140:1709–17.

7. Shiraishi K, Matsuyama H, Takihara H. Pathophysiology of varicocele in male infertility in the era of assisted reproductive technology. Int J Urol. 2012;19: 538–50.

8. Steger K. Haploid spermatids exhibit translationally repressed mRNAs. Anat Embryol (Berl). 2001;203(5):323–34.

9. Eddy EM. Male germ cell gene expression. Recent Prog Horm Res. 2002;57: 103–28.

10. Iguchi N, Tobias JW, Hecht NB. Expression profiling reveals meiotic male germ cell mRNAs that are translationally up- and down-regulated. Proc Natl Acad Sci. 2006;103:7712–7.

11. Xiao P, Tang A, Yu Z, Gui Y, Cai Z. Gene expression profile of 2058 spermatogenesis-related genes in mice. Biol Pharm Bull. 2008;31:201–6.

12. Waldman Ben-Asher H, Shahar I, Yitzchak A, Mehr R, Don J. Expression and chromosomal organization of mouse meiotic genes. Mol Reprod Dev. 2010; 77:241–8.

13. Yu Z, Guo R, Ge Y, Ma J, Guan J, Li S, Sun X, Xue S, Han D. Gene expression profiles in different stages of mouse spermatogenic cells. Biol Reprod. 2003; 69:37–47.

14. Geisinger A, Rodríguez-Casuriaga R. Flow cytometry for gene expression studies in mammalian spermatogenesis. Cytogenet Genome Res. 2010;128:46–56.

15. Johnston DS, Wright WW, Dicandeloro P, Wilson E, Kopf GS, Jelinsky SA. Stage-specific gene expression is a fundamental characteristic of rat spermatogenic cells and Sertoli cells. Proc Natl Acad Sci. 2008;10524:8315–20.

16. Schultz N, Hamra FK, Garbers DL. A multitude of genes expressed solely in meiotic or postmeiotic spermatogenic cells offers a myriad of contraceptive targets. Proc Natl Acad Sci. 2003;100:12201–6.

17. Schlecht U, Demougin P, Koch R, Hermida L, Wiederkehr C, Descombes P, Pineau C, Jégou B, Primig M. Expression profiling of mammalian male meiosis and gametogenesis identifies novel candidate genes for roles in the regulation of fertility. Molec Biol Cell. 2004;15:1031–43.

18. Xu Q, Modrek B, Lee C. Genome-wide detection of tissue-specific alternative splicing in the human transcriptome. Nucleic Acids Res. 2002;30:3754–66.

19. Huang X, Li J, Lu L, Xu M, Xiao J, Yin L, Zhu H, Zhou Z, Sha J. Novel development-related alternative splices in human testis identified by cDNA microarrays. J Androl. 2005;26:189–96.

20. Laiho A, Kotaja N, Gyenesei A, Sironen A. Transcriptome profiling of the murine testis during the first wave of spermatogenesis. PLoS One. 2013;8: e61558.

21. Soumillon M, Necsulea A, Weier M, Brawand D, Zhang X, Gu H, Barthès P, Kokkinaki M, Nef S, Gnirke A, Dym M, de Massy B, Mikkelsen TS, Kaessmann H. Cellular source and mechanisms of high transcriptome complexity in the mammalian testis. Cell Rep. 2013;3:2179–90.

22. Margolin G, Khil PP, Kim J, Bellani MA, Camerini-Otero RD. Integrated transcriptome analysis of mouse spermatogenesis. BMC Genomics. 2014;15:39.

23. da Cruz I, Rodríguez-Casuriaga R, Santiñaque FF, Farías J, Curti G, Capoano CA, Folle GA, Benavente R, Sotelo-Silveira JR, Geisinger A. Transcriptome analysis of highly purified mouse spermatogenic cell populations: gene expression signatures switch from meiotic-to postmeiotic-related processes at pachytene stage. BMC Genomics. 2016;17:294.

24. Meistrich ML, Longtin J, Brock WA, Grimes SR, Macc ML. Purification of rat spermatogenic cells and preliminary biochemical analysis of these cells. Biol Reprod. 1981;25:1065–77.

25. Vogeli M. Contraception through temporary male sterilization. Lancet. 1956; http://www.puzzlepiece.org/bcontrol/voegeli1956.txt.

26. Lue YH, Sinha Hikim AP, Swerdloff RS, Im P, Taing KS, Bui T, Leung A, Wang

C. Single exposure to heat induces stage-specific germ cell apoptosis in rats: role of intratesticular testosterone on stage specificity. Endocrinology. 1999 Apr 1;140(4):1709–17.

27. Reuter K, Schlatt S, Ehmcke J, Wistuba J. Fact or fiction: in vitro spermatogenesis. Spermatogenesis. 2012;2:245–52.

28. Lam DMK, Furrer R, Bruce WR. The separation, physical characterization, and differentiation kinetics of spermatogonial cells of the mouse. Proc Natl Acad Sci. 1970;65:192–9.

29. Go VLW, Vernon RG, Fritz IB. Studies on spermatogenesis in rats. I. Application of the sedimentation velocity technique to an investigation of spermatogenesis. Can J Biochem. 1971;49:753–60.

30. Romrell LJ, Bellvé AR, Fawcet DW. Separation of mouse spermatogenic cells by sedimentation velocity. Dev Biol. 1976;19:119–31.

31. Meistrich ML. Separation of spermatogenic cells and nuclei from rodent testes. Methods Cell Biol. 1977;15:15–54.

32. Levy-Rimler G, Viitanen P, Weiss C, Sharkia R, Greenberg A, Niv A, Lustig A, Delarea Y, Azem A. The effect of nucleotides and mitochondrial chaperonin 10 on the structure and chaperone activity of mitochondrial chaperonin 60. Eur J Biochem. 2001;268:3465–72.

33. Yunoki T, Kariya A, Kondo T, Hayashi A, Tabuchi Y. Gene expression analysis of heat shock protein a family members responsive to hyperthermic treatments in normal human fibroblastic cells. Therm Med. 2012;28:73–85.

34. Yoshihisa Y, Hassan MA, Furusawa Y, Tabuchi Y, Kondo T, Shimizu T. Alkannin, HSP70 inducer, protects against UVB-induced apoptosis in human keratinocytes. PLoS One. 2012;7(10):e47903.

35. Boussouar F, Benahmed M. Lactate and energy metabolism in male germ cells. Trends Endocrinol Metab. 2004;15:345–50.

36. Mita M, Hall PF. Metabolism of round spermatids from rats: lactate as the preferred substrate. Biol Reprod. 1982;26:445–55.

37. Goldberg E, Eddy EM, Duan C, Odet F. LDHc the ultimate testis specific gene. J Androl. 2010;31(1):86–94.

38. Odet F, Duan C, Willis WD, Goulding EH, Kung A, Eddy EM, Goldberg E. Expression of the gene for mouse lactate dehydrogenase C (Ldhc) is required for male fertility. Biol Reprod. 2008;79(1):26–34.

39. Millan JL, Driscoll CE, LeVan KM, Goldberg E. Epitopes of human testis-specific lactate dehydrogenase deduced from a cDNA sequence. Proc Natl Acad Sci. 1987;84:5311–5.

40. Murdoch FE, Goldberg E. Male contraception: another holy grail. Bioorg Med Chem Lett. 2014;24(2):419–24.

41. Kishimoto A, Ishiguro-Oonuma T, Takahashi R, Maekawa M, Toshimori K, Watanabe M, Iwanaga T. Immunohistochemical localization of GLUT3, MCT1, and MCT2 in the testes of mice and rats: the use of different energy sources in spermatogenesis. Biomed Res. 2015;36(4):225–34.

42. Galardo MN, Regueira M, Riera MF, Pellizzari EH, Cigorraga SB, Meroni SB. Lactate regulates rat male germ cell function through reactive oxygen species. PLoS One. 2014;9(1):e88024.

43. Lin R, Tao R, Gao X, Li T, Zhou X, Guan KL, Xiong Y, Lei QY. Acetylation stabilizes ATP-citrate lyase to promote lipid biosynthesis and tumor growth. Mol Cell. 2013;51(4):506–18.

44. Migita T, Okabe S, Ikeda K, Igarashi S, Sugawara S, Tomida A, Taguchi R, Soga T, Seimiya H. Inhibition of ATP citrate lyase induces an anticancer effect via reactive oxygen species: AMPK as a predictive biomarker for therapeutic impact. Am J Pathol. 2013;182(5):1800–10.

45. Hatzivassiliou G, Zhao F, Bauer DE, Andreadis C, Shaw AN, Dhanak D, Hingorani SR, Tuveson DA, Thompson CB. ATP citrate lyase inhibition can suppress tumor cell growth. Cancer Cell. 2005;8(4):311–21.

## 14

Role of hormonal and inflammatory alterations in obesity-related reproductive dysfunction at the level of the hypothalamic-pituitary-ovarian axis

Michelle Goldsammler[1], Zaher Merhi[2,3] and Erkan Buyuk[1*]

Abstract

Background: Besides being a risk factor for multiple metabolic disorders, obesity could affect female reproduction. While increased adiposity is associated with hormonal changes that could disrupt the function of the hypothalamus and the pituitary, compelling data suggest that obesity-related hormonal and inflammatory changes could directly impact ovarian function.

Objective: To review the available data related to the mechanisms by which obesity, and its associated hormonal and inflammatory changes, could affect the female reproductive function with a focus on the hypothalamic-pituitary-ovarian (HPO) axis.

Methods: PubMed database search for publications in English language until October 2017 pertaining to obesity and female reproductive function was performed.

Results: The obesity-related changes in hormone levels, in particular leptin, adiponectin, ghrelin, neuropeptide Y and agouti-related protein, are associated with reproductive dysfunction at both the hypothalamic-pituitary and the ovarian levels. The pro-inflammatory molecules advanced glycation end products (AGEs) and monocyte chemotactic protein-1 (MCP-1) are emerging as relatively new players in the pathophysiology of obesity-related ovarian dysfunction.

Conclusion: There is an intricate crosstalk between the adipose tissue and the inflammatory system with the HPO axis function. Understanding the mechanisms behind this crosstalk could lead to potential therapies for the common obesity-related reproductive dysfunction.

Keywords: Obesity, Ovary, HPO, Advanced glycation end products, Monocyte chemotactic protein-1

Background

According to a recent population study, approximately 39% of the population over the age of 20 and 18% of children between the ages of 2–19 are obese [1]. Obesity causes a huge economic burden where it is estimated that obesity will add 48–66 billion dollars in related health care expenditures by the year 2030 [2]. This is due to obesity-related comorbidities such as diabetes mellitus, hypertension, dyslipidemia, and cardiovascular disease [3]. Besides these chronic disorders, obesity is also associated with reproductive and obstetric complications such as menstrual irregularities, subfertility, endometrial hyperplasia and cancer, as well as poor obstetrical and perinatal outcomes [4–7]. This review will focus on the relationship between obesity and female reproductive function with a focus on alterations in the hypothalamic pituitary ovarian (HPO) axis and the direct effect of obesity-related inflammatory processes on ovarian function.

Normal HPO Axis

The female reproductive physiology is a complex interaction between neuroendocrine and endocrine signaling

* Correspondence: erbuyuk@yahoo.com
[1]Montefiore's Institute for Reproductive Medicine and Health, Department of Obstetrics & Gynecology and Women's Health, Albert Einstein College of Medicine, Montefiore Medical Center, Hartsdale, NY, USA
Full list of author information is available at the end of the article

affecting the hypothalamus, the pituitary gland and the ovaries. At the level of the hypothalamus, gonadotropin releasing hormone (GnRH) pulses activate the pituitary release of the two gonadotropins, follicle-stimulating hormone (FSH) and luteinizing hormone (LH) [8, 9]. FSH and LH in turn act on the ovaries to stimulate follicular growth and result in the production of estradiol and, following ovulation, progesterone [10]. Estradiol, together with ovarian inhibin B, acts primarily in a negative feedback loop on the hypothalamus suppressing the release of FSH. When estradiol reaches a sustained threshold in concentration and duration, for at least 24–48 h [11–13], it provides a positive feedback that increases the frequency and decreases the amplitude of GnRH pulses thereby activating increased pituitary release of LH surge for ovulation to occur [14]. There are multiple regulators of this cycle and our review is limited to those regulators, which are altered, directly or indirectly, in overweight and obese women.

The HPO axis plays a crucial role in pubertal transition. Normal pubertal development is under two main controls, adrenal and hypothalamic [15]. The adrenal glands participate in adrenarche, which often precedes the remainder of pubertal events. Adrenarche is independent of the hypothalamic pubertal changes as observed in several disorders of sexual differentiation [16]. The hypothalamus, with its GnRH pulse generator responsible for the initiation of puberty, is quiescent in childhood, likely under GABAergic (gamma-aminobutyric acid) inhibitory control [17, 18]. Normal central activation of the hypothalamus via kisspeptin and glutamate neurons in the arcuate nucleus results in nocturnal increases in low frequency LH pulses [19]. These pulses become more prevalent throughout the day until the GnRH pulse generator achieves the frequency and amplitude sufficient for cyclic ovarian hormonal function and ultimately menarche. During normal puberty, there is a physiologic insulin resistance that helps achieve the anticipated pubertal weight gain and growth [20–22]. The insulin resistance leads to decreased hepatic derived circulating sex hormone-binding globulin (SHBG), which in turn increases circulating free estradiol levels. This may also contribute to a parallel adrenal activation resulting in more androgen production and ultimately adrenarche [17, 18]. Increasing estradiol levels, in turn, are significantly associated with growth velocity, [23] possibly through the stimulation of the growth hormone – Insulin like growth factor 1 (IGF-1) axis [24, 25].

Obesity and the HPO axis

It has been thought that obesity changes the expected time course of puberty and leads to earlier thelarche, adrenarche and menarche [26–28]. Adiposity, and specifically the distribution of the adipose tissue, contributes to fluctuations in peripheral steroid hormone secretion, thereby impacting pubertal development [29]. For instance, the adipocytes contain aromatase, that both assists in the production [30] and the conversion of steroid hormones, mainly androgens to estrogens. Population studies have demonstrated a trend for earlier menarche, due to the obesity epidemic, over the past 30 years [31], highlighting the potential for significant increase in health care risks and cost for these young girls. Increased adipose tissue quantity rather than increased sensitization or increased aromatase activity during aging [32] and therefore increased peripheral production of estrogens leads to increased rate of serious hormone dependent cancers, such as endometrial and breast cancer [33, 34].

Obesity decreases pituitary LH pulse amplitude and mean LH release without changing its frequency, leading to impaired luteal phase [35]. Additionally, obesity may affect various components of the HPO axis, and may have direct effect on ovarian function independent of hypothalamic pituitary function. We will elucidate in the following sections the changes that occur in the metabolic and inflammatory systems that are related to ovarian dysfunction.

Leptin

Leptin is a 16-kDa adipokine secreted primarily by white adipose tissue, although it can be secreted from other tissues, such as gastric mucosa [36]. Serum leptin levels positively correlate with the amount of adipose tissue in the body [37]. Leptin has several functions, which in concert reflect body energy homeostasis. It acts to stimulate energy expenditure and suppresses appetite via its signaling at the level of the hypothalamus [18, 38]. These findings were confirmed with mouse knockout model where leptin receptor knockout mice become obese with a rapid and persistent weight gain [39]. Because leptin suppresses appetite, it was studied as a potential target for weight loss drug development [40]. However, it has been shown that increased exogenous leptin does not necessarily induce weight loss [41, 42] suggesting that there is a resistance state to the action of leptin at the level of the hypothalamus. Indeed, high circulating leptin levels observed in obese women supports the concept of leptin resistance [37]. This desensitization to leptin is not a complete blockage of leptin signaling and can possibly be reversed with weight loss [43].

Leptin's energy homeostatic function in part contributes to its effect on puberty. Puberty requires a certain energy balance to proceed [22, 44]. Leptin has a permissive action for pubertal progression, but it is not the initiator or the sole mechanism by which puberty occurs [45]. Conversely, hyperleptinemia may initially cause earlier reproductive maturation, and prolonged high leptin levels could lead to ovulatory dysfunction [46]. On the other hand, low leptin levels observed in energy-deficient states are associated with delayed or lack of puberty, when puberty is not physiologically desired [47].

Leptin affects GnRH pulse neurons indirectly though GABA or kisspeptin [39, 48]. Both GABA and kisspeptin neurons have a focus in the arcuate nucleus, where leptin receptors are readily available [39, 49, 50]. Knockout models for the leptin receptor that is found on GABA specific neurons display delayed puberty and decreased fecundability in animal models [39]. Similarly, loss of function gene mutation in the kisspeptin gene results in delayed or absent puberty [51]. Hypothalamic kisspeptin levels often correlate with leptin levels [50] in line with low energy states, making this an alternate pathway for leptin signaling [52]. Both low serum, and therefore hypothalamic, leptin levels and low hypothalamic kisspeptin levels decrease LH secretion by the pituitary, ultimately affecting ovulation [52].

Studies on the effect of leptin on ovarian folliculogenesis and ovulation have shown conflicting results. Leptin has been isolated in both mural and cumulus granulosa cells and within the follicular fluid of pre-ovulatory follicles in women undergoing in vitro fertilization (IVF) [53]. Serum leptin levels increase after ovulation and have peak levels in the mid-secretory phase, possibly contributing to the implantation window within the endometrium [54]. Some studies suggested an inhibitory effect of leptin, especially on early follicular development, while others suggested that leptin could induce ovulation, independent of LH [55] since there seems to be an interaction between estradiol and leptin [55, 56]. In a mouse model, leptin administration increased LH levels and follicular development corresponding to an increase in ovarian tissue weight [57]. In addition, IVF outcome studies pointed to leptin as negatively correlated to reproductive outcome. In one study of serum leptin levels in patients undergoing IVF, higher leptin:BMI ratio was associated with a decreased number of good quality embryos and lower implantation and pregnancy rates [58]. At the ovarian level [46], supraphysiologic levels of leptin inhibits androstenedione and progesterone production [59, 60]. Additionally, human granulosa and cumulus cells exposed to leptin in vitro lead to a downregulation in anti-Müllerian hormone (AMH) gene expression via the JAK/STAT pathway [61] potentially leading to ovulatory dysfunction. In summary, normal leptin homeostasis is required for normal physiologic functions at the level of the hypothalamus and the ovaries. While low levels of leptin could disrupt the GnRH pulsatility, supraphysiologic levels of leptin could disrupt ovarian folliculogenesis [46, 55, 62].

Ghrelin

Ghrelin is an orexigenic enterokine composed of 28 amino acids related to the oxyntomodulin family of intestinal peptides [63]. It is predominantly produced by the stomach, but is also detectable in many other tissues, like bowel, pancreas, hypothalamus and pituitary [64]. Ghrelin is increased in fasting states and stimulates appetite to compensate for decreased nutritional intake [65]. Mouse models confirm that ghrelin increases food consumption as an immediate and short-term effect [66] by acting on the arcuate nucleus in the hypothalamus and stimulates appetite via neuropeptide Y (NPY) and agouti related protein (AgRP) neurons [67]. One of ghrelin's targets is the hypothalamic arcuate nucleus where it increases the expression of NPY/AgRP mRNA [68] resulting in increased body weight and inhibiting proopiomelanocortin (POMC) neurons [69]. Double knockout (NPY-/AgRP-) mouse models, or other NPY/AgRP deficient models demonstrated suppression of ghrelin-induced appetite stimulation as compared to wild type control animals. Deficiency of both NPY and AgRP is necessary to abolish the effect of ghrelin while knockout of only one of these mediators is not sufficient to suppress ghrelin's effect [66].

In the hypothalamus, ghrelin can decrease both GnRH secretion and pulsatility [70–73] possibly through NPY- and AgRP- mediated mechanisms [74]. Vulliémoz et al. suggested that this effect is part of the homeostatic control of reproductive function in response to nutritional changes. In low energy states, such as fasting, ghrelin levels are increased, thereby altering the HPO axis cyclic activity [73]. Ghrelin also stimulates other pituitary hormone release, such as adrenocorticotropic hormone and prolactin [75]. In low energy states where ghrelin levels are elevated, prolactin levels may be increased potentially leading to disruption of ovarian cyclicity. Ghrelin has not clearly been shown to have a direct effect on pubertal transition. However, ghrelin levels decrease throughout childhood as puberty approaches [75]. Given its inverse relationship to adiposity, decreasing ghrelin levels may be a reflection of the increasing weight gain observed in the pre-pubertal stage [76].

Studies on the effect of ghrelin on ovarian steroidogenesis have shown mixed results [74, 77]. Animal studies suggest that ghrelin could induce estradiol and/or progesterone production, [78] or could inhibit estradiol release via inhibiting CYP19A1 (aromatase enzyme) expression [74, 79, 80]. These effects may be dose-dependent [81] or related to the activated portion of the ghrelin molecule [79]. The full-length ghrelin molecule stimulates estradiol secretion while certain amino acid fragments of ghrelin are inhibitory for estradiol secretion [79]. Ghrelin could affect folliculogenesis by increasing cell proliferation and decreasing apoptosis and follicular atresia [82, 83]. Similarly, chronic ghrelin infusion leads to increase in follicle number and decrease in corpus luteum number in a rat model [84]. Additionally, ghrelin, with its connection to obesity, is related to insulin regulation and insulin resistance where it decreases insulin secretion and sensitivity [64, 85, 86] ultimately leading to insulin resistance [87].

Thus, these findings suggest that ghrelin may indirectly contribute to puberty through general energy homeostasis such as insulin action, and it acts at the level of the hypothalamus, pituitary and ovary leading to alterations in normal reproductive function.

Neuropeptide Y and Agouti-related protein: (NPY/AgRP)

The connection between peripherally circulating adipokines, enterokines and the HPO axis centers on a collection of neurons within the arcuate nucleus, which secrete the neuropeptides NPY and AgRP [88]. NPY is a 36 amino acid neurotransmitter peptide predominantly expressed in sympathetic neurons. It stimulates fat angiogenesis and proliferation via both a central hypothalamic and peripheral mechanism [49, 89]. AgRP is a 112 amino acid neuropeptide expressed in the arcuate nucleus [90, 91] and stimulates appetite [91]. Both NPY and AgRP are orexigenic neurons and interact with ghrelin to promote appetite [66].

Under normal physiologic conditions, NPY concentration increases in the portal capillary blood during the ovulatory surge to potentiate the action of GnRH on pituitary gonadotropin secretion [92, 93]. Similarly, AgRP engages the GnRH pulse generator neurons within the hypothalamus and regulates gonadotropin release. Both NPY and AgRP have tonic inhibitory effects where they could be stimulated by ghrelin in order to decrease GnRH pulse frequency and amplitude [94]. Infusion of NPY, independent of ghrelin, also decreases pituitary LH secretion [95]. NPY could have a negative regulatory impact on ovarian folliculogenesis where it could have a pro-apoptotic and an anti-proliferative effect [96]. NPY has been shown to have no effect on progesterone secretion [97], but it recently has been found to stimulate estradiol and testosterone secretion in catfish [98]. Data pertaining to the direct effect of NPY and AgRP on ovarian steroidogenesis and folliculogenesis are still limited and further studies are required.

Adiponectin

Adiponectin is a 30-kDa adipokine secreted by the adipose tissue [99]. Opposite to leptin, adiponectin levels increase with starvation [99]. Adiponectin acts in the brain by binding to the adiponectin receptor 1 (AdipoR1) in the arcuate nucleus. This binding leads to activation of AMPK resulting in increased food intake and reduced energy expenditure [100]. Adiponectin production increases insulin sensitivity and is inversely correlated with adiposity [101]. Knockout studies demonstrated that the absence of adiponectin causes severe insulin resistance that is reversible

with administration of exogenous adiponectin [102]. Low adiponectin levels, as seen in certain genetic polymorphisms, have been linked to insulin resistance, metabolic syndrome and type 2 diabetes mellitus [103–105]. Interestingly, the adiponectin gene is located at 3q27, near the diabetes susceptibility gene locus [103, 106]. Adiponectin is structurally similar to the pro-inflammatory TNF- α family, however it functions as an anti-inflammatory adipokine, inhibiting the production of TNF-α within the adipocyte [102]. Conversely, pro-inflammatory agents such as TNF-α, IL-6 and IL-8 are implicated in the development of insulin resistance via hypothalamic inflammation [107]. This inflammation in turn contributes to both insulin and leptin resistance, promoting further obesity and subsequently diabetes [107]. In fact, in obese women adiponectin levels are low and pro-inflammatory markers, such as TNF-α, IL-6, and CRP are increased [46].

Adiponectin and its receptors are found in many organs including the ovaries [108–111]. Adiponectin acts in concert with insulin and IGF-1 to mediate changes within the granulosa cells during the periovulatory phase. Through IGF-1, it increases ovarian production of estradiol and progesterone in rat ovaries [108] possibly by up-regulating StAR gene [109]. It also causes vasodilation with the upregulation of VEGF and COX-2 expression in the periovulatory ovary [109]. Adiponectin knockout mice show ovarian dysfunction reflected by fewer oocytes, more atretic follicles, prolonged diestrus cycles and decreased LH receptor activity [112]. In a retrospective case-controlled analysis, adiponectin levels were higher in women who conceived after IVF and positively correlated with the number of oocytes retrieved, independent of BMI [113]. Similarly, while adiponectin levels are low or minimal in human and mouse granulosa cells, its presence enhances fertilization rates and embryo development [114, 115].

These findings suggest that adiponectin is notable for its action in mediating insulin sensitivity, with its receptors found at every level of the reproductive axis making it a great therapeutic target for ovulatory dysfunction.

Insulin

Insulin is a 51 amino acid protein synthesized in the beta islet cells of the pancreas. Its release is stimulated by glucose in the gastrointestinal tract from ingestion, as well as various amino acids directly [116]. Insulin levels rise and its sensitivity decreases with obesity [116]. Insulin resistance, in conjunction with obesity, impacts reproduction. While not a direct adipokine, adipose tissue stimulates pancreatic beta islet cells to release insulin. Hyperinsulinemia acts on the liver to cause a decrease in SHBG production [117]. This in turn leads to increased free circulating steroid hormone levels, such as estrogens and androgens. Insulin increases androgen production by two independent pathways; first by up-regulating CYP17A1 enzymes, which increase androgen production in both the adrenal gland and the ovary [118]. Second, insulin augments LH action on the ovary to increase androgen production and secretion [118, 119]. Insulin resistance is associated with higher leptin levels [38]. As noted previously, higher circulating leptin levels lead to leptin resistance which in turn leads to greater insulin resistance.

Insulin acts on the pituitary to modulate the GnRH receptor and increases LH secretion after GnRH stimulation [120]. Insulin augments FSH activity by increasing ovarian steroidogenesis and inducing LH responsiveness [121]. Hyperinsulinemia is consequently associated with elevated basal LH levels and hyperandrogenism [119]. Insulin alone does not have an effect on ovarian response to gonadotropic hyperstimulation during IVF in women without underlying insulin resistance [122]. Rather, the changes seen during IVF stimulation are due to insulin resistance [122]. Syndromic severe insulin resistance, as seen in some genetic disorders, is associated with enlarged ovaries and hyperandrogenism independent of gonadotropin levels. Elevated insulin levels over a long period of time can lead to increased autophosphorylation of its receptor, which can inactivate one of its downstream transducers, GSK3. This inactivation can lead to spindle disruption within growing oocytes [123, 124]. Additionally high insulin levels during oocyte development disrupt chromatin remodeling within mouse oocytes, thereby contributing to poorer oocyte quality [123]. Mouse models show that the pituitary is still sensitive to changes in insulin levels despite peripheral insulin resistance and basal hyperinsulinemia [120].

Disruption of insulin signaling in diet-induced obesity improves reproductive cyclicity in mice, suggesting that insulin represents a mediator for pituitary LH dysregulation in obesity [120]. Further study of insulin at the level of the ovary, specifically in insulin receptor knockout mice in theca cells, also demonstrates improved cyclic reproduction in mice, showing a coordinated effect of insulin along the HPO axis to disrupt cyclicity but not pubertal onset [118]. In summary, insulin's action is known to be necessary for changes in food intake and body weight. Its well-studied actions on the HPO axis and its relationship to adipokines such as leptin and adiponectin makes it a major player in female reproduction.

AGEs and MCP-1

Obesity is a state of chronic inflammation with macrophage infiltration into various tissues. Macrophage infiltration into adipose tissue is directly correlated to both the degree of adiposity as well as chemokine/adipokine production, such as MCP-1 [125]. The pattern of macrophage infiltration is similar to that found in disorders associated with chronic inflammation such as rheumatoid arthritis [125]. In addition to elevated circulating inflammatory markers, such as TNF-α, IL-6, and CRP [46], obese women have elevated levels of circulating AGEs [126] and MCP-1 [127]. In animal studies, obese mice have higher MCP-1 levels, which correlate with insulin resistance [128].

The pro-inflammatory AGEs may be part of the link between diet-induced obesity and inflammation, with AGEs inducing MCP-1 gene expression [129] thus forming the AGEs/MCP-1 axis. AGEs are highly reactive molecules formed by non-enzymatic cross-linking of proteins, lipids and nucleic acids with glucose [130, 131]. They may be formed endogenously or exogenously ingested as part of diet or through smoking [132]. AGE levels are elevated in chronic diseases such as type 2 Diabetes Mellitus, metabolic syndrome, cardiovascular disease, and neurodegenerative disorders [133–135]. AGEs have also been studied for their effect on reproduction [135–137].

Kandaraki et al. has demonstrated in human immortalized granulosa cells (KGN cell line) that AGEs attenuate LH- and FSH-induced ERK signaling needed for cell proliferation and proper follicular growth [138], one possible mechanism for AGE-induced ovulatory dysfunction. Similarly, AGEs interfere with glucose transport within granulosa cells [136]. Our recent data have shown that high-AGE diet could induce ovulatory dysfunction in a mouse model, as reflected by prolonged diestrus phase (unpublished data). We have also shown that high-fat diet induced obesity leads to ovulatory dysfunction in mice, as demonstrated by fewer oocytes ovulated following superovulation compared to mice on normal chow diet (controls) [139]. This ovarian dysfunction was not observed in MCP-1 knockout mice that became obese following ingestion of a high-fat diet, suggesting that lack of MCP-1 may be protective against high-fat- and obesity-induced ovarian dysfunction. Further supporting this hypothesis, we showed that elevated serum MCP-1 levels were associated with poorer outcome in women undergoing IVF [140], an effect that is pronounced in women with already diminished ovarian reserve. Additionally, AGE levels in follicular fluid were negatively correlated with IVF outcome parameters: fewer oocytes retrieved and fertilized, fewer embryos and lower ongoing pregnancy rate [137]. Taken together, these observations suggest that obesity may have direct deleterious effects on the ovaries partly through activation of inflammatory AGE/MCP-1 axis.

Relationship between obesity and assisted reproductive technology (ART) outcome

Population studies on the clinical sequelae of obesity provide a connection between obesity and subfertility.

Several studies indicated that obesity is a risk factor for ovulatory dysfunction [141–143]. For women who ovulate regularly, obesity increases the time to conception; for instance, a high waist- height ratio decreases fecundity by 30% [144]. Van der Steeg et al. found that in ovulatory infertile women (who underwent fertility evaluation but did not yet receive treatment), for every BMI unit over 29, there was a 5% decrease in the probability of a conception [145]. This increased time to conception is not only in the infertile population. Even in obese fertile women there was an increased time to conception from 3 to 5 months [146]. Other population studies have shown that 33% of obese women at age 23 did not conceive spontaneously when trying to conceive for 12 months [147]. This increases the number of couples meeting criteria for infertility and therefore for potential ART interventions [147]. Obesity could also impact ovarian reserve markers. Studies have shown that obesity is negatively correlated with serum AMH [148, 149], FSH, LH and inhibin B levels [150]. These markers provide added support for a clinician's analysis of a couple's fertility potential and may guide treatment options [151].

Obesity does not only affect spontaneous pregnancy rates in fertile patients, but it also confers a risk for poorer ART outcome. While earlier data could not demonstrate adequate convincing evidence of poorer ART outcome parameters, recent data supports this correlation. Large national cohort studies as well as systemic reviews and meta-analyses suggest that increasing BMI is negatively correlated with implantation, clinical pregnancy, and live birth rates [152–154]. Obese patients require higher doses of gonadotropins but achieve lower serum estradiol levels and lower number of oocytes retrieved [152, 155]. The oocytes of obese women tend to be smaller with decreased fertilization potential, leading to a decreased blastocyst formation and decreased trophectoderm cell number [156]. Additionally, obese women have higher cycle cancellation rates, possibly due to changes in pharmacodynamics of GnRH antagonists (clinically used to inhibit ovulation) leading to early LH surge and premature ovulation [157]. While not all studies identified these specific adverse ART outcome measures (i.e. smaller oocytes, decreased embryo quantity and quality), they still demonstrated a lower clinical pregnancy and live birth rates– up to 50% decrease compared to control women with normal BMI [152, 158].

The poorer IVF outcomes observed in obese patients are quite intriguing. These observations suggest that the effect of obesity on ovarian function is not solely dependent on the HPO axis, since gonadotropins are supplied exogenously during IVF cycles, thus bypassing the HPO axis. Obesity adversely impacts ART outcome differently in different ethnic populations [159–161]. However, these findings were inconsistent in the literature [162–164]

and may actually be in part due to ethnic variations in BMI rather than difference in ethnicity itself [159, 161].

Obesity could disrupt endometrial receptivity leading to poorer implantation rates [158, 165, 166], arguably due to endometrial inflammation. Inflammatory markers such as IL-6 and TNF-α have been implicated in lower implantation rates [46]. Similar to macrophage infiltration in the adipose tissue [125], we have shown that there is increased expression of macrophage markers in the ovaries of obese mice following the ingestion of a high-fat diet [167]. Moreover, mice given high-fat diet ovulated fewer oocytes following superovulation, further supporting the notion that obesity may have direct effect on ovaries, independent of HPO axis. Clearly the data to date demonstrates that obesity affects ART outcome in women undergoing IVF possibly via actions on all aspects: oocyte, embryo and endometrium.

Conclusion

With the uncurbed obesity epidemic, more reproductive-aged women will face metabolic and reproductive complications. Body energy hemostasis is closely linked to reproductive function through many hormones, adipokines, cytokines, and growth factors that act at the level of the brain and the ovaries. Obesity is also a state of chronic inflammation, which may directly affect ovarian function possibly by increased macrophage infiltration in the ovaries through MCP-1 mediated pathways. The elevation of AGEs in the serum and tissues of obese women may exacerbate the reproductive dysfunction associated with adiposity and may provide, along with MCP-1, a crucial link between obesity and ovarian macrophage infiltration. Each of these molecules and their prospective pathways may represent potential therapeutic targets in order to improve the overall reproductive health of overweight/obese women. Obesity, with its alterations in the AGEs/MCP-1 axis, could disrupt the ovarian microenvironment potentially compromising oocyte competence, formation of healthy embryos and ultimately conception.

Finally, this review underscores a critical need to uncover the mechanistic actions of molecules that affect almost every level of the HPO axis. Obesity, a significant and growing public health problem, is an overwhelming condition that causes reproductive disturbances in women in part due to ovarian dysfunction. Losing weight is commonly challenging and often not sustainable. Thus there is a need to establish therapies for ovarian dysfunction and to improve ovarian health in the obese patient population.

Authors' contributions
All authors contributed to the collection of literature data and writing of the manuscript. All authors read and approved the final manuscript.

Competing interests

The authors declare that they have no competing interests.

Author details

[1]Montefiore's Institute for Reproductive Medicine and Health, Department of Obstetrics & Gynecology and Women's Health, Albert Einstein College of Medicine, Montefiore Medical Center, Hartsdale, NY, USA. [2]Department of Obstetrics and Gynecology, Division of Reproductive Biology, NYU School of Medicine, New York, NY, USA. [3]Department of Biochemistry, Albert Einstein College of Medicine, Bronx, NY, USA.

References

1. Hales CM, Carroll MD, Fryar CD, Ogden CL. Prevalence of obesity among adults and youth: United States, 2015-2016. NCHS Data Brief. 2017;(288):1–8.
2. Wang YC, McPherson K, Marsh T, Gortmaker SL, Brown M. Health and economic burden of the projected obesity trends in the USA and the UK. Lancet. 2011;378(9793):815–25.
3. Tzeng CR, Chang YC, Chang YC, Wang CW, Chen CH, Hsu MI. Cluster analysis of cardiovascular and metabolic risk factors in women of reproductive age. Fertil Steril. 2014;101(5):1404–10.
4. Wei S, Schmidt MD, Dwyer T, Norman RJ, Venn AJ. Obesity and menstrual irregularity: associations with SHBG, testosterone, and insulin. Obesity (Silver Spring). 2009;17(5):1070–6.
5. Wise MR, Jordan V, Lagas A, Showell M, Wong N, Lensen S, Farquhar CM. Obesity and endometrial hyperplasia and cancer in premenopausal women: a systematic review. Am J Obstet Gynecol. 2016;214(6):689.e681–17.
6. Catalano PM, Ehrenberg HM. The short- and long-term implications of maternal obesity on the mother and her offspring. BJOG. 2006;113(10): 1126–33.
7. Massetti GM, Dietz WH, Richardson LC. Excessive weight gain, obesity, and Cancer: opportunities for clinical intervention. JAMA. 2017;318(20):1975–6.
8. Belchetz PE, Plant TM, Nakai Y, Keogh EJ, Knobil E. Hypophysial responses to continuous and intermittent delivery of hypopthalamic gonadotropin-releasing hormone. Science (New York, NY). 1978;202(4368):631–3.
9. Haisenleder DJ, Dalkin AC, Ortolano GA, Marshall JC, Shupnik MA. A pulsatile gonadotropin-releasing hormone stimulus is required to increase transcription of the gonadotropin subunit genes: evidence for differential regulation of transcription by pulse frequency in vivo. Endocrinology. 1991; 128(1):509–17.
10. Adashi EY. Endocrinology of the ovary. Hum Reprod. 1994;9(5):815–27.
11. Evans NP, Dahl GE, Mauger DT, Padmanabhan V, Thrun LA, Karsch FJ. Does estradiol induce the preovulatory gonadotropin-releasing hormone (GnRH) surge in the ewe by inducing a progressive change in the mode of operation of the GnRH neurosecretory system. Endocrinology. 1995;136(12):5511–9.
12. Xia L, Van Vugt D, Alston EJ, Luckhaus J, Ferin M. A surge of gonadotropin-releasing hormone accompanies the estradiol-induced gonadotropin surge in the rhesus monkey. Endocrinology. 1992;131(6):2812–20.
13. Knobil E. The neuroendocrine control of ovulation. Hum Reprod. 1988;3(4): 469–72.
14. Marshall JC, Griffin ML. The role of changing pulse frequency in the regulation of ovulation. Hum Reprod. 1993;8(Suppl 2):57–61.
15. Baker ER. Body weight and the initiation of puberty. Clin Obstet Gynecol. 1985;28(3):573–9.
16. Counts DR, Pescovitz OH, Barnes KM, Hench KD, Chrousos GP, Sherins RJ, Comite F, Loriaux DL, Cutler GB Jr. Dissociation of adrenarche and gonadarche in precocious puberty and in isolated hypogonadotropic hypogonadism. J Clin Endocrinol Metab. 1987;64(6):1174–8.
17. Jasik CB, Lustig RH. Adolescent obesity and puberty: the "perfect storm". Ann N Y Acad Sci. 2008;1135:265–79.
18. Burt Solorzano CM, McCartney CR. Obesity and the pubertal transition in girls and boys. Reproduction. 2010;140(3):399–410.
19. Cortés ME, Carrera B, Rioseco H, Pablo del Río J, Vigil P. The role of Kisspeptin in the onset of puberty and in the ovulatory mechanism: a mini-review. J Pediatr Adolesc Gynecol. 2015;28(5):286–91.
20. Bloch CA, Clemons P, Sperling MA. Puberty decreases insulin sensitivity. J Pediatr. 1987;110(3):481–7.
21. Kelsey MM, Zeitler PS. Insulin resistance of puberty. Curr Diab Rep. 2016; 16(7):64.
22. Frisch RE, Revelle R. Height and weight at menarche and a hypothesis of critical body weights and adolescent events. Science (New York, NY). 1970; 169(3943):397–9.
23. Goji K. Twenty-four-hour concentration profiles of gonadotropin and estradiol (E2) in prepubertal and early pubertal girls: the diurnal rise of E2 is opposite the nocturnal rise of gonadotropin. J Clin Endocrinol Metab. 1993; 77(6):1629–35.
24. Decensi A, Robertson C, Ballardini B, Paggi D, Guerrieri-Gonzaga A, Bonanni B, Manetti L, Johansson H, Barreca A, Bettega D, et al. Effect of tamoxifen on lipoprotein(a) and insulin-like growth factor-I (IGF-I) in healthy women. Eur J Cancer. 1999;35(4):596–600.
25. van den Berg G, Veldhuis JD, Frölich M, Roelfsema F. An amplitude-specific divergence in the pulsatile mode of growth hormone (GH) secretion underlies the gender difference in mean GH concentrations in men and premenopausal women. J Clin Endocrinol Metab. 1996;81(7):2460–7.
26. Chen C, Zhang Y, Sun W, Chen Y, Jiang Y, Song Y, Lin Q, Zhu L, Zhu Q, Wang X, et al. Investigating the relationship between precocious puberty and obesity: a cross-sectional study in shanghai, China. BMJ Open. 2017;7(4): e014004.
27. Kaplowitz PB, Slora EJ, Wasserman RC, Pedlow SE, Herman-Giddens ME. Earlier onset of puberty in girls: relation to increased body mass index and race. Pediatrics. 2001;108(2):347–53.
28. Rosenfield RL, Lipton RB, Drum ML. Thelarche, pubarche, and menarche attainment in children with normal and elevated body mass index. Pediatrics. 2009;123(1):84–8.
29. de Ridder CM, Bruning PF, Zonderland ML, Thijssen JH, Bonfrer JM, Blankenstein MA, Huisveld IA, Erich WB. Body fat mass, body fat distribution, and plasma hormones in early puberty in females. J Clin Endocrinol Metab. 1990;70(4):888–93.
30. Li J, Daly E, Campioli E, Wabitsch M, Papadopoulos V. De novo synthesis of steroids and oxysterols in adipocytes. J Biol Chem. 2014;289(2):747–64.
31. Freedman DS, Khan LK, Serdula MK, Dietz WH, Srinivasan SR, Berenson GS. Relation of age at menarche to race, time period, and anthropometric dimensions: the Bogalusa heart study. Pediatrics. 2002;110(4):e43.
32. Cleland WH, Mendelson CR, Simpson ER. Effects of aging and obesity on aromatase activity of human adipose cells. J Clin Endocrinol Metab. 1985; 60(1):174–7.
33. Zhao H, Zhou L, Shangguan AJ, Bulun SE. Aromatase expression and regulation in breast and endometrial cancer. J Mol Endocrinol. 2016;57(1): R19–33.
34. Nelson LR, Bulun SE. Estrogen production and action. J Am Acad Dermatol. 2001;45(3 Suppl):S116–24.
35. Jain A, Polotsky AJ, Rochester D, Berga SL, Loucks T, Zeitlian G, Gibbs K, Polotsky HN, Feng S, Isaac B, et al. Pulsatile luteinizing hormone amplitude and progesterone metabolite excretion are reduced in obese women. J Clin Endocrinol Metab. 2007;92(7):2468–73.
36. Cammisotto PG, Bendayan M. Leptin secretion by white adipose tissue and gastric mucosa. Histol Histopathol. 2007;22(2):199–210.
37. Considine RV, Sinha MK, Heiman ML, Kriauciunas A, Stephens TW, Nyce MR, Ohannesian JP, Marco CC, McKee LJ, Bauer TL, et al. Serum immunoreactive-leptin concentrations in normal-weight and obese humans. N Engl J Med. 1996;334(5):292–5.
38. Bozkurt L, Gobl CS, Rami-Merhar B, Winhofer Y, Baumgartner-Parzer S, Schober E, Kautzky-Willer A. The cross-link between Adipokines, insulin resistance and obesity in offspring of diabetic pregnancies. Horm Res Paediatr. 2016;86(5):300–8.
39. Zuure WA, Roberts AL, Quennell JH, Anderson GM. Leptin signaling in GABA neurons, but not glutamate neurons, is required for reproductive function. J Neurosci. 2013;33(45):17874–83.
40. Heymsfield SB, Greenberg AS, Fujioka K, Dixon RM, Kushner R, Hunt T, Lubina JA, Patane J, Self B, Hunt P, et al. Recombinant leptin for weight loss in obese and lean adults: a randomized, controlled, dose-escalation trial. JAMA. 1999;282(16):1568–75.
41. Liu AG, Smith SR, Fujioka K, Greenway FL. The effect of leptin, caffeine/ephedrine, and their combination upon visceral fat mass and weight loss. Obesity (Silver Spring). 2013;21(10):1991–6.
42. Zelissen PM, Stenlof K, Lean ME, Fogteloo J, Keulen ET, Wilding J, Finer N, Rossner S, Lawrence E, Fletcher C, et al. Effect of three treatment schedules of recombinant methionyl human leptin on body weight in obese adults: a randomized, placebo-controlled trial. Diabetes Obes Metab. 2005;7(6):755–61.
43. Baver SB, Hope K, Guyot S, Bjorbaek C, Kaczorowski C, O'Connell KM. Leptin

modulates the intrinsic excitability of AgRP/NPY neurons in the arcuate nucleus of the hypothalamus. J Neurosci. 2014;34(16):5486–96.

44. Frisch RE. Body fat, menarche, fitness and fertility. Hum Reprod. 1987;2(6): 521–33.

45. Cheung CC, Thornton JE, Kuijper JL, Weigle DS, Clifton DK, Steiner RA. Leptin is a metabolic gate for the onset of puberty in the female rat. Endocrinology. 1997;138(2):855–8.

46. Gosman GG, Katcher HI, Legro RS. Obesity and the role of gut and adipose hormones in female reproduction. Hum Reprod Update. 2006;12(5):585–601.

47. Egan OK, Inglis MA, Anderson GM. Leptin signaling in AgRP neurons modulates puberty onset and adult fertility in mice. J Neurosci. 2017;37(14): 3875–86.

48. Sanchez-Garrido MA, Tena-Sempere M. Metabolic control of puberty: roles of leptin and kisspeptins. Horm Behav. 2013;64(2):187–94.

49. Backholer K, Smith JT, Rao A, Pereira A, Iqbal J, Ogawa S, Li Q, Clarke IJ. Kisspeptin cells in the ewe brain respond to leptin and communicate with neuropeptide Y and proopiomelanocortin cells. Endocrinology. 2010; 151(5):2233–43.

50. Smith JT, Acohido BV, Clifton DK, Steiner RA. KiSS-1 neurones are direct targets for leptin in the Ob/Ob mouse. J Neuroendocrinol. 2006;18(4):298–303.

51. de Roux N, Genin E, Carel JC, Matsuda F, Chaussain JL, Milgrom E. Hypogonadotropic hypogonadism due to loss of function of the KiSS1-derived peptide receptor GPR54. Proc Natl Acad Sci U S A. 2003;100(19): 10972–6.

52. Castellano JM, Bentsen AH, Mikkelsen JD, Tena-Sempere M. Kisspeptins: bridging energy homeostasis and reproduction. Brain Res. 2010;1364:129–38.

53. Cioffi JA, Van Blerkom J, Antczak M, Shafer A, Wittmer S, Snodgrass HR. The expression of leptin and its receptors in pre-ovulatory human follicles. Mol Hum Reprod. 1997;3(6):467–72.

54. Hardie L, Trayhurn P, Abramovich D, Fowler P. Circulating leptin in women: a longitudinal study in the menstrual cycle and during pregnancy. Clin Endocrinol. 1997;47(1):101–6.

55. Tena-Sempere M. Roles of ghrelin and leptin in the control of reproductive function. Neuroendocrinology. 2007;86(3):229–41.

56. Brannian JD, Hansen KA. Leptin and ovarian folliculogenesis: implications for ovulation induction and ART outcomes. Semin Reprod Med. 2002;20(2):103–12.

57. Barash IA, Cheung CC, Weigle DS, Ren H, Kabigting EB, Kuijper JL, Clifton DK, Steiner RA. Leptin is a metabolic signal to the reproductive system. Endocrinology. 1996;137(7):3144–7.

58. Brannian JD, Schmidt SM, Kreger DO, Hansen KA. Baseline non-fasting serum leptin concentration to body mass index ratio is predictive of IVF outcomes. Hum Reprod. 2001;16(9):1819–26.

59. Spicer LJ, Chamberlain CS, Francisco CC. Ovarian action of leptin: effects on insulin-like growth factor-I-stimulated function of granulosa and thecal cells. Endocrine. 2000;12(1):53–9.

60. Spicer LJ, Francisco CC. Adipose obese gene product, leptin, inhibits bovine ovarian thecal cell steroidogenesis. Biol Reprod. 1998;58(1):207–12.

61. Merhi Z, Buyuk E, Berger DS, Zapantis A, Israel DD, Chua S Jr, Jindal S. Leptin suppresses anti-Mullerian hormone gene expression through the JAK2/STAT3 pathway in luteinized granulosa cells of women undergoing IVF. Hum Reprod. 2013;28(6):1661–9.

62. Carro E, Pinilla L, Seoane LM, Considine RV, Aguilar E, Casanueva FF, Dieguez C. Influence of endogenous leptin tone on the estrous cycle and luteinizing hormone pulsatility in female rats. Neuroendocrinology. 1997;66(6):375–7.

63. Kojima M, Hosoda H, Date Y, Nakazato M, Matsuo H, Kangawa K. Ghrelin is a growth-hormone-releasing acylated peptide from stomach. Nature. 1999; 402(6762):656–60.

64. Dezaki K, Sone H, Yada T. Ghrelin is a physiological regulator of insulin release in pancreatic islets and glucose homeostasis. Pharmacol Ther. 2008; 118(2):239–49.

65. Asakawa A, Inui A, Kaga T, Yuzuriha H, Nagata T, Ueno N, Makino S, Fujimiya M, Niijima A, Fujino MA, et al. Ghrelin is an appetite-stimulatory signal from stomach with structural resemblance to motilin. Gastroenterology. 2001; 120(2):337–45.

66. Chen HY, Trumbauer ME, Chen AS, Weingarth DT, Adams JR, Frazier EG, Shen Z, Marsh DJ, Feighner SD, Guan XM, et al. Orexigenic action of peripheral ghrelin is mediated by neuropeptide Y and Agouti-related protein. Endocrinology. 2004;145(6):2607–12.

67. Kojima M, Kangawa K. Ghrelin: structure and function. Physiol Rev. 2005; 85(2):495–522.

68. Kamegai J, Tamura H, Shimizu T, Ishii S, Sugihara H, Wakabayashi I. Chronic central infusion of ghrelin increases hypothalamic neuropeptide Y and Agouti-related protein mRNA levels and body weight in rats. Diabetes. 2001; 50(11):2438–43.

69. Williams KW, Elmquist JK. From neuroanatomy to behavior: central integration of peripheral signals regulating feeding behavior. Nat Neurosci. 2012;15(10): 1350–5.

70. Fernandez-Fernandez R, Tena-Sempere M, Navarro VM, Barreiro ML, Castellano JM, Aguilar E, Pinilla L. Effects of ghrelin upon gonadotropin-releasing hormone and gonadotropin secretion in adult female rats: in vivo and in vitro studies. Neuroendocrinology. 2005;82(5–6):245–55.

71. Furuta M, Funabashi T, Kimura F. Intracerebroventricular administration of ghrelin rapidly suppresses pulsatile luteinizing hormone secretion in ovariectomized rats. Biochem Biophys Res Commun. 2001;288(4):780–5.

72. Kluge M, Schussler P, Schmidt D, Uhr M, Steiger A. Ghrelin suppresses secretion of luteinizing hormone (LH) and follicle-stimulating hormone (FSH) in women. J Clin Endocrinol Metab. 2012;97(3):E448–51.

73. Vulliémoz NR, Xiao E, Xia-Zhang L, Germond M, Rivier J, Ferin M. Decrease in luteinizing hormone pulse frequency during a five-hour peripheral ghrelin infusion in the Ovariectomized rhesus monkey. J Clin Endocrinol Metab. 2004;89(11):5718–23.

74. Rak-Mardyla A. Ghrelin role in hypothalamus-pituitary-ovarian axis. J Physiol Pharmacol. 2013;64(6):695–704.

75. Broglio F, Benso A, Castiglioni C, Gottero C, Prodam F, Destefanis S, Gauna C, van der Lely AJ, Deghenghi R, Bo M, et al. The endocrine response to ghrelin as a function of gender in humans in young and elderly subjects. J Clin Endocrinol Metab. 2003;88(4):1537–42.

76. Whatmore AJ, Hall CM, Jones J, Westwood M, Clayton PE. Ghrelin concentrations in healthy children and adolescents. Clin Endocrinol. 2003;59(5):649–54.

77. Gaytan F, Barreiro ML, Chopin LK, Herington AC, Morales C, Pinilla L, Casanueva FF, Aguilar E, Dieguez C, Tena-Sempere M. Immunolocalization of ghrelin and its functional receptor, the type 1a growth hormone secretagogue receptor, in the cyclic human ovary. J Clin Endocrinol Metab. 2003;88(2):879–87.

78. Sirotkin AV, Grossmann R, Maria-Peon MT, Roa J, Tena-Sempere M, Klein S. Novel expression and functional role of ghrelin in chicken ovary. Mol Cell Endocrinol. 2006;257-258:15–25.

79. Sirotkin AV, Grossmann R. Effects of ghrelin and its analogues on chicken ovarian granulosa cells. Domest Anim Endocrinol. 2008;34(2):125–34.

80. Tropea A, Tiberi F, Minici F, Orlando M, Gangale MF, Romani F, Miceli F, Catino S, Mancuso S, Sanguinetti M, et al. Ghrelin affects the release of luteolytic and luteotropic factors in human luteal cells. J Clin Endocrinol Metab. 2007;92(8):3239–45.

81. Viani I, Vottero A, Tassi F, Cremonini G, Sartori C, Bernasconi S, Ferrari B, Ghizzoni L. Ghrelin inhibits steroid biosynthesis by cultured granulosa-lutein cells. J Clin Endocrinol Metab. 2008;93(4):1476–81.

82. Rak A, Gregoraszczuk EL. Modulatory effect of ghrelin in prepubertal porcine ovarian follicles. J Physiol Pharmacol. 2008;59(4):781–93.

83. Tilly JL, Kowalski KI, Johnson AL, Hsueh AJ. Involvement of apoptosis in ovarian follicular atresia and postovulatory regression. Endocrinology. 1991; 129(5):2799–801.

84. Kheradmand A, Roshangar L, Taati M, Sirotkin AV. Morphometrical and intracellular changes in rat ovaries following chronic administration of ghrelin. Tissue Cell. 2009;41(5):311–7.

85. Muller TD, Nogueiras R, Andermann ML, Andrews ZB, Anker SD, Argente J, Batterham RL, Benoit SC, Bowers CY, Broglio F, et al. Ghrelin. Mol Metab. 2015;4(6):437–60.

86. Sun Y, Asnicar M, Saha PK, Chan L, Smith RG. Ablation of ghrelin improves the diabetic but not obese phenotype of Ob/Ob mice. Cell Metab. 2006; 3(5):379–86.

87. Ikezaki A, Hosoda H, Ito K, Iwama S, Miura N, Matsuoka H, Kondo C, Kojima M, Kangawa K, Sugihara S. Fasting plasma ghrelin levels are negatively correlated with insulin resistance and PAI-1, but not with leptin, in obese children and adolescents. Diabetes. 2002;51(12):3408–11.

88. Hahn TM, Breininger JF, Baskin DG, Schwartz MW. Coexpression of Agrp and NPY in fasting-activated hypothalamic neurons. Nat Neurosci. 1998;1(4):271–2.

89. Kuo LE, Kitlinska JB, Tilan JU, Li L, Baker SB, Johnson MD, Lee EW, Burnett MS, Fricke ST, Kvetnansky R, et al. Neuropeptide Y acts directly in the periphery on fat tissue and mediates stress-induced obesity and metabolic syndrome. Nat Med. 2007;13(7):803–11.

90. Bures EJ, Hui JO, Young Y, Chow DT, Katta V, Rohde MF, Zeni L, Rosenfeld

RD, Stark KL, Haniu M. Determination of disulfide structure in agouti-related protein (AGRP) by stepwise reduction and alkylation. Biochemistry. 1998; 37(35):12172–7.

91. Cansell C, Denis RG, Joly-Amado A, Castel J, Luquet S. Arcuate AgRP neurons and the regulation of energy balance. Front Endocrinol. 2012;3:169.

92. Sutton SW, Toyama TT, Otto S, Plotsky PM. Evidence that neuropeptide Y (NPY) released into the hypophysial-portal circulation participates in priming gonadotropes to the effects of gonadotropin releasing hormone (GnRH). Endocrinology. 1988;123(2):1208–10.

93. Sahu A, Crowley WR, Kalra SP. Hypothalamic neuropeptide-Y gene expression increases before the onset of the ovarian steroid-induced luteinizing hormone surge. Endocrinology. 1994;134(3):1018–22.

94. Vulliémoz NR, Xiao E, Xia-Zhang L, Wardlaw SL, Ferin M. Central infusion of Agouti-related peptide suppresses pulsatile luteinizing hormone release in the Ovariectomized rhesus monkey. Endocrinology. 2005;146(2):784–9.

95. McDonald JK. Role of neuropeptide Y in reproductive function. Ann N Y Acad Sci. 1990;611:258–72.

96. Sirotkin AV, Kardosova D, Alwasel SH, Harrath AH. Neuropeptide Y directly affects ovarian cell proliferation and apoptosis. Reprod Biol. 2015;15(4):257–60.

97. Keator CS, Custer EE, Hoagland TA, Schreiber DT, Mah K, Lawson AM, Slayden OD, McCracken JA. Evidence for a potential role of neuropeptide Y in ovine corpus luteum function. Domest Anim Endocrinol. 2010;38(2):103–14.

98. Priyadarshini, Lal B. Seasonal ovarian immunolocalization of neuropeptide Y and its role in steriodogenesis in Asian catfish, Clarias batrachus. Gen Comp Endocrinol. 2018;255:32–9.

99. Lee B, Shao J. Adiponectin and energy homeostasis. Rev Endocr Metab Disord. 2014;15(2):149–56.

100. Kubota N, Yano W, Kubota T, Yamauchi T, Itoh S, Kumagai H, Kozono H, Takamoto I, Okamoto S, Shiuchi T, et al. Adiponectin stimulates AMP-activated protein kinase in the hypothalamus and increases food intake. Cell Metab. 2007;6(1):55–68.

101. Arita Y, Kihara S, Ouchi N, Takahashi M, Maeda K, Miyagawa J, Hotta K, Shimomura I, Nakamura T, Miyaoka K, et al. Paradoxical decrease of an adipose-specific protein, adiponectin, in obesity. Biochem Biophys Res Commun. 1999;257(1):79–83.

102. Maeda N, Shimomura I, Kishida K, Nishizawa H, Matsuda M, Nagaretani H, Furuyama N, Kondo H, Takahashi M, Arita Y, et al. Diet-induced insulin resistance in mice lacking adiponectin/ACRP30. Nat Med. 2002;8(7):731–7.

103. Kondo H, Shimomura I, Matsukawa Y, Kumada M, Takahashi M, Matsuda M, Ouchi N, Kihara S, Kawamoto T, Sumitsuji S, et al. Association of adiponectin mutation with type 2 diabetes: a candidate gene for the insulin resistance syndrome. Diabetes. 2002;51(7):2325–8.

104. Ohashi K, Ouchi N, Kihara S, Funahashi T, Nakamura T, Sumitsuji S, Kawamoto T, Matsumoto S, Nagaretani H, Kumada M, et al. Adiponectin I164T mutation is associated with the metabolic syndrome and coronary artery disease. J Am Coll Cardiol. 2004;43(7):1195–200.

105. Kadowaki T, Yamauchi T, Kubota N, Hara K, Ueki K, Tobe K. Adiponectin and adiponectin receptors in insulin resistance, diabetes, and the metabolic syndrome. J Clin Invest. 2006;116(7):1784–92.

106. Vionnet N, Hani EH, Dupont S, Gallina S, Francke S, Dotte S, De Matos F, Durand E, Lepretre F, Lecoeur C, et al. Genomewide search for type 2 diabetes-susceptibility genes in French whites: evidence for a novel susceptibility locus for early-onset diabetes on chromosome 3q27-qter and independent replication of a type 2-diabetes locus on chromosome 1q21-q24. Am J Hum Genet. 2000;67(6):1470–80.

107. Thaler JP, Schwartz MW. Minireview: inflammation and obesity pathogenesis: the hypothalamus heats up. Endocrinology. 2010;151(9):4109–15.

108. Chabrolle C, Tosca L, Dupont J. Regulation of adiponectin and its receptors in rat ovary by human chorionic gonadotrophin treatment and potential involvement of adiponectin in granulosa cell steroidogenesis. Reproduction. 2007;133(4):719–31.

109. Ledoux S, Campos DB, Lopes FL, Dobias-Goff M, Palin M-F, Murphy BD. Adiponectin induces Periovulatory changes in ovarian follicular cells. Endocrinology. 2006;147(11):5178–86.

110. Chabrolle C, Tosca L, Crochet S, Tesseraud S, Dupont J. Expression of adiponectin and its receptors (AdipoR1 and AdipoR2) in chicken ovary: potential role in ovarian steroidogenesis. Domest Anim Endocrinol. 2007; 33(4):480–7.

111. Campos DB, Palin MF, Bordignon V, Murphy BD. The 'beneficial' adipokines in reproduction and fertility. Int J Obes (Lond). 2008;32(2):223–31.

112. Cheng L, Shi H, Jin Y, Li X, Pan J, Lai Y, Lin Y, Jin Y, Roy G, Zhao A, et al.

Adiponectin deficiency leads to female subfertility and ovarian dysfunctions in mice. Endocrinology. 2016;157(12):4875–87.

113. Liu YH, Tsai EM, Wu LC, Chen SY, Chang YH, Jong SB, Chan TF. Higher basal adiponectin levels are associated with better ovarian response to gonadotropin stimulation during in vitro fertilization. Gynecol Obstet Investig. 2005;60(3):167–70.

114. Richards JS, Liu Z, Kawai T, Tabata K, Watanabe H, Suresh D, Kuo FT, Pisarska MD, Shimada M. Adiponectin and its receptors modulate granulosa cell and cumulus cell functions, fertility, and early embryo development in the mouse and human. Fertil Steril. 2012;98(2):471–9. e471

115. Chang HJ, Lee JH, Lee JR, Jee BC, Suh CS, Kim SH. Relationship between follicular fluid adipocytokines and the quality of the oocyte and corresponding embryo development from a single dominant follicle in in vitro fertilization/intracytoplasmic sperm injection cycles. Clin Exp Reprod Med. 2014;41(1):21–8.

116. Lundon JR. Insulin-some current concepts. Can Fam Physician. 1970;16(7):58–61.

117. Preziosi P, Barrett-Connor E, Papoz L, Roger M, Saint-Paul M, Nahoul K, Simon D. Interrelation between plasma sex hormone-binding globulin and plasma insulin in healthy adult women: the telecom study. J Clin Endocrinol Metab. 1993;76(2):283–7.

118. Wu S, Divall S, Nwaopara A, Radovick S, Wondisford F, Ko C, Wolfe A. Obesity-induced infertility and hyperandrogenism are corrected by deletion of the insulin receptor in the ovarian theca cell. Diabetes. 2014;63(4):1270–82.

119. Barbieri RL, Makris A, Ryan KJ. Effects of insulin on steroidogenesis in cultured porcine ovarian theca. Fertil Steril. 1983;40(2):237–41.

120. Brothers KJ, Wu S, DiVall SA, Messmer MR, Kahn CR, Miller RS, Radovick S, Wondisford FE, Wolfe A. Rescue of obesity-induced infertility in female mice due to a pituitary-specific knockout of the insulin receptor. Cell Metab. 2010;12(3):295–305.

121. Willis D, Mason H, Gilling-Smith C, Franks S. Modulation by insulin of follicle-stimulating hormone and luteinizing hormone actions in human granulosa cells of normal and polycystic ovaries. J Clin Endocrinol Metab. 1996;81(1):302–9.

122. La Marca A, Pati M, Giulini S, Levratti P, Caretto S, Volpe A. Does plasma insulin level affect ovarian response to exogenous administration of follicle-stimulating hormone in women without polycystic ovary syndrome? Gynecol Endocrinol. 2005;21(5):292–4.

123. Acevedo N, Ding J, Smith GD. Insulin signaling in mouse Oocytes1. Biol Reprod. 2007;77(5):872–9.

124. Ou XH, Li S, Wang ZB, Li M, Quan S, Xing F, Guo L, Chao SB, Chen Z, Liang XW, et al. Maternal insulin resistance causes oxidative stress and mitochondrial dysfunction in mouse oocytes. Hum Reprod. 2012;27(7):2130–45.

125. Weisberg SP, McCann D, Desai M, Rosenbaum M, Leibel RL, Ferrante AW Jr. Obesity is associated with macrophage accumulation in adipose tissue. J Clin Invest. 2003;112(12):1796–808.

126. Van Puyvelde K, Mets T, Njemini R, Beyer I, Bautmans I. Effect of advanced glycation end product intake on inflammation and aging: a systematic review. Nutr Rev. 2014;72(10):638–50.

127. Vazzana N, Guagnano MT, Cuccurullo C, Ferrante E, Lattanzio S, Liani R, Romano M, Davi G. Endogenous secretory RAGE in obese women: association with platelet activation and oxidative stress. J Clin Endocrinol Metab. 2012;97(9):E1726–30.

128. Sartipy P, Loskutoff DJ. Monocyte chemoattractant protein 1 in obesity and insulin resistance. Proc Natl Acad Sci U S A. 2003;100(12):7265–70.

129. Gu L, Hagiwara S, Fan Q, Tanimoto M, Kobata M, Yamashita M, Nishitani T, Gohda T, Ni Z, Qian J, et al. Role of receptor for advanced glycation end-products and signalling events in advanced glycation end-product-induced monocyte chemoattractant protein-1 expression in differentiated mouse podocytes. Nephrol Dial Transplant. 2006;21(2):299–313.

130. Grandhee SK, Monnier VM. Mechanism of formation of the Maillard protein cross-link pentosidine. Glucose, fructose, and ascorbate as pentosidine precursors. J Biol Chem. 1991;266(18):11649–53.

131. Monnier VM, Sell DR, Nagaraj RH, Miyata S, Grandhee S, Odetti P, Ibrahim SA. Maillard reaction-mediated molecular damage to extracellular matrix and other tissue proteins in diabetes, aging, and uremia. Diabetes. 1992; 41(Suppl 2):36–41.

132. Horiuchi S, Araki N, Morino Y. Immunochemical approach to characterize advanced glycation end products of the Maillard reaction. Evidence for the presence of a common structure. J Biol Chem. 1991;266(12):7329–32.

133. Yamagishi S, Nakamura K, Imaizumi T. Advanced glycation end products (AGEs) and diabetic vascular complications. Curr Diabetes Rev. 2005;1(1):93–106.

134. Tatone C, Amicarelli F, Carbone MC, Monteleone P, Caserta D, Marci R, Artini

PG, Piomboni P, Focarelli R. Cellular and molecular aspects of ovarian follicle ageing. Hum Reprod Update. 2008;14(2):131–42.

135. Diamanti-Kandarakis E, Piperi C, Patsouris E, Korkolopoulou P, Panidis D, Pawelczyk L, Papavassiliou AG, Duleba AJ. Immunohistochemical localization of advanced glycation end-products (AGEs) and their receptor (RAGE) in polycystic and normal ovaries. Histochem Cell Biol. 2007;127(6):581–9.

136. Diamanti-Kandarakis E, Chatzigeorgiou A, Papageorgiou E, Koundouras D, Koutsilieris M. Advanced glycation end-products and insulin signaling in granulosa cells. Exp Biol Med. 2016;241(13):1438–45.

137. Jinno M, Takeuchi M, Watanabe A, Teruya K, Hirohama J, Eguchi N, Miyazaki A. Advanced glycation end-products accumulation compromises embryonic development and achievement of pregnancy by assisted reproductive technology. Hum Reprod. 2011;26(3):604–10.

138. Kandaraki EA, Chatzigeorgiou A, Papageorgiou E, Piperi C, Adamopoulos C, Papavassiliou AG, Koutsilieris M, Diamanti-Kandarakis E. Advanced glycation end products interfere in luteinizing hormone and follicle stimulating hormone signaling in human granulosa KGN cells. Exp Biol Med. 2018; 243(1):29–33. 1535370217731288.

139. Asemota OA, Berger DS, Seki Y, Jindal SK, Charron MJ, Buyuk E. MCP-1, a central mediator of obesity and diet-induced ovarian dysfunction. Fertil Steril. 2014;102(3):e259.

140. Buyuk E, Asemota OA, Merhi Z, Charron MJ, Berger DS, Zapantis A, Jindal SK. Serum and follicular fluid monocyte chemotactic protein-1 levels are elevated in obese women and are associated with poorer clinical pregnancy rate after in vitro fertilization: a pilot study. Fertil Steril. 2017; 107(3):632–40. e633

141. Grodstein F, Goldman MB, Cramer DW. Body mass index and ovulatory infertility. Epidemiology. 1994;5(2):247–50.

142. Rich-Edwards JW, Spiegelman D, Garland M, Hertzmark E, Hunter DJ, Colditz GA, Willett WC, Wand H, Manson JE. Physical activity, body mass index, and ovulatory disorder infertility. Epidemiology. 2002;13(2):184–90.

143. Green BB, Weiss NS, Daling JR. Risk of ovulatory infertility in relation to body weight. Fertil Steril. 1988;50(5):721–6.

144. Zaadstra BM, Seidell JC, Van Noord PA, te Velde ER, Habbema JD, Vrieswijk B, Karbaat J. Fat and female fecundity: prospective study of effect of body fat distribution on conception rates. BMJ. 1993;306(6876):484–7.

145. van der Steeg JW, Steures P, Eijkemans MJ, Habbema JD, Hompes PG, Burggraaff JM, Oosterhuis GJ, Bossuyt PM, van der Veen F, Mol BW. Obesity affects spontaneous pregnancy chances in subfertile, ovulatory women. Hum Reprod. 2008;23(2):324–8.

146. Gesink Law DC, Maclehose RF, Longnecker MP. Obesity and time to pregnancy. Hum Reprod. 2007;22(2):414–20.

147. Lake JK, Power C, Cole TJ. Women's reproductive health: the role of body mass index in early and adult life. Int J Obes Relat Metab Disord. 1997;21(6): 432–8.

148. Moy V, Jindal S, Lieman H, Buyuk E. Obesity adversely affects serum anti-mullerian hormone (AMH) levels in Caucasian women. J Assist Reprod Genet. 2015;32(9):1305–11.

149. Freeman EW, Gracia CR, Sammel MD, Lin H, Lim LC, Strauss JF 3rd. Association of anti-mullerian hormone levels with obesity in late reproductive-age women. Fertil Steril. 2007;87(1):101–6.

150. De Pergola G, Maldera S, Tartagni M, Pannacciulli N, Loverro G, Giorgino R. Inhibitory effect of obesity on gonadotropin, estradiol, and inhibin B levels in fertile women. Obesity (Silver Spring). 2006;14(11):1954–60.

151. Practice Committee of the American Society for Reproductive Medicine. Testing and interpreting measures of ovarian reserve: a committee opinion. Fertil Steril. 2015;103(3):e9–e17.

152. Shah DK, Missmer SA, Berry KF, Racowsky C, Ginsburg ES. Effect of obesity on oocyte and embryo quality in women undergoing in vitro fertilization. Obstet Gynecol. 2011;118(1):63–70.

153. Provost MP, Acharya KS, Acharya CR, Yeh JS, Steward RG, Eaton JL, Goldfarb JM, Muasher SJ. Pregnancy outcomes decline with increasing body mass index: analysis of 239,127 fresh autologous in vitro fertilization cycles from the 2008–2010 Society for Assisted Reproductive Technology registry. Fertil Steril. 2016;105(3):663–9.

154. Maheshwari A, Stofberg L, Bhattacharya S. Effect of overweight and obesity on assisted reproductive technology–a systematic review. Hum Reprod Update. 2007;13(5):433–44.

155. Zhang D, Zhu Y, Gao H, Zhou B, Zhang R, Wang T, Ding G, Qu F, Huang H, Lu X. Overweight and obesity negatively affect the outcomes of ovarian stimulation and in vitro fertilisation: a cohort study of 2628 Chinese women.

Gynecol Endocrinol. 2010;26(5):325–32.

156. Leary C, Leese HJ, Sturmey RG. Human embryos from overweight and obese women display phenotypic and metabolic abnormalities. Hum Reprod. 2015;30(1):122–32.

157. Roth LW, Bradshaw-Pierce EL, Allshouse AA, Lesh J, Chosich J, Bradford AP, Polotsky AJ, Santoro N. Evidence of GnRH antagonist escape in obese women. J Clin Endocrinol Metab. 2014;99(5):E871–5.

158. Bellver J, Ayllon Y, Ferrando M, Melo M, Goyri E, Pellicer A, Remohi J, Meseguer M. Female obesity impairs in vitro fertilization outcome without affecting embryo quality. Fertil Steril. 2010;93(2):447–54.

159. Sharara FI, McClamrock HD. Differences in in vitro fertilization (IVF) outcome between white and black women in an inner-city, university-based IVF program. Fertil Steril. 2000;73(6):1170–3.

160. Mitwally MF, Leduc MM, Ogunleye O, Albuarki H, Diamond MP, Abuzeid M. The effect of body mass index (BMI) on the outcome of IVF and embryo transfer in women of different ethnic backgrounds. Fertility Sterility. 2006;86: S68–9.

161. Patel AP, Patel JA, Cruz M, Gupte-Shah A, Garcia Velasco JA, Banker MR. Ethnicity is an independent predictor of IVF-ICSI outcome: a study of 5,549 cycles in Spain and India. Gynecol Endocrinol. 2016;32(10):819–22.

162. Dayal MB, Gindoff P, Dubey A, Spitzer TL, Bergin A, Peak D, Frankfurter D. Does ethnicity influence in vitro fertilization (IVF) birth outcomes? Fertil Steril. 2009;91(6):2414–8.

163. Lashen H, Afnan M, Sharif K. A controlled comparison of ovarian response to controlled stimulation in first generation Asian women compared with white Caucasians undergoing in vitro fertilisation. Br J Obstet Gynaecol. 1999;106(5):407–9.

164. Nichols JE Jr, Higdon HL 3rd, Crane MM, Boone WR. Comparison of implantation and pregnancy rates in African American and white women in an assisted reproductive technology practice. Fertil Steril. 2001;76(1):80–4.

165. Bellver J, Melo MA, Bosch E, Serra V, Remohi J, Pellicer A. Obesity and poor reproductive outcome: the potential role of the endometrium. Fertil Steril. 2007;88(2):446–51.

166. Loveland JB, McClamrock HD, Malinow AM, Sharara FI. Increased body mass index has a deleterious effect on in vitro fertilization outcome. J Assist Reprod Genet. 2001;18(7):382–6.

167. Thornton KAO, Jindal S, Charron M, Buyuk E. High fat diet and aging are associated with macrophage infiltration in the ovaries. Fertil Steril. 2015; 104(3):e104–5.

## 15

Probabilistic cost-effectiveness analysis of controlled ovarian stimulation with recombinant FSH plus recombinant LH vs. human menopausal gonadotropin for women undergoing IVF

F. S. Mennini[1,2], A. Marcellusi[1,2], R. Viti[1], C. Bini[1*], A. Carosso[3], A. Revelli[3,4] and C. Benedetto[3]

Abstract

Background: The association of recombinant FSH plus recombinant LH in 2:1 ratio may be used not only to induce ovulation in anovulatory women with hypogonadotropic hypogonadism but also to achieve multiple follicular developments in human IVF. The aim of this analysis was to estimate the cost-effectiveness of Controlled Ovarian Stimulation (COS) with recombinant FSH (rFSH) plus recombinant LH (rLH) in comparison with highly purified human menopausal gonadotropin (HP-hMG) in the woman undergoing in vitro fertilization (IVF) in Italy.

Methods: A probabilistic decision tree was developed to simulate patients undergoing IVF, either using r-FSH + r-LH or HP-hMG to obtain COS. The model considers the National Health System (NHS) perspective and a time horizon equal to two years. Simulations were reported considering the number of retrieved oocytes (5–9, 10–15 and > 15) and transition probabilities were estimated through specific analyses carried out on the population of 848 women enrolled in the real-life.

Results: The model estimated that patients undertaking therapeutic protocol with r-FSH + r-LH increase the general success rate (+ 6.6% for pregnancy). The incremental cost-effectiveness ratio (ICER) per quality-adjusted life year (QALY) of r-FSH + r-LH was below the willingness to pay set at €20,000 for all the considered scenarios.

Conclusions: The cost-utility analysis demonstrated that the r-FSH + r-LH is a cost-effective option for the Italian National Health System (NHS).

Keywords: Real world data, Retrieved oocytes, Cost-utility, QALYs

Background

The twentieth century witnessed the discovery of pituitary gonadotropins follicle-stimulating hormone (FSH) and luteinising hormone (LH) that were made available as medication after the extraction and purification from the urine of menopausal women [1]. The combination of urinary FSH (u-FSH) and human chorionic gonadotropin (u-hCG), a placental hormone displaying LH activity, has been available for the last forty years under the name of "human Menopausal Gonadotropin" (hMG) About twenty-five years ago, genetic engineering developed recombinant FSH (r-FSH) and recombinant LH (r-LH) by inserting the corresponding human DNA into Chinese hamster cells and then extracting and purifying the final molecules from their supernatant [2, 3]. Nowadays a highly purified hMG (HP-hMG, Meropur, Ferring Germany) has been introduced.

Urinary-derived and recombinant gonadotropins have been widely used to treat women with infertility due to chronic anovulation [4], or to provide a therapeutic stimulation to spermatogenesis [5]. In most cases, however, these are administered to obtain the so-called

* Correspondence: chiara.stat@gmail.com
[1]Economic Evaluation and HTA (CEIS- EEHTA) - Faculty of Economics, University of Rome "Tor Vergata", Via Columbia, 2, 00133 Rome, Italy
Full list of author information is available at the end of the article

Controlled Ovarian Stimulation (COS), that is the multiple follicular developments aimed at getting the number of oocytes needed to perform in vitro fertilization (IVF). Several studies, as well as systematic reviews, have compared the effectiveness of urinary gonadotropins (u-FSH or HP-hMG) vs. r-FSH for COS, showing the superiority of r-FSH over u-FSH [4, 6, 7] and a substantial equivalence of r-FSH and HP-hMG [8–13]. Also, only in few countries the combination of r-FSH + r-LH in a 2:1 ratio (Pergoveris, Merck, Germany) for the treatment of patients with hypogonadotropic hypogonadism [14], is also licensed for COS. Comparative studies vs. hMG are rare and substantial do information are still missing [15, 16]. To date, the largest study comparing r-FSH + r-LH vs. HP-hMG in human IVF was conducted retrospectively on real-life data from clinical practice that were obtained in the IVF Unit of a University Hospital and in a private IVF Clinic [17]. In this context the r-FSH + r-LH association was demonstrated: (1) as effective as HP-hMG when the retrieved oocytes were less than 4, slightly (but not significantly); (2) superior when the retrieved oocytes were 5–8 and (3) significantly more effective in terms of pregnancy rate per embryo transfer (PR/ET) when they were 9 or more [17]. Moreover, in the same study, the advantage of using the r-FSH + r-LH therapy was even more pronounced when only mature oocytes were considered [17]. In support of the mentioned results, a multivariate logistic regression model confirmed that both the use of recombinant gonadotropins and the number of retrieved oocytes were increasing significantly the probability of a pregnancy, with an odds ratio (OR) of 1.628 and 1.083, respectively [17].

In another paper, a comparative analysis of legal restrictions on access to IVF was conducted in 13 EU countries. This study demonstrated as countries with the most generous public financing scheme tended to restrict access to IVF to a greater degree. Contrarily, no link was established between IVF utilization and the manner in which coverage was regulated or the level of public financing was set [18]. As a result of that, regulations seem generally more restrictive compared to the eligibility criteria in order to limit, through the reduced size of the covered population the budgetary outlays [18].

Nowadays the cost of pharmacological therapies represent a major issue [19] at international level and it is often considered as important as the effectiveness. Based on these premises, in the present study we aimed at performing a pharmaco economic analysis to estimate the cost-effectiveness of COS with r-FSH + r-LH in comparison with HP-hMG, considering the effectiveness of r-FSH + r-LH or HP-hMG (number of pregnancy, Positive or negative hCG test, Clinical pregnancy, Miscarriage, Cycle with embryo freezing, and Dropout) in terms of the Quality Adjusted Life Years (QALYs).

Methods

Model

A probabilistic decision tree was developed to simulate the therapeutic path of two homogeneous cohorts of 1000 patients undergoing IVF, either using r-FSH + r-LH or HP-hMG and to obtain COS. Also, the pharmacological treatment was analyzed (Fig. 1). The study was performed in 2017.

The outcomes considered in the analysis were: (a) urinary hCG pregnancy test (performed 15 days after embryo transfer), (b) clinical pregnancy (foetal heartbeat at transvaginal ultrasound performed 2–4 weeks after an hCG+ test), (c) miscarriage (absence of foetal heartbeat at transvaginal ultrasound in a patient with hCG+), and (d) dropout from IVF program. The time horizon considered in the simulation was assumed to be equal to two years, with a simulation of one IVF cycle every 6 months for a maximum of 3 cycles. It was coherent with the literature [18] that underline how the most developed countries established public financing coverage limits for three or four cycles [18]. In Italy, most couples are submitted to a maximum of three IVF attempts during a two-year period, after which they can continue to undergo IVF, but without any reimbursement by the healthcare system.

In detail, once the COS with r-FSH + r-LH or HP-hMG had started, the patient was considered to have a different probability of incurring in a positive or negative hCG test according to the results previously published by Revelli et al. [17]. In case of a positive pregnancy test, the patient could have an US-detectable clinical pregnancy, in turn becoming an ongoing pregnancy or a miscarriage within the third month of pregnancy. In case of a negative test, the patient could undergo an additional IVF cycle using or not frozen embryos or decide to abandon the therapeutic program (dropout). The model assumes that patients without frozen embryos repeated the same COS used in the previous fresh cycle.

The population considered in the model was the one previously described by Revelli et al. [17], but we carried out sub-analyses grouping patients in a different way, and the following groups were created: 5–9 retrieved oocytes, 10–15 retrieved oocytes, and > 15 retrieved oocytes.

In order to estimate the QALYs of the two patient populations undertaking the therapeutic path with r-FSH + r-LH or HP-hMG, the utilities reported in Table 1 were considered. Due to the lack of precise information on the impact of various events on the quality of life of patients undergoing COS and IVF, the annual utility measures used in the model were obtained through the opinion of IVF experts.

The utilities reported in Table 1 and obtained through the support of expert clinicians were transformed into monthly utilities to perform the analysis.

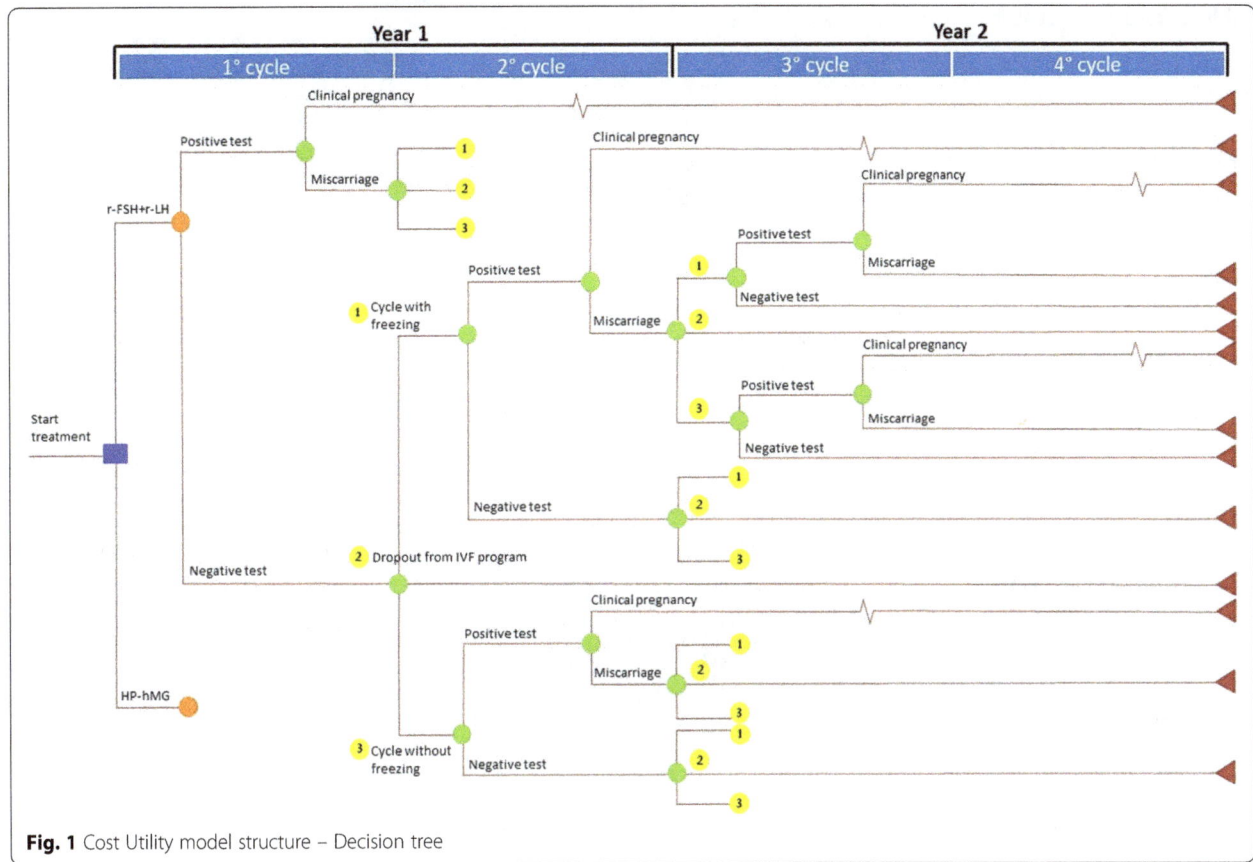

Fig. 1 Cost Utility model structure – Decision tree

Each monthly utility was applied and weighed according to the reference period reported in Table 1. The two COS protocols were considered to have a priori identical impact on the quality of life.

Transition probabilities

The probability of obtaining a positive hCG test and, later on, having or not a miscarriage was obtained through specific analyses carried out on the population of 848 women enrolled in the real-life, previously published in a clinical study [17]. Such probabilities were

calculated stratifying the population of patients according to the type of COS therapy and to the number of retrieved oocytes (Table 2). The statistical significance was evaluated with a chi-square test and Fisher's exact test when appropriate.

Analysing the general characteristics of the patients, it was observed that by increasing the patients' age, the number of retrieved oocytes would decrease. In particular, the average age of the patients (36.7 years for the whole sample) was 36.4 for women with less than 5 retrieved oocytes, 36.6 for women with 5–9 retrieved oocytes, 36 for women with 10–15 retrieved oocytes, and 35.6 for women with more than 15 retrieved oocytes. Therefore, the model assumed that the probability of obtaining a positive hCG pregnancy test was likely to decrease with age with an odds ratio of 0.901 (95% CI: 0.863–0.940) [17].

The transition probabilities of obtaining embryo freezing as well as the probability of dropping-out from the IVF program were assumed to be independent from the number of retrieved oocytes, independent from the medication used for COS, and were estimated through the expertise of clinical practice.

Table 1 Utilities considered in the model

Therapeutic path	Utility	Months	Source
r-FSH + r-LH (MIN - MAX)	0.8 (0.72–0.88)	1	Expert opinion
HP-hMG (MIN - MAX)	0.8 (0.72–0.88)	1	Expert opinion
Positive hCGtest (MIN - MAX)	0.9 (0.81–0.99)	3	Expert opinion
Negative hCGtest (MIN - MAX)	0.7 (0.63–0.77)	5	Expert opinion
Clinical pregnancy (MIN - MAX)	1 (0.90–1.00)	2	Expert opinion
Miscarriage (MIN - MAX)	0.5 (0.45–0.55)	2	Expert opinion
Cycle with embryo freezing (MIN - MAX)	0.9 (0.81–0.99)	1	Expert opinion
Cycle without embryo freezing (MIN - MAX)	0.8 (0.72–0.88)	1	Expert opinion
Dropout (MIN - MAX)	0.4 (0.36–0.44)	6	Expert opinion

Cost parameters

The costs considered in the model refer only to the direct costs covered by the Italian NHS for IVF treatment

Table 2 Transition probabilities used in the model

	r-FSH + r-LH	HP-hMG	p-value for comparison	Source
≥ 5 Oocytes				
Positive hCG test (MIN - MAX)	0.34 (0.31–0.37)	0.23 (0.21–0.25)	0.007	Analyses from [17]
Negative hCG test (MIN - MAX)	0.66 (0.60–0.73)	0.77 (0.69–0.84)		
Clinical pregnancy (MIN - MAX)	0.84 (0.76–0.92)	0.82 (0.74–0.90)	0.790	
Miscarriage (MIN - MAX)	0.16 (0.15–0.18)	0,18 (0.16–0.19)		
5–9 oocytes				
Positive hCG test (MIN - MAX)	0.28 (0.26–0.31)	0.22 (0.20–0.24)	0.158	Analyses from [17]
Negative hCG test (MIN - MAX)	0.72 (0.65–0.79)	0.78 (0.70–0.86)		
Clinical pregnancy (MIN - MAX)	0.82 (0.74–0.90)	0.79 (0.71–0.86)	0.646	
Miscarriage (MIN - MAX)	0.18 (0.16–0.19)	0.21 (0.19–0.24)		
10–15 oocytes				
Positive hCG test (MIN - MAX)	0.43 (0.39–0.48)	0.24 (0.22–0.27)	0.025	Analyses from [17]
Negative hCG test (MIN - MAX)	0.57 (0.51–0.62)	0.76 (0.68–0.83)		
Clinical pregnancy (MIN - MAX)	0.88 (0.80–0.97)	0.87 (0.78–0.95)	1.000	
Miscarriage (MIN - MAX)	0.12 (0.10–0.13)	0.13 (0.12–0.15)		
> 15 oocytes				
Positive hCG test (MIN - MAX)	0.56 (0.50–0.61)	0.33 (0.30–0.37)	0.202	Analyses from [17]
Negative hCG test (MIN - MAX)	0.44 (0.40–0.49)	0.67 (0.60–0.73)		
Clinical pregnancy (MIN - MAX)	0.80 (0.72–0.88)	1.00 (0.90–1.00)	0.524	
Miscarriage (MIN - MAX)	0.20 (0.18–0.22)	0.00 (0.00–0.00)		
Transition probabilities valid for all the sample				
Cycle with embryo freezing (MIN - MAX)	0.30 (0.27–0.33)	0.30 (0.27–0.33)		Expert opinion
Cycle without embryo freezing (MIN - MAX)	0.40 (0.36–0.44)	0.40 (0.36–0.44)		Expert opinion
Dropout (MIN - MAX)	0.30 (0.27–0.33)	0.30 (0.27–0.33)		Expert opinion

(Table 3). For the cost estimates related to pregnancy and miscarriage, we referred to the range of fees of hospital health care for acute patients [20]. Specifically, assuming that 60% of patients would have a vaginal delivery and the remaining 40% a caesarean section (expert opinion based on the general trend in Italy for IVF patients), such cost was obtained through a weighted average of the Italian diagnosis-related group (DRG) 371 (cesarean section without complications) and 373 (vaginal delivery without complications) rates. As far as miscarriage is concerned, the cost was obtained as a simple average between DRG 376 (spontaneous miscarriage without surgery) and 377 (spontaneous miscarriage with dilatation and curettage) rates.

The COS therapy medication cost was estimated on the ex-factory price, that is the price set at the level of the manufacturer, net of the discounts provided by law, the formulation and the total dose observed in the reference study [17]. The cost of the monitoring before and

during COS was derived from the work of Papaleo et al. [14] integrated by indications supplied by expert opinions (Table 3).

Cost-effectiveness analysis

Cost-effectiveness analysis as applied to health economics provides an approach to medical decision making [21]. A cost-effectiveness analysis is a type of economic evaluation in which cost is expressed over some unit of benefit (life years gained, symptom free months, etc.) [21]. A cost-utility analysis is a type of cost-effectiveness analysis in which the benefit is expressed in utility [21]. The most commonly used measure of benefit in a cost-utility analysis is the QALY [21].

Quality-adjusted life years (QALYs) has become increasingly used as a healthcare outcome measure and as an integral part of cost-utility analysis [22, 23]. It combines length of life and quality of life into a single index number [24]. It is calculated as the area under the curve when measuring utility over time [22]. The utility can be

Table 3 Input data to calculate costs

Medications	Dose (IU)	Formulation (IU)	Ex-factory price	Source
r-FSH + r-LH	2453.46	150	€ 72.55	[27]
HP-hMG	2801.49	75	€ 16.10	[27]
Pre-treatment tests	Frequency		Unit cost	Source
Hysterosalpingography	1		€ 116.10	[14], expert opinion
Transvaginal ultrasound	1		€ 45.90	[14], expert opinion
Gynaecological consultation	1		€ 21.30	[14], expert opinion
Serum oestradiol (E2)	1		€ 14.30	[14], expert opinion
Follicle-stimulating Hormone (FSH)	1		€ 11.90	[14], expert opinion
Fertility test of the seminal fluid	1		€ 7.90	[14], expert opinion
Luteinising Hormone (LH)	1		€ 12.90	[14], expert opinion
Prolactin (PLR)	1		€ 12.70	[14], expert opinion
Thyroid-stimulating Hormone (TSH)	1		€ 12.40	[14], expert opinion
Free thyroxine (FT4)	1		€ 12.60	[14], expert opinion
Free triiodothyronine (FT3)	1		€ 12.70	[14], expert opinion
Blood samples drawing	1		€ 2.70	[14], expert opinion
Tests during each IVF cycle	Frequency		Unit cost	Source
Transvaginal ultrasound	3		€ 45.90	[14], expert opinion
Gynaecological consultation	3		€ 21.30	[14], expert opinion
Serum oestradiol (E2)	3		€ 14.30	[14], expert opinion
Blood samples	3		€ 2.70	[14], expert opinion

IU International Unit

thought of as the preference for a particular health state: the greater the preference, the greater the utility associated with it [22]. Health state utilities are used to quantify health-related quality of life and are ranked on a scale 0–1, with 0 being equivalent to death and 1 being a state of perfect health. Health state utilities measured over time can be used to generate QALYs by multiplying the duration in a particular health state by the utility associated with that state.

Most health conditions lie somewhere in between, although it is possible for the lower bound to have a negative value [25]. The effectiveness of r-FSH + r-LH vs HP-hMG was expressed has incremental QALY gained. Results were expressed as an incremental cost-effectiveness ratio (ICER). Mathematically, it can be described as ICER = (C1 – C2)/(E1 – E2), where C1 and E1 are the cost and effect in the intervention or treatment group and where C2 and E2 are the cost and effect in the control care group [21].

Sensitivity analysis

In order to consider the variability of the results based on the model parameters, two sensitivity analyses were conducted.

The first one (*deterministic analysis*) used a one-way deterministic approach in which the model results were obtained changing one parameter of the model at a time, based on the variability found in the literature or assumed by the authors. In this specific case, the following scenarios were considered:

(a) probability to undergo an IVF cycle without embryo freezing (base case = 0.4): Min = 0, Max = 1;
(b) probability to dropout from the therapeutic program (base case = 0.3): Min = 0, Max = 1;
(c) change of transition probabilities based on the assumed variability of ±5% compared to the base case (Table 2);
(d) change of utilities associated with different health conditions of a given patient based on an assumed variability of ±5% compared to the base case (Table 1);
(e) change of pregnancy and miscarriage costs (pregnancy base case = € 1600.00, miscarriage base case = € 1525.50): Min pregnancy (DRG 373) = € 1272.00, Max pregnancy (DRG 371) = € 2092.00; Min miscarriage (DRG 376) = € 1264.00, Max miscarriage (DRG 377) = € 1787.00;
(f) probability to undergo an IVF cycle with embryo freezing (base case = 0.3): Min = 0, Max = 1.
(g) follow-up (base case = 2 years): 1, 2 and 3 IVF cycles.

The second analysis (*probabilistic analysis*) was conducted using a probabilistic sensitivity approach [Probabilistic Sensitivity Analysis (PSA)], modeling all the parameters through Montecarlo simulations, each of them according to a specific probabilistic distribution. The probabilistic distribution was chosen applying what is generally reported for the development of the probabilistic models in the economic evaluations, distinguishing between costs (gamma distribution) and epidemiological parameters (beta distribution) [19].

The results of the deterministic analysis were presented through a tornado chart, while the results of the probabilistic analysis were presented through the Cost-Effectiveness Acceptability Curve (CEAC).

Results

Epidemiological results

Based on the model simulations, the patients undergoing a therapeutic protocol with r-FSH + r-LH had a lower time to pregnancy (TTP) than the women receiving HP-hMG (7.2 vs. 7.5 months for positive hCG test and 13.2 vs. 13.5 months for clinical pregnancy, respectively) (Table 4). Furthermore, the general success rate over the time horizon established in the analysis (2 years) was higher for patients treated with r-FSH + r-LH, compared to HP-hMG, both in terms of positive hCG test (28.2% vs. 20.6%, respectively) and of clinical pregnancy (23.6% vs. 17.0%, respectively) (Table 4).

These data were also confirmed after the stratification of the results according to the number of retrieved

oocytes when patients with at least 5 oocytes were considered (Fig. 2).

Cost-effectiveness results

Table 5 reports the results in terms of quality of life (QALYs) and costs for each ongoing pregnancy (clinical pregnancy without miscarriage) in the NHS perspective.

In particular, the cost of the drug and miscarriage/pregnancy resulted to be higher in the r-FSH + r-LH scenario (+€ 801,570 and + € 239,601 respectively), whereas the monitoring cost was lower (–€ 67,552). This was due to two main factors: (a) the number of pregnancies using the r-FSH + r-LH approach was higher than with HP-hMG, with a higher absolute cost, but a lower cost per pregnancy (€ 7375 vs € 7400 respectively) and (b) the higher number of pregnancies and hCG positive tests involved a higher cost for the NHS with an improvement of the quality of life of over 4 QALYs gained for 100 women (Table 6).

With reference to the cost-effectiveness, Table 6 reports the average cost-utility values per patient obtained for the whole time horizon considered in the analysis, stratified according to the number of retrieved oocytes. The results indicate that, at the end of the analyzed period, the ICER per QALY values were below a willingness to pay of € 20,000 – 40,000.

Sensitivity analysis results

Figure 3 reports the results of the one-way deterministic sensitivity analysis, for patients with ≥5 retrieved oocytes. The parameters mostly influencing results are represented by the variation of the transition probabilities concerning the possibility for the patient to undergo an IVF cycle without embryo freezing and to quit the therapeutic program. In all the considered scenarios, the ICER values never exceeded € 20,000 per QALY gained, showing a good robustness of the results.

The probabilistic sensitivity analysis conducted according to the number of retrieved oocytes, corresponding to the population of patients with 10–15 retrieved oocytes, confirmed that at the end of the observation period the r-FSH + r-LH therapeutic protocol was cost-effective compared with HP-hMG. Considering a willingness to pay of about € 15,000, the probability that the r-FSH + r-LH therapeutic protocol could result to be advantageous with respect to HP-hMG resulted to be higher than 80% (Fig. 4).

The results of the probabilistic analysis reported in Fig. 5 confirm the above calculation, showing higher uncertainty in the short term (blue line). As the time horizon - and consequently the number of IVF cycles - extends, the cost-effectiveness probability increases. At the end of the observation period, with a willingness to pay of about

Table 4 Epidemiological parameters from 1000 patients' simulation – patients having at least 5 retrieved oocytes

	HP-hMG	r-FSH + r-LH
Cycle 1 clinical pregnancies	191	284
Cycle 2 clinical pregnancies	97	128
Cycle 3 clinical pregnancies	51	60
Clinical pregnancies	339	473
Average time at clinical pregnancy (months)	*13.5*	*13.2*
Clinical pregnancy rate	*17.0%*	*23.6%*
	HP-hMG	r-FSH + r-LH
Cycle 1 positive hCGtest	232	339
Cycle 2 positive hCG test	118	153
Cycle 3 positive hCG test	62	72
Positive hCG tests	413	563
Average time at positive hCG test (months)	*7.5*	*7.2*
Positive hCG test rate	*20.6%*	*28.2%*
	HP-hMG	r-FSH + r-LH
Miscarriages	37	45

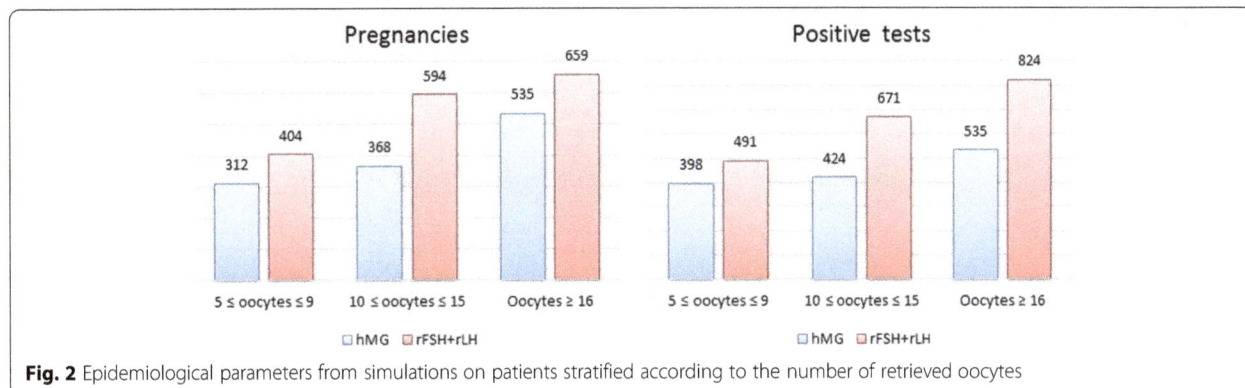

Fig. 2 Epidemiological parameters from simulations on patients stratified according to the number of retrieved oocytes

€ 35,000, the r-FSH + r-LH therapeutic protocol appeared to be the most cost-effective with a probability higher than 70%.

Discussion

The association of recombinant FSH plus recombinant LH in 2:1 ratio (Pergoveris, Merck, Germany) may be used not only to induce ovulation in anovulatory women with hypogonadotropic hypogonadism [14], but also to achieve multiple follicular developments in human IVF. To date, there are still scarce or poorly informative data that compared the COS using r-FSH + r-LH with that obtained using other medications (e.g.HP-hMG) in the IVF setting. Indeed in several studies [8–13] the urinary-derived HP-hMG was compared to r-FSH alone, without taking into account that HP-hMG contains not only FSH, but also LH and hCG that act on the same receptor of LH and have a powerful LH activity.

A randomized controlled trial (RCT) comparing HP-hMG and r-FSH + r-LH in patients undergoing IVF included only 122 women and showed comparable outcomes in terms of pregnancy rate [16]. Unfortunately, this study was clearly underpowered as it was designed to assess the difference in oocyte rather than in the pregnancy rates. Another RCT study on 579 patients, included patients submitted to intrauterine insemination (IUI) rather than to IVF [15]. This showed comparable outcomes, but without enough observations to show a significant difference of effectiveness between medication. In fact, IUI allows to get a much lower pregnancy rate than the expected when using IVF in patients of the same age (17.3% in the cited study [15] vs. approximately 30–40%).

To the best of our knowledge, the wider study comparing HP-hMG and r-FSH + r-LH in IVF patients is a retrospective analysis of real-life data that included 848 women classified as expected "poor" or "normal" responders to gonadotropins [17]. Data were collected under real-life practice circumstances in IVF Unit in S. Anna Hospital (Torino, Italy), and the pregnancy rate with fresh embryo transfer was calculated by stratifying patients according to the number of retrieved oocytes, in order to exclude that a difference in the results could be due to oocyte availability [17]. The study showed an improvement in pregnancy rate according to the increasing number of retrieved oocytes. However, when comparing patients within the same oocyte, the two medications obtained comparable results when up to 4 oocytes, and a slight/ not significant advantage with 5–8 oocytes. However, the PR/ET became significantly higher when 9 or more oocytes were available [17]. The multivariable logistic regression analysis confirmed that both the use of r-FSH + r-LH and the total number of retrieved oocytes increased the probability of pregnancy, with an odds ratio (OR) of 1.628 and 1.083, respectively, showing that the medication used for COS was even more influent than the number of oocytes itself.

Despite the contribution yielded by the previous literature in the field, the cost of COS, is still a major issue in times of global economic restrictions. This is relevant both in health systems where the patients cover the costs with their own resources and in countries where the National Health Service (NHS) takes care, partially or completely, of the expenses. Due to the evidenced gap of knowledge and the relevance of the proposed subject, the present study represents the

Table 5 Average cost and effectiveness results per 1000 patients – 2 years base case follow-up (patients with ≥5 retrieved oocytes)

	Medication cost	Monitoring cost	Miscarriage/pregnancy cost	Overall cost	Pregnancies	Cost per pregnancy
HP-hMG	€ 889,012	€ 967,508	€ 654,635	€ 2,511,155	339	€ 7400
r-FSH + r-LH	€ 1,690,582	€ 899,956	€ 894,236	€ 3,484,774	473	€ 7375
Difference	+€ 801,570	-€ 67,552	+€ 239,601	+€ 973,618	*+ 133*	-€ 25

Table 6 Cost-effectiveness table per number of retrieved oocytes (average results per treated patient)

	Cost	QALYs	Incremental Cost	Incremental QALYs	ICER per QALYs
≥ 5 oocytes					
HP-hMG	€ 1256	0.71			
r-FSH + r-LH	€ 1742	0.76	€ 487	0.04	€ 11,365
5 ≤ oocytes ≤ 9					
HP-hMG	€ 1254	0.70			
r-FSH + r-LH	€ 1726	0.73	€ 472	0.03	€ 16,309
10 ≤ oocytes ≤ 15					
HP-hMG	€ 1254	0.72			
r-FSH + r-LH	€ 1751	0.80	€ 497	0.08	€ 6569
≥ 16 oocytes					
HP-hMG	€ 1272	0.78			
r-FSH + r-LH	€ 1824	0.82	€ 551	0.04	€ 12,274

first attempt to evaluate the cost-effectiveness of COS when recombinant gonadotropins in 2:1 combination (Pergoveris) or HP-hMG are used in a large series of patients undergoing IVF. Precisely we aimed to measure, through a sophisticated economic analysis the overall cost-effectiveness of IVF cycles based on the previously published database [17].

As a result, the present analysis demonstrates that r-FSH + r-LH therapy showed higher cost-effectiveness than HP-hMG in the considered two-years observation periods with a slightly lower overall cost per pregnancy despite a higher cost per medication. The cost-effectiveness acceptability curve (CEAC) showed that the observed difference between the two medications was likely to further increase if the time horizon was prolonged and the number of IVF cycles rose. The advantage given by recombinant gonadotropins vs. HP-hMG was not linked to a higher number of retrieved oocytes because calculations were

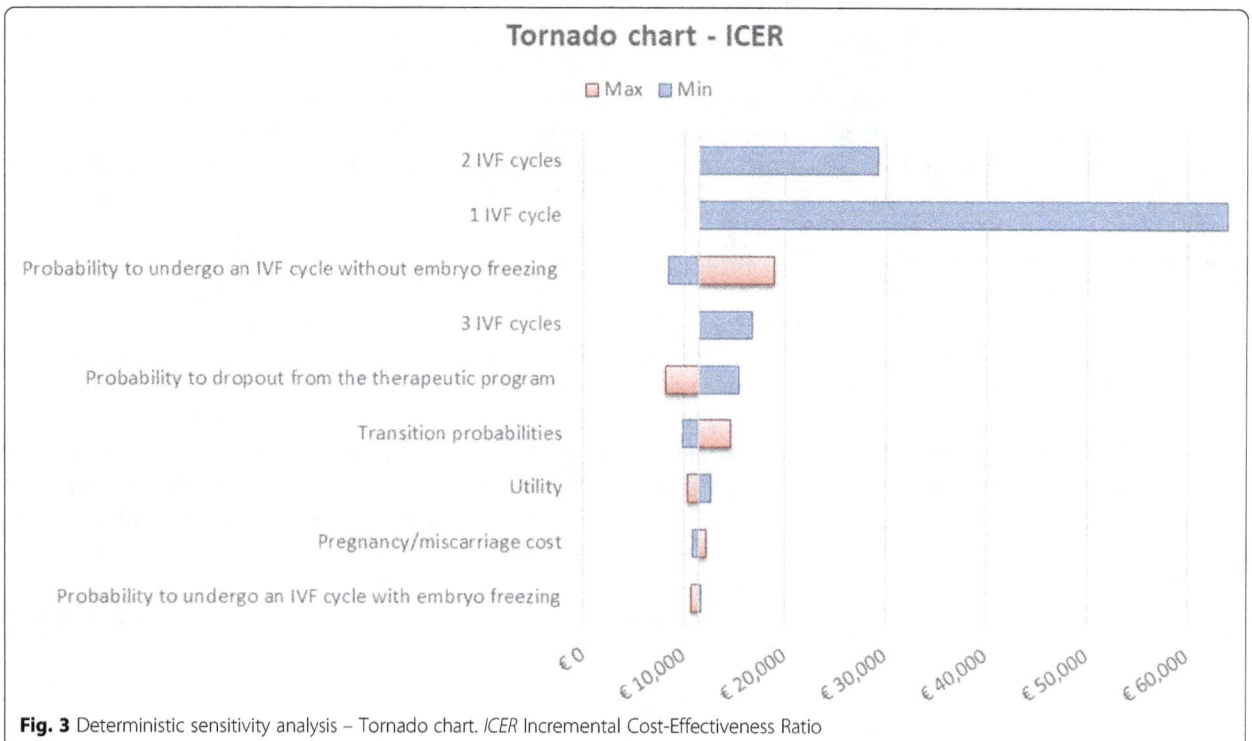

Fig. 3 Deterministic sensitivity analysis – Tornado chart. *ICER* Incremental Cost-Effectiveness Ratio

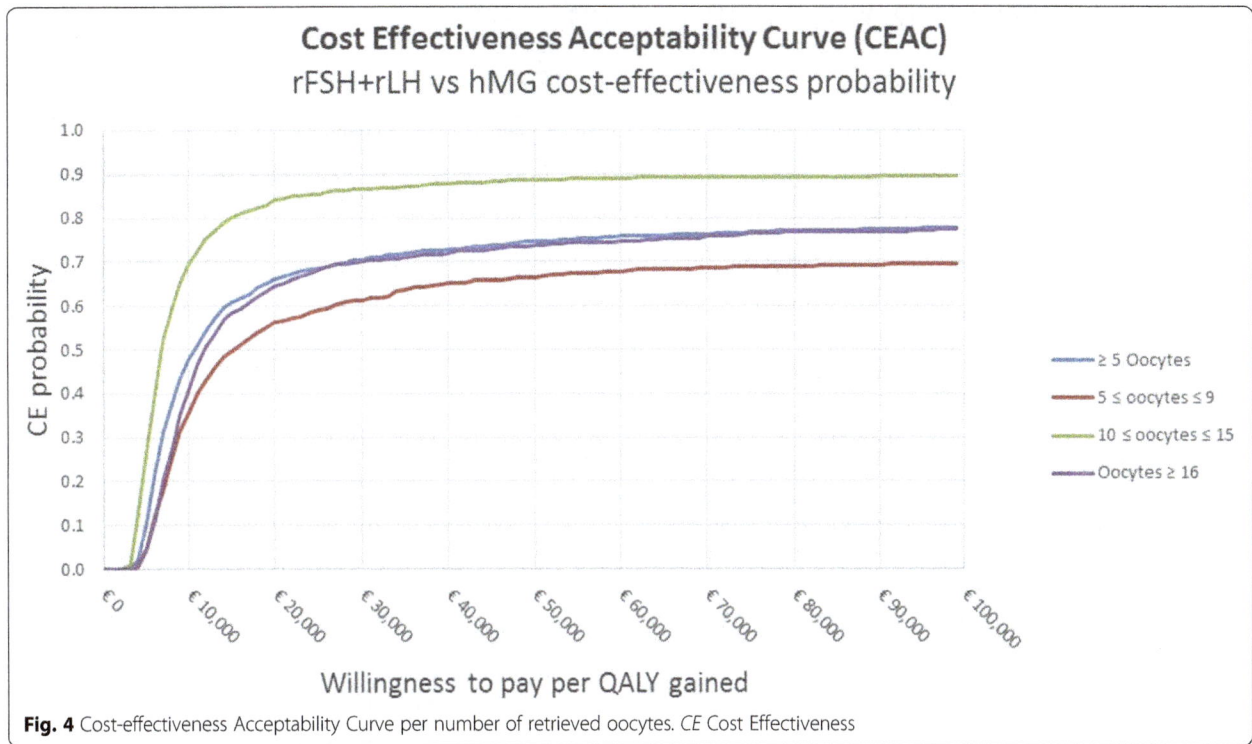

Fig. 4 Cost-effectiveness Acceptability Curve per number of retrieved oocytes. *CE* Cost Effectiveness

performed after patients' stratification in subgroups and having the same number of available oocytes. In detail, for the population of patients obtaining 5 or more oocytes, the r-FSH + r-LH therapy resulted to be highly cost-effective compared with HP-hMG, with an ICER period equal to €11,365 per QALY. Interestingly the patients that obtained the highest advantage from being treated with r-FSH + r-LH instead of HP-hMG were those with 10–15 retrieved oocytes, who had an ICER of € 6569 per QALY. According to the medical

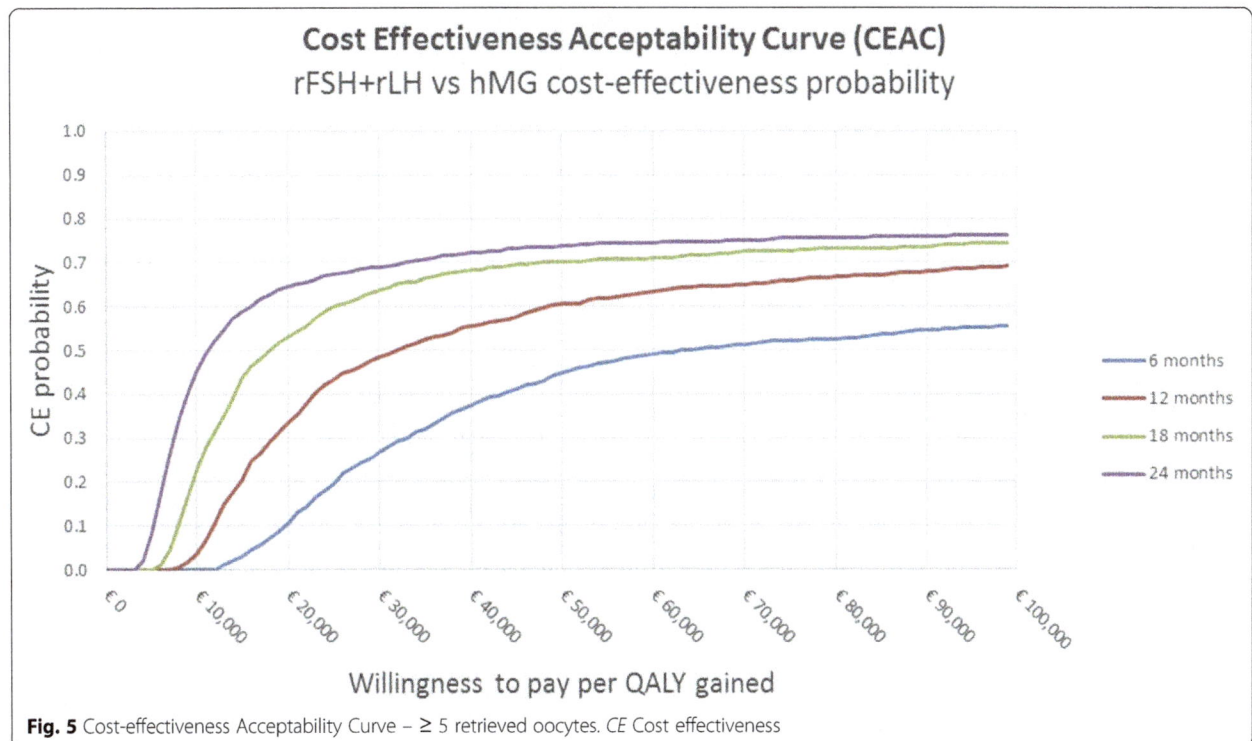

Fig. 5 Cost-effectiveness Acceptability Curve – ≥ 5 retrieved oocytes. *CE* Cost effectiveness

literature, patients getting 10–15 retrieved oocytes are among those with the best prognosis after fresh embryo transfer [26] and may be considered "normal responders" to gonadotropin stimulation, representing approximately 40–50% of the overall population undergoing IVF.

Our analysis, showed two main limitations: (a) the lack of reports on the quality of life of patients undergoing IVF did not allow an exact quantification of the utility measures used in the model, some of which were obtained considering the opinion of IVF experts; (b) the database on which our analysis was based did not report about embryo freezing and dropouts from the program. Even in this case, their incidence was estimated according to the opinion of IVF experts. However, the one-way sensitivity analyses allow to take this uncertainty into account, and therefore these two limits should not have affected the validity of our results. A final limitation, c) regards the generalisability of our results on other countries. This study was specifically settled on the Italian general practice and the model was populated with Italian costs and tariffs different than what happens in other European countries. However, the regulation in Europe demonstrates a difference in term of access to IVF [18]. Contrarily, no link was established between IVF utilization and the manner in which coverage was regulated or the level of public financing was set [18]. As a result of that, we can assume that the general management of these patients could be homogeneous around Europe and the model structure represents a general approach for other countries. Further analysis, could consider the same model structure adapting the specific economic parameters and evaluate the cost-effectiveness results for each country perspective. The National Healthcare Assistance in Italy covers the complete cost for gonadotropin treatment in IVF, provided that the patient is younger than 45 and her basal FSH circulating level is below 30 U/l. Not all countries have such a system, but in general, most healthcare systems help patients to face a percentage (variable in different countries) of the economic cost of IVF medications and procedure. Although the results found herein are not perfectly applicable to other countries due to such differences in the healthcare assistance reimbursement, the relative proportion of the cost of ovarian stimulation with recombinant FSH and LH vs. hMG is rather constant everywhere, and therefore the general concepts expressed in this study may be of interest even outside Italy.

The strength point of this analysis is that is based on real-world data [17]; the transition probabilities used to perform the model have been obtained from an Italian study which collected data from clinical charts of IVF Unit in S. Anna Hospital (Torino, Italy).

Conclusions

In conclusion, the present cost-utility analysis demonstrated that the r-FSH + r-LH combination, although more expensive than HP-hMG when medication costs are considered, may be effectively used to obtain COS in IVF patients without increasing the overall costs for the patients or the NHS. On the contrary, the r-FSH + r-LH association allows getting slightly reduced costs for pregnancy, improved cost-effectiveness and quality of life, especially when the so-called "normal-responders", who represent the majority of IVF patients, are considered.

Funding

The authors declare that they have no received funding for this study. This research did not receive any specific grant from funding agencies in the public, commercial, or not-for-profit sectors.

Authors' contributions

FSM provided the conception and design of the study. AM design the study, performed the statistical analysis and wrote the manuscript. RV and CB performed the statistical analysis and wrote the manuscript. AR provided the interpretation of data and critically reviewed the manuscript. AC and CB critically reviewed the manuscript and helped draft the final version. All authors approved the final manuscript.

Competing interests

The authors declare that they have no competing interests.

Author details

[1]Economic Evaluation and HTA (CEIS- EEHTA) - Faculty of Economics, University of Rome "Tor Vergata", Via Columbia, 2, 00133 Rome, Italy. [2]Institute for Leadership and Management in Health - Kingston Hill Campus, Kingston Hill, Kingston upon Thames KT2 7LB, UK. [3]Gynecology and Obstetrics I, Physiopathology of Reproduction and IVF Unit, Department of Surgical Sciences, University of Torino, S. Anna Hospital, Via Ventimiglia 3, 10126 Torino, Italy. [4]LIVET Infertility and IVF Clinic, Via Tiziano Vecellio, 3, 10126 Torino, Italy.

References

1. Lunenfeld B. Historical perspectives in gonadotrophin therapy. Hum Reprod Update. 2004;10(6):453–67.
2. Loumaye E, Campbell R, Salat-Baroux J. Human follicle-stimulating hormone produced by recombinant DNA technology: a review for clinicians. Hum Reprod Update. 1995;1(2):188–99.
3. Hull M, et al. Recombinant human luteinising hormone: an effective new gonadotropin preparation. Lancet. 1994;344:334–5.
4. Baker VL, et al. Clinical efficacy of highly purified urinary FSH versus recombinant FSH in volunteers undergoing controlled ovarian stimulation for in vitro fertilization: a randomized, multicenter, investigator-blind trial. Fertil Steril. 2009;91(4):1005–11.
5. Shiraishi K, Matsuyama H. Gonadotoropin actions on spermatogenesis and hormonal therapies for spermatogenic disorders [review]. Endocr J. 2017;64(2):123–31.
6. Liu X, Hao C, Wang J. Efficacy of highly purified urinary FSH versus recombinant FSH in Chinese women over 37 years undergoing assisted reproductive techniques. International Journal of Fertility & Sterility. 2015;8(4):385–92.

7. Daya S. Updated meta-analysis of recombinant follicle-stimulating hormone (FSH) versus urinary FSH for ovarian stimulation in assisted reproduction. Fertil Steril. 2002;77(4):711–4.

8. Andersen AN, Devroey P, Arce JC. Clinical outcome following stimulation with highly purified hMG or recombinant FSH in patients undergoing IVF: a randomized assessor-blind controlled trial. Hum Reprod. 2006;21(12):3217–27.

9. Hompes PG, et al. Effectiveness of highly purified human menopausal gonadotropin vs. recombinant follicle-stimulating hormone in first-cycle in vitro fertilization-intracytoplasmic sperm injection patients. Fertil Steril. 2008;89(6):1685–93.

10. Bosch E, et al. Highly purified hMG versus recombinant FSH in ovarian hyperstimulation with GnRH antagonists--a randomized study. Hum Reprod. 2008;23(10):2346–51.

11. Frydman R, Howles CM, Truong F. A double-blind, randomized study to compare recombinant human follicle stimulating hormone (FSH; Gonal-F) with highly purified urinary FSH (Metrodin) HP in women undergoing assisted reproductive techniques including intracytoplasmic sperm injection. The French Multicentre Trialists Human Reproduction. 2000;15(3):520–5.

12. Devroey P, et al. A randomized assessor-blind trial comparing highly purified hMG and recombinant FSH in a GnRH antagonist cycle with compulsory single-blastocyst transfer. Fertil Steril. 2012;97(3):561–71.

13. van Wely M, et al. Effectiveness of human menopausal gonadotropin versus recombinant follicle-stimulating hormone for controlled ovarian hyperstimulation in assisted reproductive cycles: a meta-analysis. Fertil Steril. 2003;80(5):1086–93.

14. Papaleo E, et al. Cost-effectiveness analysis on the use of rFSH + rLH for the treatment of anovulation in hypogonadotropic hypogonadal women. Ther Clin Risk Manag. 2014;10:479–84.

15. Moro F, et al. Highly purified hMG versus recombinant FSH plus recombinant LH in intrauterine insemination cycles in women >/=35 years: a RCT. Hum Reprod. 2015;30(1):179–85.

16. Pacchiarotti A, et al. Urinary hMG (Meropur) versus recombinant FSH plus recombinant LH (Pergoveris) in IVF: a multicenter, prospective, randomized controlled trial. Fertil Steril. 2010;94(6):2467–9.

17. Revelli R, et al. Controlled ovarian stimulation with recombinant-FSH plus recombinant-LH vs. human menopausal gonadotropin based on the number of retrieved oocytes: results from a routine clinical practice in a real-life population. Reprod Biol Endocrinol. 2015;13:77.

18. Berg Brigham K, Cadier B, Chevreul K. The diversity of regulation and public financing of IVF in Europe and its impact on utilization. Hum Reprod. 2013;28(3):666–75.

19. Briggs A, Claxton K, Sculpher M. Decision Modelling for Health Economic Evaluation. N Y: O.U.P. Inc; 2007.

20. Decreto del Ministero della Salute 18 ottobre 2012, Tariffe delle prestazioni di assistenza ospedaliera per acuti. Gazzetta Ufficiale n. 23 del 28 gennaio 2013.

21. Patel RR, Albert TJ, Rihn JA. Cost-effectiveness, QALYs, and incremental cost-effectiveness ratios. Seminars in Spine Surgery. 2014;26:2–7.

22. Prieto L, Sacristan JA. Problems and solutions in calculating quality-adjusted life years (QALYs). Health Qual Life Outcomes. 2003;1:80.

23. Patrick DL, Erickson P. Health Status and Health Policy: Quality of Life in Health Care Evaluation and Resource Allocation. N Y: O.U. Press; 1993.

24. Drummond, M.F., et al., Methods for the Economic Evaluation of Health Care Programmes. 2nd ed. ed, ed. O.M. Publications. 1997, Oxford.

25. Wouters OJ, Naci H, Samani NJ. QALYs in cost-effectiveness analysis: an overview for cardiologists. Heart. 2015;101(23):1868–73.

26. Sunkara SK, et al. Association between the number of eggs and live birth in IVF treatment: an analysis of 400 135 treatment cycles. Hum Reprod. 2011;26(7):1768–74.

27. Agenzia Italiana del Farmaco. Liste di trasparenza e rimborsabilità. Available from: http://www.agenziafarmaco.gov.it/content/liste-di-trasparenza-e-rimborsabilit%C3%A0.

## 16

Exogenous leptin affects sperm parameters and impairs blood testis barrier integrity in adult male mice

Xiaotong Wang[1], Xiaoke Zhang[1,2], Lian Hu[1*] and Honggang Li[1*]

Abstract

Background: Serum leptin levels are augmented in obese infertile men and in men with azoospermia. They also correlate inversely with sperm concentration, motility and normal forms. The mechanisms underlying the adverse effects of excess leptin on male reproductive function remain unclear. The present study aimed to evaluate the effects of exogenous leptin on sperm parameters in mice and to explore the underlying mechanisms.

Methods: We treated normal adult male mice with saline, 0.1, 0.5 or 3 mg/kg leptin daily for 2 weeks. After treatment, serum leptin levels, serum testosterone levels, sperm parameters and testicular cell apoptosis were evaluated. Blood testis barrier integrity and the expression of tight junction-associated proteins in testes were also assessed. We further verified the direct effects of leptin on tight junction-associated proteins in Sertoli cells and the possible leptin signaling pathways involved in this process.

Results: After treatment, there were no significant differences in body weights, reproductive organ weights, serum leptin levels and serum testosterone levels between leptin-treated mice and control mice. Administration of 3 mg/kg leptin reduced sperm concentration, motility and progressive motility while increasing the percentage of abnormal sperm and testicular cell apoptosis. Mice treated with 3 mg/kg leptin also had impaired blood testis barrier integrity, which was related to decreased tight junction-associated proteins in testes. Leptin directly reduced tight junction-associated proteins in Sertoli cells, JAK2/STAT, PI3K and ERK pathways were suggested to be involved in this process.

Conclusions: Exogenous leptin negatively affects sperm parameters and impairs blood testis barrier integrity in mice. Leptin reduced tight junction-associated proteins in Sertoli cells, indicating that leptin has a direct role in impairing blood testis barrier integrity. Given the function of blood testis barrier in maintaining normal spermatogenesis, leptin-induced blood testis barrier impairment may be one of the mechanisms contributing to male subfertility and infertility.

Keywords: Obesity, Leptin, Male infertility, Mice, Sertoli cell, Blood testis barrier

Background

Leptin is a 16 kDa peptide product of the *ob* gene and is secreted by the adipose tissue [1]. It binds to leptin receptors (OB-R) to mediate several signaling pathways, including Janus kinase 2/signal transducers and activators of transcription (JAK2/STAT), extracellular signal-regulated kinase (ERK) and phosphoinositide 3-kinase (PI3K) [2]. Leptin has a role in energy homeostasis, glucose and lipid metabolism, and immune and neuroendocrine function that has been shown in both humans and rodents [3]. Leptin is able to restore fertility in *ob/ob* mice which are leptin deficient, obese and infertile, indicating that leptin serves as a permissive signal to the reproductive system [4, 5]. Certainly, there is increasing evidence that leptin participates in many events in reproduction [1].

Serum leptin levels are higher in most obese people and in rodents that have ingested the high-fat diet for a long-term [6, 7]. Obese men also have higher seminal leptin levels which are associated with increased serum leptin levels [8]. Body mass index (BMI) has positive correlations with serum leptin levels; both BMI and

* Correspondence: hulian02@163.com; lhgyx@hotmail.com
[1]Family Planning Research Institute/Center of Reproductive Medicine, Tongji Medical College, Huazhong University of Science and Technology, Wuhan 430030, China
Full list of author information is available at the end of the article

serum leptin levels correlate positively with abnormal sperm morphology, and correlate negatively with sperm concentration and motility [9, 10]. This supports the concept that serum leptin mediates a link between obesity and male infertility [10]. Moreover, serum leptin levels are also increased in azoospermic men compared with normozoospermic fertile men [11]. This elevation is not gonadotropin dependent, indicating that leptin has a direct effect on testis function, especially on spermatogenesis [11]. Animal studies have provided evidence that leptin negatively affects male reproduction. Hyperleptinemia has been found to inhibit testicular steroidogenesis and halt testicular maturation in rodents [12, 13].

Administration of exogenous leptin decreased sperm count and increased the percentage of abnormal sperm in nonobese rodents, suggesting that leptin plays a role in the negative correlations between BMI and sperm quantity and quality [14]. In nonobese rodents, some studies have also shown that exogenous leptin can increase the percentage of abnormal sperm and the DNA fragmentation level while decreasing sperm count and motility, histone to protamine transition during spermatogenesis, and the ability to generate offspring [15–19]. Leptin may exhibit a direct effect on testicular tissues or spermatozoa leading to abnormal sperm parameters [14]. It may also induce reactive oxygen species (ROS) production and hormone profile modulation to affect male fertility [15]. However, additional research is needed to further clarify the mechanisms of leptin's negative effects on male reproductive function.

Leptin secreted by visceral adipose tissue has been reported to increase the permeability of the intestinal epithelial barrier by reducing the expression of tight junction (TJ)-associated proteins such as zona occludens-1 (ZO-1), zona occludens-3 (ZO-3), claudin 5 and occludin [20–22]. In addition to be the primary structure of the intestinal epithelial barrier, TJ is also a vital structure of the blood testis barrier (BTB). The BTB is comprised of coexisting TJ, basal ectoplasmic specialization, gap junction and desmosome [23]. TJ in the BTB has two main functions, restricting the passage of molecules and dividing the seminiferous epithelium into basal and apical compartments [24]. In mice, the contribution of occludin and claudins to BTB integrity are determined by deletion of occludin gene or genes for transcription factors that are upstream regulators of claudins [25]. The BTB creates a specialized microenvironment that is necessary for germ cells development and movement [24]. Damage to the BTB can cause germ cell loss, reduced sperm count, male infertility or subfertility [23, 26–28]. As leptin impairs TJ integrity in the intestinal epithelium, and because the impact of leptin on BTB integrity has not been addressed in previous

studies, we supposed that leptin might affect male reproduction by impairing BTB integrity.

In this study, we administered different doses of leptin or same volume of saline as a control to adult male mice for 2 weeks. We examined the effects of exogenous leptin on serum leptin levels, serum testosterone levels, sperm parameters and testicular cell apoptosis, as well as BTB integrity and TJ-associated proteins. To evaluate whether leptin had a direct effect on TJ-associated proteins, we treated TM4 cells (a mouse Sertoli cell line) with leptin and further investigated the possible leptin-mediated signaling pathways involved in this process.

Methods

Animals and treatments

Seven-week-old male C57BL/6 mice were purchased from Hubei Research Center of Laboratory Animals. Mice were kept under a 12 h light and 12 h darkness cycle at 24 °C and allowed to adapt for 1 week before the experiments. At the age of 8 weeks, mice received daily intraperitoneal injections with 0.1, 0.5 or 3 mg/kg leptin (recombinant mouse leptin, Prospec, Israel) dissolved in saline or same volume of saline as a control for 2 weeks. The weights of mice and food in each cage were measured every 2 days.

Mice were sacrificed by exsanguination under anesthesia the day after treatment ended. Reproductive organs including testes and epididymides were weighed immediately and used for further experiments. Blood samples were collected and stored at room temperature for 1 h to clot, before centrifuging at 3000 rpm for 15 min to obtain serum for ELISA.

All animal experiments were approved by the Tongji Medical College Committee on the Use and Care of Animals and were conducted according to the Committee's guidelines.

Cell culture and treatment

TM4 cells were obtained from ATCC and stored in Family Planning Research Institute of Tongji Medical College. TM4 cells were cultured in DMEM/F12 supplemented with 2.5% fetal bovine serum and 5% equine serum at 37 °C and 5% CO_2.

To detect the direct effects of leptin on TJ-associated proteins in TM4 cells, cells were seeded at a density of 1×10^5/ml in 6-well dishes, cultured with low-serum medium containing 0, 10 or 100 nM leptin for 48 h and then harvested for further experiments. Inhibitors of leptin signaling mediators were employed to determine the possible leptin-mediated signaling pathways in vitro. Cells were pretreated with low-serum medium containing 10 μM AG490, LY294002 or U0126 (the inhibitors of JAK2, PI3K and ERK, respectively) (MCE, USA) dissolved in dimethyl sulfoxide (DMSO) for 4 h (the final concentration of DMSO was 0.1%). The inhibitors were removed, and cells were washed with pre-warmed phosphate buffered saline (PBS). Low-serum medium containing 100 nM leptin was then added to cells. After cultivation for 48 h, cells were harvested for further experiments. The concentration of AG490, LY294002 and U0126 was chosen according to earlier studies [29–31].

Measurement of serum leptin and testosterone levels

Mouse serum leptin and testosterone levels were measured using commercial ELISA kits from Boster Biological Technology (Wuhan, China) and Cusabio (Wuhan, China), respectively. The measurements were processed according to the manufacturer's protocols.

Assessment of sperm parameters

Cauda epididymides from each mouse were dissected in 1 ml pre-warmed Ham' s F10 buffer (Sigma-Aldrich, USA) and incubated at 37 °C for 15 min to allow spermatozoa to swim out. Sperm concentration, motility and progressive motility were determined according to the 5th WHO laboratory manual guidelines [32]. For the detection of sperm with abnormal morphology, sperm suspensions were smeared on glass slides, allowed to dry, and then fixed and stained using a Diff-Quick kit (Phygene, Fuzhou, China) according to the manufacturer's protocol. The slides were viewed under a light microscope. At least 200 spermatozoa from each sample were assessed. Abnormalities in sperm morphology including head, tail and head-neck connection abnormalities were determined according to Ward et al. [33].

Apoptosis of testicular cells

TUNEL assay was conducted to detect testicular cell apoptosis. Sections (5 μm) from frozen testes were deproteinized using proteinase K for 25 min at 37 °C. After blocking with 0.1% Triton X-100 for 20 min at room temperature, sections were incubated with TUNEL working solutions (Roche, Germany) in the dark at 37 °C for 1 h and then stained with DAPI and mounted in glycerin. Sections were observed using a fluorescent microscope, and TUNEL positive nuclei which indicated apoptosis were counted in at least 40 seminiferous tubules from three non-consecutive testis sections from each mouse.

Biotin tracer experiment

The biotin tracer experiment was used to determine BTB integrity according to the method of Meng et al. [34], with a minor modification. EZ-Link Sulfo-NHS-LC-Biotin (Thermo Scientific, USA) was freshly diluted in PBS containing 1 mM $CaCl_2$ at a final concentration of 10 mg/ml. Mice were anesthetized, and their testes were exposed. A 30G needle was used to gently inject 30 μl of biotin solution into the testes. After 30 min, mice were euthanized, and their testes were immediately removed and frozen. Sections (5 μm) from frozen testes were blocked with 5% albumin from bovine serum in PBS containing 0.1% Triton X-100 for 1 h, and then incubated with streptavidin conjugate-Alexa Fluor 568 (1: 3000, Invitrogen, USA) for 30 min at room temperature. Finally, sections were stained with DAPI, mounted in glycerin and observed using a fluorescent microscope. At least 30 seminiferous tubules from three non-consecutive testis sections from each mouse were examined.

Western blot

Western blot was used to detect the expression of TJ-associated proteins both in testes and in TM4 cells, and was performed according to the standard procedure. Antibodies against claudin 5 (Invitrogen, USA), occludin (Proteintech, USA), ZO-1 (Proteintech, USA) and β-Actin (Proteintech, USA) were used with the details given in Additional file 1: Table S1. Immunopositive bands were detected using the enhanced chemiluminescence (ECL) (Beyotime, Beijing, China). β-Actin served as the loading control. The densitometric analysis was performed using ImageJ software.

Immunofluorescence

Immunofluorescence was used to detect the expression and localization of TJ-associated proteins in sections (5 μm) from frozen testes, and was conducted according to the standard procedure. Antibodies against claudin 5 (Invitrogen, USA), occludin (Proteintech, USA) and ZO-1 (Proteintech, USA) were used with the details given in Additional file 1: Table S1. After incubated with Alexa Fluor 488-conjugated secondary antibodies (1:200, Proteintech, USA), sections were stained with DAPI, mounted in glycerin and observed by a fluorescent microscope.

RNA isolation and PCR

Total RNA in TM4 cells and testes was extracted using TRIzol reagent (Invitrogen, USA), and was then reversed-transcribed into cDNA using a PrimeScript RT reagent kit (TAKARA, Japan). To detect leptin receptor mRNA in TM4 cells, synthesized cell cDNA was subjected to PCR using Premix Taq (TAKARA, Japan). PCR products were run in 1.5% agarose gel electrophoresis (120 V, 30 min) and visualized using an imaging system (Bio-Rad, USA). To determine the expression of steroidogenic genes (*Sf-1*, *Star* and *Cyp11a1*) and androgen receptor in testes, synthesized testicular cDNA was subjected to real time quantitative PCR using SYBR ® Premix Ex Taq II (TAKARA, Japan). The primer sequences were listed in Additional file 2: Table S2. Primers for leptin receptor and *Sf-1* have been reported by El-Hefnawy et al. [35] and Woods et al. [36], respectively.

Statistical analysis

All data were analyzed using SPSS (ver.21) software. Differences between groups were determined using Kruskal-Wallis test, one-way ANOVA followed by Dunnett test, chi-square test or Student's t test. Data were expressed as mean ± SD, and differences were considered significant when $p < 0.05$. Graphs were made using Graphpad Prism 7.

Results

Leptin administration did not significantly alter serum leptin and testosterone levels in mice

After 2 weeks of leptin administration, serum leptin and testosterone levels in the leptin-treated groups showed no significant differences compared with the control group (Fig. 1a and b). However, the expression of testicular steroidogenic genes such as steroidogenic factor 1 (*Sf-1*), steroidogenic acute regulatory protein (*Star*) and cytochrome P450 family 11 subfamily A member 1

(*Cyp11a1*) were significantly downregulated in mice treated with a relatively high dose of leptin (3 mg/kg) compared with control mice ($p < 0.05$) (Additional file 3: Figure S1 E).

Throughout the experiment, there were no significant differences in body weights, food intake or reproductive organ weights between the leptin-treated groups and the control group (Additional file 3: Figure S1 A–D).

Leptin administration altered sperm parameters and increased testicular cell apoptosis

Sperm concentration in the 3 mg/kg leptin-treated group decreased by 50.90% compared with the control group (3.26 ± 1.27 vs. $6.41 \pm 2.06 \times 10^6$/ml, $p < 0.05$) (Fig. 1c). Sperm motility was $68.38 \pm 1.87\%$ in the control group but was lower at $58.57 \pm 6.24\%$ in the 0.5 mg/kg leptin-treated group and $56.60 \pm 6.32\%$ in the 3 mg/kg leptin-treated group (both $p < 0.05$) (Fig. 1d). Sperm progressive motility in the 0.5 ($24.71 \pm 7.49\%$) and 3 mg/kg ($20.93 \pm 4.43\%$) leptin-treated groups also decreased significantly compared with the control group ($40.84 \pm 4.55\%$) (both $p < 0.05$) (Fig. 1e). The 0.5 and 3 mg/kg

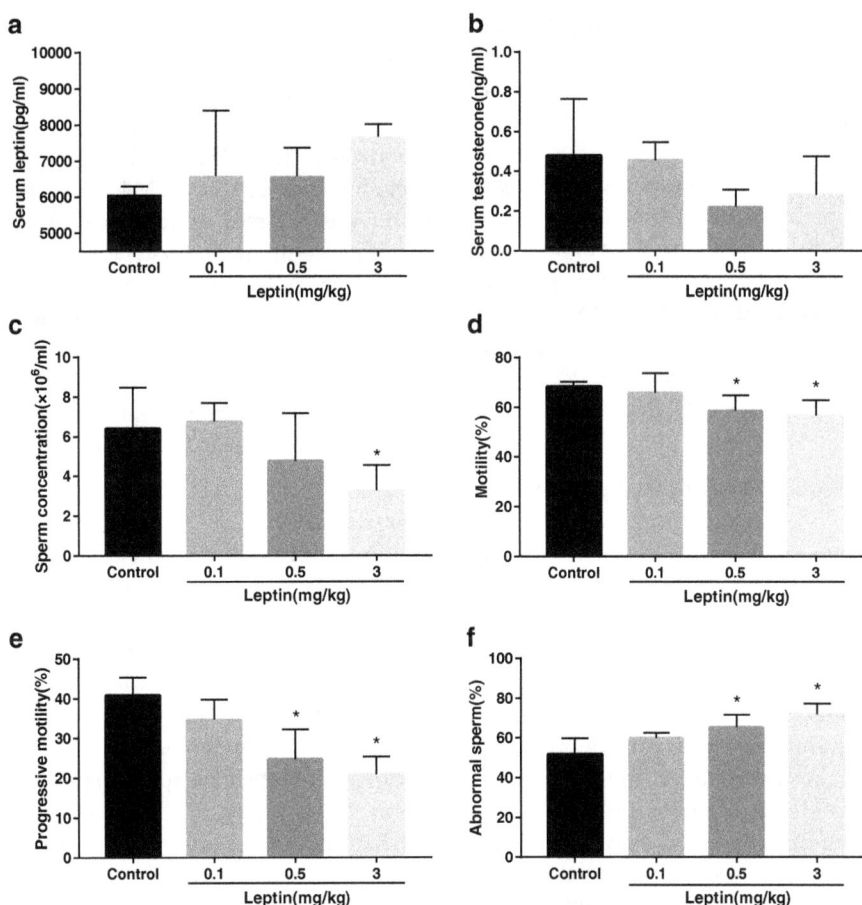

Fig. 1 Serum leptin, serum testosterone and sperm parameters in mice. **a** serum leptin. **b** serum testosterone. Data are expressed as mean ± SD, $n = 5$. **c** sperm concentration. **d** sperm motility. **e** sperm progressive motility. **f** percentage of abnormal sperm (sperm with abnormal morphology). Data are expressed as mean ± SD, $n = 8$. * versus control, $p < 0.05$

leptin-treated groups both had higher proportions of spermatozoa with abnormal morphology, which were 1.25-fold ($65.31 \pm 6.51\%$) and 1.38-fold ($72.05 \pm 5.30\%$) compared with the control group ($51.80 \pm 8.01\%$), respectively (both $p < 0.05$) (Fig. 1f). Administration of 0.1 mg/kg leptin did not alter sperm parameters significantly.

TUNEL was conducted to detect whether leptin treatment induced testicular cell apoptosis. The number of TUNEL positive nuclei (indicating apoptotic cells) per seminiferous tubule increased significantly in the 3 mg/kg leptin-treated group compared with the control group ($p < 0.05$), and it seemed that apoptosis mainly occurred in germ cells in seminiferous tubules. The number of apoptotic cells per seminiferous tubule in the control, 0.1 and 0.5 mg/kg leptin-treated groups were similar (Fig. 2a and b).

Leptin administration impaired BTB integrity

We used a biotin tracer to assess if BTB integrity was affected in leptin-treated mice. Biotin passed through the BTB and accumulated visibly in the adluminal compartments of most seminiferous tubules in 3 mg/kg leptin-treated mice, indicating impaired BTB integrity in these mice. In contrast, biotin was restricted to the interstitial and seminiferous tubule-basal compartments in control mice, as well as in 0.1 and 0.5 mg/kg leptin-treated mice (Fig. 2c).

Interestingly, we also observed that seminiferous tubules at stage VIII, of which the BTB undergoes restructuring to allow the transit of preleptotene spermatocytes, more often have the biotin in the adluminal compartments compared with seminiferous tubules at other stages. The proportion of seminiferous tubules that have the biotin in the adluminal compartments in all observed seminiferous tubules at stage VIII and other stages were 66.67% and 39.77%, respectively ($\chi^2 = 10.323$, $p < 0.05$) (Fig. 2d).

Leptin administration reduced TJ-associated proteins in testes

We determined whether impaired BTB integrity was related to decreased expression of TJ-associated proteins, as TJ restricts the passage of molecules at this barrier. Western blot results demonstrated that the expression of testicular claudin 5, occludin and ZO-1 in 3 mg/kg leptin-treated mice, which had impaired BTB integrity, decreased significantly compared with control mice ($p < 0.05$) (Fig. 3a and b). In control mice, immunofluorescence showed that claudin 5, occludin and ZO-1 were located at the basal compartments of seminiferous tubules, consistent with their expression locations at BTB area, and claudin 5 was simultaneously expressed in germ cells and in vascular endothelium. However, the immunofluorescent stains of these proteins at BTB area became thin and irregular in

3 mg/kg leptin-treated mice (Fig. 3c). In addition, androgen receptor (AR) is reported to be an upstream factor affecting BTB integrity. We found that testicular AR expression in 3 mg/kg leptin-treated mice decreased significantly compared with control mice ($p < 0.05$) (Additional file 3: Figure S1 F).

Leptin directly reduced TJ-associated proteins in TM4 cells

To identify whether leptin could directly reduce TJ-associated proteins in Sertoli cells in vitro, we treated TM4 cells, an OB-R expressing mouse Sertoli cell line (Fig. 4a), with 0 (control), 10 or 100 nM leptin for 48 h. We found that the expression of claudin 5, occludin and ZO-1 decreased significantly in cells treated with 100 nM leptin compared with control cells ($p < 0.05$). The presence of 10 nM leptin showed no significant influence on the expression of TJ-associated proteins in TM4 cells (Fig. 4b and c).

Leptin's effect on TJ-associated proteins in TM4 cells was attenuated by leptin signaling pathway inhibitors

We further investigated the requirement of leptin-mediated signaling pathways for reducing TJ-associated proteins in TM4 cells. Various inhibitors of leptin signaling mediators were used in this study: AG490, LY294002 and U0126 (the inhibitors of JAK2, PI3K and ERK, respectively). The decreased expression of claudin 5, occludin and ZO-1 in TM4 cells induced by 100 nM leptin was reversed in various degrees when cells were pretreated with inhibitors. Leptin's effect on claudin 5 was significantly reduced by LY294002, and U0126 was the most effective inhibitor to abolish leptin's effect on occludin and ZO-1 (both $p < 0.05$) (Fig. 4d and e). The results indicated that JAK2/STAT, PI3K and ERK pathways were involved in leptin-induced decline in TJ-associated proteins in TM4 cells.

Discussion

Leptin is a well-known protein secreted by adipose tissue that maintains normal reproductive function. This is proven by administering leptin to *ob/ob* mice to restore fertility [4, 5]. However, leptin seems to have adverse impacts on male fertility when serum leptin levels are higher than normal and in nonobese rodents given exogenous leptin. The present study highlighted the effects of exogenous leptin on sperm parameters and the role of leptin in damaging BTB integrity, which could be a mechanism for leptin-related male subfertility and infertility.

It is evident that leptin treatment restores reproductive function in *ob/ob* mice [4, 5, 37]. However, the effects of leptin treatment on normal rodents are negative [14–19]. In our study, sperm concentration,

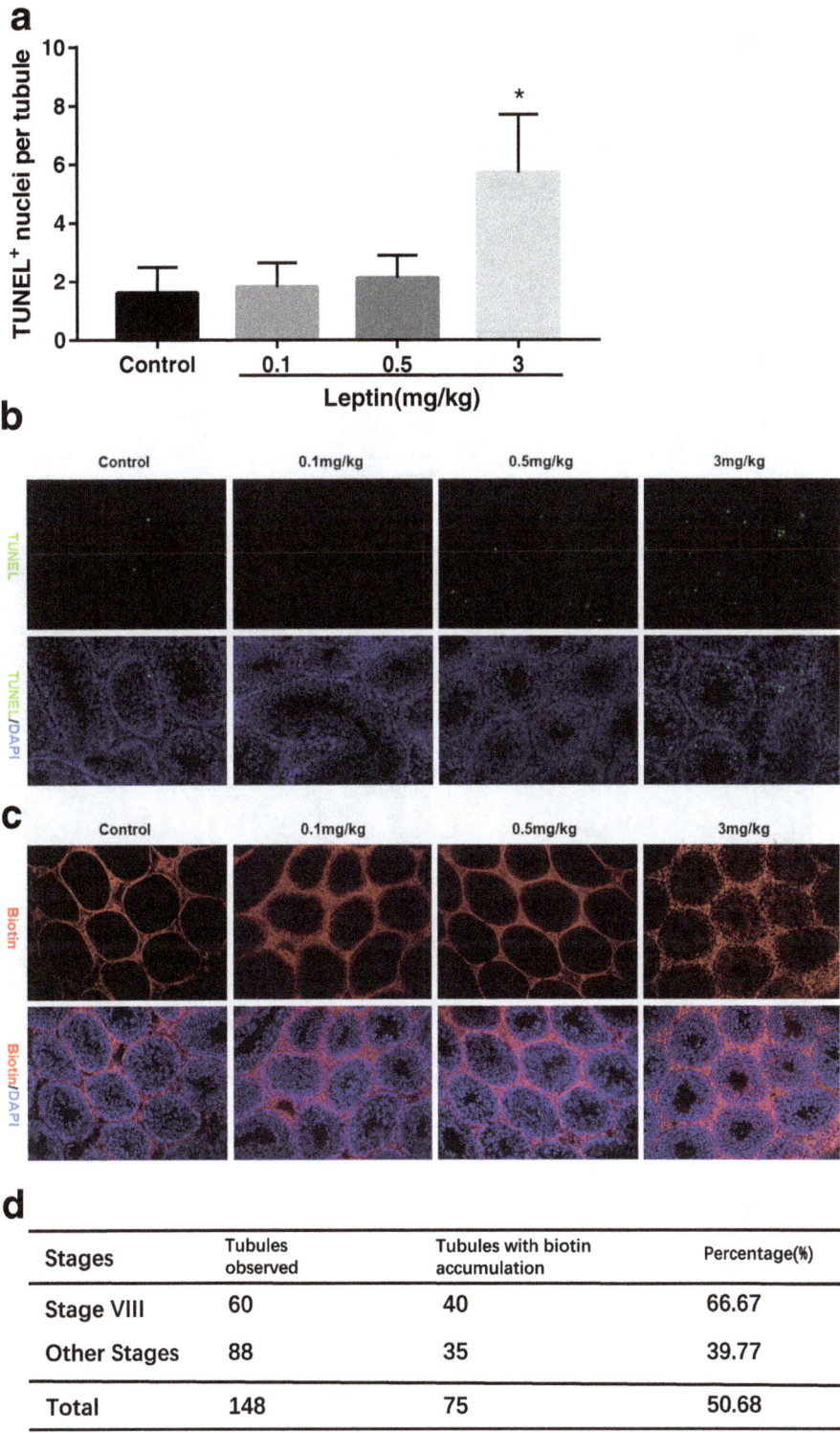

Stages	Tubules observed	Tubules with biotin accumulation	Percentage(%)
Stage VIII	60	40	66.67
Other Stages	88	35	39.77
Total	148	75	50.68

Fig. 2 Evaluation of testicular cell apoptosis and BTB integrity. **a** the number of TUNEL positive nuclei per seminiferous tubule. Data are expressed as mean ± SD, $n = 3$. * versus control, $p < 0.05$. **b** TUNEL positive nuclei (green) which indicated apoptosis were mainly localized in germ cells in seminiferous tubules. Cell nuclei were stained with DAPI (blue). **c** biotin (red) only passed through the BTB and accumulated in the adluminal compartments of seminiferous tubules in 3 mg/kg leptin-treated mice. Cell nuclei were stained with DAPI (blue). **d** proportion of seminiferous tubules that have the biotin in the adluminal compartments in all observed seminiferous tubules at stage VIII and other stages. $n = 4$. $\chi^2 = 10.323$, $p < 0.05$

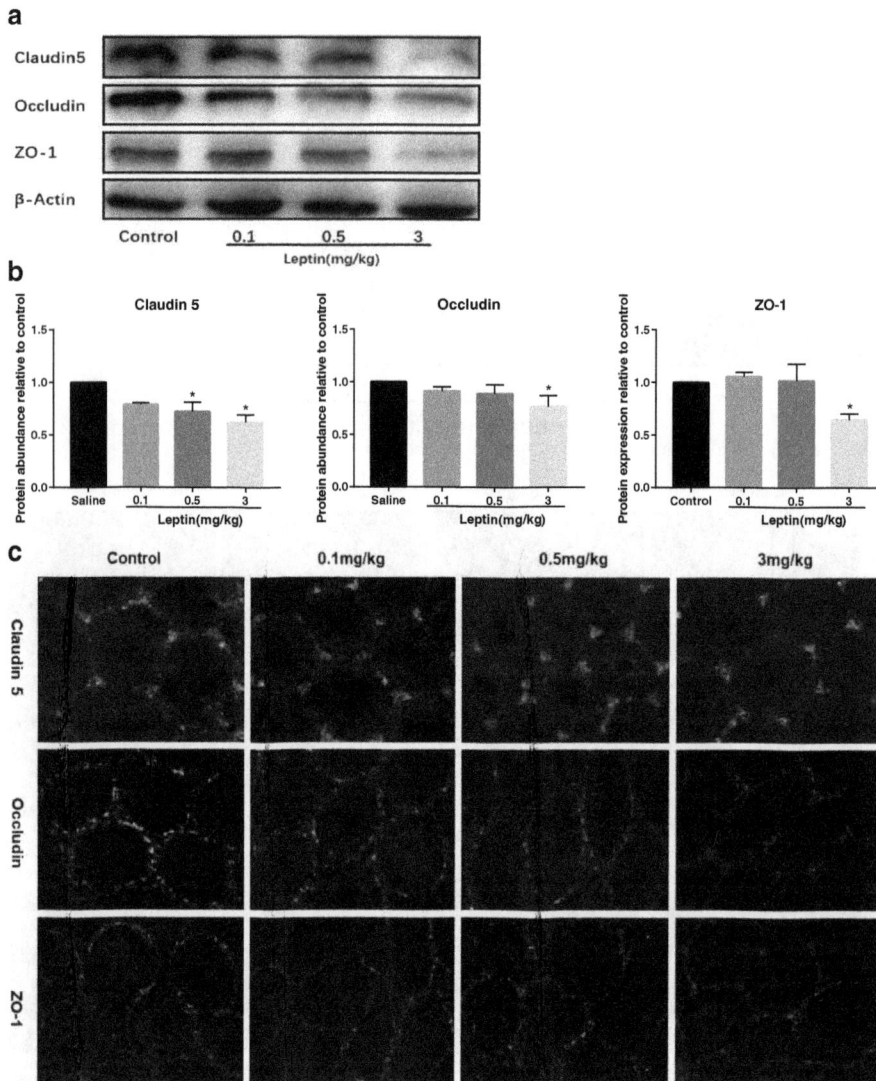

Fig. 3 Expression and localization of TJ-associated proteins in testes. **a** western blot analysis of claudin 5, occludin and ZO-1 in testes. **b** densitometric analysis for immunopositive bands of claudin 5, occludin and ZO-1 in testes. Data are expressed as mean ± SD, $n = 6$. * versus control, $p < 0.05$. **c** immunofluorescence showed the expression and localization of claudin 5, occludin and ZO-1 (green) in testes

motility and progressive motility decreased whereas the percentage of abnormal sperm and the number of apoptotic testicular cells increased in 3 mg/kg leptin-treated mice. Using a biotin tracer, we showed that these mice also had impaired BTB integrity. Haron et al. suggested that decreased sperm count and increased abnormal spermatozoa in leptin-treated rodents were likely due to a direct effect of leptin on spermatozoa or testicular tissues [14]; Abbasihormozi et al. proposed that exogenous leptin suppressed male fertility by sperm ROS production or hormone modulation [15]. Here, we showed that altered sperm parameters in normal mice exposed to exogenous leptin had a relationship with impaired BTB integrity. The BTB acts as a physical and immunological barrier

to protect spermatogenic cells from toxicants, and from being recognized and attacked by the immune system [23]. Exposure to some environmental toxicants can induce injury to the BTB and elicit subsequent damage as germ cell loss, reduced sperm count, male infertility or subfertility [23, 26–28]. Impaired BTB might alter the microenvironment for spermatogenesis in 3 mg/kg leptin-treated mice leading to germ cell apoptosis and compromised sperm quantity and quality. The biotin tracer assay also showed that biotin was more often observed in the adluminal compartments of seminiferous tubules at stage VIII. Although the BTB disassembles and reconstructs to facilitate the transit of preleptotene spermatocytes into the apical compartments at this stage,

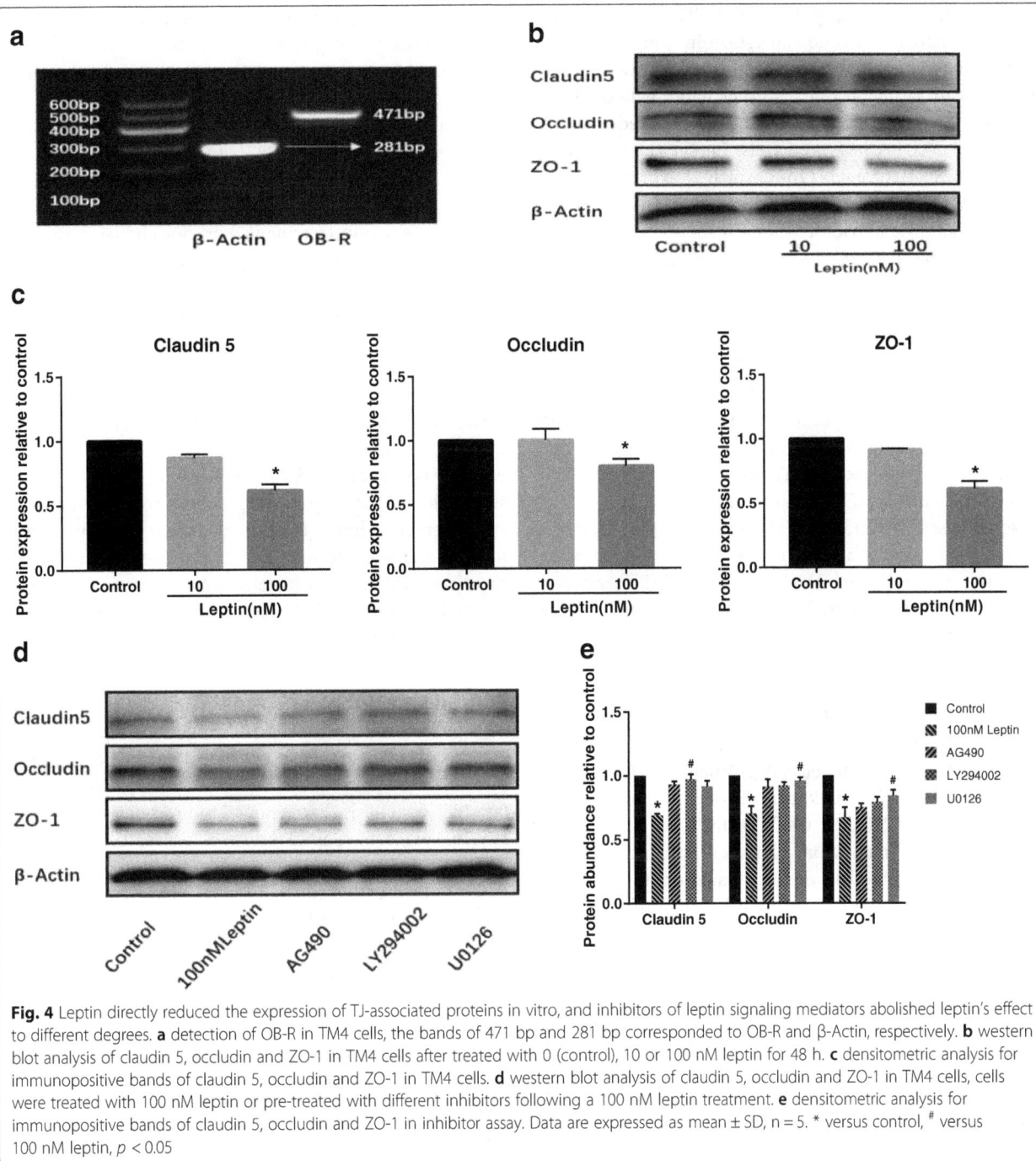

Fig. 4 Leptin directly reduced the expression of TJ-associated proteins in vitro, and inhibitors of leptin signaling mediators abolished leptin's effect to different degrees. **a** detection of OB-R in TM4 cells, the bands of 471 bp and 281 bp corresponded to OB-R and β-Actin, respectively. **b** western blot analysis of claudin 5, occludin and ZO-1 in TM4 cells after treated with 0 (control), 10 or 100 nM leptin for 48 h. **c** densitometric analysis for immunopositive bands of claudin 5, occludin and ZO-1 in TM4 cells. **d** western blot analysis of claudin 5, occludin and ZO-1 in TM4 cells, cells were treated with 100 nM leptin or pre-treated with different inhibitors following a 100 nM leptin treatment. **e** densitometric analysis for immunopositive bands of claudin 5, occludin and ZO-1 in inhibitor assay. Data are expressed as mean ± SD, n = 5. * versus control, # versus 100 nM leptin, $p < 0.05$

it still holds intact function due to its distinctive structure under normal condition [23]. The results of biotin tracer assay suggested that leptin might interfere with the reconstruction process of the BTB at stage VIII, and thus the BTB was more often impaired at this stage.

The BTB is formed largely by TJ between Sertoli cells, which serves as a barrier and boundary in the seminiferous epithelium. We hypothesized that impaired BTB integrity was associated with decreased expression of TJ-associated proteins. As expected, in 3 mg/kg leptin-treated mice, which had impaired BTB integrity, the expression of claudin 5, occludin and ZO-1 decreased significantly and the immunofluorescent stains of these proteins became thin and irregular at BTB area. Further studies are needed to fully understand the mechanisms underlying leptin's disruption to the BTB as other junctions in the BTB have not yet been evaluated. Fan et al. determined AR expression using testicular proteins in diet-induced obese mice and suggested AR as an upstream factor affecting BTB integrity [38]. The decreased testicular AR gene expression in 3 mg/kg leptin-treated mice suggested that it could contribute to inducing BTB impairment. On the other hand, we could not rule out the possibility that leptin directly reduced TJ-associated proteins in Sertoli cells. Leptin carries out its biological effects through OB-R which is expressed in rat Sertoli cells and human Sertoli cells [39, 40]. Since leptin can modulate the nutritional support for spermatogenesis by altering the metabolic behavior of human Sertoli cells [40], we treated TM4 cells with low (10 nM) and high concentration (100 nM) of leptin to test the direct effect of leptin on TJ-associated proteins. We first confirmed the presence of OB-R, which allows leptin to interact with TM4 cells. We then found that 100 nM leptin reduced the expression of claudin 5, occludin and ZO-1 in TM4 cells. Taken together, our in vitro experiments confirmed that leptin alone directly reduced TJ-associated proteins, which could contribute to BTB impairment in vivo.

Leptin uses JAK2/STAT3 as its principle signaling pathway [41], and it also activates ERK and PI3K pathways [2]. Inhibition of JAK2, ERK and PI3K reversed leptin-induced decline in TJ-associated proteins in TM4 cells to different extents (Fig. 4e). However, AG490, an inhibitor of JAK2, was not the most effective inhibitor to rescue the decrease of TJ-associated proteins in TM4 cells. Activation of JAK2/STAT3, along with the activation of PI3K and ERK, is involved in leptin-induced TJ dysfunction in intestinal cells [20]. When SUMO-2/3 specific protease (SENP3) is knocked down, it compromises the activation of STAT3, resulting in TJ dysfunction in Sertoli cells [42]. In addition, a high level of leptin has also been found to upregulate the expression of suppressor of cytokine signaling 3 (SOCS3), which can inhibit STAT3 phosphorylation [12]. The role of the JAK2/STAT3 pathway in leptin-induced decline in TJ-associated proteins required further investigation. In this study, JAK2/STAT, PI3K and ERK pathways were suggested to be involved in leptin-induced decline in TJ-associated proteins.

Leptin treatment causes body weight loss and increases reproductive organ weights in *ob/ob* mice [4]. However, leptin treatment hardly alters body weights or reproductive organ weights in normal rodents [14, 16–19, 43], also shown in this study, indicating that the effect on sperm parameters after leptin administration is unlikely due to leptin resistance [14]. Previous studies have reported that leptin treatment has no influence on serum leptin levels in normal rodents [14, 18]. Although circulating leptin levels at 1 h after administration of 3 mg/kg leptin show a 170-fold increase in fasted mice and a 13-fold increase in fed mice, the half-life of mouse leptin is found to be 40.2 min [44]. This could explain why serum leptin levels in our leptin-treated mice were not significantly different compared with control mice.

The relationship between leptin treatment and testosterone has been investigated in many studies. In *ob/ob* mice, leptin treatment increases intratesticular testosterone via improved Leydig cell function [37]. However, serum testosterone is negatively correlated with serum leptin in humans and rodents [45–47]. In vitro experiments also show that leptin can directly reduce testosterone secretion and the expression of steroidogenic genes [12, 39, 48]. In normal rats, leptin treatment does not change serum testosterone significantly [14, 18], although parenchymal testosterone decreases by about 49% compared with control rats [18]. Our study showed that 3 mg/kg leptin treatment repressed testicular steroidogenesis genes expression in vivo but did not produce a significant decrease in serum testosterone levels. The conflicting findings observed in various studies are most likely due to different experimental objectives and variable study designs such as the different doses of leptin used and experiment durations. In our study, altered sperm parameters and impaired BTB integrity observed in leptin-treated mice were unlikely to be related to the alterations in serum testosterone levels since the decreases were not statistically different. Instead, it seemed to be leptin that exerted critical and direct effects on male reproductive tissues.

Conclusions

The present study shows that exogenous leptin exhibits significant adverse effects on sperm parameters, induces testicular cell apoptosis, and possibly suppresses testicular steroidogenesis. Exogenous leptin impairs BTB integrity in vivo, which is likely to be a result of decreased TJ-associated proteins. We have further verified that leptin can directly reduce TJ-associated proteins in Sertoli cells in vitro, and identified that JAK2/STAT, PI3K and ERK pathways may be involved in this process. Given the pivotal role of BTB integrity in maintaining an appropriate microenvironment for normal spermatogenesis, BTB impairment may cause male subfertility and infertility. We have proposed a mechanism for leptin's adverse effects on male reproductive function, which will help to have a deeper insight into subfertility and infertility in the context of obesity and azoospermia.

Abbreviations

AR: Androgen receptor; BMI: Body mass index; BTB: Blood testis barrier; *Cyp11a1*: Cytochrome P450 family 11 subfamily A member 1; ERK: Extracellular signal-regulated kinase; JAK2: Janus kinase 2; OB-R: Leptin receptor; PI3K: Phosphoinositide 3-kinase; ROS: Reactive oxygen species; *Sf-1*: Steroidogenic factor 1; SOCS3: Suppressor of cytokine signaling 3; *Star*: Steroidogenic acute regulatory protein; STAT3: Signal transducer and activator of transcription 3; TJ: Tight junction; TUNEL: TdT-mediated dUTP Nick End Labeling; ZO-1: Zona occludens-1; ZO-3: Zona occludens-3

Acknowledgments

We would like to thank Liling Wang, Na Fang, and Yuanyuan Li of the Family

Planning Research Institute/Center of Reproductive Medicine, Tongji Medical College, HUST, for their excellent technical assistance.

Funding
This study was supported by National Key Research and Development Program of China 2017YFC1002001, Integrated Innovative Team for Major Human Diseases Program of Tongji Medical College, HUST; the Fundamental Research Funds for the Central Universities,2015MS130.

Authors' contributions
All authors participated in study design. WXT and ZXK performed experiments and data analysis. WXT wrote the manuscript. HL and LHG revised and commented the manuscript. All authors read and approved the final version of the manuscript.

Competing interests
The authors declare that they have no competing interests.

Author details
[1]Family Planning Research Institute/Center of Reproductive Medicine, Tongji Medical College, Huazhong University of Science and Technology, Wuhan 430030, China. [2]Center for Reproductive Medicine, The Third Affiliated Hospital of Zhengzhou University, Zhengzhou 450052, China.

References
1. González RR, Simón C, Caballero-Campo P, Norman R, Chardonnens D, Devoto L, Bischof P. Leptin and reproduction. Hum Reprod Update. 2000; 6(3):290–330.
2. Zhou Y, Rui L. Leptin signaling and leptin resistance. Front Med. 2013;7(2): 207–22.
3. Ahima RS. Adipose tissue as an endocrine organ. Obesity. 2006;14(S8):242S–9S.
4. Barash IA, Cheung CC, Weigle DS, Ren H, Kabigting EB, Kuijper JL, Clifton DK, Steiner RA. Leptin is a metabolic signal to the reproductive system. Endocrinology. 1996;137(7):3144–7.
5. Mounzih K, Lu R, Chehab FF. Leptin treatment rescues the sterility of genetically obese Ob/Ob males. Endocrinology. 1997;138(3):1190–3.
6. Considine RV, Sinha MK, Heiman ML, Kriauciunas A, Stephens TW, Nyce MR, et al. Serum immunoreactive-leptin concentrations in normal-weight and obese humans. N Engl J Med. 1996;334(5):292–5.
7. Handjieva-Darlenska T, Boyadjieva N. The effect of high-fat diet on plasma ghrelin and leptin levels in rats. J Physiol Biochem. 2009;65(2):157–64.
8. Leisegang K, Bouic PJ, Menkveld R, Henkel RR. Obesity is associated with increased seminal insulin and leptin alongside reduced fertility parameters in a controlled male cohort. Reprod Biol Endocrinol. 2014;12:34.
9. Einollahi N, Dashti N, Emamgholipour S, Zarebavani M, Sedighi-Gilani MA, Choobineh H. Evidence for alteration in serum concentrations of leptin in infertile men categorized based on BMI. Clin Lab. 2016;59:2361–6.
10. Hofny ER, Ali ME, Abdel-Hafez HZ, Eel-D K, Mohamed EE, Abd El-Azeem HG, Mostafa T. Semen parameters and hormonal profile in obese fertile and infertile males. Fertil Steril. 2010;94(2):581–4.
11. Steinman N, Gamzu R, Yogev L, Botchan A, Schreiber L, Yavetz H. Serum leptin concentrations are higher in azoospermic than in normozoospermic men. Fertil Steril. 2001;75(4):821–2.
12. Yuan M, Huang G, Li J, Zhang J, Li F, Li K, et al. Hyperleptinemia directly affects testicular maturation at different sexual stages in mice, and suppressor of cytokine signaling 3 is involved in this process. Reprod Biol Endocrinol. 2014;12:15.
13. Giovambattista A, Suescun MO, Nessralla CC, França LR, Spinedi E, Calandra RS. Modulatory effects of leptin on leydig cell function of normal and hyperleptinemia rats. Neuroendocrinology. 2003;78(5):270–9.
14. Haron MN, D'Souza UJ, Jaafar H, Zakaria R, Singh HJ. Exogenous leptin administration decreases sperm count and increases the fraction of abnormal sperm in adult rats. Fertil Steril. 2010;93(1):322–4.
15. Abbasihormozi S, Shahverdi A, Kouhkan A, Cheraghi J, Akhlaghi AA, Kheimeh A. Relationship of leptin administration with production of reactive oxygen species, sperm DNA fragmentation, sperm parameters and hormone profile in the adult rat. Arch Gynecol Obstet. 2013;287(6):1241–9.
16. Almabhouh FA, Osman K, Ibrahim SF, Gupalo S, Gnanou J, Ibrahim E, Singh HJ. Melatonin ameliorates the adverse effects of leptin on sperm. Asian J Androl. 2016;19(6):647–54.
17. Almabhouh FA, Singh HJ. Adverse effects of leptin on histone- to-protamine transition during spermatogenesis are prevented by melatonin in Sprague- Dawley rats. Andrologia. 2018;50(1):e12814.
18. Fernandez CD, Fernandes GS, Favareto AP, Perobelli JE, Sanabria M, Kempinas WD. Decreased implantation number after in utero artificial insemination can reflect an impairment of fertility in adult male rats after exogenous leptin exposure. Reprod Sci. 2017;24(2):234–41.
19. Almabhouh FA, Osman K, Siti Fatimah I, Sergey G, Gnanou J, Singh HJ. Effects of leptin on sperm count and morphology in Sprague-Dawley rats and their reversibility following a 6-week recovery period. Andrologia. 2015;47(7):751–8.
20. Kim CY, Kim KH. Curcumin prevents leptin-induced tight junction dysfunction in intestinal Caco-2 BBe cells. J Nutr Biochem. 2014;25(1):26–35.
21. Le Dréan G, Haure-Mirande V, Ferrier L, Bonnet C, Hulin P, de Coppet P, Segain JP. Visceral adipose tissue and leptin increase colonic epithelial tight junction permeability via a RhoA-ROCK-dependent pathway. FASEB J. 2014;28(3):1059–70.
22. Le Dréan G, Segain JP. Connecting metabolism to intestinal barrier function: the role of leptin. Tissue Barriers. 2014;2(4):e970940.
23. Cheng CY, Mruk DD. The blood-testis barrier and its implications for male contraception. Pharmacol Rev. 2012;64(1):16–64.
24. Mruk DD, Cheng CY. Sertoli-Sertoli and Sertoli-germ cell interactions and their significance in germ cell movement in the seminiferous epithelium during spermatogenesis. Endocr Rev. 2004;25(5):747–806.
25. Morrow CM, Mruk D, Cheng CY, Hess RA. Claudin and occludin expression and function in the seminiferous epithelium. Philos Trans R Soc Lond Ser B Biol Sci. 2010;365(1546):1679–96.
26. Cao XN, Shen LJ, Wu SD, Yan C, Zhou Y, Xiong G, et al. Urban fine particulate matter exposure causes male reproductive injury through destroying blood-testis barrier (BTB) integrity. Toxicol Lett. 2017;266:1–12.
27. Zhang J, Li Z, Qie M, Zheng R, Shetty J, Wang J. Sodium fluoride and sulfur dioxide affected male reproduction by disturbing blood-testis barrier in mice. Food Chem Toxicol. 2016;94:103–11.
28. Qiu L, Zhang X, Zhang X, Zhang Y, Gu J, Chen M, et al. Sertoli cell is a potential target for perfluorooctane sulfonate-induced reproductive dysfunction in male mice. Toxicol Sci. 2013;135(1):229–40.
29. Ahn JH, Choi YS, Choi JH. Leptin promotes human endometriotic cell migration and invasion by up-regulating MMP-2 through the JAK2/STAT3 signaling pathway. Mol Hum Reprod. 2015;21(10):792–802.
30. Rossi SP, Windschüttl S, Matzkin ME, Rey-Ares V, Terradas C, Ponzio R, et al. Reactive oxygen species (ROS) production triggered by prostaglandin D2 (PGD2) regulates lactate dehydrogenase (LDH) expression/activity in TM4 Sertoli cells. Mol Cell Endocrinol. 2016;434:154–65.
31. Choi MS, Park HJ, Oh JH, Lee EH, Park SM, Yoon S. Nonylphenol-induced apoptotic cell death in mouse TM4 Sertoli cells via the generation of reactive oxygen species and activation of the ERK signaling pathway. J Appl Toxicol. 2014;34(6):628–36.
32. World Health Organization, editor. WHO laboratory manual for the examination and processing of human semen. 5th ed. Geneva: World Health Organization; 2010.
33. Ward MA. Intracytoplasmic sperm injection effects in infertile azh mutant mice. Biol Reprod. 2005;73(1):193–200.
34. Meng J, Holdcraft RW, Shima JE, Griswold MD, Braun RE. Androgens regulate the permeability of the blood–testis barrier. Proc Natl Acad Sci. 2005;102(46):16696–700.
35. El-Hefnawy T, Ioffe S, Dym M. Expression of the leptin receptor during germ cell development in the mouse testis. Endocrinology. 2000;141(7):2624–30.
36. Woods DC, White YA, Niikura Y, Kiatpongsan S, Lee HJ, Tilly JL. Embryonic stem cell–derived granulosa cells participate in ovarian follicle formation in vitro and in vivo. Reprod Sci. 2013;20(5):524–35.
37. Hoffmann A, Manjowk GM, Wagner IV, Klöting N, Ebert T, Jessnitzer B, et al. Leptin within the subphysiological to physiological range dose-dependently improves male reproductive function in an obesity mouse model. Endocrinology. 2016;157(6):2461–8.
38. Fan Y, Liu Y, Xue K, Gu G, Fan W, Xu Y, Ding Z. Diet-induced obesity in male

C57BL/6 mice decreases fertility as a consequence of disrupted blood-testis barrier. PLoS One. 2015;10(4):e0120775.

39. Tena-Sempere M, Manna PR, Zhang FP, Pinilla L, González LC, Diéguez C, Huhtaniemi I, Aguilar E. Molecular mechanisms of leptin action in adult rat testis: potential targets for leptin-induced inhibition of steroidogenesis and pattern of leptin receptor messenger ribonucleic acid expression. J Endocrinol. 2001;170(2):413–23.

40. Martins AD, Moreira AC, Sá R, Monteiro MP, Sousa M, Carvalho RA, et al. Leptin modulates human Sertoli cell acetate production and glycolytic profile: a novel mechanism of obesity-induced male infertility? Biochim Biophys Acta. 2015;1852(9):1824–32.

41. Peelman F, Zabeau L, Moharana K, Savvides SN, Tavernier J. 20 years of leptin: insights into signaling assemblies of the leptin receptor. J Endocrinol. 2014;223(1):T9–23.

42. Wu D, Huang CJ, Khan FA, Jiao XF, Liu XM, Pandupuspitasari NS, Brohi RD, Huo LJ. SENP3 grants tight junction integrity and cytoskeleton architecture in mouse Sertoli cells. Oncotarget. 2017;8(35):58430–42.

43. Donahoo WT, Stob NR, Ammon S, Levin N, Eckel RH. Leptin increases skeletal muscle lipoprotein lipase and postprandial lipid metabolism in mice. Metabolism. 2011;60(3):438–43.

44. Burnett LC, Skowronski AA, Rausch R, LeDuc CA, Leibel RL. Determination of the half-life of circulating leptin in the mouse. Int J Obes. 2017;41(3):355–9.

45. Luukkaa V, Pesonen U, Huhtaniemi I, Lehtonen A, Tilvis R, Tuomilehto J, Koulu M, Huupponen R. Inverse correlation between serum testosterone and leptin in men. J Clin Endocrinol Metab. 1998;83(9):3243–6.

46. Söderberg S, Olsson T, Eliasson M, Johnson O, Brismar K, Carlström K, Ahrén B. A strong association between biologically active testosterone and leptin in non-obese men and women is lost with increasing (central) adiposity. Int J Obes Relat Metab Disord. 2001;25(1):98–105.

47. Vigueras-Villaseñor RM, Rojas-Castañeda JC, Chávez-Saldaña M, Gutiérrez-Pérez O, García-Cruz ME, Cuevas-Alpuche O, et al. Alterations in the spermatic function generated by obesity in rats. Acta Histochem. 2011;113(2):214–20.

48. Landry DA, Sormany F, Haché J, Roumaud P, Martin LJ. Steroidogenic genes expressions are repressed by high levels of leptin and the JAK/STAT signaling pathway in MA-10 Leydig cells. Mol Cell Biochem. 2017;433(1–2):79–95.

## 17

Reactive oxygen species and male reproductive hormones

Mahsa Darbandi[1†], Sara Darbandi[1†], Ashok Agarwal[2*] (iD), Pallav Sengupta[3], Damayanthi Durairajanayagam[4], Ralf Henkel[5] and Mohammad Reza Sadeghi[6]

Abstract

Reports of the increasing incidence of male infertility paired with decreasing semen quality have triggered studies on the effects of lifestyle and environmental factors on the male reproductive potential. There are numerous exogenous and endogenous factors that are able to induce excessive production of reactive oxygen species (ROS) beyond that of cellular antioxidant capacity, thus causing oxidative stress. In turn, oxidative stress negatively affects male reproductive functions and may induce infertility either directly or indirectly by affecting the hypothalamus-pituitary-gonadal (HPG) axis and/or disrupting its crosstalk with other hormonal axes. This review discusses the important exogenous and endogenous factors leading to the generation of ROS in different parts of the male reproductive tract. It also highlights the negative impact of oxidative stress on the regulation and cross-talk between the reproductive hormones. It further describes the mechanism of ROS-induced derangement of male reproductive hormonal profiles that could ultimately lead to male infertility. An understanding of the disruptive effects of ROS on male reproductive hormones would encourage further investigations directed towards the prevention of ROS-mediated hormonal imbalances, which in turn could help in the management of male infertility.

Keywords: Antioxidants, Hypothalamic-pituitary-gonadal axis, Male infertility, Oxidative stress, Reactive oxygen species, Testosterone

Background

Over the past 40 years, reports regarding the decline in semen quality [1–4] and its probable consequences on male fertility have encouraged studies about the effects of environment and lifestyle factors on the male reproductive potential. Reactive oxygen species (ROS) produced by exogenous and endogenous factors are highly reactive oxygen derivatives with half-lives in the nano- to milliseconds range. These molecules reportedly play a key role in altering male reproductive functions [5, 6]. Lifestyle modifications, technological advancements, escalating levels of pollution, alcohol consumption, smoking of cigarettes and vaping, and physical stress are among the prime exogenous causes of ROS production [7–9]. Also, multiple mechanisms involving metabolism in the cell

membrane, mitochondria, peroxisomes, and endoplasmic reticulum can produce endogenous ROS [7, 9].

Antioxidants defend against excessive ROS levels through enzymatic (superoxide dismutase, catalases, and peroxidases) and non-enzymatic (vitamins, steroids etc.) mechanisms [7, 10]. In cases where the imbalance between oxidants (ROS) and antioxidants leans towards the oxidants, oxidative stress (OS) occurs, which puts the cells and the body under stress. As a result, excessive ROS can induce lipid peroxidation, disrupt DNA, RNA as well as protein functions in the spermatozoa and other testicular cells [10].

High ROS levels can increase the possibility of infertility not only directly by inducing OS, but also indirectly by acting through the hypothalamic axes of hormone release [11–13]. ROS reduce male sex hormone levels and disrupt the hormonal balance that regulates male reproductive functions [14], and thus causes infertility. These "endocrine disruptors" not only interfere in the communication between testis and the hypothalamic-pituitary unit, they also disrupt the cross-talk between the

* Correspondence: agarwaa@ccf.org
[†]Mahsa Darbandi and Sara Darbandi contributed equally to this work.
[2]American Center for Reproductive Medicine, Cleveland Clinic, Cleveland, Ohio 44195, USA
Full list of author information is available at the end of the article

hypothalamic-pituitary-gonadal (HPG) axis with other hypothalamic hormonal axes [15, 16]. The testis, as the primary male sex organ, is not only concerned with spermatogenesis, but also with the secretion of several hormones [17] which are required for regulation of gonadotropin secretion, spermatogenesis, formation of male phenotype during sexual differentiation, and normal sexual behaviour [18]. Hence, by interfering with normal hormonal release, ROS disrupt these essential reproductive functions.

Therefore, this review precisely elucidates (a) the role of ROS, generated by various exogenous and endogenous factors, in disrupting hormone secretion by interfering in the endocrine pathways, as well as in their cross-talk, (b) hormonal regulation of the oxidative status of male reproduction, and (c) a possible mechanism of action of ROS-induced disruption of the male reproductive hormonal profile.

Endocrinology of male fertility

The gonadotropin releasing hormone (GnRH) secreted by the hypothalamus regulates the release and secretion of gonadotropins, luteinizing hormone (LH) and follicle-stimulating hormone (FSH) from anterior pituitary that in turn regulate testicular functions [17]. These gonadal steroids as well as the pituitary gonadotropins, via feedback regulatory mechanisms, further establish physiological homeostasis and maintains normal reproductive functions [14, 17, 19]. FSH receptors are located on the membrane of Sertoli cells, while those of LH are on the Leydig cells. They coordinate to synthesize testosterone, maintain normal spermatogenesis, sperm health and density [19–21].

Moreover, other hormones like estradiol (E2) and prolactin (PRL) also take part in the management of male reproductive function. E2, produced both by the testis and via the peripheral conversion of androgenic precursors, is a potent inhibitor of LH and FSH [18, 19] (Fig. 1). PRL-inhibiting GnRH secretion via modulation of dopaminergic pathway may also reduce LH and testosterone level and thus is associated with hypogonadism [22]. Dehydroepiandrosterone (DHEA) is another male reproduction ameliorating, steroid hormone secreted by the adrenal cortex [23, 24]. Inhibin A and B, dimeric hormones produced by Sertoli cells, exhibit negative feedback on FSH secretion and thus also on testicular functions [25]. Moreover, melatonin (MLT), a tryptophan-derived hormone of the pineal gland, positively regulates gonadotropin and testosterone secretion, and thus aid male reproductive functions [26, 27]. Anti-Mullerian hormone (AMH), a dimeric glycoprotein hormone produced in embryonic Sertoli cells, is structurally related to inhibin and is responsible for regression of Mullerian ducts during the first 8 weeks of embryogenesis. It reflects Sertoli cell

functions and is inhibited by testosterone under the influence of LH [28–30]. Interactions between the hypothalamo-pituitary-thyroid (HPT) and HPG axes potentially influence testicular development, mostly by the participation of thyroid hormones and FSH [31].

Thus, besides the central control through the HPG axis, the major male reproductive hormones act either individually or via the cross-talks among different endocrine axes to influence male reproductive functions. Consequently, any disruption to these networks may adversely affect male fertility.

Generation of ROS in the male reproductive tract

Reactive oxygen species (ROS), which are short-lived, unstable, and highly reactive species containing at least one oxygen atom, are able to snatch electrons from other molecules to achieve an electronically-stable state. In this process, the other molecule loses an electron following which a new radical is formed. Subsequently, this radical reacts with another neighbouring molecule, thus passing on the radical status via a reaction called 'radical-chain reaction' until two radicals react with one another forming a stable bond. These reactions amplify the degree of alterations in the cellular structures [32–34].

Human spermatozoa contain abundant mitochondria, particularly in its midpiece [35]. An NADH-dependent oxidoreductase (in the inner mitochondrial membrane) and NAD (P) H-oxidase (in the plasma membrane) are two main sources of superoxide ($O_2^{\bullet-}$) [32, 33, 36]. The majority of ROS generated in human spermatozoa is $O_2^{\bullet-}$ which is a product of oxidative phosphorylation by addition of an electron to intracellular oxygen and is created between complex I and III of the electron transport chain [37]. H_2O_2 is an uncharged, membrane permeable molecule which has been found to be the major initiator of peroxidative damage of the plasma membranes of germ cells [34]. In the presence of transition metals, such as iron (Fe^{3+}) and copper, $O_2^{\bullet-}$ and H_2O_2 can generate the extremely reactive $OH^{\bullet}$ through the Haber-Weiss reaction, which consist of a reduction of ferric (Fe^{3+}) to ferrous ion (Fe^{2+}) [38]. In a subsequent second step, called Fenton reaction, Fe^{2+} is oxidized by H_2O_2 to Fe^{3+} whereby hydroxide (OH^-) and the most reactive hydroxyl radical ($OH^{\bullet}$) are formed. Furthermore, $O_2^{\bullet-}$ has the ability to interact with nitric oxide (NO) to form peroxynitrite ($ONOO^-$), subsequent reactions of which may lead to either apoptotic or necrotic cell death [39]. In the male reproductive tract, ROS finally can be generated by one of these sources according to the above-mentioned mechanisms.

In order to produce the immense amount of energy needed for motility, spermatozoa possess numerous mitochondria in the mid-piece of the flagellum. In the mitochondria, disruption of the membrane potential

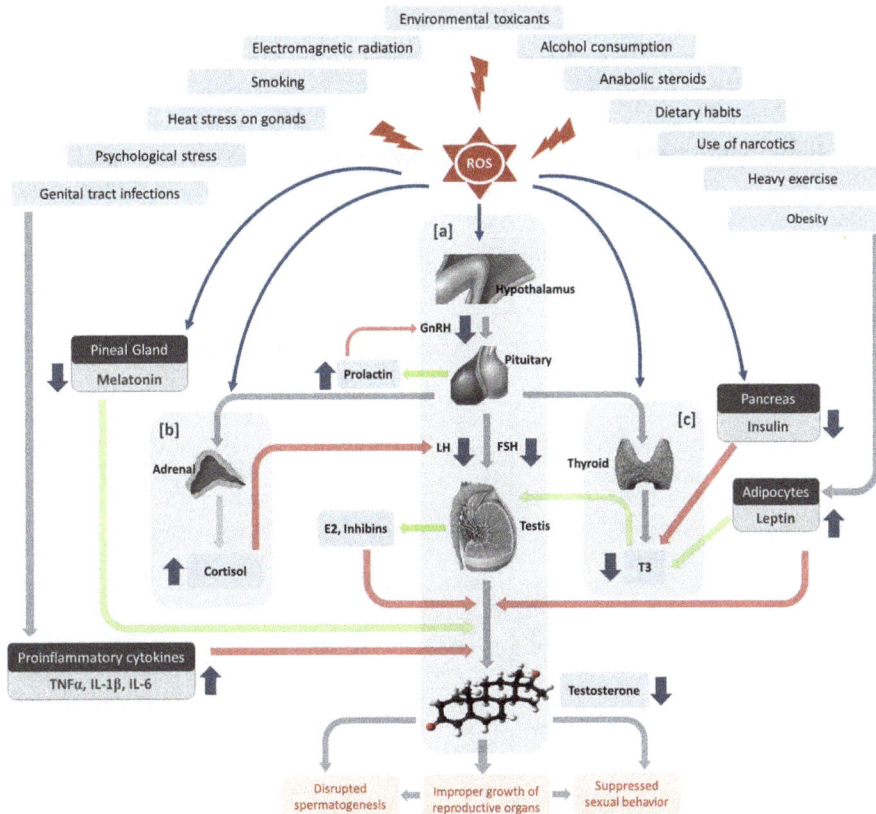

Fig. 1 Sources of reactive oxygen species (ROS) and their impact on the complex endocrine network regulating male reproduction. **a** High levels of ROS impact upon the HPG axis which results in decreased secretion of male reproductive hormones. **b** Through the HPA axis, ROS increases the release of the stress hormone cortisol, which through the HPA-HPG axes cross-talk, further decreases LH secretion. **c** Elevated ROS also affects the HPT axis which results in decreased T3 production from the thyroid gland, which through the cross-talk between HPT and HPG axes, again decreases testosterone synthesis. ROS also affects the other endocrine glands which interfere with these endocrine axes to result in decreased testosterone production. Increased oxidative stress (OS), in different conditions, decreases insulin production from the pancreas which again reduces T3 production from the thyroid gland and through HPT-HPG axes cross-talk decreases testosterone biosynthesis. ROS production in obesity also increases circulating leptin levels which directly reduces testosterone synthesis in the testis. Reduced melatonin in OS, and increased production of pro-inflammatory cytokines during reproductive tract infections, affects the HPG axis to reduce testosterone biosynthesis. OS also increases prolactin secretion from the anterior pituitary and E2 synthesis from the testis. These two hormones reduce GnRH secretion from the hypothalamus and testosterone biosynthesis from the testis, respectively

leads to electron leakage in the electron transfer chain and subsequently produces ROS. The Ca^{2+}-dependent NADPH oxidase, called NOX5 (encoded by the *NOX5* gene) was initially detected in the human testis, but was also found to be present in the acrosomal and mid-piece regions of human spermatozoa [40]. NOX5 is a major generator of ROS and could subsequently induce OS. This enzyme is activated when Ca^{2+} binds to its cytosolic N-terminal EF-hand and causes conformational changes to the cell through OS [41]. Moreover, during spermatogenesis, the developing spermatozoa extrude their cytoplasm. When spermiogenesis is disrupted and/or excess cytoplasm is not completely extruded (excess residual cytoplasm), the excess cytoplasm will be retained around the mid-piece. Since cytoplasm contains the enzymatic machinery to produce ROS, any hindrance in the elimination of excess cytoplasm would trigger the production

of intrinsic amounts of ROS in excess, which, in turn, would lead to oxidative damage of the plasma membrane and sperm DNA [42].

The prostate and seminal vesicles are the major sources of peroxidase-positive leukocytes (polymorpho-nuclear leukocytes (50 ~ 60%) as well as macrophages (20 ~ 30%)) [43, 44]. Inflammatory responses trigger these cells to generate ROS about 100-times more than it is produced under normal conditions [34, 45, 46]. This elevated ROS production is a part of the natural defense mechanisms of these cells, whereby NADPH-production through the hexose monophosphate shunt is elevated. Leukocyte participation in inflammation is closely connected with the accompanying leukocytospermia [47], a condition defined by the World Health Organization (WHO) as semen samples containing more than one million peroxidase-positive leukocytes per milliliter of semen [48]. Varicocele, a condition caused by an abnormal dilation of veins in the pampiniform plexus surrounding the spermatic cord [49], is also associated with elevated levels of seminal ROS [50].

ROS and male reproductive hormones

ROS generation, which can be elicited through various exogenous and endogenous pathways, may adversely affect the male reproductive potential by interfering with the endocrine axes both individually and via their cross-talks (Table 1).

Exogenous factors
Psychological stress
Psychological stress has been demonstrated as a cause of idiopathic male infertility and several studies have

described a correlation between stress and impaired semen parameters [51–53]. It was reported that psychological stress can increase the circulating levels of cortisol and norepinephrine [54]. These hormones have a significant impact on increasing intracellular levels of ROS/reactive nitrogen species (RNS) to have damaging effects on cellular microstructures and activation of the immune and inflammatory systems [54, 55]. Psychological stress inhibits male reproductive functions by directly affecting the action of glucocorticoids on Leydig cells [11]. As a result, circulating testosterone levels decrease through suppression of androgen synthesis and induction of apoptosis of Leydig cells [56]. Psychological stress can also increase the serum levels of corticosterone (in animals) and cortisol (in humans), which then enhance the apoptotic frequency of Leydig cells

Table 1 Sources of reactive oxygen species (ROS), their mechanism of generation and effects on male reproductive hormones

Sources of ROS	Mechanism of ROS generation	Effects on male reproductive hormones
Exogenous sources		
Psychological stress	By increasing stress hormone (cortisol) levels and activating the immune–inflammatory system	Decreases serum testosterone and LH levels by suppressing androgen synthesis and inducing Leydig cells apoptosis
Heat stress	By decreasing antioxidant enzyme activities, increasing NADPH oxidase activity and disrupting mitochondrial homeostasis	Disrupts Sertoli cell functions, decreases testosterone and LH levels
Environmental toxicants	By activating inflammatory mechanisms and cellular death	Decreases Leydig and Sertoli cell functions, hormonal biosynthesis
Electromagnetic radiations	By decreasing total antioxidant capacity	Decreases serum testosterone and LH levels
Long-term heavy exercise	By stimulating mitochondrial enzymes including NOX and XO	Decreases LH, FSH, and testosterone levels
Obesity	By increasing leptin levels in human endothelial cells and increasing mitochondrial fatty acid oxidation	Activation of the HPG axis stimulates FSH and LH release. Leptin can directly affect the gonads due to its receptor isoforms in gonadal tissue and stimulate steroid secretion, through increasing the GnRH
High-fat and high-protein food	By decreasing natural food antioxidants and free radical scavengers	Decreases testosterone biosynthesis, LH secretion and androgen profile
Alcohol	By stimulating cytochrome P450s enzyme activities in the liver, altering levels of necessary metals in the body, and reducing antioxidant levels	Increases Sertoli cells and Leydig cells apoptosis, reduces serum testosterone, LH and FSH levels
Marijuana and narcotic drugs	By increasing inflammation and cytochrome p53-induced apoptotic cell death	Inhibits GnRH release and LH production, inhibits HPG axis, reduces testosterone level, and increases SHBG level
Smoking	By decreasing oxygen delivery to the testis and the high metabolic requirements of spermatogenesis, releasing a large number of mutagens and metabolites, weakening of the antioxidant defense systems. Stimulation of NOX enzymes	Alters plasma levels of testosterone, prolactin, estradiol, FSH, LH and SHBG by affecting the Leydig and Sertoli cells
Anabolic steroids	By stimulating mitochondrial respiratory chain complexes, inflammatory cytokine release and cellular apoptosis	Disrupts Leydig cell functions, suppresses HPG axis, reduces LH release and thus testicular testosterone biosynthesis
Endogenous sources		
Aging	By decreasing the activities of antioxidant enzymes, alteration in the mitochondrial membrane potential	Increases lipid peroxidation of Leydig cells, LH sensitivity by diminishing LH receptors, reduces the rate of steroidogenesis, testosterone biosynthesis and secretion
Infections of the reproductive tract	Bacterial strains that colonize the male reproductive tract causes inflammatory damage by inducing leukocyte migration, release of cytokines and other inflammatory mediators, activation of macrophages, lymphocytes and other immunoreactive cells	Reduces serum testosterone levels by disrupting the hormonal axis, increase in LH and FSH levels

[57]. Furthermore, during glucocorticoid production by 11β-hydroxysteroid dehydrogenase-1 (11βHSD-1), NADPH was produced as a cofactor that is used for the biosynthesis of steroidogenic enzymes and testosterone [58].

Stress adversely affects steroidogenesis, since changes in the autonomic catecholaminergic activities during stress may suppress Leydig cell functions, thus inhibiting steroidogenic enzyme activities and testosterone production [11]. Stress-induced elevations of glucocorticoid levels can directly decrease testosterone levels without altering LH levels [59–61]. Further, in case of chronic stress, a decrease in LH and GnRH levels becomes apparent [62, 63].

Heat stress on gonads

In males, testes are suspended in a scrotum outside the body in order to keep the temperature 2 to 4 °C lower than that of core body temperature. This is a requirement for normal spermatogenesis [64]. However, heat stress to the testes not only decreases semen quality but also indirectly lowers embryo quality after fertilization as the spermatozoa produced in overheated testis exhibits damage [65–67]. In this context, heat stress is responsible for enhancing ROS production as well as decreasing antioxidant enzyme activities, increasing NADPH oxidase activity and disrupting mitochondrial homeostasis [68, 69]. Numerous reports have documented that factors such as fever, sauna or steam room use, sleeping posture, long time sitting or driving, polyester-lined athletic supports, using a laptop on the lap and electric blankets impose negative effects on scrotal temperatures and subsequently spermatogenesis [70, 71]. Studies have also reported that clinical conditions such as cryptorchidism, varicocele, and acute febrile illness can increase testicular temperature and suppress spermatogenesis [70].

Activation of the hypothalamic–pituitary–adrenal (HPA) axis and the consequent increase in plasma glucocorticoid concentrations are two of the most important responses to heat stress. Heat stress imparts detrimental effects on male reproduction partly by disrupting the normal release of GnRH from the hypothalamus as well as LH and FSH from the anterior pituitary gland [72]. Several studies have indicated that testicular heat stress leads to a decline in the circulating levels of testosterone and LH but increases serum cortisol levels [73, 74]. Testicular heat stress also leads to Leydig cell apoptosis and a reduction in testosterone biosynthesis in adult rat testes [75]. Moreover, increased testicular temperature adversely affects Sertoli cell function, production of testicular androgen-binding protein, spermatogenesis and semen parameters [76]. Thus, increased heat stress elevates the generation of ROS in the male reproductive tract by directly affecting cellular metabolism [69] and by influencing stress hormone levels [77].

The resulting increase in ROS production, in turn, damages testicular germ cells and other endocrine cells to disrupt the hormonal balance, thereby curbing male fertility [34].

Environmental toxicants

Exposure to environmental contaminants adversely affects the male reproductive potential [78, 79]. Male infertility caused by exposure to environmental toxicants such as cadmium [80, 81], mercury [82, 83], bisphenol A (BPA) [84, 85] and dioxin [86] is a worldwide problem. Even chemical components of air pollution can induce OS by triggering redox-sensitive pathways subsequently leading to various malaise, such as inflammation and cell death [87].

These contaminations deteriorate semen parameters, DNA integrity via disrupting Leydig and Sertoli cell function, hormone biosynthesis, gene expression and epigenetic modifications [12, 88, 89]. These toxicants commonly act as 'endocrine disrupting chemicals' (EDCs) that interfere with normal hormonal functions [90], enhance the level of circulating cortisol owing to OS induction [91] and reduces circulating testosterone levels [92, 93]. Increased cortisol decreases LH secretion through crosstalk between the HPG-HPA axes. Decreased LH concentration fails to stimulate the Leydig cells resulting in decreased testosterone production, whereas decreased FSH affects normal Sertoli cell functions [94]. These toxicants also interfere with the cellular communications and adhesions between Sertoli–Sertoli cells and Sertoli–germ cells via the phosphatidylinositol 3-kinase (PI3K)/c-Src/focal adhesion kinase (FAK) signalling pathway which leads to reproductive dysfunction [95] and disrupted hormonal secretion. Thus, these toxicants disrupt normal male reproductive hormonal balance by their disruptive influence upon the endocrine and reproductive organs as well as by interfering in the cross-talk among different endocrine axes [96].

Electromagnetic radiations

Since the last few decades, it has been widely reported that long-term exposure to electromagnetic radiations can generate ROS in reproductive organs, which not only declines motility, viability, and normal morphology of functional spermatozoa [97, 98], but also disorients reproductive hormonal profiles. The use of cell phones [99], wireless internet [100] and other occupational or environmental radiations [101] are found to be major causative factors directly augmenting ROS generation in male reproductive organs [102, 103]. Electromagnetic radiation affects the HPA axis and increases adrenocorticotropic hormone (ACTH) secretion from the anterior pituitary thereby increasing the production of cortisol from adrenal cortex [104]. These radiations can also decrease testosterone secretion from Leydig cells by disrupting the male reproductive hormonal axis [105]. Electromagnetic radiation significantly affect LH levels but not FSH and PRL levels [106]. It has also been reported that exposure to electromagnetic waves directly affects the pineal gland, thereby deteriorating the biological effect of melatonin on GnRH pulse in the hypothalamus [107]. Thus, altered GnRH levels influence FSH and LH secretion and negatively affects testosterone synthesis in the testis [108].

Exercise

Contrary to regular exercise that enhances antioxidant defences in the body, unaccustomed and/or exhaustive exercise can lead to the undesirable generation of excessive ROS [109]. Although the exact redox mechanisms remain elusive, it seems that mitochondria, NADPH oxidase (NOX), and xanthine oxidase (XO) are the major endogenous sources of ROS in skeletal muscle [109]. Some studies showed that moderate physical activity can increase FSH, LH, and testosterone levels [110], which is widely associated with increased energy and muscle strength [111, 112]. Despite the impact of moderate exercise, data suggest that vigorous exercise may decrease LH, FSH, and testosterone levels as well as semen parameters [113, 114]. However, other investigators have reported that testosterone levels remain unaltered following heavy exercise [115, 116].

Obesity

Obesity is a complex health disorder that severely affects hormonal balance [117]. Obesity disrupts serum levels of leptin [118], ghrelin [119], adiponectin [120], orexin [121], obestatin [122] and other metabolic hormone profiles [117]. Reportedly, leptin correlates positively with body fat mass [123, 124] and a leptin-induced generation of ROS in human endothelial cells result from increased mitochondrial fatty acid oxidation [123, 124]. The activation of the HPG axis could be enhanced by leptin and thus stimulate the release of GnRH, FSH and LH [125]. Moreover, leptin can directly affect the gonads due to its receptor isoforms in gonadal tissue [125].

Though the impact of ghrelin on serum testosterone level is contentious [126–128], it is reported that ghrelin receptors are present in the testis and that ghrelin plays a key role in testosterone production, but not directly in spermatogenesis [126]. Increased ROS levels appear to cause increased levels of ghrelin [129] which may, in turn, result in obesity and further ROS production.

Serum adiponectin level is negatively correlated with both testosterone [130] and ROS production [131]. Orexin (hypocretin) is known to stimulate testosterone production by enhancing the activities of steroidogenic enzymes in Leydig cells [132]. It is also reported to attenuate ROS-induced cell damage [133]. All these metabolic hormones either directly or indirectly reduce the androgen profile in men.

The complex cross-talk among these hormones is interrupted in obesity, thus causing a massive annihilation of the hormonal milieu, which in turn affects male reproductive functions. Although there is a body of evidence highlighting the complexity and the multifactorial effects that obesity has on certain male reproductive functions, the correlation between obesity and semen parameters is still debated [134, 135].

Food intake

There is an inverse relationship between the dietary intake of antioxidant-rich food and incidence of human diseases [136]. Many naturally-occurring antioxidant compounds from plant sources have been identified as free radicals or active oxygen scavengers [136]. Studies show that men who consume high dietary fish, fruits, vegetables, legumes, whole grains and omega-3- and omega-6-fatty acids have better semen parameters compared with men consuming high fat, caffeine (> 800 mg/day), red meat, processed meat, pizza, sugary drinks, and sweets in their diet [137, 138]. Therefore, in order to compensate for poor nutritional vitamin intake, food and medicine are routinely supplemented with synthetic and natural food antioxidants.

It is well-known that chronic high-fat and high-protein diets lead to an increase in ROS generation and subsequently OS [139, 140] by disrupting the antioxidant defence [140] and mitochondrial metabolism [139, 141]. This in turn negatively impacts semen quality through alteration of hormone levels [142, 143]. Antioxidant therapies may possibly have a beneficial impact on semen parameters, probably by protecting semen from ROS, reducing OS and improving basic sperm parameters. This improvement can be established by stimulation of testosterone biosynthesis, FSH and LH secretion, inhibin B and enhancement of androgen profile [144]. Investigators have showed that mainly selenium, coenzyme Q10 (CoQ10), and N-acetyl-cysteine can affect semen parameters by increasing testosterone and inhibin B [145]. However, further research is warranted to determine if there are any appropriate antioxidant compounds as well as suitable doses that could potentially be used in clinical practice.

Alcohol

Alcohol consumption promotes the generation of ROS through its metabolism pathway in the liver by stimulating the activity of cytochrome P450 enzymes, alteration of certain levels of metals (particularly free iron or copper ions) in the body, and finally, reduction in the antioxidant levels [146]. Due to the critical contribution of certain metals (particularly iron and copper) to the production of hydroxyl radical, anything that increases the levels of these metals can also promote ROS generation and OS [147]. It has been reported that alcohol increases iron levels in the body not only by iron-rich alcoholic beverages, such as red wine, but also by enhancing the absorption of iron from food [148].

Evidences in both animals and humans show that alcohol is also associated with high levels of estradiol and this finds relevance in the fact that estradiol enhances beta-endorphin release that is conventionally linked with the effects of alcohol consumption [149]. Chronic alcohol consumption can reduce serum testosterone, LH, and FSH levels by affecting the interactions between the neural and endocrine systems [149, 150]. Alcohol disrupts the cleavage of GnRH molecule from its precursor pre-pro GnRH and prevents the movement of protein kinase C15 which is necessary for the GnRH-stimulation of LH and FSH [151, 152]. Eventually, this disrupts the endocrine balance and subsequently affects semen parameters [153].

Among testicular cells, Sertoli cells are those that are most affected by chronic alcohol consumption [154]. Since Sertoli cells contribute the most to testicular size, chronic alcohol abuse eventually causes testicular atrophy, degeneration of germ cells, decreased size of lumen of seminiferous tubules, an abundance of lipid droplets, vacuoles, dilatation of the blood vessels, variation in seminal vesicle diameter as well as apoptosis of Sertoli cells. Due to the intratesticular cross-talk between Sertoli and Leydig cells, Leydig cells are eventually also affected by these changes [154, 155]. Though the correlation between alcohol consumption and infertility seems to be dose-dependent, the threshold of alcohol consumption beyond which would affect male fertility remains ambiguous [156].

Opioids, narcotics and recreational drugs

Opioids administration is associated with disrupted spermatogenesis and reduced sexual performance [157]. Both endogenous and exogenous opioids inhibit GnRH secretion, by disrupting the functions of HPG axis [158]. They reportedly generate ROS [159], induce inflammation as well as aid DNA/chromosomal damages and apoptosis in cells by p53 [160, 161]. Opioid consumption leads to increase in serum concentrations of sex hormone binding globulin (SHBG), a protein which tightly binds testosterone and E2 thus restricting the levels of unbound testosterone [162, 163]. Therefore, for opioid users, the level of total testosterone and E2 remain subnormal [162, 163]. Consequently, decreased testosterone levels also result in the decrease of LH levels. The loss of integrity of the HPG axis via opioid actions on sex hormones and LH levels, lead to clinical hypogonadism [162, 164]. The opioid methadone is also reported to

significantly reduce testosterone levels by directly affecting steroidogenesis [158].

Marijuana contains the cannabinoid, delta-9-tetrahydrocannabinol (THC), which inhibits GnRH release and LH production [164]. Thus, THC, by imposing adversities upon the HPG axis and causing dose-dependent reduction in testosterone production, impairs spermatogenesis [164, 165] at different mitotic and meiotic stages, resulting in several morphogenetic sperm defects as well as gynecomastia, impaired libido, erectile and ejaculatory dysfunction [166].

Studies showed that heroin can decrease gonadotropin and testosterone levels by affecting the HPG axis [158]. Similarly, cocaine exposure can also disrupt normal gonadal functions and are associated with decreased testosterone production and HPG axis dysregulation [167].

Non-medical use of drug narcotics, such as hydrocodone and oxycodone can interfere with spermatogenesis through their effects on the hypothalamus, and suppress LH release [164].

Smoking

Smoking is a well-known cause of male subfertility/infertility [168]. A major mechanism for this effect appears to be ROS production by the interference of oxygen delivery to the testis which compromises the high metabolic requirements of spermatogenesis [168–170]. Smoking also releases a large number of mutagens and metabolites (including radioactive polonium, cadmium, benzopyrene, carbon monoxide, tar, naphthalene, and aromatic hydrocarbons) which disrupt the normal structure and function of the male reproductive organs [168, 169]. It may enhance OS not only directly through the production of reactive oxygen radicals in cigarette smoke, but also indirectly through the weakening of the antioxidant defence systems [171–173]. Studies have indicated that exposure to smoke can change plasma levels of testosterone, PRL, E2, FSH, LH and SHBG by effects on Leydig and Sertoli cells [171–173]. Studies have also shown that smoking is associated with alterations in semen quality of both fertile and infertile men by affecting pituitary, thyroid, adrenal and testicular functions [174].

Anabolic steroids

Regular consumption of exogenous steroids can produce ROS by disrupting mitochondrial respiratory chain complexes and lead to the release of inflammatory cytokines and apoptosis [175]. Exogenous steroid hormones inhibit spermatogenesis by suppressing the HPG axis, thus limiting the release of FSH and LH and in turn decreasing testosterone biosynthesis in the testis [176, 177]. Hypogonadism associated with anabolic androgenic steroid (AAS) abuse is usually reversible within 3–6 months after discontinuation. However, complete recovery takes more than 3 years or may even be impossible to achieve [164]. AAS abuse primarily produces Leydig cell alterations which lead to a decrease in testosterone synthesis [177]. However, disruption in the end stage of spermatogenesis with a lack of mature spermatozoa (oligozoospermia/ azoospermia), testicular atrophy, and morphologically-abnormal sperm have been reported in AAS consumers [178]. Following AAS discontinuation, Leydig cells start further proliferation but cellular counts generally remain less than normal, accounting for delayed recovery of testosterone levels and the occasional irreversible effects of AAS [179].

Endogenous factors

Though endogenous ROS is necessary for normal male reproductive functions, its excessive production may interfere with the endocrine axes and their cross-talk.

Aging

In the aged male, Leydig cells are oxidatively damaged due to excessive generation of endogenous ROS and decreased concentration and activity of antioxidant enzymes [180]. As a result of excessive ROS generation, oxidative modifications of DNA and alterations in the mitochondrial membrane potential required for testosterone synthesis take place [181, 182]. Alongside these changes, an increase in LH sensitivity due to diminishing LH receptors per cell and a reduced ability of LH to activate steroidogenic acute regulatory (StAR) protein, which transport cholesterol from the outer mitochondrial membrane to the inner, occurs [183, 184]. Thus, overproduction of ROS may play a role in age-related testicular degeneration associated with male infertility [185].

The steroidogenic steps regulated by the P450 enzymes are the most likely sites of ROS action [186, 187]. FSH and human chorionic gonadotropin (hCG) together have been reported to stimulate ROS-producing cellular metabolisms affecting differentiation processes in germ cells [185, 188, 189]. Furthermore, following ROS production, the activities of several enzymes of the testosterone biosynthetic pathway are reduced, resulting in further decrease in testosterone synthesis and secretion [190, 191].

Reproductive tract infections

Reproductive tract infections is an important cause of disrupted male reproductive function and infertility [47]. Many immunoregulatory and pro-inflammatory cytokines are produced by testicular spermatogenic and somatic cells, both under normal conditions as well as during an inflammatory scenario [192]. Cytokines (such as IL–1, IL–6 or TNF-α) are even produced by non-immune cells like Leydig cells and Sertoli cells, that appear as typical components of seminal plasma to maintain normal spermatogenesis [192, 193]. Reproductive tract infections can be caused by ejaculatory duct inflammation, epididymitis, sexually transmitted infections (e.g. gonorrhoea, *Chlamydia trachomatis*, *Escherichia coli*, mycobacteria and *Ureaplasma urealyticum*), urethritis, testicular torsion, varicocele and several other causes like chronic prostatitis, inflammation of one or both testes (orchitis), and even by some drug therapy (escitalopram, tramadol, levonorgestrel etc.) [47, 194]. With the progression of inflammatory damage and weakening of antioxidant defence, as a mitigation strategy against the colonised bacterial strains, there can be increased ROS levels in the male genital tract, affecting the prostate gland, seminal vesicles or the epididymis [47, 195].

Reproductive tract infections indirectly cause germ cell degeneration and disruption of spermatogenesis through either of the following occurrences [196]: (i) changes in testicular temperature following high fever; (ii) congestion of seminiferous tubule following interstitial oedema; or (iii) modification of testosterone production. Though studies on male sex hormones and reproductive tract infections are scanty, some investigators observed the reduction of testosterone together with an increase in LH and FSH levels in patients with reproductive tract infections [196–198]. It has been reported that in patients with chronic prostatitis, corticosterone level decreases, while testosterone level increases compared to normal controls [199]. Whereas in mumps orchitis, increased corticosterone level decreases both LH and FSH levels which results in reduced production of testosterone from Leydig cells [200].

Hormonal influence on the oxidative status of male reproduction

OS that occurs due to either the enhanced production of ROS or reduced availability of antioxidants may cause lipid peroxidation in Leydig cells and germ cells, damage to lipoproteins, protein aggregation and fragmentation, and steroidogenic enzyme inhibition [10]. Testicular OS causes a reduction in testosterone production, either as a result of the injury to the Leydig cells or to other endocrine structures like the anterior pituitary [201, 202]. Reportedly, normal steroidogenesis also generates ROS, which are largely produced by mitochondrial respiration and the catalytic reactions of the steroidogenic cytochrome P450 enzymes [186]. ROS generated in this way, in turn, have been identified to inhibit subsequent steroid productions, and to damage mitochondrial membranes of spermatozoa [203]. OS is associated with increased numbers of immature spermatozoa via an indirect effect on the male hormone production that is correlated with spermatogenesis [204, 205].

It has been reported that systemic hormones (FSH, LH, testosterone, E2, PRL) may regulate seminal total antioxidant capacity (TAC) [206, 207]. A positive relationship between PRL or free T4 (fT4) and a negative correlation between gonadotropins or gonadal steroids with TAC have also been shown [22]. It is evident that some hormones like testosterone and MLT may act as antioxidants to protect sperm and other testicular cells from damage induced by ROS [208, 209]. Other metabolites of the steroidogenic pathway like DHEA are reported to enhance the level of cellular antioxidants, but the proper mechanism is still unclear [210]. Direct and indirect relationships between testosterone and antioxidant levels like selenium and/or CoQ10 and between testosterone and zinc in infertile men, respectively, have been observed [207, 211]. CoQ10 can decrease FSH and LH levels [212]. A negative relationship has been found between serum level of testosterone, E2, fT4 and sperm DNA damage [213, 214]. Also, the antioxidant inhibition could affect triiodothyronine (T3), thyroxine (T4), neurotransmitter noradrenaline and increase sperm DNA damage [215]. Intramuscular or subcutaneous injection of highly purified FSH to idiopathic infertile men reduces ROS production [216] and the subsequent sperm DNA damage [217]. Although it has been reported that testosterone could produce DNA fragmentation in Sertoli and germ cells by stimulating caspase activities in Sertoli cells [218], long-term effects of antioxidants can alter FSH, testosterone, and inhibin B levels [219].

Mechanism of action

Innumerable exogenous and endogenous factors, as discussed above, can produce ROS in the male reproductive system by disrupting the balance of oxidants and antioxidants. Following the generation of ROS, the HPA axis becomes activated and releases corticosterone (in animals) and cortisol (in humans) in response to stress. These stress hormones, through the cross-talk between the HPG and HPA axes, negatively affect LH secretion from the anterior pituitary. Decreased LH fails to stimulate Leydig cells to produce enough testosterone. Decreased FSH diminishes the release of androgen-binding protein (ABP) from the Sertoli cells, and thus, an overall decline in circulating testosterone occurs during severe OS.

ROS also affect HPT axis to reduce T3 and T4 secretion. Decreased T3 reduces the levels of the StAR mRNA and protein in Leydig cells, as well as testosterone production [220]. Increased OS also decreases the secretion of insulin from the pancreas which further negatively affects T3 release from the thyroid gland and thereby testosterone biosynthesis.

Conditions such as obesity not only involve the HPA and HPT axes, it also includes several metabolic hormones that manifest ROS-induced alterations in male reproductive functions. Obesity-induced ROS can affect adipocytes to secrete more leptin, which together with insulin, negatively regulate T3-release and thereby inhibit testicular functions. Leptin, secreted by adipocytes also inhibit GnRH release from the hypothalamus.

Testicular E2 and inhibin are produced intensely during OS, which then inhibit testosterone release. Following ROS exposure, aromatase activity increases which result in more E2 production. ROS exposure is also reported to increase PRL secretion from anterior pituitary which causes decreased GnRH release. Infections in the reproductive tract can lead to the production of pro-inflammatory cytokines (TNF-α, IL-1b, and IL-6) which again inhibit both GnRH release and testosterone secretion.

Thus, through its actions on an individual hormonal axis and/or by disrupting the cross-talk among different endocrine systems, ROS can lead to decreased testosterone production as the outcome of endocrine disruption. Decreased testosterone fails to regulate spermatogenesis properly to produce enough mature spermatozoa. It also fails to maintain the normal growth of accessory reproductive organs which play crucial roles in sperm maturation. As a prime regulator of male reproductive behaviour, testosterone deficiency may lead to suppressed sexual behaviour among men. Thus, by disrupting the endocrine reproductive functions, ROS may result in male infertility (Fig. 1).

Conclusion

This review summarizes the alterations of the reproductive endocrinological status by numerous endogenous and exogenous sources of ROS. Pivotal hormonal regulators of male reproductive functions can be affected by the disruption of the balance between ROS production and the antioxidant defence mechanism in the male reproductive system. Uncontrolled generation of ROS may directly damage reproductive tissues or can interfere with the normal regulatory mechanisms of the HPG axis and its crosstalk with other endocrine axes, to adversely affect male reproductive functioning, thereby inducing male infertility.

Abbreviations

11β-HSD: 11β-hydroxysteroid dehydrogenase; AAS: Anabolic androgenic steroid; AMH: Anti-Mullerian hormone; CORT: Corticosterone; delta-9-THC: Delta-9-tetrahydrocannabinol; DHEA: Dehydroepiandrosterone; E2: Estradiol; FSH: Follicle-stimulating hormone; fT4: Free T4; GC: Glucocorticoid; GnRH: Gonadotropin releasing hormone; HPG: Hypothalamic-pituitary-gonadal; LH: Luteinizing hormone; MLT: Melatonin; NOX: NADPH oxidase; OS: Oxidative stress; PRL: Prolactin; ROS: Reactive oxygen species; SHBG: Sex hormone binding globulin; TAC: Total antioxidant capacity; XO: Xanthine oxidase

Acknowledgements
Authors acknowledge the support by the American Center for Reproductive Medicine, Cleveland Clinic, USA.

Authors' contributions

MD and SD drafted this article and contributed equally in the writing of the manuscript. AA conceived the original design for this study and supervised the project. PS, DD and RH revised the article critically for its scientific content and edited the manuscript and MRS helped supervise the writing of the manuscript. All authors read and approved the final manuscript.

Competing interests

The authors declare that they have no competing interests.

Author details

¹Reproductive Biotechnology Research Center, Avicenna Research Institute, Academic Center for Education, Culture and Research, Tehran, Iran. ²American Center for Reproductive Medicine, Cleveland Clinic, Cleveland, Ohio 44195, USA. ³Department of Physiology, Faculty of Medicine, MAHSA University, Jalan SP2, Bandar Saujana Putra, 42610 Jenjarom, Selangor, Malaysia. ⁴Department of Physiology, Faculty of Medicine, Universiti Teknologi MARA, Sungai Buloh Campus, Jalan Hospital, 47000 Sungai Buloh, Selangor, Malaysia. ⁵Department of Medical Biosciences, University of the Western Cape, Bellville, Cape Town 7535, South Africa. ⁶Reproductive Immunology Research Center, Avicenna Research Institute, Academic Center for Education, Culture and Research, Tehran, Iran.

References

1. Carlsen E, Giwercman A, Keiding N, Skakkebaek NE. Evidence for decreasing quality of semen during past 50 years. Bmj. 1992;305(6854):609–13.

2. Swan SH, Elkin EP, Fenster L. The question of declining sperm density revisited: an analysis of 101 studies published 1934-1996. Environ Health Perspect. 2000;108(10):961.

3. Rolland M, Le Moal J, Wagner V, Royère D, De Mouzon J. Decline in semen concentration and morphology in a sample of 26 609 men close to general population between 1989 and 2005 in France. Hum Reprod. 2012;28(2):462–70.

4. Sengupta P, Dutta S, Krajewska-Kulak E. The disappearing sperms: analysis of reports published between 1980 and 2015. Am J Mens Health. 2017;11(4): 1279–1304.

5. Sikka SC. Relative impact of oxidative stress on male reproductive function. Curr Med Chem. 2001;8(7):851–62.

6. Agarwal A, Prabakaran SA. Mechanism, measurement, and prevention of oxidative stress in male reproductive physiology. Indian J Exp Biol. 2005; 43(11):963–74.

7. Rakhit M, Gokul SR, Agarwal A, du Plessis SS. Antioxidant strategies to overcome OS in IVF-embryo transfer. In: Studies on Women's Health. Editors: Agarwal, A., Aziz, N. and Rizk, B. Humana Press, Springer Science +Business Media, New York; 2013. p. 237–262.

8. Barazani Y, Katz BF, Nagler HM, Stember DS. Lifestyle, environment, and male reproductive health. Urol Clin North Am. 2014;41(1):55–66.

9. Sullivan LB, Chandel NS. Mitochondrial reactive oxygen species and cancer. Cancer Metab. 2014;2:17.

10. Darbandi S, Darbandi M. Lifestyle modifications on further reproductive problems. Cresco J Reprod Sci. 2016;1(1):1–2.

11. Hardy MP, Gao H-B, Dong Q, Ge R, Wang Q, Chai WR, et al. Stress hormone and male reproductive function. Cell Tissue Res. 2005;322(1):147–53.

12. Diamanti-Kandarakis E, Bourguignon J-P, Giudice LC, Hauser R, Prins GS, Soto AM, et al. Endocrine-disrupting chemicals: an Endocrine Society scientific statement. Endocr Rev. 2009;30(4):293–342.

13. Spiers JG, Chen HJ, Sernia C, Lavidis NA. Activation of the hypothalamic-pituitary-adrenal stress axis induces cellular oxidative stress. Front Neurosci. 2014;8:456.

14. Appasamy M, Muttukrishna S, Pizzey A, Ozturk O, Groome N, Serhal P, et al. Relationship between male reproductive hormones, sperm DNA damage and markers of oxidative stress in infertility. Reprod BioMed Online. 2007; 14(2):159–65.

15. Baker H, Burger H, de Kretser D, Hudson B (1986) Relative incidence of etiologic disorders in male infertility. In: Santen RJ, Swerdloff RS (eds) Male reproductive dysfunction: diagnosis and management of hypogonadism, infertility and impotence. Marcel Dekker, New York, pp 341–372.

16. Santen R, Paulsen C. Hypogonadotropic eunuchoidism. I. Clinical study of the mode of inheritance. J Clin Endocrinol Metab. 1973;36(1):47–54.

17. Kavoussi P, Costabile RA, Salonia A. Clinical urologic endocrinology: principles for Men's health. London: Springer; 2012.

18. Jameson JL. Harrison's endocrinology, 4E. New York: McGraw-Hill Education; 2016.

19. Patton PE, Battaglia DE. Office andrology. New York: Humana Press; 2007.

20. Byrd W, Bennett MJ, Carr BR, Dong Y, Wians F, Rainey W. Regulation of biologically active dimeric inhibin a and B from infancy to adulthood in the male. J Clin Endocrinol Metab. 1998;83(8):2849–54.

21. Raivio T, Perheentupa A, McNeilly AS, Groome NP, Anttila R, Siimes MA, et al. Biphasic increase in serum inhibin B during puberty: a longitudinal study of healthy Finnish boys. Pediatr Res. 1998;44(4):552–6.

22. Mancini A, Festa R, Silvestrini A, Nicolotti N, Di Donna V, La Torre G, et al. Hormonal regulation of total antioxidant capacity in seminal plasma. J Androl. 2009;30(5):534–40.

23. Parker CR. Dehydroepiandrosterone and dehydroepiandrosterone sulfate production in the human adrenal during development and aging. Steroids. 1999;64(9):640–7.

24. Jacob MH, DdR J, Belló-Klein A, Llesuy SF, Ribeiro MF. Dehydroepiandrosterone modulates antioxidant enzymes and Akt signaling in healthy Wistar erat hearts. J Steroid Biochem Mol Biol. 2008;112(1):138–44.

25. Lu C, Yang W, Chen M, Liu T, Yang J, Tan P, et al. Inhibin a inhibits follicle-stimulating hormone (FSH) action by suppressing its receptor expression in cultured rat granulosa cells. Mol Cell Endocrinol. 2009;298(1–2):48–56.

26. Li C, Zhou X. Melatonin and male reproduction. Clin Chim Acta. 2015;446:175–80.

27. Awad H, Halawa F, Mostafa T, Atta H. Melatonin hormone profile in infertile males. Int J Androl. 2006;29(3):409–13.

28. La Marca A, Sighinolfi G, Radi D, Argento C, Baraldi E, Artenisio AC, et al. Anti-Müllerian hormone (AMH) as a predictive marker in assisted reproductive technology (ART). Hum Reprod Update. 2010;16(2):113–30.

29. Holdcraft RW, Braun RE. Hormonal regulation of spermatogenesis. Int J Androl. 2004;27(6):335–42.

30. Trigo RV, Bergadá I, Rey R, Ballerini MG, Bedecarrás P, Bergadá C, et al. Altered serum profile of inhibin B, pro-αC and anti-Müllerian hormone in prepubertal and pubertal boys with varicocele. Clin Endocrinol. 2004;60(6): 758–64.

31. Castañeda Cortés DC, Langlois VS, Fernandino JI. Crossover of the hypothalamic pituitary–adrenal/Interrenal, –thyroid, and –gonadal axes in testicular development. Front Endocrinol. 2014;5:139.

32. Bisht S, Faiq M, Tolahunase M, Dada R. Oxidative stress and male infertility. Nat Rev Urol. 2017;14(8):470–85.

33. Gosalvez J, Tvrda E, Agarwal A. Free radical and superoxide reactivity detection in semen quality assessment: past, present, and future. J Assist Reprod Genet. 2017;34:697–707.

34. Agarwal A, Virk G, Ong C, du Plessis SS. Effect of oxidative stress on male reproduction. World J Men's Health. 2014;32(1):1–17.

35. Ramalho-Santos J, Varum S, Amaral S, Mota PC, Sousa AP, Amaral A. Mitochondrial functionality in reproduction: from gonads and gametes to embryos and embryonic stem cells. Hum Reprod Update. 2009;15(5):553–72.

36. Kussmaul L, Hirst J. The mechanism of superoxide production by NADH: ubiquinone oxidoreductase (complex I) from bovine heart mitochondria. Proc Natl Acad Sci U S A. 2006;103(20):7607–12.

37. Vinogradov AD, Grivennikova VG. Generation of superoxide-radical by the NADH:ubiquinone oxidoreductase of heart mitochondria. Biochem Mosc. 2005;70(2):120–7.

38. Kehrer JP. The Haber-Weiss reaction and mechanisms of toxicity. Toxicology. 2000;149(1):43–50.

39. Blaylock MG, Cuthbertson BH, Galley HF, Ferguson NR, Webster NR. The effect of nitric oxide and peroxynitrite on apoptosis in human polymorphonuclear leukocytes. Free Radic Biol Med. 1998;25(6):748–52.

40. Sabeur K, Ball B. Characterization of NADPH oxidase 5 in equine testis and spermatozoa. Reprod. 2007;134(2):263–70.

41. Petrushanko IY, Lobachev VM, Kononikhin AS, Makarov AA, Devred F, Kovacic H, et al. Oxidation of capital ES, Cyrillicsmall a, Cyrillic2+-binding domain of NADPH oxidase 5 (NOX5): toward understanding the mechanism of inactivation of NOX5 by ROS. PLoS One. 2016;11(7):e0158726.

42. Rengan AK, Agarwal A, van der Linde M, du Plessis SS. An investigation of excess residual cytoplasm in human spermatozoa and its distinction from the cytoplasmic droplet. Reprod Biol Endocrinol. 2012;10(1):92.

43. Saleh RA, Agarwal A, Nada EA, El-Tonsy MH, Sharma RK, Meyer A, et al. Negative effects of increased sperm DNA damage in relation to seminal

oxidative stress in men with idiopathic and male factor infertility. Fertil Steril. 2003;79:1597–605.

44. Gharagozloo P, Aitken RJ. The role of sperm oxidative stress in male infertility and the significance of oral antioxidant therapy. Hum Reprod. 2011;26(7):1628–40.

45. Lavranos G, Balla M, Tzortzopoulou A, Syriou V, Angelopoulou R. Investigating ROS sources in male infertility: a common end for numerous pathways. Reprod Toxicol. 2012;34(3):298–307.

46. Agarwal A, Saleh RA, Bedaiwy MA. Role of reactive oxygen species in the pathophysiology of human reproduction. Fertil Steril. 2003;79(4):829–43.

47. Azenabor A, Ekun AO, Akinloye O. Impact of inflammation on male reproductive tract. J Reprod Infertil. 2015;16(3):123.

48. World Health Organization. WHO laboratory manual for the examination and processing of human semen. Fifth Edition. WHO: Geneva, 2010.

49. Agarwal A, Prabakaran S, Allamaneni SS. Relationship between oxidative stress, varicocele and infertility: a meta-analysis. Reprod BioMed Online. 2006;12(5):630–3.

50. Shiraishi K, Matsuyama H, Takihara H. Pathophysiology of varicocele in male infertility in the era of assisted reproductive technology. Int J Urol. 2012; 19(6):538–50.

51. Clarke RN, Klock SC, Geoghegan A, Travassos DE. Relationship between psychological stress and semen quality among in-vitro fertilization patients. Hum Reprod. 1999;14(3):753–8.

52. Lampiao F. Variation of semen parameters in healthy medical students due to exam stress. Malawi Med J. 2009;21(4):166–7.

53. Gollenberg AL, Liu F, Brazil C, Drobnis EZ, Guzick D, Overstreet JW, et al. Semen quality in fertile men in relation to psychosocial stress. Fertil Steril. 2010;93(4):1104–11.

54. Flaherty RL, Owen M, Fagan-Murphy A, Intabli H, Healy D, Patel A, et al. Glucocorticoids induce production of reactive oxygen species/reactive nitrogen species and DNA damage through an iNOS mediated pathway in breast cancer. Breast Cancer Res. 2017;19(1):35.

55. Bakunina N, Pariante CM, Zunszain PA. Immune mechanisms linked to depression via oxidative stress and neuroprogression. Immunol. 2015;144(3): 365–73.

56. O'Hara L, McInnes K, Simitsidellis I, Morgan S, Atanassova N, Slowikowska-Hilczer J, et al. Autocrine androgen action is essential for Leydig cell maturation and function, and protects against late-onset Leydig cell apoptosis in both mice and men. FASEB J. 2015;29(3):894–910.

57. Gao HB, Tong MH, Hu YQ, Guo QS, Ge R, Hardy MP. Glucocorticoid induces apoptosis in rat leydig cells. Endocrinol. 2002;143(1):130–8.

58. MacAdams MR, White RH, Chipps BE. Reduction of serum testosterone levels during chronic glucocorticoid therapy. Ann Intern Med. 1986;104(5):648–51.

59. Norman R. Effects of corticotropin-releasing hormone on luteinizing hormone, testosterone, and cortisol secretion in intact male rhesus macaques. Biol Reprod. 1993;49(1):148–53.

60. Orr T, Taylor M, Bhattacharyya A, Collins D, Mann D. Acute immobilization stress disrupts testicular steroidogenesis in adult male rats by inhibiting the activities of 17α-hydroxylase and 17, 20-Lyase without affecting the binding of LH/hCG receptors. J Androl. 1994;15(4):302–8.

61. Gao H-B, Tong M-H, Hu Y-Q, You H-Y, Guo Q-S, Ge R-S, et al. Mechanisms of glucocorticoid-induced Leydig cell apoptosis. Mol Cell Endocrinol. 2003; 199(1):153–63.

62. Almeida S, Anselmo-Franci J, Silva AR e, Carvalho TL. Chronic intermittent immobilization of male rats throughout sexual development: a stress protocol. Exp Physiol. 1998;83(05):701–4.

63. Wagenmaker ER, Breen KM, Oakley AE, Tilbrook AJ, Karsch FJ. Psychosocial stress inhibits amplitude of gonadotropin-releasing hormone pulses independent of cortisol action on the type II glucocorticoid receptor. Endocrinol. 2009;150(2):762–9.

64. Ivell R. Lifestyle impact and the biology of the human scrotum. Reprod Biol Endocrinol. 2007;5(1):15.

65. Paul C, Murray AA, Spears N, Saunders PT. A single, mild, transient scrotal heat stress causes DNA damage, subfertility and impairs formation of blastocysts in mice. Reprod. 2008;136(1):73–84.

66. Paul C, Teng S, Saunders PT. A single, mild, transient scrotal heat stress causes hypoxia and oxidative stress in mouse testes, which induces germ cell death. Biol Reprod. 2009;80(5):913–9.

67. Yaeram J, Setchell BP, Maddocks S. Effect of heat stress on the fertility of male mice in vivo and in vitro. Reprod Fertil Dev. 2006;18(6):647–53.

68. Moon EJ, Sonveaux P, Porporato PE, Danhier P, Gallez B, Batinic-Haberle I,

et al. NADPH oxidase-mediated reactive oxygen species production activates hypoxia-inducible factor-1 (HIF-1) via the ERK pathway after hyperthermia treatment. Proc Natl Acad Sci. 2010;107(47):20477–82.

69. Belhadj Slimen I, Najar T, Ghram A, Dabbebi H, Ben Mrad M, Abdrabbah M. Reactive oxygen species, heat stress and oxidative-induced mitochondrial damage. Rev Int J Hyperthermia. 2014;30(7):513–23.

70. Jung A, Schuppe HC. Influence of genital heat stress on semen quality in humans. Andrologia. 2007;39(6):203–15.

71. Garolla A, Torino M, Sartini B, Cosci I, Patassini C, Carraro U, et al. Seminal and molecular evidence that sauna exposure affects human spermatogenesis. Hum Reprod. 2013;28(4):877–85.

72. Aggarwal A, Upadhyay R. Heat stress and hormones, in heat stress and animal productivity. India: Springer; 2013. p. 27–51.

73. Rhynes W, Ewing L. Testicular endocrine function in Hereford bulls exposed to high ambient temperature 1. Endocrinology. 1973;92(2):509–15.

74. Hansen PJ. Effects of heat stress on mammalian reproduction. Philosophical transactions of the Royal Society of London B. Biol Sci. 2009;364(1534):3341–50.

75. Li Z, Tian J, Cui G, Wang M, Yu D. Effects of local testicular heat treatment on Leydig cell hyperplasia and testosterone biosynthesis in rat testes. Reproduction, fertility. Development. 2016;28(9):1424–32.

76. Hagenas L, Ritzen EM, Svensson J, Hansson V, Purvis K. Temperature dependence of Sertoli cell function. Int J Androl. 1978;1(Supplement 2): 449–58.

77. Megahed G, Anwar M, Wasfy S, Hammadeh M. Influence of heat stress on the cortisol and oxidant-antioxidants balance during Oestrous phase in buffalo-cows (Bubalus bubalis): Thermo-protective role of antioxidant treatment. Reprod Domest Anim. 2008;43(6):672–7.

78. Coutts SM, Fulton N, Anderson RA. Environmental toxicant-induced germ cell apoptosis in the human fetal testis. Hum Reprod. 2007;22(11):2912–8.

79. Wong W, Yan H, Li W, Lie P, Mruk D, Cheng C. Cell junctions in the testis as targets for toxicants. In: Richburg J, Hoyer P, editors. Comprehensive toxicology. Oxford: Elsevier; 2010. p. 167–88.

80. Benoff S, Hauser R, Marmar JL, Hurley IR, Napolitano B, Centola GM. Cadmium concentrations in blood and seminal plasma: correlations with sperm number and motility in three male populations (infertility patients, artificial insemination donors, and unselected volunteers). Mol Med. 2009; 15(7–8):248–62.

81. Luparello C, Sirchia R, Longo A. Cadmium as a transcriptional modulator in human cells. Crit Rev Toxicol. 2011;41(1):75–82.

82. Choy CM, Yeung QS, Briton-Jones CM, Cheung CK, Lam CW, Haines CJ. Relationship between semen parameters and mercury concentrations in blood and in seminal fluid from subfertile males in Hong Kong. Fertil Steril. 2002;78(2):426–8.

83. Mocevic E, Specht IO, Marott JL, Giwercman A, Jonsson BA, Toft G, et al. Environmental mercury exposure, semen quality and reproductive hormones in Greenlandic Inuit and European men: a cross-sectional study. Asian J Androl. 2013;15(1):97–104.

84. Welshons WV, Nagel SC, Vom Saal FS. Large effects from small exposures. III. Endocrine mechanisms mediating effects of bisphenol a at levels of human exposure. Endocrinology. 2006;147(6 Suppl):S56–69.

85. Calafat AM, Ye X, Wong LY, Reidy JA, Needham LL. Exposure of the U.S. population to bisphenol a and 4-tertiary-octylphenol: 2003-2004. Environ Health Perspect. 2008;116(1):39–44.

86. Galimova EF, Amirova ZK, Galimov Sh N. Dioxins in the semen of men with infertility. Environ Sci Pollut Res Int. 2015;22(19):14566–9.

87. Lodovici M, Bigagli E. Oxidative stress and air pollution exposure. Journal of toxicology. 2011;2011:1–9.

88. Pacey A. Environmental and lifestyle factors associated with sperm DNA damage. Hum Fertil. 2010;13(4):189–93.

89. Skinner MK, Manikkam M, Guerrero-Bosagna C. Epigenetic transgenerational actions of environmental factors in disease etiology. Trends Endocrinol Metab. 2010;21(4):214–22.

90. Sengupta P, Dutta S. Metals. In M. K. Skinner (Ed.), Encyclopedia of Reproduction. vol. 1, pp. 579–587. Academic Press: Elsevier, Cambridge, Massachusetts, United States.

91. Güven M, Bayram F, Ünlühizarci K, Kelestimur F. Endocrine changes in patients with acute organophosphate poisoning. Hum Exp Toxicol. 1999;18(10):598–601.

92. Herath CB, Jin W, Watanabe G, Arai K, Suzuki AK, Taya K. Adverse effects of environmental toxicants, octylphenol and bisphenol a, on male reproductive functions in pubertal rats. Endocrine. 2004;25(2):163–72.

93. Meeker JD, Rossano MG, Protas B, Padmanahban V, Diamond MP, Puscheck E, et al. Environmental exposure to metals and male reproductive hormones: circulating testosterone is inversely associated with blood molybdenum. Fertil Steril. 2010;93(1):130–40.

94. Shimon I, Lubina A, Gorfine M, Ilany J. Feedback inhibition of gonadotropins by testosterone in men with hypogonadotropic hypogonadism: comparison to the intact pituitary-testicular axis in primary hypogonadism. J Androl. 2006;27(3):358–64.

95. Sharma RP, Schuhmacher M, Kumar V. Review on crosstalk and common mechanisms of endocrine disruptors: scaffolding to improve PBPK/PD model of EDC mixture. Environ Int. 2017;99:1–14.

96. Sengupta P, Banerjee R. Environmental toxins: alarming impacts of pesticides on male fertility. Hum Exp Toxicol. 2014;33(10):1017–39.

97. Vignera S, Condorelli RA, Vicari E, D'Agata R, Calogero AE. Effects of the exposure to mobile phones on male reproduction: a review of the literature. J Androl. 2012;33(3):350–6.

98. Darbandi M, Darbandi S, Agarwal A, Henkle R, Sadeghi MR. The effects of exposure to low frequency electromagnetic fields on male fertility. Altern Ther Health Med. 2017;23

99. Agarwal A, Singh A, Hamada A, Kesari K. Cell phones and male infertility: a review of recent innovations in technology and consequences. Int Braz J Urol. 2011;37(4):432–54.

100. Yildirim ME, Kaynar M, Badem H, Cavis M, Karatas OF, Cimentepe E. What is harmful for male fertility: cell phone or the wireless internet? Kaohsiung J Med Sci. 2015;31(9):480–4.

101. Al-Quzwini OF, Al-Taee HA, Al-Shaikh SF. Male fertility and its association with occupational and mobile phone towers hazards: an analytic study. Middle East Fertil Soc J. 2016;21(4):236–40.

102. Agarwal A, Deepinder F, Sharma RK, Ranga G, Li J. Effect of cell phone usage on semen analysis in men attending infertility clinic: an observational study. Fertil Steril. 2008;89(1):124–8.

103. Agarwal A, Desai NR, Makker K, Varghese A, Mouradi R, Sabanegh E, et al. Effects of radiofrequency electromagnetic waves (RF-EMW) from cellular phones on human ejaculated semen: an in vitro pilot study. Fertil Steril. 2009;92(4):1318–25.

104. Mahdavi SM, Sahraei H, Yaghmaei P, Tavakoli H. Effects of electromagnetic radiation exposure on stress-related behaviors and stress hormones in male wistar rats. Biomolecules Ther. 2014;22(6):570.

105. Meo SA, Al-Drees AM, Husain S, Khan MM, Imran MB. Effects of mobile phone radiation on serum testosterone in Wistar albino rats. Saudi Med J. 2010;31(8):869–73.

106. Merhi ZO. Challenging cell phone impact on reproduction: a review. J Assist Reprod Genet. 2012;29(4):293–7.

107. Stevens RG, Davis S. The melatonin hypothesis: electric power and breast cancer. Environ Health Perspect. 1996;104(Suppl 1):135.

108. Malpaux B, Daveau A, Maurice F, Gayrard V, Thiery J-C. Short-day effects of melatonin on luteinizing hormone secretion in the ewe: evidence for central sites of action in the mediobasal hypothalamus. Biol Reprod. 1993;48(4):752–60.

109. Adefuye AO, Adeola HA, Sales KJ, Katz AA. Seminal fluid-mediated inflammation in physiology and pathology of the female reproductive tract. J Immunol Res. 2016;2016:1–13.

110. Vaamonde D, Da Silva-Grigoletto ME, García-Manso JM, Barrera N, Vaamonde-Lemos R. Physically active men show better semen parameters and hormone values than sedentary men. Eur J Appl Physiol. 2012;112(9):3267–73.

111. Grandys M, Majerczak J, Duda K, Zapart-Bukowska J, Kulpa J, Zoladz J. Endurance training of moderate intensity increases testosterone concentration in young, healthy men. Int J Sports Med. 2009;30(07):489–95.

112. Fahrner C, Hackney AC. Effects of endurance exercise on free testosterone concentration and the binding affinity of sex hormone binding globulin (SHBG). Int J Sports Med. 1998;19(01):12–5.

113. Flynn M, Pizza F, Brolinson P. Hormonal responses to excessive training: influence of cross training. Int J Sports Med. 1997;18(03):191–6.

114. Safarinejad MR, Azma K, Kolahi AA. The effects of intensive, long-term treadmill running on reproductive hormones, hypothalamus–pituitary–testis axis, and semen quality: a randomized controlled study. J Endocrinol. 2009; 200(3):259–71.

115. Kindermann W, Schnabel A, Schmitt W, Biro G, Cassens J, Weber F. Catecholamines, growth hormone, cortisol, insulin, and sex hormones in anaerobic and aerobic exercise. Eur J Appl Physiol Occup Physiol. 1982; 49(3):389–99.

116. Jurimae J, Jurimae T. Responses of blood hormones to the maximal rowing ergometer test in college rowers. J Sports Med Phys Fitness. 2001;41(1):73.

117. Kopelman PG. Hormones and obesity. Baillieres Clin Endocrinol Metab. 1994; 8(3):549–75.

118. Ahima RS. Revisiting leptin's role in obesity and weight loss. J Clin Invest. 2008;118(7):2380.

119. Álvarez-Castro P, Pena L, Cordido F. Ghrelin in obesity, physiological and pharmacological considerations. Mini Rev Med Chem. 2013;13(4):541–52.

120. Kawano J, Arora R. The role of adiponectin in obesity, diabetes, and cardiovascular disease. J Cardiometab Syndr. 2009;4(1):44–9.

121. Perez-Leighton C, Butterick-Peterson T, Billington C, Kotz C. Role of orexin receptors in obesity: from cellular to behavioral evidence. Int J Obes. 2013; 37(2):167–74.

122. Ren A-J, Guo Z-F, Wang Y-K, Lin L, Zheng X, Yuan W-J. Obestatin, obesity and diabetes. Peptides. 2009;30(2):439–44.

123. Bouloumie A, Marumo T, Lafontan M, Busse R. Leptin induces oxidative stress in human endothelial cells. FASEB J. 1999;13(10):1231–8.

124. Yamagishi SI, Edelstein D, Du XL, Kaneda Y, Guzman M, Brownlee M. Leptin induces mitochondrial superoxide production and monocyte chemoattractant protein-1 expression in aortic endothelial cells by increasing fatty acid oxidation via protein kinase a. J Biol Chem. 2001; 276(27):25096–100.

125. Wauters M, Considine RV, Van Gaal LF. Human leptin: from an adipocyte hormone to an endocrine mediator. Eur J Endocrinol. 2000;143(3):293–311.

126. Ishikawa T, Fujioka H, Ishimura T, Takenaka A, Fujisawa M. Ghrelin expression in human testis and serum testosterone level. J Androl. 2007;28(2):320–4.

127. Wang L, Fang F, Li Y, Zhang Y, Pu Y, Zhang X. Role of ghrelin on testosterone secretion and the mRNA expression of androgen receptors in adult rat testis. Systems Biol Reprod Med. 2011;57(3):119–23.

128. Greenman Y, Rouach V, Limor R, Gilad S, Stern N. Testosterone is a strong correlate of ghrelin levels in men and postmenopausal women. Neuroendocrinology. 2009;89(1):79–85.

129. Suzuki H, Matsuzaki J, Hibi T. Ghrelin and oxidative stress in gastrointestinal tract. J Clin Biochem Nutr. 2010;48(2):122–5.

130. Page ST, Herbst KL, Amory JK, Coviello AD, Anawalt BD, Matsumoto AM, et al. Testosterone administration suppresses adiponectin levels in men. J Androl. 2005;26(1):85–92.

131. Yuan F, Li Y-N, Liu Y-H, Yi B, Tian J-W, Liu F-Y. Adiponectin inhibits the generation of reactive oxygen species induced by high glucose and promotes endothelial NO synthase formation in human mesangial cells. Mol Med Rep. 2012;6(2):449–53.

132. Zheng D, Zhao Y, Shen Y, Chang X, Ju S, Guo L. Orexin A-mediated stimulation of 3β-HSD expression and testosterone production through MAPK signaling pathways in primary rat Leydig cells. J Endocrinol Investig. 2014;37(3):285–92.

133. Duffy CM, Nixon JP, Butterick TA. Orexin a attenuates palmitic acid-induced hypothalamic cell death. Mol Cell Neurosci. 2016;75:93–100.

134. Aggerholm AS, Thulstrup AM, Toft G, Ramlau-Hansen CH, Bonde JP. Is overweight a risk factor for reduced semen quality and altered serum sex hormone profile? Fertil Steril. 2008;90(3):619–26.

135. Al-Ali B M, Gutschi T, Pummer K, Zigeuner R, Brookman-May S, Wieland W, et al. Body mass index has no impact on sperm quality but on reproductive hormones levels. Andrologia. 2014;46(2):106–11.

136. Lobo V, Patil A, Phatak A, Chandra N. Free radicals, antioxidants and functional foods: impact on human health. Pharmacognosy Rev. 2010;4(8):118.

137. Chavarro JE, Toth TL, Sadio SM, Hauser R. Soy food and isoflavone intake in relation to semen quality parameters among men from an infertility clinic. Hum Reprod. 2008;23(11):2584–90.

138. Mendiola J, Torres-Cantero AM, Moreno-Grau JM, Ten J, Roca M, Moreno-Grau S, et al. Food intake and its relationship with semen quality: a case-control study. Fertil Steril. 2009;91(3):812–8.

139. Ruggiero C, Ehrenshaft M, Cleland E, Stadler K. High-fat diet induces an initial adaptation of mitochondrial bioenergetics in the kidney despite evident oxidative stress and mitochondrial ROS production. Am J Physiol Endocrinol Metab. 2011;300(6):8.

140. Kolodziej U, Maciejczyk M, Niklinska W, Waszkiel D, Zendzian-Piotrowska M, Zukowski P, et al. Chronic high-protein diet induces oxidative stress and alters the salivary gland function in rats. Arch Oral Biol. 2017;84:6–12.

141. Kahle M, Schafer A, Seelig A, Schultheiss J, Wu M, Aichler M, et al. High fat diet-induced modifications in membrane lipid and mitochondrial-membrane protein signatures precede the development of hepatic insulin

142. Chakraborty TR, Donthireddy L, Adhikary D, Chakraborty S. Long-term high fat diet has a profound effect on body weight, hormone levels, and estrous cycle in mice. Med Sci Monit. 2016;22:1601–8.

143. Attaman JA, Toth TL, Furtado J, Campos H, Hauser R, Chavarro JE. Dietary fat and semen quality among men attending a fertility clinic. Hum Reprod. 2012; 27(5):1466–74.

144. Agarwal A, Sekhon LH. The role of antioxidant therapy in the treatment of male infertility. Hum Fertil (Camb). 2010;13(4):217–25.

145. Ahmadi S, Bashiri R, Ghadiri-Anari A, Nadjarzadeh A. Antioxidant supplements and semen parameters: an evidence based review. Int J Reprod Biomed. 2016; 14(12):729–36.

146. Wu D, Cederbaum AI. Alcohol, oxidative stress, and free radical damage. Alcohol Res Health. 2003;27:277–84.

147. Qureshi GA, Memon SA, Memon AB, Ghouri RA, Memon JM, Parvez SH. The emerging role of iron, zinc, copper, magnesium and selenium and oxidative stress in health and diseases. Brill Online. 2005;19(2):147–69.

148. Whitfield JB, Zhu G, Heath AC, Powell LW, Martin NG. Effects of alcohol consumption on indices of iron stores and of iron stores on alcohol intake markers. Alcohol Clin Exp Res. 2001;25(7):1037–45.

149. Emanuele MA, Emanuele N. Alcohol and the male reproductive system. Alcohol Res Health. 2001;25(4):282–7.

150. Maneesh M, Dutta S, Chakrabarti A, Vasudevan D. Alcohol abuse-duration dependent decrease in plasma testosterone and antioxidants in males. Indian J Physiol Pharmacol. 2006;50(3):291.

151. Uddin S, Wilson T, Emanuele M, Williams D, Kelley M, Emanuele N. Ethanol-induced alterations in the posttranslational processing, but not secretion of luteinizing hormone-releasing hormone in vitro. Alcohol Clin Exp Res. 1996; 20(3):556–60.

152. Kim JH, Kim HJ, Noh HS, Roh GS, Kang SS, Cho GJ, et al. Suppression by ethanol of male reproductive activity. Brain Res. 2003;989(1):91–8.

153. Salonen I, Huhtaniemi I. Effects of chronic ethanol diet on pituitary-testicular function of the rat. Biol Reprod. 1990;42(1):55–62.

154. Zhu Q, Van Thiel DH, Gavaler JS. Effects of ethanol on rat Sertoli cell function: studies in vitro and in vivo. Alcohol Clin Exp Res. 1997;21(8):1409–17.

155. Zhu Q, Meisinger J, Emanuele NV, Emanuele MA, LaPaglia N, Thiel DH. Ethanol exposure enhances apoptosis within the testes. Alcohol Clin Exp Res. 2000;24(10):1550–6.

156. Pajarinen J, Karhunen PJ, Savolainen V, Lalu K, Penttilä A, Laippala P. Moderate alcohol consumption and disorders of human spermatogenesis. Alcohol Clin Exp Res. 1996;20(2):332–7.

157. Subiran N, Casis L, Irazusta J. Regulation of male fertility by the opioid system. Mol Med. 2011;17(7–8):846–53.

158. Brown TT, Wisniewski AB, Gonadal DAS. Adrenal abnormalities in drug users: cause or consequence of drug use behavior and poor health outcomes. Am J Infect Dis. 2006;2(3):130–5.

159. Sarafian TA, Magallanes JAM, Shau H, Tashkin D, Roth MD. Oxidative stress produced by marijuana smoke: an adverse effect enhanced by cannabinoids. Am J Respir Cell Mol Biol. 1999;20(6):1286–93.

160. Kim HR, Son BH, Lee SY, Chung KH, Oh SM. The role of p53 in marijuana smoke condensates-induced genotoxicity and apoptosis. Environ Health Toxicol. 2012;27:e2012017.

161. Faux SP, Tai T, Thorne D, Xu Y, Breheny D, Gaca M. The role of oxidative stress in the biological responses of lung epithelial cells to cigarette smoke. Biomarkers. 2009;1:90–6.

162. Abs R, Verhelst J, Maeyaert J, Van Buyten J-P, Opsomer F, Adriaensen H, et al. Endocrine consequences of long-term intrathecal administration of opioids. J Clin Endocrinol Metab. 2000;85(6):2215–22.

163. Daniell HW. Hypogonadism in men consuming sustained-action oral opioids. J Pain. 2002;3(5):377–84.

164. Fronczak CM, Kim ED, Barqawi AB. The insults of illicit drug use on male fertility. J Androl. 2012;33(4):515–28.

165. Park B, McPartland JM, Glass M. Cannabis, cannabinoids and reproduction. Prostaglandins Leukot Essent Fatty Acids. 2004;70(2):189–97.

166. Patra P, Wadsworth R. Quantitative evaluation of spermatogenesis in mice following chronic exposure to cannabinoids. Andrologia. 1991;23(2):151–6.

167. Heesch CM, Negus BH, Bost JE, Keffer JH, Snyder RW 2nd, Eichhorn EJ. Effects of cocaine on anterior pituitary and gonadal hormones. J Pharmacol Exp Ther. 1996;278(3):1195–200.

168. Meri ZB, Irshid IB, Migdadi M, Irshid AB, Mhanna SA. Does cigarette smoking affect seminal fluid parameters? A comparative study. Oman Med J. 2013;

28(1):12–6.

169. Sheynkin Y, Gioia K. Environmental and lifestyle considerations for the infertile male. AUA Update Ser. 2013;32(4):30–8.

170. Tostes RC, Carneiro FS, Lee AJ, Giachini FR, Leite R, Osawa Y, et al. Cigarette smoking and erectile dysfunction: focus on NO bioavailability and ROS generation. J Sex Med. 2008;5(6):1284–95.

171. Halmenschlager G, Rossetto S, Lara GM, Rhoden EL. Endocrinology: evaluation of the effects of cigarette smoking on testosterone levels in adult men. J Sex Med. 2009;6(6):1763–72.

172. Shiels MS, Rohrmann S, Menke A, Selvin E, Crespo CJ, Rifai N, et al. Association of cigarette smoking, alcohol consumption, and physical activity with sex steroid hormone levels in US men. Cancer Causes Control. 2009; 20(6):877–86.

173. Trummer H, Habermann H, Haas J, Pummer K. The impact of cigarette smoking on human semen parameters and hormones. Hum Reprod. 2002; 17(6):1554–9.

174. Kapoor D, Jones TH. Smoking and hormones in health and endocrine disorders. Eur J Endocrinol. 2005;152(4):491–9.

175. Neri M, Bello S, Bonsignore A, Cantatore S, Riezzo I, Turillazzi E, et al. Anabolic androgenic steroids abuse and liver toxicity. Mini Rev Med Chemist. 2011;11(5):430–7.

176. Buchanan JF, Davis LJ. Drug-induced infertility. Drug Intell Clin Pharm. 1984; 18(2):122–32.

177. de Souza GL, Hallak J. Anabolic steroids and male infertility: a comprehensive review. BJU Int. 2011;108(11):1860–5.

178. El Osta R, Almont T, Diligent C, Hubert N, Eschwege P, Hubert J. Anabolic steroids abuse and male infertility. Basic Clin Androl. 2016;26:1–8.

179. Foster ZJ, Housner JA. Anabolic-androgenic steroids and testosterone precursors: ergogenic aids and sport. Curr Sports Med Rep. 2004;3(4):234–41.

180. Fujii J, Iuchi Y, Matsuki S, Ishii T. Cooperative function of antioxidant and redox systems against oxidative stress in male reproductive tissues. Asian J Androl. 2003;5(3):231–42.

181. Allen JA, Shankara T, Janus P, Buck S, Diemer T, Held Hales K, et al. Energized, polarized, and actively respiring mitochondria are required for acute Leydig cell steroidogenesis. Endocrinology. 2006;147(8):3924–35.

182. Chen H, Zhou L, Lin C-Y, Beattie MC, Liu J, Zirkin BR. Effect of glutathione redox state on Leydig cell susceptibility to acute oxidative stress. Mol Cell Endocrinol. 2010;323(2):147–54.

183. Veldhuis JD. Recent insights into neuroendocrine mechanisms of aging of the human male hypothalamic-pituitary-gonadal Axis. J Androl. 1999;20(1):1–18.

184. Diemer T, Allen JA, Hales KH, Hales DB. Reactive oxygen disrupts mitochondria in MA-10 tumor Leydig cells and inhibits steroidogenic acute regulatory (StAR) protein and steroidogenesis. Endocrinology. 2003;144(7):2882–91.

185. Koksal I, Usta M, Orhan I, Abbasoglu S, Kadioglu A. Potential role of reactive oxygen species on testicular pathology associated with infertility. Asian J Androl. 2003;5(2):95–100.

186. Hanukoglu I. Antioxidant protective mechanisms against reactive oxygen species (ROS) generated by mitochondrial P450 systems in steroidogenic cells. Drug Metab Rev. 2006;38(1–2):171–96.

187. Peltola V, Huhtaniemi I, Metsa-Ketela T, Ahotupa M. Induction of lipid peroxidation during steroidogenesis in the rat testis. Endocrinology. 1996; 137(1):105–12.

188. Perheentupa A, De Jong F, Huhtaniemi I. Biphasic effect of exogenous testosterone on follicle-stimulating hormone gene expression and synthesis in the male rat. Mol Cell Endocrinol. 1993;93(2):135–41.

189. Perheentupa A, Huhtaniemi I. Gonadotropin gene expression and secretion in gonadotropin-releasing hormone antagonist-treated male rats: effect of sex steroid replacement. Endocrinology. 1990;126(6):3204–9.

190. Aitken RJ, Roman SD. Antioxidant systems and oxidative stress in the testes. Oxidative Med Cell Longev. 2008;1(1):15–24.

191. Chigurupati S, Son TG, Hyun D-H, Lathia JD, Mughal MR, Savell J, et al. Lifelong running reduces oxidative stress and degenerative changes in the testes of mice. J Endocrinol. 2008;199(2):333–41.

192. Loveland KL, Klein B, Pueschl D, Indumathy S, Bergmann M, Loveland BE, et al. Cytokines in male fertility and reproductive pathologies: Immunoregulation and beyond. Front Endocrinol. 2017;8:1–16.

193. Maegawa M, Kamada M, Irahara M, Yamamoto S, Yoshikawa S, Kasai Y, et al. A repertoire of cytokines in human seminal plasma. J Reprod Immunol. 2002;54(1–2):33–42.

194. Joki-Korpela P, Sahrakorpi N, Halttunen M, Surcel HM, Paavonen J, Tiitinen A. The role of Chlamydia trachomatis infection in male infertility. Fertil

Steril. 2009;91(4 Suppl):1448–50.

195. Ochsendorf F. Infections in the male genital tract and reactive oxygen species. Hum Reprod Update. 1999;5(5):399–420.

196. Dejucq N, Jegou B. Viruses in the mammalian male genital tract and their effects on the reproductive system. Microbiol Mol Biol Rev. 2001;65(2):208–31.

197. Aiman J, Brenner PF, MacDonald PC. Androgen and estrogen production in elderly men with gynecomastia and testicular atrophy after mumps orchitis. J Clin Endocrinol Metab. 1980;50(2):380–6.

198. Adamopoulos DA, Lawrence DM, Vassilopoulos P, Contoyiannis PA, Swyer GI. Pituitary-testicular interrelationships in mumps orchitis and other viral infections. Br Med J. 1978;1(6121):1177–80.

199. Dimitrakov J, Joffe HV, Soldin SJ, Bolus R, Buffington CT, Nickel JC. Adrenocortical hormone abnormalities in men with chronic prostatitis/chronic pelvic pain syndrome. Urology. 2008;71(2):261–6.

200. Lane TM, Hines J. The management of mumps orchitis. BJU Int. 2006;97(1):1–2.

201. Zirkin BR, Chen H. Regulation of Leydig cell steroidogenic function during aging. Biol Reprod. 2000;63(4):977–81.

202. Turner TT, Bang HJ, Lysiak JJ. Experimental testicular torsion: reperfusion blood flow and subsequent testicular venous plasma testosterone concentrations. Urology. 2005;65(2):390–4.

203. Luo L, Chen H, Trush MA, Show MD, Anway MD, Zirkin BR. Aging and the brown Norway rat leydig cell antioxidant defense system. J Androl. 2006; 27(2):240–7.

204. Aitken RJ, Baker MA, Sawyer D. Oxidative stress in the male germ line and its role in the aetiology of male infertility and genetic disease. Reprod BioMed Online. 2003;7(1):65–70.

205. Agarwal A, Said TM. Role of sperm chromatin abnormalities and DNA damage in male infertility. Hum Reprod Update. 2003;9(4):331–45.

206. Meucci E, Milardi D, Mordente A, Martorana GE, Giacchi E, De Marinis L, et al. Total antioxidant capacity in patients with varicoceles. Fertil Steril. 2003;79:1577–83.

207. Mancini A, Leone E, Festa R, Grande G, Silvestrini A, Marinis L, et al. Effects of testosterone on antioxidant systems in male secondary hypogonadism. J Androl. 2008;29(6):622–9.

208. Chainy G, Samantaray S, Samanta L. Testosterone-induced changes in testicular antioxidant system. Andrologia. 1997;29(6):343–9.

209. Shang X, Huang Y, Ye Z, Yu X, Gu W. Protection of melatonin against damage of sperm mitochondrial function induced by reactive oxygen species. Zhonghua Nan Ke Xue. 2004;10(8):604–7.

210. Lakpour N, Mahfouz RZ, Akhondi MM, Agarwal A, Kharrazi H, Zeraati H, et al. Relationship of seminal plasma antioxidants and serum male hormones with sperm chromatin status in male factor infertility. Syst Biol Reprod Med. 2012;58(5):236–44.

211. Oluboyo A, Adijeh R, Onyenekwe C, Oluboyo B, Mbaeri T, Odiegwu C, et al. Relationship between serum levels of testosterone, zinc and selenium in infertile males attending fertility clinic in Nnewi, south East Nigeria. Afr J Med Med Sci. 2012;41:51–4.

212. Safarinejad MR. Efficacy of coenzyme Q10 on semen parameters, sperm function and reproductive hormones in infertile men. J Urol. 2009;182(1): 237–48.

213. Richthoff J, Spano M, Giwercman Y, Frohm B, Jepson K, Malm J, et al. The impact of testicular and accessory sex gland function on sperm chromatin integrity as assessed by the sperm chromatin structure assay (SCSA). Hum Reprod. 2002;17(12):3162–9.

214. Meeker JD, Singh NP, Hauser R. Serum concentrations of estradiol and free T4 are inversely correlated with sperm DNA damage in men from an infertility clinic. J Androl. 2008;29(4):379–88.

215. Dobrzyńska MM, Baumgartner A, Anderson D. Antioxidants modulate thyroid hormone-and noradrenaline-induced DNA damage in human sperm. Mutagenesis. 2004;19(4):325–30.

216. Palomba S, Falbo A, Espinola S, Rocca M, Capasso S, Cappiello F, et al. Effects of highly purified follicle-stimulating hormone on sperm DNA damage in men with male idiopathic subfertility: a pilot study. J Endocrinol Investig. 2011;34(10):747–52.

217. Colacurci N, Monti MG, Fornaro F, Izzo G, Izzo P, Trotta C, et al. Recombinant human FSH reduces sperm DNA fragmentation in men with idiopathic oligoasthenoteratozoospermia. J Androl. 2012;33(4):588–93.

218. Tesarik J, Martinez F, Rienzi L, Iacobelli M, Ubaldi F, Mendoza C, et al. In-vitro effects of FSH and testosterone withdrawal on caspase activation and DNA fragmentation in different cell types of human seminiferous epithelium. Hum Reprod. 2002;17(7):1811–9.

216. Palomba S, Falbo A, Espinola S, Rocca M, Capasso S, Cappiello F, et al. Effects of highly purified follicle-stimulating hormone on sperm DNA damage in men with male idiopathic subfertility: a pilot study. J Endocrinol Investig. 2011;34(10):747–52.

217. Colacurci N, Monti MG, Fornaro F, Izzo G, Izzo P, Trotta C, et al. Recombinant human FSH reduces sperm DNA fragmentation in men with idiopathic oligoasthenoteratozoospermia. J Androl. 2012;33(4):588–93.

218. Tesarik J, Martinez F, Rienzi L, Iacobelli M, Ubaldi F, Mendoza C, et al. In-vitro effects of FSH and testosterone withdrawal on caspase activation and DNA fragmentation in different cell types of human seminiferous epithelium. Hum Reprod. 2002;17(7):1811–9.

## 18

Meta-analysis of ART outcomes in women with different preconception TSH levels

T. Zhao[1], B. M. Chen[2], X. M. Zhao[3] and Z. Y. Shan[1*]

Abstract

Background: To assess whether elevated thyroid-stimulating hormone (TSH) levels before conception can predict poor outcomes of assisted reproductive technology (ART).

Methods: Prior to July 2018, we searched the PubMed, EMBASE, COCHRANE, Google Scholar, and CNKI databases for studies. Retrospective or prospective reports that compared ART results in patients with subclinical hypothyroidism (SCH) with normal thyroid function were selected. Two reviewers separately reviewed each potential article for qualification, analyzed the quality of the studies according to the Newcastle-Ottawa scale, and extracted the data. The PRISMA guidelines were adopted.

Results: We selected a total of 18 publications that included 14,846 participants for this meta-analysis. When the TSH cut-off value for SCH was set at 2.5 mIU/L, no significant differences were observed in ART-related outcomes between SCH patients and normal women. The evaluated outcomes included the live birth rate (LBR) (OR: 0.93; 95% CI (0.77,1.12), $P = 0.43$), clinical pregnancy rate (CPR) (OR:1.02; 95% CI (0.90,1.17); $P = 0.74$), pregnancy rate (PR) (OR: 1.00; 95% CI (0.89,1.12); $P = 0.99$), and miscarriage rate (MR) (OR:1.24; 95% CI (0.85, 1.80); $P = 0.26$). Furthermore, when a higher TSH level was used as the cut-off value to diagnose SCH (i.e., 3.5–5 mIU/L), a significant difference was found in the MR (OR: 1.91; 95% CI (1.09, 3.35); $P = 0.02$) between the two groups of ART-treated women. However, when a broader cut-off value was used to define SCH, no significant differences were observed in the LBR (OR: 0.72; 95% CI (0.47,1.11); $P = 0.14$), CPR (OR: 0.82; 95% CI (0.66,1.00); $P = 0.052$), or PR (OR: 1.07; 95% CI (0.72,1.60); $P = 0.74$) between the two groups of ART-treated women.

Conclusion: No difference was observed in ART outcomes when a TSH cut-off value of 2.5 mIU/L was used. However, when a broader TSH cut-off value was used, preconception SCH resulted in a higher miscarriage rate than in normal women.

Keywords: Thyroid-stimulating hormone, Pregnancy, Clinical pregnancy, Live birth, Miscarriage, Assisted reproduction technology

Background

SCH affects 2–5% of all pregnant women in the United States. This disease is characterized by abnormalities in the hypothalamic-pituitary-thyroid axis that are reflected by alter standard serum thyroxine (T4) levels and increased serum TSH levels [1]. Opinions vary regarding the different guidelines available related to the treatment of women with SCH seeking to use ART because the optimal therapy for these patients remains unknown. This is partly because of limitations related to a lack of consequence data on miscarriages that occur in early pregnancy.

Overt hypothyroidism (OH) is defined as a high level of TSH and a low level of T4 and is related to infertility as well as adverse pregnancy outcomes [2], including early pregnancy miscarriage, stillbirth and preterm delivery [3–5]. Recently, many studies have emerged that have evaluated the association between SCH during pregnancy and multiple poor maternal outcomes [6–8]. However, their conclusions have not been consistent. One meta-analysis demonstrated that SCH during pregnancy is related to multiple adverse neonatal and maternal consequences [9].

The relationship between ART outcomes and thyroid function has been a hot topic and the subject of a great deal of debate in recent years [10]. The reason for this

* Correspondence: shanzhongyan@medmail.com.cn
[1]Department of Endocrinology and Metabolism, Institute of Endocrinology, First Affiliated Hospital, China Medical University, Shenyang, Liaoning, China
Full list of author information is available at the end of the article

interest seems obvious, at least from an epidemiological point of view, because ART is continually being performed and thyroid disorders are highly prevalent in women of reproductive age. In accordance with the results described in a recent report by the European Society of Human Reproduction and Embryology (ESHRE), between 0.8 and 4.1% of children born in Europe are the result of in vitro fertilization (IVF) [11]. Until recently, societies governing the use of human reproductive technologies did not recommend measuring TSH levels in asymptomatic ovulatory women [12, 13]. However, the new guidelines reported by the American Society for Reproductive Medicine (ASRM) endorse measuring TSH concentrations in infertile women seeking to become pregnant [14]. The prevalence of thyroid disorders has increased in subfertile women, and this has been recognized by the American Thyroid Association (ATA) [15] and the Endocrine Society. These organizations have consequently produced recommendations regarding the measurement of TSH levels in woman at "high-risk" of thyroid disease, including asymptomatic infertile patients [16].

During a pregnancy, variations occur in the normal range of TSH levels, and this has led to the introduction of SCH, a more vaguely defined complication observed in pregnant patients [17]. While the lower range of normal serum TSH levels has remained consistent, the upper limit for normal TSH levels has changed dramatically in recent years [18]. The ATA and The National Association of Clinical Biochemistry (NACB) [19] have lowered the upper limit for normal TSH levels in the first trimester of pregnancy from 4.5 mIU/L to 2.5 mIU/L. [15] Other clinical institutions, such as the American Association for Clinical Chemistry (AACC), have traditionally set 5.0 mIU/L as the upper limit for normal TSH levels [20].

ART patients experience many barriers when attempting to achieve conception, and identifying the optimal range of pregestational TSH levels is now specifically recognized as an important parameter. Furthermore, the superovulation caused by ART generates a rapid increase in E2 levels [21] that increases the hepatic synthesis of thyroid-binding globulin and leads to a reduction in free, unbound T4 [22–24]. These events can potentially aggravate the condition of a patient with underlying SCH. The risk of poor iatrogenic-related reproductive outcomes in ART has made SCH a special focus in the ART population.

Though obstetricians can correct TSH in patients who are already pregnant, by inspecting data associated with a large cohort of ART patients, in this study, we attempt to determine whether elevated TSH levels in the preconception period predict adverse outcomes in ART patients. We seek to address whether it is appropriate to apply traditional TSH criteria in patients about to undergo ART (i.e., are these criteria associated with any clinical benefit) and to prompt reproductive medical organizations to develop methods to increase the ability of practitioners to identify and treat ART patients whose TSH status puts them at high risk of adverse results.

Methods

Eligibility criteria

The included studies were limited to prospective or retrospective studies that compared ART consequences in patients with SCH with normal thyroid function. Publications were excluded if (1) only women with SCH were described without a comparison group consisting of women without SCH, (2) the included women had overt hypothyroidism or hyperthyroidism (3) TSH was not evaluated before the ovarian stimulation cycle we begun, (4) the number of IVF/ICSI cycles was not specified, (5) no specific TSH cut-off value was used to define SCH.

Information sources and search

These searches were performed in the Medline, PubMed, EMBASE and COCHRANE, Google Scholar, CNKI databases. For instance, Medline was searched using the following search string for articles published from January 1990 to July 2018: (((("insemination"[MeSH Terms] OR "insemination"[All Fields]) OR ("fertilization in vitro"[All Fields] OR "fertilization in vitro"[MeSH Terms] OR ("fertilization"[All Fields] AND "vitro"[All Fields]) OR "fertilization in vitro"[All Fields])) OR ("reproductive techniques"[MeSH Terms] OR ("reproductive"[All Fields] AND "techniques"[All Fields]) OR "reproductive techniques"[All Fields])) AND ((((("hypothyroidism"[MeSH Terms] OR "hypothyroidism"[All Fields]) OR (("thyroid gland"[MeSH Terms] OR ("thyroid"[All Fields] AND "gland"[All Fields]) OR "thyroid gland"[All Fields] OR "thyroid"[All Fields] OR "thyroid (usp)"[MeSH Terms] OR ("thyroid"[All Fields] AND "(usp)"[All Fields]) OR "thyroid (usp)"[All Fields]) AND ("physiopathology"[Subheading] OR "physiopathology"[All Fields] OR "dysfunction"[All Fields]))) OR ("thyroid diseases"[MeSH Terms] OR ("thyroid"[All Fields] AND "diseases"[All Fields]) OR "thyroid diseases"[All Fields] OR ("thyroid"[All Fields] AND "disorder"[All Fields]) OR "thyroid disorder"[All Fields])) OR ("thyroid diseases"[MeSH Terms] OR ("thyroid"[All Fields] AND "diseases"[All Fields]) OR "thyroid diseases"[All Fields] OR ("thyroid"[All Fields] AND "disease"[All Fields]) OR "thyroid disease"[All Fields])). We included all published retrospective or prospective studies. All relevant publications were retrieved. We also systematically reviewed the reference lists of the identified articles to identify additional reports that could be included in the meta-analysis. We made no attempt to identify unpublished reports.

Study selection and Data Collection Processes.

Two authors (Zhao T and Chen BM) performed the original screening of the titles and abstracts of all studies, and citations considered irrelevant by both observers were excluded. The PRISMA flow diagram (Fig. 1) provided more detailed information on the selection process of articles. Two authors (Zhao T and Chen BM) independently extracted all research data into normative forms. When there was a difference of opinion, the third author (Zhao XM) consulted with the two authors to achieve consensus. The year of publication, country, setting, study design, number of participants, clinical characteristics of the study subjects, thyroid function assays used, and ART (IVF, ICSI or intrauterine insemination (IUI)) implemented in the comparable groups were recorded.

Quality assessment

We evaluated the quality of the articles according to the Newcastle–Ottawa scale, which is an effective method for scoring observational and non-randomized studies. All articles were evaluated independently by two authors.

Discrepancies were solved by consensus. The Newcastle–Ottawa scale employs a score system based on the following three primary criteria: the selection of participants, the comparability of study groups, and outcome or, for case-control studies, an assessment of exposure. While 'comparability of cohorts' was scored as 2, 1 or 0; the other two primary criteria were scored based on eight items, each scored as either 0 or 1. Accordingly, the quantitative estimation of the total quality of each individual article ranged from 0 to 9. In the meta-analysis, articles were considered high quality if they obtained seven or more scores, those obtaining four to six scores were believed medium quality, and those obtaining three or less scores were believed low quality.

Data items

We extracted information related to the research characteristics, the quality of the publications and the test results from each included article. The primary outcome was the LBR per woman, which was defined as the number of childbirths that led to one live born baby. The

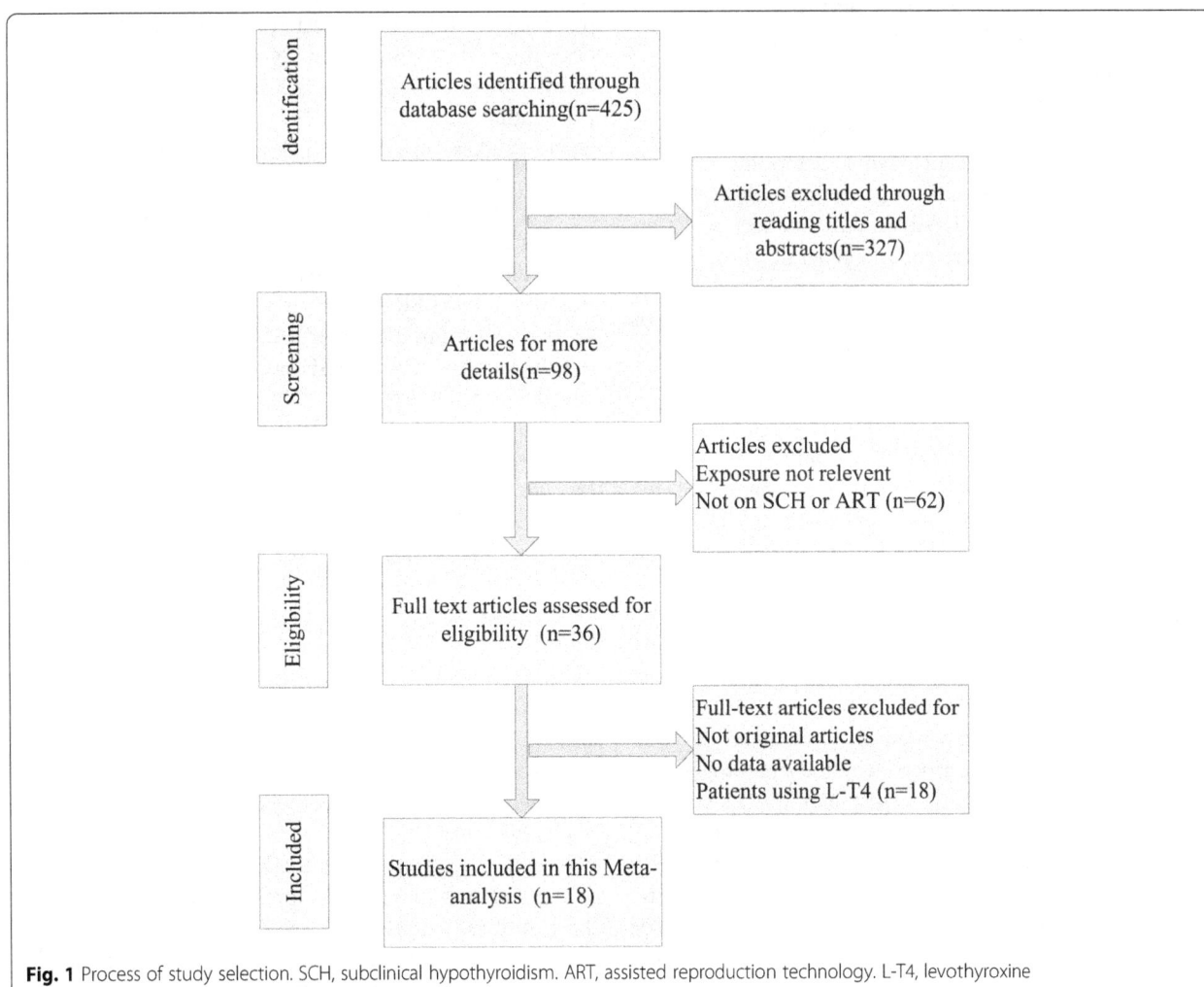

Fig. 1 Process of study selection. SCH, subclinical hypothyroidism. ART, assisted reproduction technology. L-T4, levothyroxine

following secondary outcomes were applied: (i) the CPR per patient, which was defined using conceptions diagnosed by ultrasonography, including cases in which there was one or more gestational sacs in the uterus; (ii) the PR per woman, with pregnancies diagnosed as serum b-hCG levels ≥5 mIU/mL within 14 days following ART; and (iii) the MR per clinical conception.

Risk of bias
We adopted the Cochrane Collaboration's tool for assessing risk of bias to evaluate the risk of bias in individual studies. We analyzed the following risk of biases: 1) selection bias (i.e., bias introduced by the selection of individuals, groups or data for analysis in such a way that proper randomization is not achieved, thereby ensuring that the sample obtained is not representative of the population intended to be analyzed) 2) performance bias (i.e., bias due to the knowledge of the allocated interventions by personnel and participants during the research) 3) detection bias (i.e., bias due to randomization of the allocated interventions is not achieved by outcome assessors) 4) attrition bias (i.e., bias due to loss of follow-up, withdrawal, and no response during the study) 5) reporting bias (i.e., selective revealing or suppression of the outcomes).

Except for the above-mentioned types of biases, other two types of biases were included 1) sampling bias (i.e., bias leading to samples can not represent all the study population, mainly associated with the subject selection problem which can undermine the generalization of outcomes) 2) measurement bias (i.e., bias resulting from inappropriate use of tests or scales to measurement of preconception TSH values and ART outcomes mainly related to inconsistent or non-validated criteria).

Summary measures and synthesis of results
We used Stata (version 11) to analyze the data. We calculated a combined odds ratio (OR) with a 95% confidence interval (CI) to assess the strength of the connection between SCH and the risk of adverse pregnancy-related outcomes. The significance of the combined OR (counted using the Mantel–Haenszel statistical approach) was identified with the Z test. We defined significance as a P value less than 0.05. Random effects and fixed effects models were used in this meta-analysis. To evaluate between-study heterogeneity, both the ×2-based Q statistic test and the I2 statistic were applied. We defined I2 values of 25%, 50%, and 75% as representing low, moderate, and high heterogeneity, respectively. We used a random effects model to pool outcomes when high heterogeneity was observed; whereas we used a fixed effects model to pool outcomes when heterogeneity was not high.

Additional analyses
We evaluated the effect of each article on the overall risk appraisal by sequentially omitting each report to validate the authenticity of the results of the meta-analysis. We utilized Begg's funnel plots and Egger's linear regression test to estimate potential publication bias. The present study fulfilled the criteria of Preferred Reporting Items for Systematic reviews and Meta-Analyses (PRISMA) (Additional file 1: Figure S1).

Results
Study selection
We selected a total of eighteen publications that included 14,846 participants for this meta-analysis. The included studies were selected from 425 potentially related articles (Fig. 1).

Study characteristics
The detailed characteristics of the involved studies are presented in Table 1. Seven of the included articles were prospective cohort studies [25–31], and 11 were retrospective cohort reports [32–41]. In all of the included publications, the authors tested serum TSH levels before beginning the stimulation protocol. The participant count varied from 98 to 3143 subjects, and the year of publication ranged from 1999 to 2017. Nine of the selected studies reported a high-limit TSH cut-off value. For all included studies, the following results were reported: PR ($n = 8$ using a stricter TSH cut-off value; $n = 6$ using a broader TSH cut-off value), CPR ($n = 13$ using a stricter TSH cut-off value; $n = 8$ using a broader TSH cut-off value), LBR ($n = 13$ using a stricter TSH cut-off value; $n = 9$ using a broader TSH cut-off value), and MR ($n = 10$ using a stricter TSH cut-off value; $n = 8$ using a broader TSH cut-off value) (Table 1).

Synthesis of results and additional analysis
Live birth rate
Thirteen of the included articles analyzed the LBR as an outcome. Outcomes were pooled from the studies, and the results showed that the LBR was non-significantly lower in women with SCH (TSH cut-off value: 2.5 mIU/L) than in women with normal thyroid function (OR: 0.93; 95% CI (0.77, 1.12), $P = 0.43$). The I^2 value (58.2%) calculated for these studies indicated high heterogeneity, and we therefore used a random effects model to evaluate the pooled effect estimate (Fig. 2a). A sensitivity analysis demonstrated no difference in the OR when each publication was individually omitted (Additional file 2: Figure S2a). Egger's test and Begg's funnel plots ($P = 0.064$) did not indicate the presence of asymmetry for these studies (Additional file 3: Figure S3a).

We also found an insignificant difference in the pooled data for LBR between women with SCH and those with

Table 1 The Characteristics of Selected Studies

Author	Year	N	Country	Study design	Assays used	TSH Cut-off	ART details	Outcomes
Coelho	2016	650	Brazil	retrospective	a third-generation assay	2.5;4.0	IVF/ICSI	PR; CPR; LBR; MR
Aghahosseini	2013	816	Iran	retrospective	NS	2.5	IVF	CPR
Mintziori	2014	158	Greece	retrospective	ELISA	2.5	IVF	PR; CPR; LBR; MR
Unuane	2017	3143	Belgium	retrospective	NS	2.5	IUI	PR; LBR; MR
Michalakis	2011	1216	USA	retrospective	NS	2.5;4.0	NS	PR; CPR; LBR; MR
Muller	1999	141	Netherlands	prospective	an immunoluminometric assay	4.5	IVF	PR; LBR; MR
Chai	2014	505	China	retrospective	Access HYPERsensitive hTSH Reagent Pack and Access Free T4 Reagent Pack	2.5;4.5	IVF/ICSI	CPR; LBR; MR
Baker	2006	146	USA	retrospective	chemiluminometric technology	2.5	IVF	LBR
Karmon	2014	1477	USA	prospective	third-generation assays	2.5	IUI	CPR; LBR
Weghofer	2015	98	USA	retrospective	Electrochemiluminescence immunoassay	2.5	IVF	CPR; LBR
Seungdamrong	2017	1306	USA	prospective	Immulite 2000 system	2.5	IUI	PR; CPR; LBR; MR
Wu	2017	138	China	prospective	NS	2.5; 5	IVF/ICSI	PR; CPR; LBR; MR
Ba	2013	413	China	prospective	NS	4.2	IVF/ICSI	PR; CPR; LBR; MR
Zhang	2012	1832	China	retrospective	NS	3.9	IVF/ICSI	PR; CPR; LBR; MR
Zeng	2014	375	China	prospective	Chemiluminescent immunoassay	2.5;3.5	IVF/ICSI	CPR; LBR; MR
Gingold	2016	1201	USA	retrospective	NS	2.5;5.0	IVF	PR; CPR; LBR
Reh	2010	1055	USA	retrospective	NS	2.5;4.5	IVF	CPR; LBR; MR
Cai	2017	176	China	prospective	electro- chemiluminescence immunoassays	2.5	IVF	CPR; LBR; MR

IVF In vitro fertilization, *ICSI* intracytoplasmatic sperm injection, *IUI* intra-uterine insemination, *ART* assisted reproduction technology, *TSH* thyroid stimulating hormone, *CPR* clinical pregnancy rate, *MR* miscarriage rate, *LBR* live birth rate, *PR* pregnancy rate, *ELISA* enzyme-linked immunosorbent assay

normal thyroid function when a TSH cut-off value of 3.5–5.0 mIU/L was used (OR: 0.72; 95% CI (0.47, 1.11); $P = 0.14$). The I^2 value (67%) indicated a high degree of heterogeneity. We therefore utilized a random effects model to pool the effect estimate (Fig. 3a). A sensitivity analysis demonstrated no variation in the OR when each trial was individually removed (Additional file 4: Figure S4a). Egger's test ($P = 0.57$) and Begg's funnel plots ($P = 0.92$) indicated no asymmetry among these studies (Additional file 5: Figure S5a).

Secondary outcomes
Clinical pregnancy rate
Thirteen of the included articles compared the CPR in participants with and without SCH (TSH cut-off value, 2.5 mIU/L). The meta-analysis indicated no association between SCH and the CPR. Comparison of the CPR between women with SCH and euthyroid women indicated no significant difference (OR: 1.02; 95% CI (0.90, 1.17); $P = 0.74$). The I^2 value was 39.9%, indicating low heterogeneity. We therefore chose a fixed effects model to pool the effect estimate (Fig. 2b). When each trial was removed, no variation

appeared in the direction of the OR (Additional file 2: Figure S2b). Egger's test ($P = 0.57$) and Begg's funnel plots ($P = 0.92$) indicated no asymmetry among these studies (Additional file 3: Figure S3b).

We also found an insignificant difference in the pooled data for the CPR between women with SCH and those with normal thyroid function when a cut-off TSH value of 3.5–5.0 mIU/L was used (OR: 0.82; 95% CI (0.66, 1.00); $P = 0.052$). The I^2 value (18.1%) indicated low heterogeneity. We therefore utilized a fixed effects model to pool the effect estimate (Fig. 3b). A sensitivity analysis demonstrated no variation in the OR when each trial was individually removed (Additional file 4: Figure S4b). Egger's test ($P = 0.61$) and Begg's funnel plots ($P = 0.39$) indicated no asymmetry among the studies (Additional file 5: Figure S5b).

Pregnancy rate
Nine reports estimated the relationship between SCH (TSH cut-off value, 2.5) and PR. We failed to find a meaningful association between the presence of SCH and the PR (OR: 1.00; 95% CI (0.89, 1.12); $P = 0.99$). The I^2 value was 0%, indicating an absence of significant heterogeneity

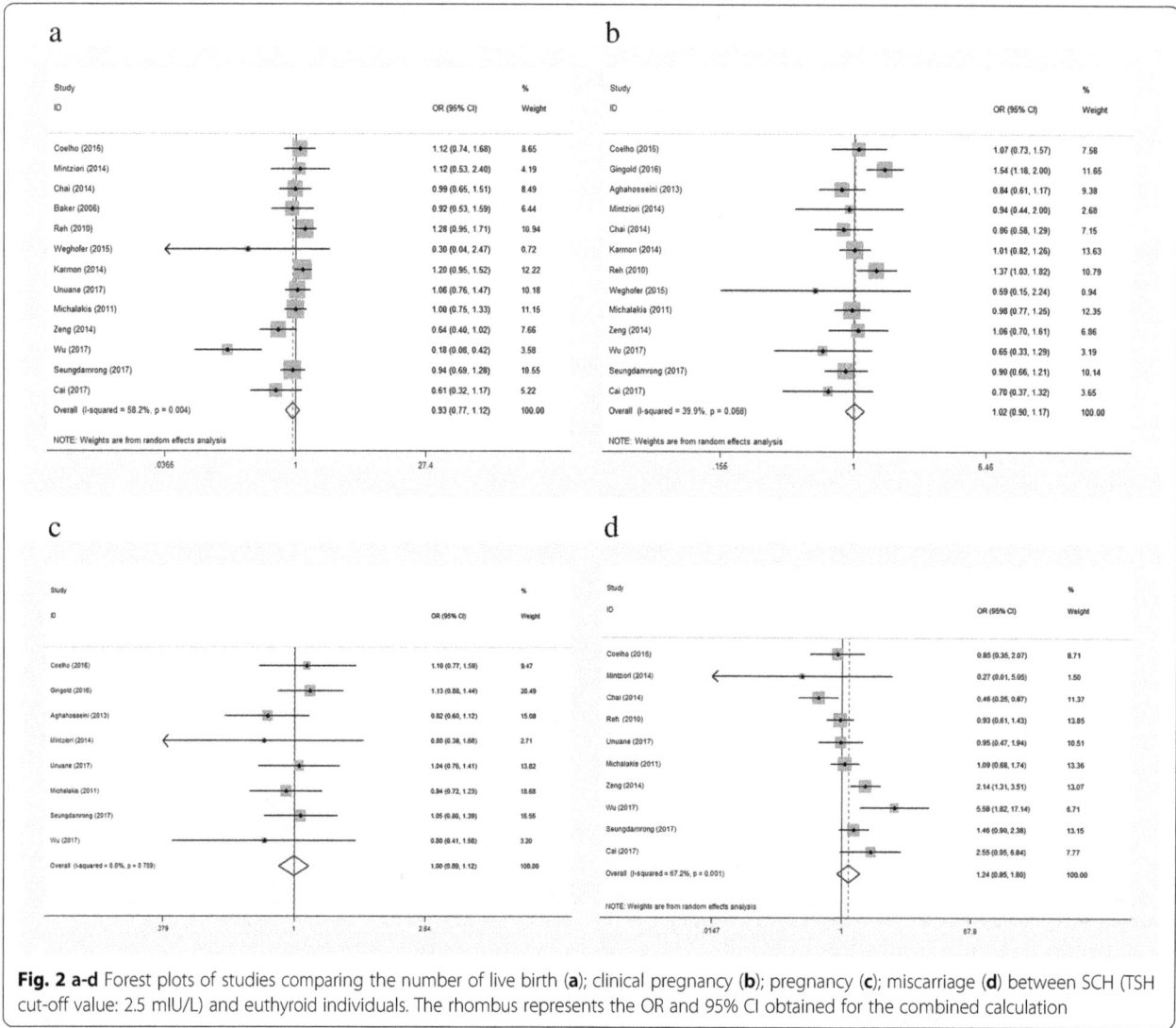

Fig. 2 a-d Forest plots of studies comparing the number of live birth (**a**); clinical pregnancy (**b**); pregnancy (**c**); miscarriage (**d**) between SCH (TSH cut-off value: 2.5 mIU/L) and euthyroid individuals. The rhombus represents the OR and 95% CI obtained for the combined calculation

(Fig. 2c). A sensitivity analysis showed no variation in the OR when each article was omitted (Additional file 2: Figure S2c). Egger's test ($P = 0.21$) and Begg's funnel plots ($P = 0.27$) did not indicate the presence of asymmetry in the involved studies (Additional file 3: Figure S3c).

We also found an insignificant difference in the pooled data for the PR between women with SCH and those with normal thyroid function when a cut-off TSH value of 3.5–5.0 mIU/L was used (OR: 1.07; 95% CI (0.72, 1.60); $P = 0.74$). The I^2 value (67.2%) indicated high heterogeneity. We therefore utilized a random effects model to pool the effect estimate (Fig. 3c). A sensitivity analysis demonstrated no variation in the OR when each trial was individually removed (Additional file 4: Figure S4c). Egger's test ($P = 0.27$) and Begg's funnel plots ($P = 0.45$) indicated no asymmetry among the studies (Additional file 5: Figure S5c).

Miscarriage rate

A total of ten publications assessed the association between SCH and miscarriage. A meta-analysis of these 7 reports indicated an insignificant difference in the risk of miscarriage between euthyroid women and SCH patients (OR: 1.24; 95% CI (0.85, 1.80); $P = 0.26$). The I^2 value was 67.2%, indicating high heterogeneity. We therefore chose a random effects model to pool the effect estimate (Fig. 2d). A sensitivity analysis showed no variation in the OR when each article was individually removed (Additional file 2: Figure S2d). Egger's test ($P = 0.85$) and Begg's funnel plots ($P = 0.59$) indicated no asymmetry in the studies (Additional file 3: Figure S3d).

We also found a significant difference in the pooled data for the MR between women with SCH and those with normal thyroid function when a TSH cut-off value of 3.5–5.0 mIU/L was used (OR: 1.91; 95% CI (1.09,

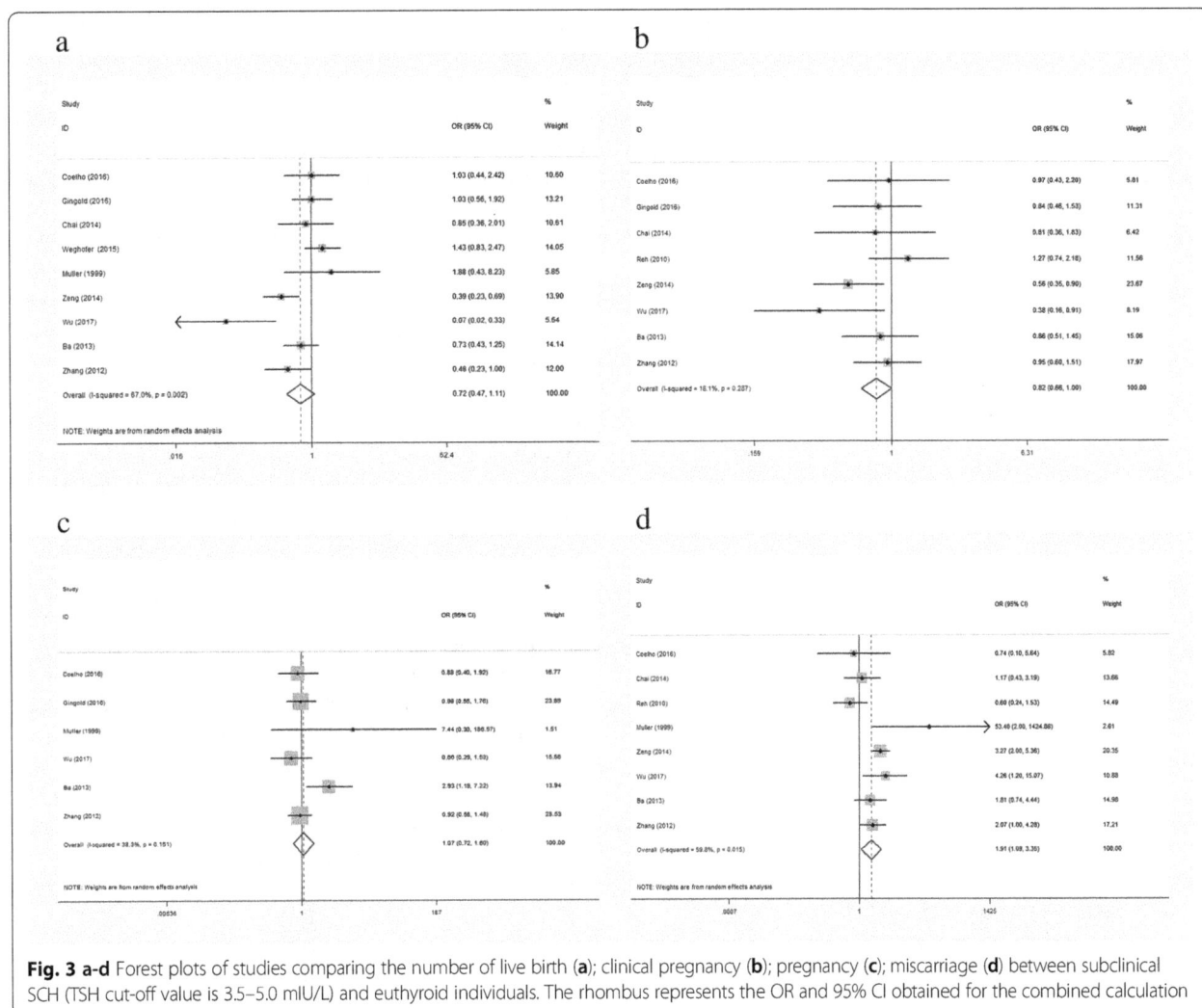

Fig. 3 a-d Forest plots of studies comparing the number of live birth (**a**); clinical pregnancy (**b**); pregnancy (**c**); miscarriage (**d**) between subclinical SCH (TSH cut-off value is 3.5–5.0 mIU/L) and euthyroid individuals. The rhombus represents the OR and 95% CI obtained for the combined calculation

3.35); $P = 0.02$). The I^2 value (59.8%) indicated high heterogeneity. We therefore utilized a random effects model to pool the effect estimate (Fig. 3d). A sensitivity analysis demonstrated no variation in the OR when each trial was individually removed (Additional file 4: Figure S4d). Egger's test ($P = 0.83$) and Begg's funnel plots ($P = 0.90$) indicated no asymmetry among these studies (Additional file 5: Figure S5d).

Quality assessment and risk of bias

The quality assessment of the studies included in the meta-analysis is shown in Table 2. An overview and summary of probable risks of bias across all included studies is showed in Table 3. Selection bias was rated as high risk across five researches. In terms of potential performance bias, five studies were found to be of high risk. Detection bias was potentially rated as high risk in eight studies. Only four studies potentially posed high risk for potential attrition bias. Reporting bias was potentially rated as high risk across five studies. Other

sources of biases included the sampling bias and measurement bias. Sampling bias was judged as high risk in one study. Furthermore, measurement bias was rated as high risk in ten studies.

Discussion

This meta-analysis was specifically aimed at evaluating the associations between preconception maternal TSH levels and ART outcomes. We found that a stricter TSH cut-off value did not seem to influence ART outcomes including the LBR, PR, CPR, and MR. Furthermore, using a broader TSH cut-off value resulted in a significant difference in poor ART outcomes including the MR.

Many previous studies have researched the association between SCH during conception and maternal outcomes, but their conclusions have been inconsistent. In 2016, a meta-analysis focused on thyroid dysfunction indicated that SCH during pregnancy is related to multiple poor neonatal and maternal outcomes, especially

Table 2 Quality of the studies on the Newcastle-Ottawa scale

Study	Selection	Comparability	Exposure/ Outcome	Total Stars
Coelho 2016	*****	*	**	8
Aghahosseini 2013	****	**	**	8
Mintziori 2014	****	**	*	7
Unuane 2017	***	**	**	7
Michalakis 2011	****	**	*	7
Muller 1999	***	**	**	7
Chai 2014	****	*	**	7
Weghofer 2015	****	**	*	7
Baker 2006	***	**	**	7
Karmon 2014	****	**	**	8
Cai 2017	****	**	**	8
Seungdamrong 2017	****	**	**	8
Zhang 2012	*****	**	*	8
Ba 2013	***	**	**	7
Reh 2010	***	**	**	7
Zeng 2014	*****	*	**	8
Gingold 2016	****	**	*	7
Wu 2017	****	**	*	7

* means 1 score

abortion [9]. However, the studies evaluated in that analysis had enrolled participants who were normal fertile woman. However, we should not ignore the fact that more and more infertile patients are undergoing ART treatment. Recently, many articles have focused on the relationship between preconception SCH in infertile patients and multiple ART outcomes. However, their conclusions have been conflicting. Nevertheless, this information is very important because most reproductive endocrinologists routinely perform preconception tests for serum TSH levels as a part of an elementary infertility workup.

Moreover, subclinical thyroid function disorder is a focus of studies evaluating patients undergoing ovarian stimulation because it has been suggested that these patients experience a decrease in thyroxin levels and an increase in TSH levels during ovulation induction.

Due to the increased subsequent risk of hypothyroidism in participants with a TSH level above 2.0 mIU/L (e.g., as demonstrated in the Whickham survey [42]), the NACB guidelines suggest that 2.5 mIU/L should be regarded as the upper limit for a normal TSH reference range [43]. In patients previously diagnosed with hypothyroidism, the Endocrine Society (TES) practice guidelines suggest that preconception TSH values should be under 2.5 mIU/ mL [44]. The ATA and the American Association of Clinical Endocrinologists co-sponsored guidelines for the treatment of hypothyroidism in patients attempting to

Table 3 Assessment of risk of bias in individual studies

Study	Selection bias	Performance bias	Detection bias	Attrition bias	Reporting bias	Other bias	
						Sampling bias	Measurement bias
Coelho 2016	−	+	−	−	−	?	−
Aghahosseini 2013	−	−	?	−	+	−	−
Mintziori 2014	+	−	+	−	−	−	+
Unuane 2017	+	−	−	−	−	+	+
Michalakis 2011	+	?	+	−	−	?	+
Muller 1999	−	+	−	+	−	?	−
Chai 2014	+	+	−	−	−	−	+
Weghofer 2015	−	?	+	+	−	?	+
Baker 2006	?	−	+	−	+	−	−
Karmon 2014	−	?	−	−	+	−	−
Cai 2017	−	−	?	−	−	?	+
Seungdamrong 2017	−	−	−	+	−	−	+
Zhang 2012	−	+	−	+	−	−	+
Ba 2013	+	−	?	−	−	−	−
Reh 2010	−	+	+	−	+	?	+
Zeng 2014	?	−	+	−	−	?	−
Gingold 2016	?	−	+	−	−	−	+
Wu 2017	−	?	+	−	+	−	−

+ high risk of bias; − low risk of bias; ? unclear risk of bias

conceive [19]. Their proposal reinforces the notion that TSH levels should be maintained at lower than 2.5 mIU/L in women with hypothyroidism, including those with overt hypothyroidism and SCH before pregnancy. Moreover, there is a lack of consistency regarding what cut-off value for serum TSH levels should be used to define SCH in individuals undergoing ART. Several studies have relied on the use of a recommended basal cut-off value of TSH < 2.5 mIU/l in individuals termed "desirable" for conception. However, we cannot ignore that some prospective and retrospective studies found no difference in IVF outcomes between women with serum TSH < 2.5 mU/L and those with mild TSH elevations, defined as a TSH level between 2.5 and 5 mU/L. The results of these studies were inconsistent with our outcomes. The underlying reason remains uncertain. One of the probable reasons is the distribution of TSH levels in infertile women. Braverman et al. found that the distribution of TSH levels in infertile individuals presented a left skew with a long tail [20]. The argument for decreasing the upper TSH reference range presumes that it conforms to a Gaussian distribution in nature. However, studies have found that in some euthyroid outliers, such as patients recovering from nonthyroidal illness, measurements that include bioactive TSH isoforms or receptor gene polymorphisms as well as occult autoimmune thyroid dysfunction show that the upper tail of the distribution is skewed [45, 46]. Additionally, TSH levels can be influenced by strenuous exercise, the timing of phlebotomy and sleep deprivation [47]. Previous publications have also indicated that the distribution of TSH levels gradually shifts toward higher values with age [48]. Hence, TSH concentrations could represent an epiphenomenon in which the above-mentioned factors account for its influence on pregnancy outcomes.

When a broader TSH cut-off value was used, we found a significant difference in the MR between SCH patients and normal women. This outcome is consistent with some random clinical trials (RCTs). These trials demonstrated that treatment of SCH patients who were defined using a broader TSH cut-off value appeared beneficial. An RCT was conducted in patients aged 20–40 years old with SCH (serum TSH > 4.5 mU/L, normal fT4) who were undergoing IVF [49]. A total of 64 participants were randomized for supplementation with LT4 (to maintain TSH levels < 2.5 mU/L) vs. placebo. The treated patients had MRs, higher CPRs, and higher LBRs. Another RCT randomized 64 infertile women with SCH (TSH > 4.2 mU/L, normal fT4) to a treatment group receiving 50 mcg/day LT4 vs. a placebo group [50]. Similar to the above trial, the study showed higher PRs, lower MRs, and higher LBRs in the treatment group than in the control group. Taken together, these data suggest that SCH likely impacts ART in a dose-dependent manner, and the impact worsens as

TSH concentrations increase. Hence, in 2017, the ATA guidelines recommended that women with SCH undergoing IVF or ICSI should be treated with LT4 with a goal of maintaining a TSH concentration < 2.5 mU/L. It is worth noting that this recommendation is focused on women who are undergoing ART. However, the effect of SCH before ART on ART outcomes remains uncertain. Our results suggest that applying a broader TSH cut-off value during the preconception period may improve ART outcomes such as the pregnancy loss rate.

In addition, we found that an increasing number of clinicians are uncertain regarding whether to perform preconception thyroid function tests, especially for women seeking ART [51]. Routine preconception testing for all women is not recommended by any relevant professional body (ATA, ACOG, RCOG) primarily because there is no high-level evidence to support its use. Our search also provided high-level evidence regarding the necessity of routine thyroid function tests before conception in women seeking to ART. We found that women with SCH defined using the broader TSH cut-off value before conception could have poor ART outcomes, such a higher MR.

In contrast to our findings, a recent prospective trial published by Negro et al. [7] included 4123 thyroid antibody–negative subjects and found that the risk of miscarriage was higher in women with TSH values between 2.5 and 5.0 mIU/L at < 11 weeks of pregnancy. The reasons for this discrepancy may include the following. For example, the subjects were individuals with spontaneous conceptions who were already in the first trimester and did not include infertile women. Therefore, TSH levels were tested only in subjects who were already pregnant, whereas in our study, all TSH concentrations were measured before conception. This difference could be partially responsible for the difference in the effect in that if TSH values decreases during early pregnancy, as suggested in a previous study [52], then individuals with TSH values above 2.5 mIU/L during the first trimester might have had higher TSH levels before pregnancy. In addition, ovarian stimulation seems to influence TSH concentrations [24, 53].

Strengths and limitations of this meta-analysis

There are several limitations to this meta-analysis. First, the sizes of the populations included in many of the original studies and the total number of patients were small. Second, because some original articles were retrospective, it is probable that other factors may account for the differences observed in outcomes. In retrospective cohort studies, it is feasible that there will be selection bias, problems with the quality of the original publications, publication bias, confounding and heterogeneity. Third, TPO, an important confounding factor, could not be eliminated in several of the original papers because of limitations associated with the studies. In spite of these limitations, the current meta-analysis has some strengths. Our methodology was rigorous, and the outcomes achieved after the results of these trials were pooled were more credible. We also comprehensively compared the CPR, PR and MR as secondary outcomes between normal women and SCH patients to explore the influence of preconception SCH on ART outcomes. Furthermore, we analyzed the data using two different cut-off values for TSH levels to explore the association between SCH and adverse ART outcomes. The results suggested a new diagnosis standard to define SCH in woman seeking ART.

Conclusions

Our data indicate no difference in ART outcomes when a TSH cut-off value of 2.5 mIU/L is used. However, using a broader cut-off value of TSH, we found a higher MR in SCH patients seeking ART than in the control group. We suggest that a thyroid function test should be a routine examination in women seeking ART.

Additional files

Additional file 1: Figure S1. PRISMA Checklist. (EPS 538 kb)

Additional file 2: Figure S2. a-d Sensitivity analysis of the studies included in the meta- analysis. The figure (a-d) shows the OR obtained by combined analysis of the remaining studies after the successive exclusion of each study individually. The excluded study is listed on the left, and the corresponding horizontal lines indicate the OR and CI obtained by re-calculation after its exclusion. The CI for the overall meta-analysis of the studies is indicated by two vertical lines. (TIF 746 kb)

Additional file 3: Figure S3. a-d Begg's funnel plot for publication bias analysis. Each point represents a separate study. (TIF 347 kb)

Additional file 4: Figure S4. a-d Sensitivity analysis of the studies included in the meta- analysis. The figure (a-d) shows the OR obtained by combined analysis of the remaining studies after the successive exclusion of each study individually. The excluded study is listed on the left, and the corresponding horizontal lines indicate the OR and CI obtained by re-calculation after its exclusion. The CI for the overall meta-analysis of the studies is indicated by two vertical lines. (TIF 587 kb)

Additional file 5: Figure S5. a-d Begg's funnel plot for publication bias analysis. Each point represents a separate study. (TIF 316 kb)

Abbreviations

AACC: American Association for Clinical Chemistry; ART: Assisted reproductive technology; ASRM: American Society for Reproductive Medicine; ATA: American Thyroid Association; CI: Confidence interval; CPR: Clinical pregnancy rate; ESHRE: European Society of Human Reproduction and Embryology; ICSI: Intra-cytoplasmic sperm injection; IUI: Intrauterine insemination; IVF: In vitro fertilization; LBR: Live birth rate; MR: Miscarriage rate; NACB: National Association of Clinical Biochemistry; OH: Overt hypothyroidism; OR: Odds ratio; PR: Pregnancy rate; SCH: Subclinical hypothyroidism; T4: Thyroxine; TES: The Endocrine Society; TSH: Thyroid-stimulating hormone

Acknowledgements

I would like to extend my sincere gratitude to American Journal Experts (AJE). AJE's editing service was used for English language editing of our manuscript.

Funding

no funding support.

Authors' contributions

ZT and CB designed the search strategies, searched for papers in the databases, assessed study quality, independently extracted data from the papers and wrote the paper. ZX, as a third reviewer, was asked for advice if a disagreement occurred. ZX participated in the revision of the paper. SZ provided advice on the discussion section of this article. All authors read and approved the final manuscript.

Competing interests

The authors declare that they have no competing interests.

Author details

[1]Department of Endocrinology and Metabolism, Institute of Endocrinology, First Affiliated Hospital, China Medical University, Shenyang, Liaoning, China. [2]The First Affiliated Hospital of Sun Yat-sen University, Guangzhou, China. [3]Chengde Medical University, Chengde, Hebei, China.

References

1. Casey BM. Subclinical hypothyroidism and pregnancy. Obstet Gynecol Surv. 2006;61(6):415–20 quiz 23.
2. Abalovich M, Gutierrez S, Alcaraz G, Maccallini G, Garcia A, Levalle O. Overt and subclinical hypothyroidism complicating pregnancy. Thyroid. 2002;12(1):63–8.
3. Lao TT. Thyroid disorders in pregnancy. Curr Opin Obstet Gynecol. 2005; 17(2):123–7.
4. Leung AS, Millar LK, Koonings PP, Montoro M, Mestman JH. Perinatal outcome in hypothyroid pregnancies. Obstet Gynecol. 1993;81(3):349–53.
5. Lao TT, Chin RK, Swaminathan R, Lam YM. Maternal thyroid hormones and outcome of pre-eclamptic pregnancies. Br J Obstet Gynaecol. 1990; 97(1):71–4.
6. Tong Z, Xiaowen Z, Baomin C, Aihua L, Yingying Z, Weiping T, et al. The Effect of Subclinical Maternal Thyroid Dysfunction and Autoimmunity on Intrauterine Growth Restriction: A Systematic Review and Meta-Analysis. Medicine. 2016;95(19):e3677.
7. Negro R, Schwartz A, Gismondi R, Tinelli A, Mangieri T, Stagnaro-Green A. Increased pregnancy loss rate in thyroid antibody negative women with TSH levels between 2.5 and 5.0 in the first trimester of pregnancy. J Clin Endocrinol Metab. 2010;95(9):E44–8.
8. Wilson KL, Casey BM, McIntire DD, Halvorson LM, Cunningham FG. Subclinical thyroid disease and the incidence of hypertension in pregnancy. Obstet Gynecol. 2012;119(2 Pt 1):315–20.
9. Maraka S, Ospina NM, O'Keeffe DT, Espinosa De Ycaza AE, Gionfriddo MR, Erwin PJ, et al. Subclinical Hypothyroidism in Pregnancy: A Systematic Review and Meta-Analysis. Thyroid. 2016;26(4):580–90.
10. Mintziori G, Anagnostis P, Toulis KA, Goulis DG. Thyroid diseases and female reproduction. Minerva Med. 2012;103(1):47–62.
11. de Mouzon J, Goossens V, Bhattacharya S, Castilla JA, Ferraretti AP, Korsak V, et al. Assisted reproductive technology in Europe, 2006: results generated from European registers by ESHRE. Hum Reprod. 2010;25(8):1851–62.
12. Pfeifer S, Goldberg J, Lobo R, McClure R, Thomas M, Widra E, et al. Diagnostic evaluation of the infertile female: a committee opinion. Fertil Steril. 2012;98(2):302–7.
13. National Collaborating Centre for Ws, Children's H. National Institute for Health and Clinical Excellence: Guidance. Fertility: Assessment and Treatment for People with Fertility Problems. London: Royal College of Obstetricians & Gynaecologists National Collaborating Centre for Women's and Children's Health.; 2013.
14. Pfeifer S, Butts S, Dumesic D, Fossum G, Goldberg J, Gracia C, et al. Subclinical hypothyroidism in the infertile female population: a guideline. Fertil Steril. 2015;104(3):545–53.

15. Stagnaro-Green A, Abalovich M, Alexander E, Azizi F, Mestman J, Negro R, et al. Guidelines of the American Thyroid Association for the diagnosis and management of thyroid disease during pregnancy and postpartum. Thyroid. 2011;21(10):1081–125.

16. De Groot L, Abalovich M, Alexander EK, Amino N, Barbour L, Cobin RH, et al. Management of thyroid dysfunction during pregnancy and postpartum: an Endocrine Society clinical practice guideline. J Clin Endocrinol Metab. 2012; 97(8):2543–65.

17. Reh A, Grifo J, Danoff A. What is a normal thyroid-stimulating hormone (TSH) level? Effects of stricter TSH thresholds on pregnancy outcomes after in vitro fertilization. Fertil Steril. 2010;94(7):2920–2.

18. Maraka S, O'Keeffe DT, Montori VM. Subclinical Hypothyroidism During Pregnancy-Should You Expect This When You Are Expecting?: A Teachable Moment. JAMA Intern Med. 2015;175(7):1088–9.

19. Garber JR, Cobin RH, Gharib H, Hennessey JV, Klein I, Mechanick JI, et al. Clinical practice guidelines for hypothyroidism in adults: cosponsored by the American Association of Clinical Endocrinologists and the American Thyroid Association. Thyroid. 2012;22(12):1200–35.

20. Hollowell JG, Staehling NW, Flanders WD, Hannon WH, Gunter EW, Spencer CA, et al. Serum TSH, T(4), and thyroid antibodies in the United States population (1988 to 1994): National Health and Nutrition Examination Survey (NHANES III). J Clin Endocrinol Metab. 2002;87(2):489–99.

21. Macklon NS, Stouffer RL, Giudice LC, Fauser BC. The science behind 25 years of ovarian stimulation for in vitro fertilization. Endocr Rev. 2006;27(2):170–207.

22. Glinoer D, Gershengorn MC, Dubois A, Robbins J. Stimulation of thyroxine-binding globulin synthesis by isolated rhesus monkey hepatocytes after in vivo beta-estradiol administration. Endocrinology. 1977;100(3):807–13.

23. Glinoer D, McGuire RA, Gershengorn MC, Robbins J, Berman M. Effects of estrogen on thyroxine-binding globulin metabolism in rhesus monkeys. Endocrinology. 1977;100(1):9–17.

24. Stuckey BG, Yeap D, Turner SR. Thyroxine replacement during super-ovulation for in vitro fertilization: a potential gap in management? Fertil Steril. 2010;93(7):2414 e1-3.

25. Muller AF, Verhoeff A, Mantel MJ, Berghout A. Thyroid autoimmunity and abortion: a prospective study in women undergoing in vitro fertilization. Fertil Steril. 1999;71(1):30–4.

26. Karmon AE, Batsis M, Chavarro JE, Souter I. Preconceptional thyroid-stimulating hormone levels and outcomes of intrauterine insemination among euthyroid infertile women. Fertil Steril. 2015;103(1):258–63 e1.

27. Seungdamrong A, Steiner AZ, Gracia CR, Legro RS, Diamond MP, Coutifaris C, et al. Preconceptional antithyroid peroxidase antibodies, but not thyroid-stimulating hormone, are associated with decreased live birth rates in infertile women. Fertil Steril. 2017;108(5):843–50.

28. Zeng X, Wang L, Shu X, Xiong Z, Dang X. Influence of basic thyroid-stimulating hormone levels on outcomes of IVF/ICSI in Qinghai. Zhonghua fu chan ke za zhi. 2014;49(10):763–7.

29. LL B. Effects of subclinical hypothyroidism on pregnancy outcomes of assisted reproductive technology. Reprod Med. 2013;22(12):905–9.

30. YJ W. The Influence of L-T4 on Patience with TBOAb Negative Subclinic Hypothyroidism Undergoing IVF/ICSI-ET [master's degree]: Lanzhou University; 2017.

31. Cai YY, Zhong LP, Guan J, Guo RJ, Niu B, Ma YP, et al. Outcome of in vitro fertilization in women with subclinical hypothyroidism. Reprod Biol Endocrinol. 2017;15(1):39.

32. Coelho Neto MA, Martins WP, Melo AS, Ferriani RA. Navarro PA. Subclinical Hypothyroidism and Intracytoplasmic Sperm Injection Outcomes. Rev Bras Ginecol Obstet. 2016;38(11):552–8.

33. Aghahosseini M, Asgharifard H, Aleyasin A, Tehrani Banihashemi A. Effects of Thyroid Stimulating Hormone (TSH) level on clinical pregnancy rate via In Vitro Fertilization (IVF) procedure. Med J Islam Repub Iran. 2014;28:46.

34. Mintziori G, Goulis DG, Gialamas E, Dosopoulos K, Zouzoulas D, Gitas G, et al. Association of TSH concentrations and thyroid autoimmunity with IVF outcome in women with TSH concentrations within normal adult range. Gynecol Obstet Invest. 2014;77(2):84–8.

35. Unuane D, Velkeniers B, Bravenboer B, Drakopoulos P, Tournaye H, Parra J, et al. Impact of thyroid autoimmunity in euthyroid women on live birth rate after IUI. Hum Reprod. 2017;32(4):915–22.

36. Michalakis KG, Mesen TB, Brayboy LM, Yu B, Richter KS, Levy M, et al. Subclinical elevations of thyroid-stimulating hormone and assisted reproductive technology outcomes. Fertil Steril. 2011;95(8):2634–7.

37. Chai J, Yeung WY, Lee CY, Li HW, Ho PC, Ng HY. Live birth rates following in vitro fertilization in women with thyroid autoimmunity and/or subclinical hypothyroidism. Clin Endocrinol (Oxf). 2014;80(1):122–7.

38. Baker VL, Rone HM, Pasta DJ, Nelson HP, Gvakharia M, Adamson GD. Correlation of thyroid stimulating hormone (TSH) level with pregnancy outcome in women undergoing in vitro fertilization. Am J Obstet Gynecol. 2006;194(6):1668–74 discussion 74-5.

39. Weghofer A, Himaya E, Kushnir VA, Barad DH, Gleicher N. The impact of thyroid function and thyroid autoimmunity on embryo quality in women with low functional ovarian reserve: a case-control study. Reprod Biol Endocrinol. 2015;13:43.

40. Gingold JA, Zafman K, Rodriguez-Purata J, Whitehouse MC, Lee JA, Sandler B, et al. Do elevated TSH levels predict early pregnancy loss in ART patients? Gynecol Endocrinol. 2016;32(12):973–6.

41. YX Z. Effect of thyroid stimulating hormone (TSH) level on IVF/ICSI outcomes. Reprod Contracept. 2012;32(1):17–23.

42. Vanderpump MP, Tunbridge WM, French JM, Appleton D, Bates D, Clark F, et al. The incidence of thyroid disorders in the community: a twenty-year follow-up of the Whickham Survey. Clin Endocrinol (Oxf). 1995;43(1):55–68.

43. Baloch Z, Carayon P, Conte-Devolx B, Demers LM, Feldt-Rasmussen U, Henry JF, et al. Laboratory medicine practice guidelines. Laboratory support for the diagnosis and monitoring of thyroid disease. Thyroid. 2003;13(1):3–126.

44. Glendenning P. Management of thyroid dysfunction during pregnancy and postpartum: an Endocrine Society Clinical Practice Guideline. Clin Biochem Rev. 2008;29(2):83–5.

45. Jensen E, Blaabjerg O, Petersen PH, Hegedus L. Sampling time is important but may be overlooked in establishment and use of thyroid-stimulating hormone reference intervals. Clin Chem. 2007;53(2):355–6.

46. Wartofsky L, Dickey RA. The evidence for a narrower thyrotropin reference range is compelling. J Clin Endocrinol Metab. 2005;90(9):5483–8.

47. Surks MI, Goswami G, Daniels GH. The thyrotropin reference range should remain unchanged. J Clin Endocrinol Metab. 2005;90(9):5489–96.

48. Surks MI, Hollowell JG. Age-specific distribution of serum thyrotropin and antithyroid antibodies in the US population: implications for the prevalence of subclinical hypothyroidism. J Clin Endocrinol Metab. 2007;92(12):4575–82.

49. Abdel Rahman AH, Aly AH, Abbassy AA. Improved in vitro fertilization outcomes after treatment of subclinical hypothyroidism in infertile women. Endocr Pract. 2010;16(5):792.

50. Kim CH, Ahn JW, Kang SP, Kim SH, Chae HD, Kang BM. Effect of levothyroxine treatment on in vitro fertilization and pregnancy outcome in infertile women with subclinical hypothyroidism undergoing in vitro fertilization/intracytoplasmic sperm injection. Fertil Steril. 2011;95(5):1650–4.

51. Maheshwari A, Bhide P, Pundir J, Bhattacharya S. Routine serum thyroid-stimulating hormone testing-optimizing pre-conception health or generating toxic knowledge? Hum Reprod. 2017;32(9):1779–85.

52. Gilbert RM, Hadlow NC, Walsh JP, Fletcher SJ, Brown SJ, Stuckey BG, et al. Assessment of thyroid function during pregnancy: first-trimester (weeks 9-13) reference intervals derived from Western Australian women. Med J Aust. 2008;189(5):250–3.

53. Gracia CR, Morse CB, Chan G, Schilling S, Prewitt M, Sammel MD, et al. Thyroid function during controlled ovarian hyperstimulation as part of in vitro fertilization. Fertil Steril. 2012;97(3):585–91.

## 19

Identification of mRNAs related to endometrium function regulated by lncRNA CD36–005 in rat endometrial stromal cells

Xueying Zhang[1], Ying Xu[1], Lulu Fu[1], Dandan Li[1], Xiaowei Dai[1], Lianlian Liu[1], Jingshun Zhang[1], Lianwen Zheng[1*] and Manhua Cui[2*]

Abstract

Background: Polycystic ovary syndrome (PCOS) is a heterogeneous endocrine disorder in women of reproductive age and is commonly complicated by adverse endometrial outcomes. Long non-coding RNAs (lncRNAs) are a class of non-protein-coding transcripts that are more than 200 nucleotides in length. Accumulating evidence indicates that lncRNAs are involved in the development of various human diseases. Among these lncRNAs, lncRNA CD36–005 (CD36–005) is indicated to be associated with the pathogenesis of PCOS. However, the mechanisms of action of CD36–005 have not yet been elucidated.

Methods: This study determined the CD36–005 expression level in the uteri of PCOS rat model and its effect on the proliferation activity of rat primary endometrial stromal cells. RNA sequencing (RNA-seq) and bioinformatics analysis were performed to detect the mRNA expression profiles and the biological pathways in which these differentially expressed mRNAs involved, after CD36–005 overexpression in the primary endometrial stromal cells. The differential expression of Hmgn5, Nr5a2, Dll4, Entpd1, Fam50a, and Brms1 were further validated by quantitative reverse transcription polymerase chain reaction (qRT-PCR).

Results: CD36–005 is highly expressed in the uteri of PCOS rat model and promotes the proliferation of rat primary endometrial stromal cells. A total of fifty-five mRNAs differentially expressed were identified in CD36–005 overexpressed stromal cells. Further analyses identified that these differentially expressed mRNAs participate in many biological processes and are associated with various human diseases. The results of qRT-PCR validation were consistent with the RNA-seq data.

Conclusions: These data provide a list of potential target mRNA genes of CD36–005 in endometrial stromal cells and laid a foundation for further studies on the molecular function and mechanism of CD36–005 in the endometrium.

Keywords: lncRNA, CD36–005, RNA sequencing, Endometrium, Stromal cells, PCOS

Background

Polycystic ovary syndrome (PCOS) is one of the most common and complex endocrine disorders in women of reproductive age, with a prevalence estimated to be 5–10% [1–4]. The clinical features of PCOS are highly heterogeneous. Patients with PCOS have reproductive dysfunction and metabolic abnormalities, and are commonly characterized by persistent ovulatory disorder, ovarian polycystic morphology, hyperandrogenism, insulin resistance (IR), hyperinsulinemia, and obesity [5, 6]. In addition, in women with PCOS, the risk of type 2 diabetes, cardiovascular disease, infertility, and some adverse endometrial outcomes increases [7–11]. The diversity of the clinical features of PCOS is attributed to the multifactorial contribution on its pathogenesis, including complex genetic and environmental factors [12]. Patients with PCOS often have endometrial abnormalities and most are anovulatory or oligo ovulatory. However, after the anovulation or oligo

---

* Correspondence: davezheng@sohu.com; jlucmh@163.com
[1]Reproductive Medical Center, Department of Obstetrics and Gynecology, The Second Hospital of Jilin University, No. 218 Ziqiang Street, Changchun 130041, Jilin, China
[2]Department of Obstetrics and Gynecology, The Second Hospital of Jilin University, No. 218 Ziqiang Street, Changchun 130041, Jilin, China

ovulation is treated, they still have lower pregnancy rates and higher spontaneous miscarriage rates, which suggest the decrease of their endometrial receptivity [10, 13]. Additionally, patients with PCOS have a significantly higher risk of having endometrial hyperplasia and developing endometrial cancer [11]. These adverse endometrial outcomes are associated with the metabolic abnormalities of PCOS including chronic unopposed estrogen, IR, hyperinsulinemia, hyperandrogenism, and obesity, and complex genetic alterations [11, 14]. However, the underlying mechanisms of PCOS in the uterus are still unclear.

Long non-coding RNAs (lncRNAs) are defined as a class of non-coding transcripts with the length of more than 200 nucleotides. Although lncRNAs lack the capacity to code for proteins, they can regulate gene expression at epigenetic, transcriptional, posttranscriptional, and other levels [15]. lncRNAs are proven to play key roles in many biological processes, including genetic imprinting, X-chromosome inactivation, gene transcription regulation, organelle biogenesis, and subcellular trafficking [16]. Dysfunctional lncRNAs contribute to the pathogenesis of many human diseases, such as diabetic nephropathy, nonalcoholic steatohepatitis, cardiomyopathy, atherosclerosis, and cancers in various systems [17–21]. The role of lncRNAs in the pathogenesis of several endometrial diseases has also been reported in recent studies, including implantation failure or spontaneous miscarriage, endometrial hyperplasia, adenomyosis, endometriosis, and endometrial cancer [11, 22–24]. However, we knew little about the role of lncRNAs in the pathogenesis of adverse endometrial outcomes of PCOS.

In our previous research, we found that lncRNA CD36–005 (CD36–005) was significantly upregulated in the ovaries of PCOS rat model by lncRNA expression profile analysis [25]. After determining that CD36–005 is also highly expressed in the uteri of PCOS rat model in the present study, we suggest that the upregulation of CD36–005 expression might be associated with the pathogenesis of PCOS in the uterus. We used primary endometrial stromal cells from rat uteri as the in-vitro model, and performed RNA sequencing (RNA-seq) technology and bioinformatics analyses after CD36–005 overexpression to investigate its potential role from a more comprehensive perspective. We also conducted CCK-8 assay to determine the effect of CD36–005 on the proliferation activity of stromal cells, which is the first step of decidualization. Our results provide insights into the underlying molecular mechanisms of CD36–005 in the regulation of endometrial stromal cells and the pathogenesis of adverse endometrial outcomes of PCOS.

Methods

Animals

All animal procedures were approved by the Institutional Animal Care and Use Committee of Jilin University, and were conducted in accordance with the Guidelines for the Care and Use of Laboratory Animals. Mature female Wistar rats (8 weeks old) were purchased for the isolation of primary endometrial stromal cells in the present study.

Animal model, vaginal smears, tissue sampling, and hormone assays

The uterine tissue used in this study was collected from the PCOS rat model in the article "Expression profiles of mRNA and long noncoding RNA in the ovaries of letrozole-induced polycystic ovary syndrome rat model through deep sequencing [25]." The middle of the uteri (body of uterus) was collected for subsequent total RNA extraction.

Isolation of endometrial stromal cells

Primary endometrial stromal cells were isolated from 8-week-old Wistar rats' uteri using previously described methods, cultured with DMEM-nutrient mixture F-12 Ham (DMEM-F12, Hyclone, USA) containing 10% heat-inactivated fetal bovine serum (FBS, Gibco, USA), and incubated at 37 °C with 5% CO_2 [26].

Cell immunofluorescence

Stromal cells were seeded on coverslips and washed with phosphate buffer saline (PBS, Hyclone, USA). Then, the confluent cells were fixed in cold methanol, permeabilized with 0.1% Triton X-100, and blocked with 1% goat serum. Stromal cells were incubated overnight at 4 °C with rabbit anti-mouse monoclonal antibody specific to vimentin and cytokeratin-19 at a 1:200 dilution in PBS (Boster, Wuhan, China) [27–29]. In order to validate the specificity of vimentin antibody, 5% nonimmune goat serum was used as negative control. After washed by PBS three times, stromal cells were incubated with goat-anti-rabbit second antibody (Boster, Wuhan, China) for 2 h at room temperature. Finally, coverslips were rinsed and mounted with DAPI. The stained stromal cells were observed using Olympus IX71 fluorescence microscope and images were analyzed by using cellSens Dimension.

Overexpression and knockdown of lncRNA CD35–005 in endometrial stromal cells

When stromal cells reached 70% confluency, they were transiently transfected with either Ad-CD36–005 or Ad-GFP designed by Hanbio Biotechnology Co., Ltd. (Shanghai, China) at the designated multiplicity of infection (MOI) of 50. The full-length sequence of CD36–005 was directly cloned into the pHBAD-EF1-MCS-3flag-CMV-GFP vector by seamless cloning. After 6 h incubation at 37 °C in 5% CO2, the medium was replaced with fresh growth medium. After transfection with Ad-CD36–005 or Ad-GFP, the stromal cells were collected at 48 h.

The small-interfering RNA (siRNA) duplexes for targeting CD36–005, as well as a scrambled sequence (control siRNA duplex, negative control) were synthesized by the RiboBio Company (Guangzhou, China). The sequences were shown as follows: 5'-UAAGGACCUCUAUUGCUUG TT and CAAGCAAUAGAGGUCCUUATT (CD36–005 siRNA); 5'-UUCUCCGAACGUGUCACGUTT and 5'-A CGUGACACGUUCGGAGAATT (nonspecific scrambled siRNA, negative control). Transfections for siRNA were performed according to Fugene HD Transfection Reagent (Promega, USA) protocol. After transfection with CD36–005 or control siRNA, stromal cells were collected at 36 h.

Cell proliferation
CCK-8 reagent (Promega, USA) was used to perform the proliferation assays according to the manufacturer's directions. Stromal cells were seeded at a density of 1×10^5 /well in 96-well plates and cultured in the DMEM/F12 medium containing 2% heat-inactivated FBS. After transfection with Ad-CD36–005, Ad-GFP, or CD36–005 siRNA, the stromal cells were cultured for 48 h. Finally, cells in each well were added with 10 μl of CCK-8 reagent and incubated for 2 h. Absorbance was measured at 490 nm using a 96-well plate reader.

RNA extraction
Total RNA from the middle of the uteri and stromal cells were extracted using TRIzol (Invitrogen/Life Technologies, USA) according to the manufacturer's protocol. The concentration and quality of RNA were determined using NanoDrop 2000 spectrophotometer (Thermo Fisher Scientific, UK) to ensure that the OD260/280 absorbance ratios of all samples were between 1.8 and 2. RNA integrity was evaluated using the Agilent 2100 Bioanalyzer (Agilent Technologies, USA).

RNA sequencing and bioinformatics analysis
RNA samples from three stromal cells in each group with RNA Integrity Number (RIN) ≥ 7 were subjected to the subsequent mRNA sequencing by Shanghai OE Biotech Co., Ltd. (Shanghai, China). The libraries were constructed using TruSeq Stranded mRNA LTSample Prep Kit (Illumina, San Diego, CA, USA) according to the manufacturer's instructions. These libraries were sequenced on the Illumina sequencing platform (HiSeqTM 2500 or Illumina HiSeq X Ten) and 125 bp/150 bp paired-end reads were generated. We used Gene Ontology (GO) to categorize the function of the differentially expressed mRNAs and Kyoto Encyclopedia of Genes and Genomes (KEGG) to predict the signaling pathways in which these differentially expressed mRNAs may be involved.

Real-time quantitative PCR analysis
Reverse transcription reactions were performed using PrimeScript RT Reagent Kit (Takara Bio) according to the manufacturer's protocol. Quantitative real-time polymerase chain reaction (qRT-PCR) analyses were performed at the following conditions: 95 °C for 2 min followed by 40 cycles of 95 °C for 15 s and 59 °C for 30 s, according to the instructions of SYBR Premix Ex Taq (TaKaRa). The mRNAs and lncRNA CD36–005 were normalized to glyceraldehyde-3-phosphate dehydrogenase (GAPDH), and the relative expression levels were analyzed by calculating the fold changes using the $2^{-\Delta\Delta Ct}$ value method. We purchased the primer sequences for qRT-PCR from RiboBio Company (Guangzhou, China).

Statistics
Significance of difference between two groups was compared by Independent-Samples T Test. Data are shown mean ± SEM. Significance of difference was considered significant at $P < 0.05$. All statistical analyses were performed using SPSS17.0 software (SPSS Inc., Chicago).

Results
Quality control of primary endometrial stromal cell cultures
The purity of the primary endometrial stromal cells was assessed using the difference in vimentin and cytokeratin expression. The absence of primary antibody was used as a negative control. Results of cell immunofluorescence show that the purity of endometrial stromal cells was more than 90%, which can be used for subsequent experiments (Fig. 1).

Expression of lncRNA CD36–005 in the uteri of PCOS model
Result of the qRT-PCR analyses showed that the expression level of CD36–005 in the uteri of PCOS rat model was significantly higher than in the normal (Fig. 2).

Overexpression and knockdown of lncRNA CD36–005 in primary endometrial stromal cells
Result of the qRT-PCR analyses showed that the expression level of CD36–005 in the Ad-CD36–005 transfected stromal cells was significantly higher compared with that of Ad-GFP transfected cells; CD36–005 expression level in the CD36–005 siRNA transfected stromal cells was significantly lower compared with that of the negative control siRNA transfected cells (Fig. 3).

Effects of lncRNA CD36–005 on primary endometrial stromal cell proliferation
Overexpression of CD36–005 could strengthen the proliferation activity of stromal cells. On the contrary, the proliferation activity of stromal cells was reduced

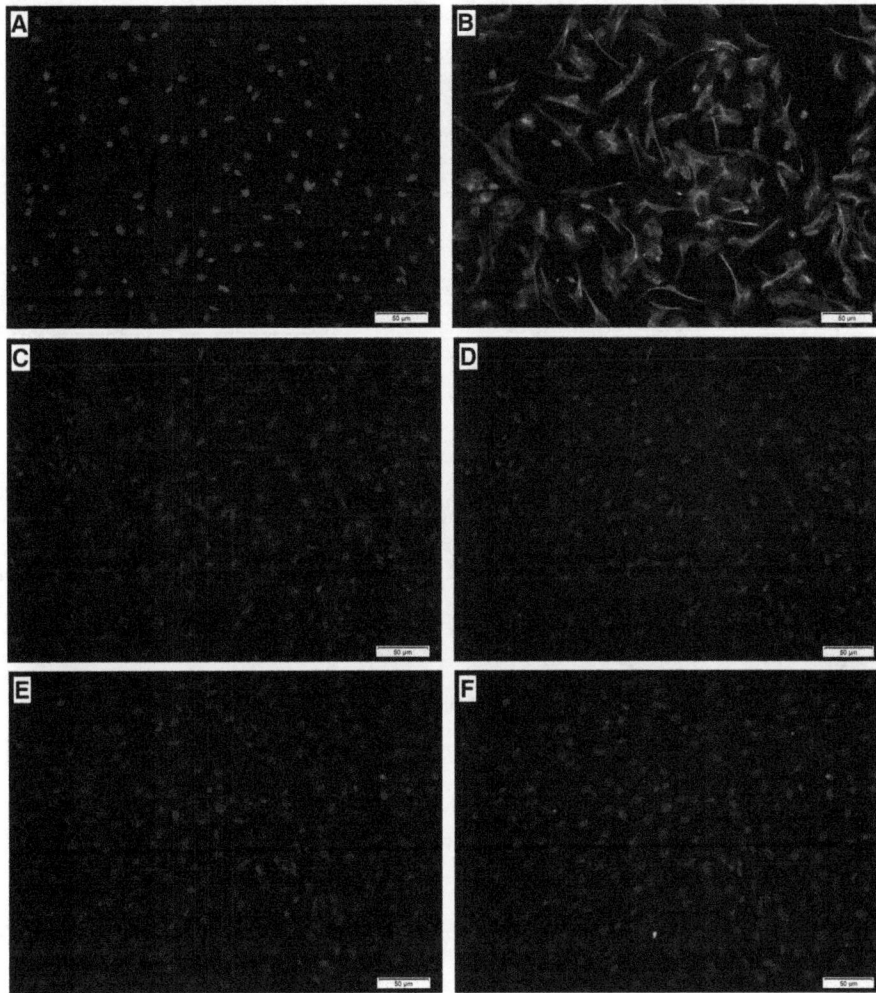

Fig. 1 Immunofluorescence for vimentin in endometrial stromal cells. **a, c, e** Only DAPI staining on endometrial stromal cell cultures. **b** Vimentin double staining on endometrial stromal cell cultures. **d** Negative control with primary antibody omitted for endometrial stromal cell cultures. **f** Cytokeratin-19 double staining on endometrial stromal cell cultures. The scale bar is shown in the lower right corner of each picture. The length of the scale bar is equivalent to 50 μm

compared with control after they were transfected with CD36–005 siRNA (Fig. 4).

Gene expression profiling following CD36–005 overexpression

A total of 55 mRNAs were differentially expressed between the Ad-CD36–005 and Ad-GFP groups (absolute $\log_2$(fold change) > 1, p < 0.05) (Fig. 5). Moreover, 22 mRNAs were differentially expressed with absolute $\log_2$(fold change) > 2. Among the 55 differentially expressed mRNAs, 28 mRNAs were upregulated and 27 mRNAs were downregulated in the Ad-CD36–005 group.

Validation of differentially expressed mRNAs

According to references and our interest, six mRNAs from the results of RNA-seq were selected for further validation by using qRT-PCR analysis. Compared with the Ad-GFP group, Hmgn5, Nr5a2, Dll4, Entpd1, and Brms1 displayed a decreased expression, and Fam50a displayed an increased expression in the Ad-CD36–005 group (p < 0.05) (Fig. 6). These results showed that the qRT-PCR results of expression levels of all six mRNAs confirmed were consistent with the RNA-seq data.

Bioinformatics analysis

Results of the GO analyses categorized the differentially expressed mRNAs into different biological processes, such as biological adhesion, reproductive process, and metabolic process (Fig. 7). KEGG pathway analyses predicted that the differentially expressed mRNAs were involved in various biochemical pathways, including cell growth and death, transport and catabolism, signal transduction, lipid metabolism, and so on (Fig. 8).

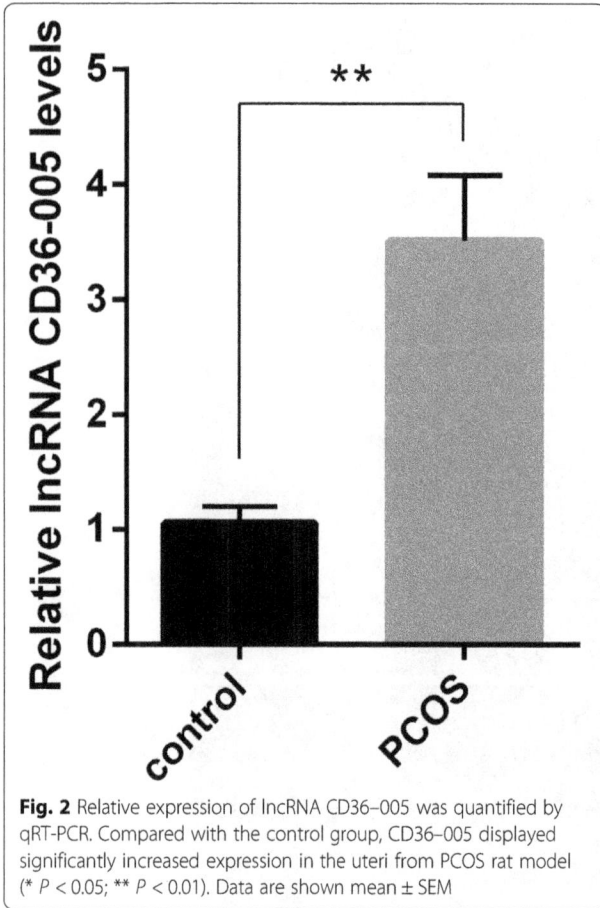

Fig. 2 Relative expression of lncRNA CD36–005 was quantified by qRT-PCR. Compared with the control group, CD36–005 displayed significantly increased expression in the uteri from PCOS rat model (* $P < 0.05$; ** $P < 0.01$). Data are shown mean ± SEM

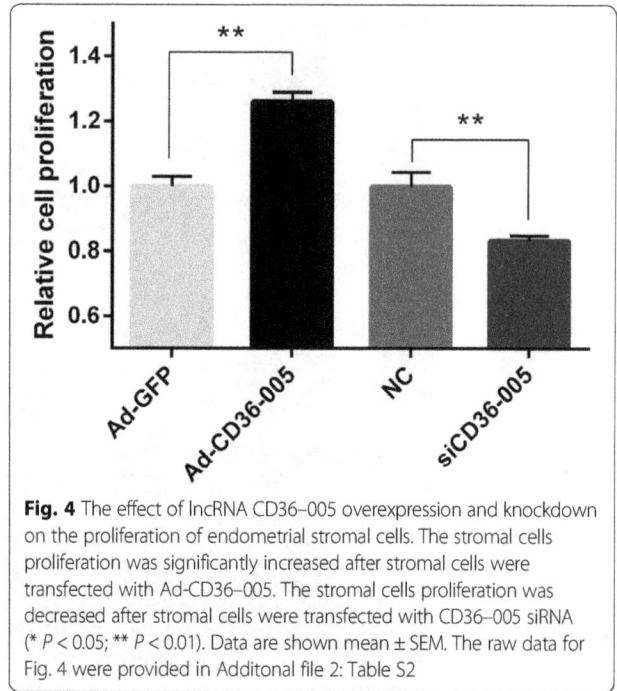

Fig. 3 Relative expression of lncRNA CD36–005 in the endometrial stromal cells after transfected with Ad-GFP, Ad-CD36–005, control siRNA and CD36–005 siRNA. The CD36–005 expression was significantly increased after stromal cells were transfected with Ad-CD36–005. The CD36–005 expression was significantly decreased after stromal cells were transfected with CD36–005 siRNA (* $P < 0.05$; ** $P < 0.01$). Data are shown mean ± SEM. The raw data for Fig. 3 were provided in Additonal file 1: Table S1

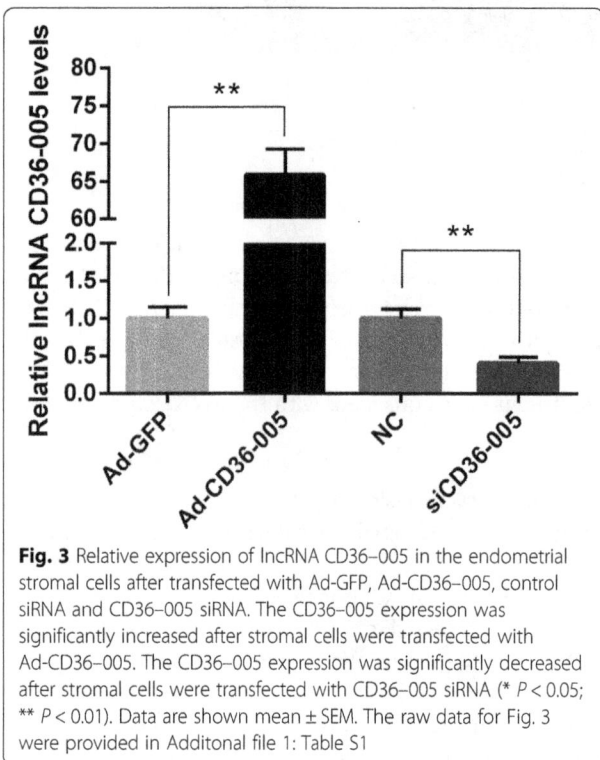

Fig. 4 The effect of lncRNA CD36–005 overexpression and knockdown on the proliferation of endometrial stromal cells. The stromal cells proliferation was significantly increased after stromal cells were transfected with Ad-CD36–005. The stromal cells proliferation was decreased after stromal cells were transfected with CD36–005 siRNA (* $P < 0.05$; ** $P < 0.01$). Data are shown mean ± SEM. The raw data for Fig. 4 were provided in Additonal file 2: Table S2

Discussion

Accumulating evidence shows that the endocrinal and metabolic disorders of PCOS have complex effects on the endometrium, leading to endometrial abnormalities [11, 14]. The endometrium is a steroid hormone-targeting tissue that undergoes cyclic secretion and proliferation dynamically in response to estrogen and progesterone produced by the ovaries [30]. Because most patients with PCOS are anovulatory or oligo ovulatory, the endometrium is continuously stimulated by unopposed estrogen in the absence of the regulatory effects of progesterone, which decrease the endometrial receptivity and promote the development of endometrial hyperplasia and even cancer in the long run [11]. In addition, patients with PCOS often have IR and obesity [6]. Insulin levels in the local endometrium affect the endometrial development and receptivity. IR can cause hyperglycemia, which further aggravates hyperandrogenism [14]. These are all high risk factors of endometrial cancer [11]. The pathogenesis of PCOS and its abnormal endometrial outcomes is a multifactorial biological process that involves a large number of genes and biological pathways, among which the role of lncRNAs has been studied in recent years [22, 31].

Owing to the abundance but low expression level of lncRNAs, they were initially considered to be transcriptional noise without any biological function [32]. With the rapid development of genomics and transcriptomics technology, researchers gradually found the regulatory

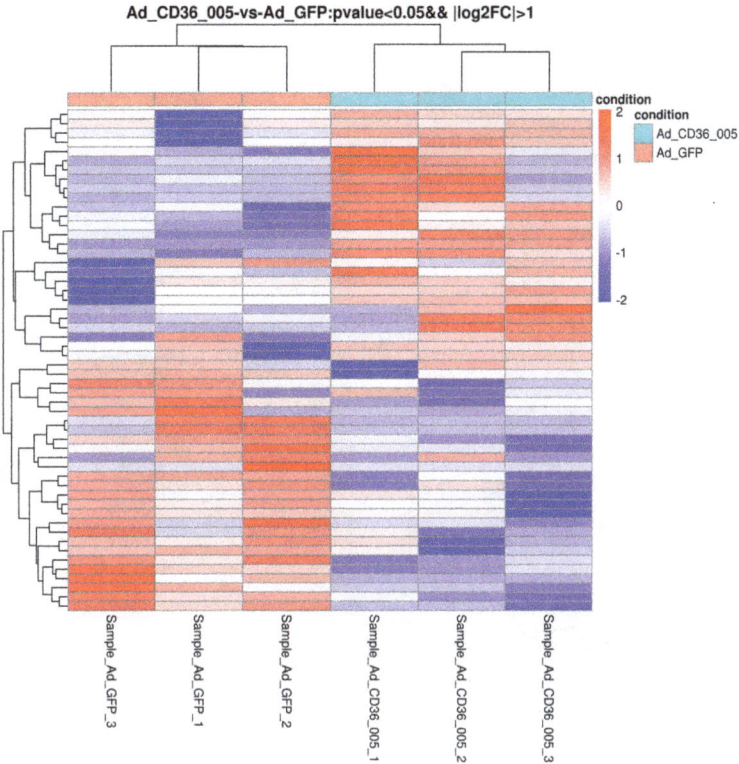

Fig. 5 Hierarchical clustering heatmaps of differentially expressed mRNAs in the endometrial stromal cells after lncRNA CD36–005 overexpression

role of lncRNAs in various human diseases [17]. In accumulating studies, only a few lncRNAs have been reported to be associated with both PCOS and various endometrial disorders. The expression of steroid receptor RNA activator (SRA) as well as lncRNA CTBP1-AS, a novel androgen receptor modulator, was significantly higher in peripheral blood leukocytes of women with PCOS. Meantime, it is known that women with PCOS show dysregulated hormone receptors expression, suggesting us a potential role of genes modulating hormone receptors in PCOS-associated endometrial disorders [33–35]. However, the functions and underlying mechanisms of these dysregulated remains unclear and need to be further studied.

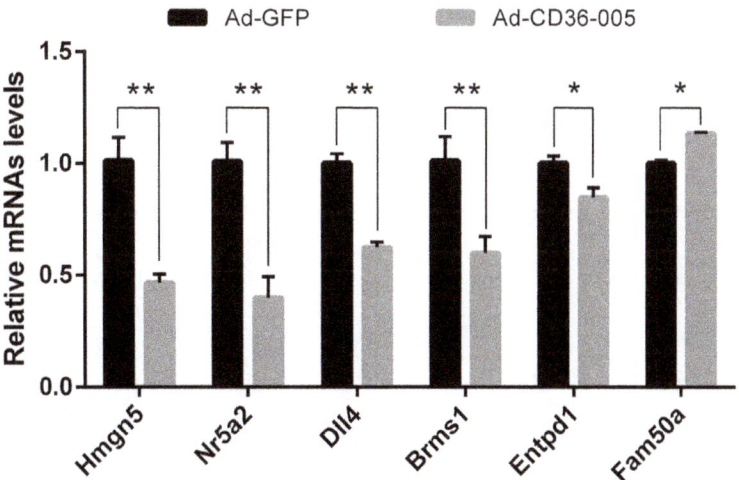

Fig. 6 Relative expression of six selected mRNA was quantified by qRT-PCR. Compared with the Ad-GFP group, Hmgn5, Nr5a2, Dll4, Entpd1, and Brms1 displayed decreased expression, whereas Fam50a displayed an increased expression in the Ad-CD36–005 group (* $P < 0.05$; ** $P < 0.01$). Data are shown mean ± SEM

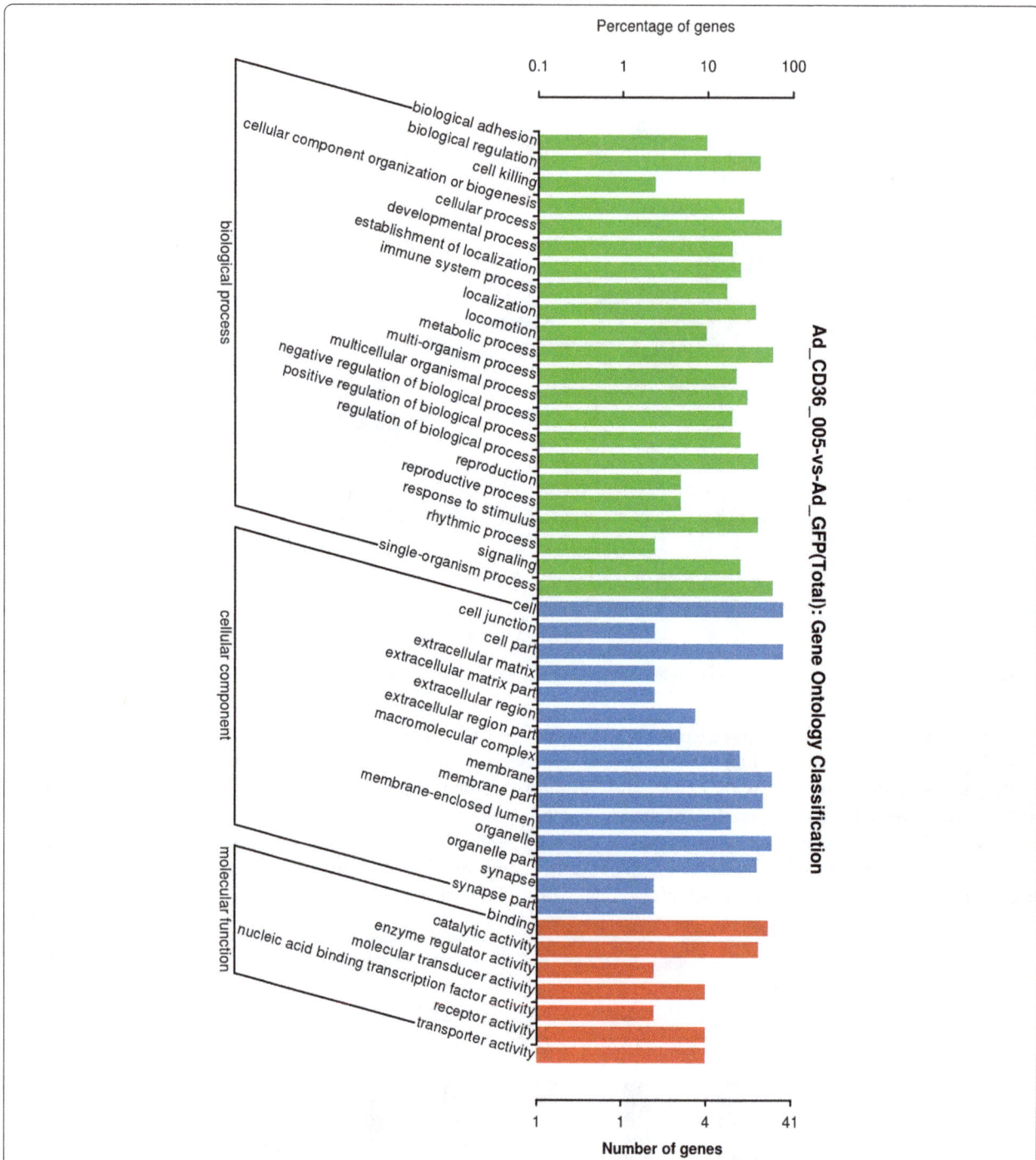

Fig. 7 Gene Ontology (GO) classification of differentially expressed mRNAs. GO annotation showed that the differentially expressed mRNAs were associated with different biological processes

The endometrial stromal cell is one of the in-vitro models of the endometrial tissue used for the study of the molecular mechanisms of endometrial diseases. Decidualization is a process of endometrial stromal cell proliferation and subsequent differentiation, during which stromal cells transform into specialized decidual cells [36, 37]. This process is essential for embryo implantation and successful pregnancy. Although many studies have focused on the molecular mechanisms of decidualization, known lncRNAs associated with decidualization were limited. HK2P1 is a lncRNA found to be decreased in the decidua of severe preeclampsia patients. In vitro results show that downregulated HK2P1 inhibited human endometrial stromal cell (HESC) proliferation and

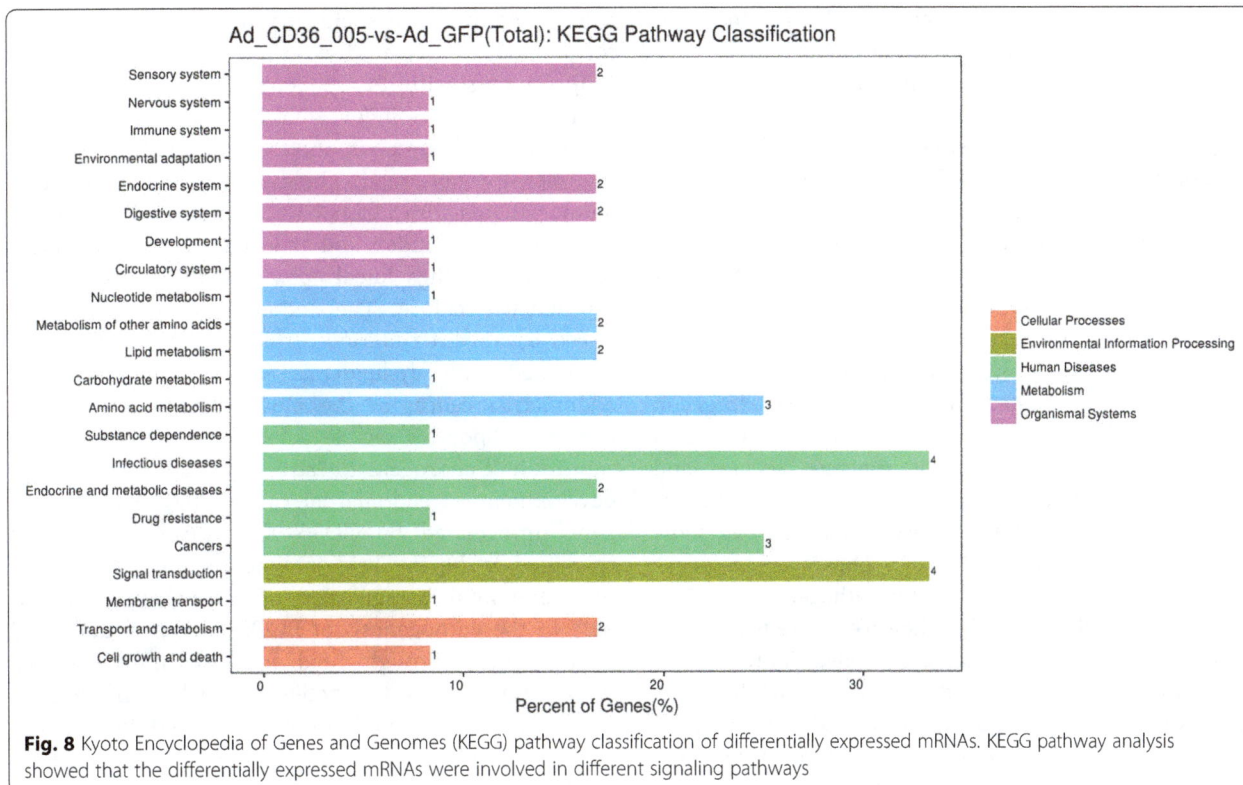

Fig. 8 Kyoto Encyclopedia of Genes and Genomes (KEGG) pathway classification of differentially expressed mRNAs. KEGG pathway analysis showed that the differentially expressed mRNAs were involved in different signaling pathways

differentiation by regulating miR-6887-3p and its target gene HK2 expression as a ceRNA [38]. The expression of another lncRNA, LINC00473, is highly induced in HESCs after decidual stimulus [39]. These studies prove a crucial role of lncRNA in stromal cell decidualization and suggest that lncRNAs participate in some endometrial diseases partly through affecting stromal cells, of which some may be caused by PCOS.

In the present study, CD36–005 was upregulated in the uteri of PCOS rat model and could promote the proliferation of stromal cells. However, the molecular mechanisms remain to be characterized. Thus, we conducted RNA-seq and found 55 known mRNAs in the primary endometrial stromal cells differentially expressed between the Ad-CD36–005 and Ad-GFP group with a threshold of $p <$ 0.05 and $|\log_2(\text{Fold-Change})| > 1$. We chose six mRNAs (Hmgn5, Nr5a2, Dll4, Entpd1, Fam50a, and Brms1) for qRT-PCR validation, and the results were consistent with the RNA-seq data. In previous studies, Qiao performed microarray analysis on the endometrial biopsies of women with PCOS during the implantation window and found down-regulated genes were associated with endometrial receptivity [40]. Similarly, Bellver performed microarray hybridization and identified an aberrant endometrial transcriptome in obese women with PCOS during the implantation window [41]. Among our RNA-seq result, several genes have been reported to be involved in endometrial disorders, but little is known whether these

endometrial disorders are related to PCOS. Hmgn5, also known as Nsbp1, regulates uterine decidualization as a downstream gene of Hoxa10 in a differentiation-specific manner [42]. Hmgn5 was also found to be hypomethylated in mouse uteri when exposed to diethylstilbestrol or fenistein neonatally [43]. Nr5a2, also known as Lrh-1, was known as a key transcriptional factor of multiple steroidogenic genes in vitro [44]. In Wang's study, Nr5a2 promotes aromatase expression in primary rat granulosa cells, indicating its potential involvement in PCOS while the ovaries of women with PCOS have abnormal steroidogenesis and folliculogenesis [45, 46]. Consistent with above report, Kevin elucidated in his review that a higher level of Lrh-1 could activate estradiol production in the endometrium of women with endometrial cancer [47]. Lrh-1 is also essential for a successful pregnancy as its indispensible roles in the luteal function, decidualization, and placental formation [48]. Combined with our result, we could speculate that the dysregulated expression of Nr5a2 may be associated with PCOS-associated endometrial disorders. Dll4, a gene involved in the delta-notch pathways, participates in the decidualization failure of stromal cells from women with endometriosis [49]. The promiscuous expression of Dll4 impaired decidual angiogenesis, and coordinated with disrupted decidual cellular proliferation and apoptosis, could be one of the causes of early miscarriages [50]. No relevant studies focus on the relationship of Entpd1, Fam50a, and Brms1 to endometrial disorders, and further studies are needed.

GO and KEGG analyses were performed to identify the potential functions and pathways of the 55 target genes of CD36–005. GO analyses revealed that these differentially expressed genes were involved in various categories, such as nitric oxide biosynthetic process and positive regulation of gene expression including toll-like receptor 7/9 (TLR-7/9) and interleukin-6/8 (IL-6/8). The nitric oxide (NO)/ nitric oxide synthase (NOS) system was presumed to locally regulate the endometrial functions, including stromal cells decidualization [51]. Nos2, a synthase involved in NO production, was upregulated by CD36–005 overexpression and predicted to be involved in the nitric oxide mediated signal transduction, nitric-oxide synthase activity, and nitric-oxide synthase binding. Nos2 was also found to participate in the inflammatory process of PCOS and some endometrial abnormalities [52, 53]. Thus, we can speculate that Nos2 may play a role in the pathogenesis of endometrial abnormalities of PCOS, however, there is no direct evidence and further studies are needed. TLR-7/9 and IL-6/8 were shown to be related to endometrial disorders. The expression of TLR-9 was increased with reduced DNA methylation in spontaneous preterm labor [54]. Higher TLR-9 transcriptional activity may be a protective factor for endometrial cancer risk [55]. According to Gu, the expression of TLR9 in cumulus cells was influenced significantly by PCOS, which may further lower the embryo quality and decrease the fertility rate of women with PCOS. These results suggest us the dysregulated expression of TLR9 may be potentially involved in the pathogenesis of PCOS and its adverse endometrial outcomes. TRL-7 is crucial in the establishment and maintenance of pregnancy in sheep [56]. IL-8 participates in the pathogenesis of endometriosis by regulating ectopic endometrial cell proliferation, invasion, and adhesion [57]. Levels of IL-6 in the mid-secretory-phase endometrium are lower in women with previous recurrent miscarriage [58]. Additionally, the aberrant IL-6 and IL-8 in endometrial stromal fibroblasts from women with PCOS was thought be related to the altered endometrial immune profile and imbalanced leukocyte migration, both of which contribute to a sub-optimal implantation of women with PCOS [59]. Thus, the regulation of these biological processes may be one of the complex mechanisms of some endometrial abnormalities, of which some might be induced by PCOS.

KEGG analyses showed that these differentially expressed genes were associated with diverse signaling pathways, including cell growth and death, transport and catabolism, signal transduction, lipid metabolism, endocrine and metabolic diseases, and cancers. Among these pathways, lipid metabolism was a biological process closely related to PCOS and its endometrial abnormalities. In previous studies, 70% of women with PCOS

were found to have dyslipidemia, which is also a risk factor for cardiovascular disease and endometrial cancer [60]. Patients with PCOS commonly suffer from increased body mass index, total cholesterol, triglyceride, low-density lipoprotein-cholesterol, and decreased high-density lipoprotein-cholesterol [61]. In Chekir's study, patients with PCOS have an increased uterine arterial pulsatility index and reduced endometrial thickness during the luteal phase, which may cause reproductive failure. The endometrial dysfunction induced by impaired uterine perfusion was thought to be correlated with dyslipidemia [61]. Nieman regarded endometrial cancer as the most relevant cancer with obesity. Adipocytes secrete adipokines and mediate the transition of androgens to estrogen, which promotes the development of endometrial cancer [62]. Mogat1 is a gene upregulated by CD36–005 overexpression and predicted to be involved in lipid metabolism. Hence, the differential upregulation of Mogat1 may participate in the pathogenesis of PCOS and its endometrial abnormalities through lipid metabolism. Above all, these results suggest a potential mechanism through which the dysregulated mRNAs involved in different categories and biological pathways contribute together to the regulation of stromal cells and the pathogenesis of endometrial abnormalities, some of which may be caused by PCOS.

Conclusion

We identified a list of 55 potential target mRNAs of CD36–005 in the primary endometrial stromal cells by RNA-seq and confirmed the relative expression levels of Hmgn5, Nr5a2, Dll4, Entpd1, Fam50a, and Brms1 using qRT-PCR. We used GO and KEGG pathway analyses, and predicted the various biochemical pathways that regulate the proliferation and decidualization of stromal cells and the pathogenesis of some endometrial abnormalities, in which these differentially expressed mRNAs may be involved in. Our results partly explained the mechanisms by which CD36–005 regulate the etiology and pathophysiology of PCOS in the uterus of rat with letrozole-induced PCOS, and laid a foundation for further studies on the molecular function and mechanism of CD36–005 in stromal cells. Further detailed studies are needed to clarify the underlying mechanisms of CD36–005 on the regulation of stromal cells and to investigate if these alterations could serve as biomarkers for the prediction of some endometrial diseases induced by PCOS.

Abbreviations

CD36–005: lncRNA CD36–005; E$_2$: 17-beta estradiol; GO: Gene Ontology; HESC: human endometrial stromal cell; IL: interleukin; IR: insulin resistance; KEGG: Kyoto Encyclopedia of Genes and Genomes; LncRNA: long non-coding

RNA; MOI: multiplicity of infection; NO: nitric oxide; NOS: nitric oxide synthase; PCOS: polycystic ovary syndrome; RNA-seq: RNA sequencing; SRA: steroid receptor RNA activator; TLR: toll-like receptor

Authors' contributions
XZ, LZ and MC designed the study; XZ, YX, LF and DL performed the experiments; XZ wrote the manuscript. All authors discussed the results, read and approved the final manuscript.

Competing interests
The authors declare that they have no competing interests.

References

1. Li R, Zhang Q, Yang D, Li S, Lu S, Wu X, et al. Prevalence of polycystic ovary syndrome in women in China: a large community-based study. Hum Reprod. 2013;28:2562–9.
2. Asuncion M, Calvo RM, San Millan JL, Sancho J, Avila S, Escobar-Morreale HF. A prospective study of the prevalence of the polycystic ovary syndrome in unselected Caucasian women from Spain. J Clin Endocrinol Metab. 2000; 85:2434–8.
3. March WA, Moore VM, Willson KJ, Phillips DI, Norman RJ, Davies MJ. The prevalence of polycystic ovary syndrome in a community sample assessed under contrasting diagnostic criteria. Hum Reprod. 2010;25:544–51.
4. Azziz R, Woods KS, Reyna R, Key TJ, Knochenhauer ES, Yildiz BO. The prevalence and features of the polycystic ovary syndrome in an unselected population. J Clin Endocrinol Metab. 2004;89:2745–9.
5. Christakou C, Diamanti-Kandarakis E. Polycystic ovary syndrome--phenotypes and diagnosis. Scand J Clin Lab Invest Suppl. 2014;244:18–22 discussion 1.
6. Ranasinha S, Joham AE, Norman RJ, Shaw JE, Zoungas S, Boyle J, et al. The association between polycystic ovary syndrome (PCOS) and metabolic syndrome: a statistical modelling approach. Clin Endocrinol. 2015;83:879–87.
7. Kakoly NS, Khomami MB, Joham AE, Cooray SD, Misso ML, Norman RJ, et al. Ethnicity, obesity and the prevalence of impaired glucose tolerance and type 2 diabetes in PCOS: a systematic review and meta-regression. Hum Reprod Update. 2018;24:455–67.
8. Bilal M, Haseeb A, Rehman A. Relationship of polycystic ovarian syndrome with cardiovascular risk factors. Diabetes Metab Syndr. 2018;12:375–80.
9. Joham AE, Teede HJ, Ranasinha S, Zoungas S, Boyle J. Prevalence of infertility and use of fertility treatment in women with polycystic ovary syndrome: data from a large community-based cohort study. J Women's Health (2002). 2015;24:299–307.
10. Shang K, Jia X, Qiao J, Kang J, Guan Y. Endometrial abnormality in women with polycystic ovary syndrome. Reprod Sci. 2012;19:674–83.
11. Giudice LC. Endometrium in PCOS: implantation and predisposition to endocrine CA. Best Pract Res Clin Endocrinol Metab. 2006;20:235–44.
12. Franks S, McCarthy MI, Hardy K. Development of polycystic ovary syndrome: involvement of genetic and environmental factors. Int J Androl. 2006;29: 278–85 discussion 86–90.
13. Bahri Khomami M, Boyle JA, Tay CT, Vanky E, Teede HJ, Joham AE, et al. Polycystic ovary syndrome and adverse pregnancy outcomes: current state of knowledge, challenges and potential implications for practice. Clin Endocrinol. 2018;88:761–9.
14. Jeanes YM, Reeves S. Metabolic consequences of obesity and insulin resistance in polycystic ovary syndrome: diagnostic and methodological challenges. Nutr Res Rev. 2017;30:97–105.
15. An S, Song JJ. The coded functions of noncoding RNAs for gene regulation. Mol Cells. 2011;31:491–6.
16. Guttman M, Amit I, Garber M, French C, Lin MF, Feldser D, et al. Chromatin signature reveals over a thousand highly conserved large non-coding RNAs in mammals. Nature. 2009;458:223–7.
17. Taft RJ, Pang KC, Mercer TR, Dinger M, Mattick JS. Non-coding RNAs: regulators of disease. J Pathol. 2010;220:126–39.
18. Alvarez ML, Distefano JK. The role of non-coding RNAs in diabetic nephropathy: potential applications as biomarkers for disease development and progression. Diabetes Res Clin Pract. 2013;99:1–11.
19. Sookoian S, Flichman D, Garaycoechea ME, San Martino J, Castano GO,

Pirola CJ. Metastasis-associated lung adenocarcinoma transcript 1 as a common molecular driver in the pathogenesis of nonalcoholic steatohepatitis and chronic immune-mediated liver damage. Hepatol Commun. 2018;2:654–65.
20. Yang W, Li Y, He F, Wu H. Microarray profiling of long non-coding RNA (lncRNA) associated with hypertrophic cardiomyopathy. BMC Cardiovasc Disord. 2015;15:62.
21. Wu G, Cai J, Han Y, Chen J, Huang ZP, Chen C, et al. LincRNA-p21 regulates neointima formation, vascular smooth muscle cell proliferation, apoptosis, and atherosclerosis by enhancing p53 activity. Circulation. 2014;130:1452–65.
22. Panir K, Schjenken JE, Robertson SA, Hull ML. Non-coding RNAs in endometriosis: a narrative review. Hum Reprod Update. 2018;24:497–515.
23. Chen MY, Liao GD, Zhou B, Kang LN, He YM, Li SW. Genome-wide profiling of long noncoding RNA expression patterns in women with repeated implantation failure by RNA sequencing. Reprod Sci. 2018: 1933719118756752. https://doi.org/10.1177/1933719118756752.
24. Wang H, Cao Q, Ge J, Liu C, Ma Y, Meng Y, et al. LncRNA-regulated infection and inflammation pathways associated with pregnancy loss: genome wide differential expression of lncRNAs in early spontaneous abortion. Am J Reprod Immunol. 2014;72:359–75.
25. Fu LL, Xu Y, Li DD, Dai XW, Xu X, Zhang JS, et al. Expression profiles of mRNA and long noncoding RNA in the ovaries of letrozole-induced polycystic ovary syndrome rat model through deep sequencing. Gene. 2018;657:19–29.
26. Tian XC, Wang QY, Li DD, Wang ST, Yang ZQ, Guo B, et al. Differential expression and regulation of Cryab in mouse uterus during preimplantation period. Reproduction. 2013;145:577–85.
27. Yuhki M, Kajitani T, Mizuno T, Aoki Y, Maruyama T. Establishment of an immortalized human endometrial stromal cell line with functional responses to ovarian stimuli. Reprod Biol Endocrinol. 2011;9:104.
28. Shen M, Liu X, Zhang H, Guo SW. Transforming growth factor beta1 signaling coincides with epithelial-mesenchymal transition and fibroblast-to-myofibroblast transdifferentiation in the development of adenomyosis in mice. Hum Reprod. 2016;31:355–69.
29. De Clercq K, Hennes A, Vriens J. Isolation of mouse endometrial epithelial and stromal cells for in vitro Decidualization. J Vis Exp. 2017. https://doi.org/10.3791/55168.
30. Gellersen B, Brosens JJ. Cyclic decidualization of the human endometrium in reproductive health and failure. Endocr Rev. 2014;35:851–905.
31. Takenaka K, Chen BJ, Modesitt SC, Byrne FL, Hoehn KL, Janitz M. The emerging role of long non-coding RNAs in endometrial cancer. Cancer Genet. 2016;209:445–55.
32. Struhl K. Transcriptional noise and the fidelity of initiation by RNA polymerase II. Nat Struct Mol Biol. 2007;14:103–5.
33. Liu Z, Hao C, Huang X, Zhang N, Bao H, Qu Q. Peripheral blood leukocyte expression level of lncRNA steroid receptor RNA activator (SRA) and its association with polycystic ovary syndrome: a case control study. Gynecol Endocrinol. 2015;31:363–8.
34. Liu Z, Hao C, Song D, Zhang N, Bao H, Qu Q. Androgen receptor Coregulator CTBP1-AS is associated with polycystic ovary syndrome in Chinese women: a preliminary study. Reprod Sci. 2015;22:829–37.
35. Piltonen TT. Polycystic ovary syndrome: endometrial markers. Best Pract Res Clin Obstet Gynaecol. 2016;37:66–79.
36. Dey SK, Lim H, Das SK, Reese J, Paria BC, Daikoku T, et al. Molecular cues to implantation. Endocr Rev. 2004;25:341–73.
37. Zhang S, Lin H, Kong S, Wang S, Wang H, Wang H, et al. Physiological and molecular determinants of embryo implantation. Mol Asp Med. 2013;34:939–80.
38. Lv H, Tong J, Yang J, Lv S, Li WP, Zhang C, et al. Dysregulated Pseudogene HK2P1 May Contribute to Preeclampsia as a Competing Endogenous RNA for Hexokinase 2 by Impairing Decidualization. Hypertension. 2018;71:648–58.
39. Liang XH, Deng WB, Liu YF, Liang YX, Fan ZM, Gu XW, et al. Non-coding RNA LINC00473 mediates decidualization of human endometrial stromal cells in response to cAMP signaling. Sci Rep. 2016;6:22744.
40. Qiao J, Wang L, Li R, Zhang X. Microarray evaluation of endometrial receptivity in Chinese women with polycystic ovary syndrome. Reprod BioMed Online. 2008;17:425–35.
41. Bellver J, Martinez-Conejero JA, Labarta E, Alama P, Melo MA, Remohi J, et al. Endometrial gene expression in the window of implantation is altered in obese women especially in association with polycystic ovary syndrome. Fertil Steril. 2011;95:2335–41 41.e1–8.
42. Li DD, Zhao SY, Yang ZQ, Duan CC, Guo CH, Zhang HL, et al. Hmgn5 functions downstream of Hoxa10 to regulate uterine decidualization in

mice. Cell Cycle. 2016;15:2792–805.

43. Tang WY, Morey LM, Cheung YY, Birch L, Prins GS, Ho SM. Neonatal exposure to estradiol/bisphenol a alters promoter methylation and expression of Nsbp1 and Hpcal1 genes and transcriptional programs of Dnmt3a/b and Mbd2/4 in the rat prostate gland throughout life. Endocrinology. 2012;153:42–55.

44. Saxena D, Escamilla-Hernandez R, Little-Ihrig L, Zeleznik AJ. Liver receptor homolog-1 and steroidogenic factor-1 have similar actions on rat granulosa cell steroidogenesis. Endocrinology. 2007;148:726–34.

45. Wang Q, Kim JY, Xue K, Liu JY, Leader A, Tsang BK. Chemerin, a novel regulator of follicular steroidogenesis and its potential involvement in polycystic ovarian syndrome. Endocrinology. 2012;153:5600–11.

46. Garg D, Merhi Z. Relationship between advanced glycation end products and steroidogenesis in PCOS. Reprod Biol Endocrinol. 2016;14:71.

47. Mouzat K, Baron S, Marceau G, Caira F, Sapin V, Volle DH, et al. Emerging roles for LXRs and LRH-1 in female reproduction. Mol Cell Endocrinol. 2013; 368:47–58.

48. Zhang C, Large MJ, Duggavathi R, DeMayo FJ, Lydon JP, Schoonjans K, et al. Liver receptor homolog-1 is essential for pregnancy. Nat Med. 2013;19: 1061–6.

49. Su RW, Strug MR, Joshi NR, Jeong JW, Miele L, Lessey BA, et al. Decreased notch pathway signaling in the endometrium of women with endometriosis impairs decidualization. J Clin Endocrinol Metab. 2015;100: E433–42.

50. Garcia-Pascual CM, Ferrero H, Zimmermann RC, Simon C, Pellicer A, Gomez R. Inhibition of Delta-like 4 mediated signaling induces abortion in mice due to deregulation of decidual angiogenesis. Placenta. 2014;35:501–8.

51. Yoshiki N, Kubota T, Matsumoto Y, Aso T. Expression of inducible nitric oxide synthase in human cultured endometrial stromal cells. Mol Hum Reprod. 1999;5:353–7.

52. Wang XR, Hao HG, Chu L. Glycyrrhizin inhibits LPS-induced inflammatory mediator production in endometrial epithelial cells. Microb Pathog. 2017; 109:110–3.

53. Schmidt J, Weijdegard B, Mikkelsen AL, Lindenberg S, Nilsson L, Brannstrom M. Differential expression of inflammation-related genes in the ovarian stroma and granulosa cells of PCOS women. Mol Hum Reprod. 2014;20:49–58.

54. Walsh SW, Chumble AA, Washington SL, Archer KJ, Sahingur SE, Strauss JF 3rd. Increased expression of toll-like receptors 2 and 9 is associated with reduced DNA methylation in spontaneous preterm labor. J Reprod Immunol. 2017;121:35–41.

55. Ashton KA, Proietto A, Otton G, Symonds I, McEvoy M, Attia J, et al. Toll-like receptor (TLR) and nucleosome-binding oligomerization domain (NOD) gene polymorphisms and endometrial cancer risk. BMC Cancer. 2010;10:382.

56. Ruiz-Gonzalez I, Minten M, Wang X, Dunlap KA, Bazer FW. Involvement of TLR7 and TLR8 in conceptus development and establishment of pregnancy in sheep. Reproduction. 2015;149:305–16.

57. Sikora J, Smycz-Kubanska M, Mielczarek-Palacz A, Kondera-Anasz Z. Abnormal peritoneal regulation of chemokine activation-the role of IL-8 in pathogenesis of endometriosis. Am J Reprod Immunol. 2017;77. https://doi.org/10.1111/aji.12622.

58. Jasper MJ, Tremellen KP, Robertson SA. Reduced expression of IL-6 and IL-1alpha mRNAs in secretory phase endometrium of women with recurrent miscarriage. J Reprod Immunol. 2007;73:74–84.

59. Piltonen TT, Chen JC, Khatun M, Kangasniemi M, Liakka A, Spitzer T, et al. Endometrial stromal fibroblasts from women with polycystic ovary syndrome have impaired progesterone-mediated decidualization, aberrant cytokine profiles and promote enhanced immune cell migration in vitro. Hum Reprod. 2015;30:1203–15.

60. Legro RS, Kunselman AR, Dunaif A. Prevalence and predictors of dyslipidemia in women with polycystic ovary syndrome. Am J Med. 2001; 111:607–13.

61. Chekir C, Nakatsuka M, Kamada Y, Noguchi S, Sasaki A, Hiramatsu Y. Impaired uterine perfusion associated with metabolic disorders in women with polycystic ovary syndrome. Acta Obstet Gynecol Scand. 2005;84:189–95.

62. Nieman KM, Romero IL, Van Houten B, Lengyel E. Adipose tissue and adipocytes support tumorigenesis and metastasis. Biochim Biophys Acta 2013;1831:1533–1541.

## 20

Rosiglitazone ameliorates palmitic acid-induced cytotoxicity in TM4 Sertoli cells

Xie Ge[†], Peng Pan[†], Jun Jing, Xuechun Hu, Li Chen, Xuhua Qiu, Rujun Ma, Kadiliya Jueraitetibaike, Xuan Huang and Bing Yao[*]

Abstract

The Sertoli cell is the only somatic cell within the seminiferous tubules, and is vital for testis development and spermatogenesis. Rosiglitazone (RSG) is a member of the thiazolidinedione family and is a peroxisome proliferator-activated receptor-γ (PPARγ) agonist. It has been reported that RSG protects various types of cells from fatty acid-induced damage. However, whether RSG serves a protective role in Sertoli cells against palmitic acid (PA)-induced toxicity remains to be elucidated. Therefore, the aim of the present study was to investigate the effect of RSG on PA-induced cytotoxicity in Sertoli cells. MTT assay and Oil Red O staining revealed that RSG ameliorated the PA-induced decrease in TM4 cell viability, which was accompanied by an alleviation of PA-induced lipid accumulation in cells. In primary mouse Sertoli cells, RSG also showed similar protective effects against PA-induced lipotoxicity. Knockdown of PPARγ verified that RSG exerted its protective role in TM4 cells through a PPARγ-dependent pathway. To evaluate the mechanism underlying the protective role of RSG on PA-induced lipotoxicity, the present study analyzed the effects of RSG on PA uptake, and the expression of genes associated with both fatty acid oxidation and triglyceride synthesis. The results demonstrated that although RSG did not affect the endocytosis of PA, it significantly elevated the expression of carnitine palmitoyltransferase (CPT)-1A, a key enzyme involved in fatty acid oxidation, which indicated that the protective effect of RSG may have an important role in fatty acid oxidation. On the other hand, the expression of CPT1B was not affected by RSG. Moreover, the expression levels of diacylglycerol O-acyltransferase (DGAT)-1 and DGAT2, both of which encode enzymes catalyzing the synthesis of triglycerides, were not suppressed by RSG. The results indicated that RSG reduced PA-induced lipid accumulation by promoting fatty acid oxidation mediated by CPT1A. The effect of RSG in protecting cells from lipotoxicity was also found to be specific to Sertoli cells and hepatocytes, and not to other cell types that do not store excess lipid in large quantities, such as human umbilical vein endothelial cells. These findings provide insights into the cytoprotective effects of RSG on Sertoli cells and suggest that PPARγ activation may be a useful therapeutic method for the treatment of Sertoli cell dysfunction caused by dyslipidemia.

Keywords: Rosiglitazone, Palmitic acid, Sertoli cells, Cytotoxicity

Background

Sertoli cells, located in the basal compartment of seminiferous tubules, play an important role in testis development and spermatogenesis. They not only secrete functional proteins for the regulation of spermatogonia proliferation and differentiation, but also secrete hormones, such as inhibin B and anti-Mullerian hormone [1, 2]. Moreover, Sertoli cells form cell junctions between themselves or with germ cells, either to construct a blood-testis barrier to provide a separated microenvironment for spermatogenesis, or to bind with germ cells to regulate their development [3, 4]. In fact, the majority of nutrients required for spermatogenesis, including lactates and lipids, are provided by Sertoli cells [5]. Therefore, the number of Sertoli cells defines the population size of germ cells, which is essential for the maintenance of spermatogenesis and consequently, male fertility [6].

In recent years, due to the increase in obesity as well as the rising rates of male infertility, the relationship between obesity and male infertility has drawn an increasing level of public attention [7]. As obesity is usually accompanied by elevated fatty acid levels,

---

* Correspondence: yaobing@nju.edu.cn
†Xie Ge and Peng Pan contributed equally to this work.
Center of Reproductive Medicine, Nanjing Jinling Hospital, Clinical School of Medical College, Nanjing University, Nanjing 210002, Jiangsu, China

especially saturated fatty acids such as palmitic acid (PA) [8], it is thought that increased levels of saturated fatty acids may be a risk factor for male infertility caused by obesity. PA is the most common type of saturated fatty acid in the plasma, and has been reported to be toxic to various types of cells, including pancreatic β-cells, hepatocytes and retinal ganglion cells [9–11]. PA is also the major saturated fatty acid in human spermatozoa; some previous studies have indicated that there may be a relationship between PA concentration in the spermatozoa and male infertility [12, 13]. An in vitro study also demonstrated the proapoptotic effect of PA on Leydig cells, which are located in the interstitial space of the testis [14]. Moreover, according to our previous study, PA decreased Sertoli cell viability by inducing apoptosis (unpublished data). Therefore, excess PA may be harmful to the testes and negatively affect spermatogenesis. Ameliorating the toxic effects of PA on testis cells, including Sertoli cells, may be an effective method to treat male infertility coupled with obesity.

Rosiglitazone (RSG) is a member of the thiazolidinedione class of drugs; it exerts anti-diabetic effects by activating peroxisome proliferator-activated receptor-γ (PPARγ). It has also been reported to have beneficial effects on lipid accumulation in the liver [15], and it previously ameliorated dyslipidemia in obese mice [16]. A number of studies have reported that RSG has protective roles in fatty acid-induced cell toxicity, including in pancreatic β-cells and skeletal muscle cells [17, 18]. In both of these types of cells, PA-induced apoptosis was ameliorated following treatment with RSG. Therefore, it is possible that RSG may protect Sertoli cells from PA-induced damage. To test this hypothesis, the present study investigated the effect of RSG on PA-induced cytotoxicity in Sertoli cells.

Methods
Materials
RSG was purchased from Aladdin Reagents (Shanghai, China), and was dissolved in dimethyl sulfoxide (DMSO; Sigma-Aldrich, Shanghai, China) to generate a 200 mM stock for subsequent use. PA was purchased from Sigma-Aldrich. For cell treatments, PA was dissolved in ethanol to create a 600 mM solution and then diluted with Dulbecco's modified Eagle's medium/Ham's nutrient mixture F12 (DMEM/F12; Yuanye, Shanghai, China) containing 2% fatty acid free-bovine serum albumin (Yeasen, Shanghai, China) to a final concentration of 10 mM, which was used as a stock for further experimentation. 3-(4,5-Dimethyl-2-thiazolyl)-2,5-diphenyl-2-H-tetrazolium bromide (MTT) was purchased from Biosharp (Hefei, China), and dissolved in phosphate buffer saline (PBS) to produce a 5 mg/ml stock. Oil Red O (ORO) was purchased from Sigma-Aldrich, and dissolved in isopropanol to generate a 5 mg/ml stock, which was diluted before use

with distilled water to produce a 3 mg/ml working solution. 4,4-Difluoro-5,7-dimethyl-4-bora-3a,4a-diaza-s-indacene-3-hexadecanoic acid (BODIPY FL C16) was purchased from Invitrogen (Thermo Fisher Scientific, Inc., Waltham, MA, USA) and dissolved in DMSO to create a 2 mM stock for subsequent use.

TM4 cell culture
The TM4 cell line was purchased from iCell Bioscience, Inc. (Shanghai, China). The HepG2 [American Type Culture Collection (ATCC)® HB-8065™] and human umbilical vein endothelial cells (HUVECs; ATCC® PCS-100-010™) cell lines were purchased from ATCC (Manassas, VA, USA). TM4 cells and HUVECs were cultured in DMEM/F12 supplemented with 10% fetal bovine serum (FBS; Gibco; Thermo Fisher Scientific, Inc.) at 37 °C in 5% CO_2. HepG2 cells were cultured in DMEM supplemented with 10% FBS at 37 °C in 5% CO_2.

Primary mouse Sertoli cell isolation and culture
Male ICR mice were purchased from Beijing Vital River Laboratory Animal Technology Co., Ltd. (Nanjing, China), which were housed on a 12 h light:12 h dark cycle at 22 ± 2 °C and had free access to food and water. The procedures of animal experiments were executed according to the NIH guide for the care and use of laboratory animals, and were approved by the Ethics Committee of the Nanjing Jinling Hospital. Primary mouse Sertoli cells were isolated from testis of 20-day old male ICR mice by a two-step enzyme digestion as previously described [19] with some modifications. Briefly, testes were decapsulated, digested with 0.25% trypsin (Gibco; Thermo Fisher Scientific, Inc.) at 37 °C in a rocking incubator for 4–6 min, and washed with PBS, so that interstitial cells can be removed. The isolated seminiferous tubules were then digested with 1 mg/ml collagenase I at 37 °C in a rocking incubator for 6–8 min to remove peritubular cells. A 200-mesh stainless steel filter was used to filter the homogenate. Following two times of PBS washing, cells were resuspended with DMEM/F12 supplemented with 10% FBS, seeded in dishes, and incubated in a humidified 34 °C, 5% CO_2 incubator. After adherence for 4 h, Sertoli cells became attached to the bottoms of dishes, while germ cells were suspended in the medium. Thus the cells were washed with PBS twice to remove most germ cells, and a hypotonic solution (0.3 × HBSS) was used to treat the cells for 3 min, so that residual germ cells can be lysed and removed. The cells were then cultured in a humidified 34 °C, 5% CO_2 incubator for 2–3 days before the experiments.

Cell viability assay
To analyze cell viability, an MTT assay was conducted. Cells were seeded in 96-well plates at a density of 5×10^3, and cultured overnight to allow for cell attachment. The

cells were pre-treated with RSG (20 μM) for 2 h and then PA (0.2 or 0.4 mM) was applied. After PA treatment for 12 or 24 h, the cell culture medium in each well was discarded and replaced with 200 μl fresh DMEM/F12 without FBS, and 20 μl MTT stock was added. The plate was incubated at 37 °C for 4 h, then the medium was discarded and 150 μl DMSO was added to each well to dissolve the formazan, which was reduced from MTT by living cells. Finally, the absorbance was measured at 450 nm using a microplate reader (Bio-Rad Laboratories, Inc., Hercules, CA, USA). For dose- and time-dependent analysis of the effect of RSG on PA-induced cytotoxicity, TM4 cells were treated with RSG at the indicated concentrations 2 h before, simultaneously with, or 2 h after the beginning of PA treatment; all of the cells were treated with PA for 24 h except for the cells in the control group. The MTT assay was then performed to analyze cell viability. For cell morphological observations, TM4 cells were seeded in 6-well plates at a density of 15×10^4 and cultured overnight for cell attachment before the indicated treatments were applied. Images were captured following cell treatments using a microscope (IX73; Olympus Corporation, Tokyo, Japan).

ORO staining
Cells were stained with ORO to assess intracellular lipid accumulation. Briefly, the cells were seeded in 6-well plates at a density of 1×10^5, and cultured overnight for cell attachment. After cell treatments, the cells were fixed with 4% paraformaldehyde and stained with the freshly diluted ORO working solution at room temperature for 1 h. After rinsing with 75% ethanol for 30 s and washing with PBS twice, the cells were counterstained with hematoxylin for 10 s. Observations were made and images were captured using a microscope (IX73; Olympus Corporation). For the quantification of lipid accumulation, the stained samples were washed with PBS and incubated at 37 °C to evaporate any remaining water. Then, 200 μl isopropanol was added to each well, and the plates were slowly agitated at room temperature for 10 min for the dissolution of ORO staining. Following this, the samples were transferred to a 96-well plate, and the absorbance was measured at 510 nm using a microplate reader (Bio-Rad Laboratories, Inc.).

Analysis of PA endocytosis
To observe PA endocytosis, a fluorescently-labeled PA analogue BODIPY FL C16 was used. TM4 cells were pretreated with or without 20 μM RSG for 24 h, and then treated with 1 μM BODIPY FL C16 for 30 min. Once washed three times with PBS, the cells were fixed with 4% paraformaldehyde. Fluorescent images were captured using a fluorescence microscope (IX73; Olympus Corporation), and the mean fluorescence intensities were

quantified using ImageJ version 1.32j software (National Institutes of Health, Bethesda, MD, USA).

RNA extraction and reverse transcription-quantitative polymerase chain reaction (RT-qPCR)
The mRNA levels of carnitine palmitoyltransferase 1A (CPT1A), carnitine palmitoyltransferase 1B (CPT1B), diacylglycerol O-acyltransferase 1 (DGAT1) and diacylglycerol O-acyltransferase 2 (DGAT2) were quantified by RT-qPCR. Briefly, total RNA was extracted from cells using a Total RNA Isolation Kit (BEI-BEI Biotech, Zhengzhou, China). The PrimeScript RT Master Mix (Takara Bio, Inc., Otsu, Japan) was used for RT-PCR. qPCR was carried out using the AceQ qPCR SYBR Green Master Mix (Vazyme Biotech, Nanjing, China) following the manufacturer's instruction. The samples were amplified and monitored using a Roche LightCycler 96 Real-time PCR system (Roche Diagnostics, Basel, Switzerland). The thermocycling conditions were: 95 °C for 10 min for initial denaturation, and 40 cycles of amplification consisting of 95 °C for 10 s and 60 °C for 30 s. The relative expression levels were calculated using the $2^{-\Delta\Delta Cq}$ method [20], and the gene 36B4 (also known as ribosomal protein lateral stalk subunit P0) was used as the internal control. The primers used were as follows: 36B4, forward 5′-GAAACTGCTGCCTCACATCCG-3′ and reverse 5′-GCTGGCACAGTGACCTCACACG-3′; CPT1A, forward 5′-CTCAGTGGGAGCGACTCTTCA-3′ and reverse 5′-GGCCTCTGTGGTACACGACAA-3′; CPT1B, forward 5′-TACAGCTTCCAAACGTCACTGCC-3′ and reverse 5′-CACCATGACTTGAGCACCAGG-3′; DGAT1, forward 5′-TCCGTCCAGGGTGGTAGTG-3′ and reverse 5′-TGAACAAAGAATCTTGCAGACGA-3′; DGAT2, forward 5′-GCGCTACTTCCGAGACTACTT-3′ and reverse 5′-GGGCCTTATGCCAGGAAACT-3′.

Western blot analysis
The cells were lysed in Radioimmunoprecipitation Assay buffer for protein extraction [21]. Protein concentrations were analyzed using the Pierce™ BCA Protein Assay Kit (Thermo Fisher Scientific, Inc.), and 20 μg protein was loaded in each lane for gel electrophoresis. The following operations were done as previously described [21]. The primary antibodies used were as follows: Rabbit polyclonal CPT1A (1:2,000; cat. no. 15184–1-AP; ProteinTech Group, Inc., Chicago, IL, USA) and mouse monoclonal GAPDH (1:2,000; cat. no. KC-5G5; KangChen Biotech, Inc., Shanghai, China). The secondary antibodies used were as follows: Goat anti-rabbit IgG (H + L) secondary antibody, horseradish peroxidase (HRP)-conjugated (1:5,000; cat. no. 31460; Invitrogen; Thermo Fisher Scientific, Inc.) and goat anti-mouse IgG (H + L) secondary antibody, HRP-conjugated (1:5,000; cat. no. 31430; Invitrogen; Thermo Fisher Scientific,

Inc.). The bands were visualized using enhanced chemiluminescence reagents (Promega Corporation, Madison, WI, USA), and images were captured using the Tanon-5200 Chemiluminescent Imaging System (Tanon Science and Technology, Co., Ltd., Shanghai, China). The relative protein expression levels were reflected by the intensities of the target bands, which were quantified using ImageJ version 1.32j software (National Institutes of Health).

PPARγ RNAi

The mouse PPARγ-specific siRNA set (siPPARγ) and non-specific siRNA (scrambled siRNA, NC-siRNA) were designed and synthesized by Ribobio (Guangzhou, China). To knockdown the expression of PPARγ, the cells were transfected with NC-siRNA or siPPARγ 6 h in advance of indicated treatments. The transfection of siRNAs were performed using Lipofectamine 3000 reagent (cat. no. L3000015, Invitrogen; Thermo Fisher Scientific, Inc.) according to the manufacturer's instructions.

Statistical analysis

GraphPad Prism 5 software (GraphPad Software, Inc., La Jolla, CA, USA) was used for graph generation. The data are presented as the mean ± standard deviation. To compare the results between different groups, one-way analysis of variance followed by the Least Significant Difference (for equal variances) or the Games-Howell (for unequal variances) post hoc test were conducted using SPSS software version 17.0 (SPSS, Inc., Chicago, IL, USA). Differences were considered to be statistically significant when $P < 0.05$, and highly significant when $P < 0.01$.

Results

RSG ameliorates the decline in Sertoli cell viability induced by PA

To validate the toxicity of PA, TM4 Sertoli cells were treated with 0.2 or 0.4 mM PA for 12 or 24 h. The concentrations of PA used in the present study are in reference to the concentration of free fatty acids in circulation [22] and the concentration of PA commonly used in other studies [23, 24]. The MTT assay results revealed that both concentrations of PA decreased cell viability (Fig. 1a and b). However, the 20 μM RSG treatment, which was added 2 h prior to PA stimulation, significantly ameliorated this decline in cell viability, thereby indicating the potential protective effect of RSG in TM4 Sertoli cells (Fig. 1a and b). To verify the effect of RSG, a dose- and time-dependent experiment was executed. A total of 5, 10 or 20 μM RSG was added to cells 2 h prior to, simultaneously with, or 2 h after the addition of 0.4 mM PA, then cells were subsequently treated with PA for 24 h. Both the results of the MTT assay and the cell status observed by a microscope

demonstrated that RSG exhibited protective effects in all these treatments (Fig. 1c and Additional file 1: Figure S1). Moreover, according to MTT results, the toxicity of PA, and the protective role of RSG, were also observed in primary mouse Sertoli cells (Fig. 1d).

RSG alleviates PA-induced lipid accumulation in Sertoli cells

To determine whether the protection from PA-induced cytotoxicity by RSG is due to reduced lipid accumulation in cells, ORO staining was performed to observe the neutral lipid droplets in cells. As was expected, treatment with PA significantly increased the levels of ORO staining in TM4 cells, indicating there was elevated lipid accumulation. When the cells were pretreated with RSG for 2 h, there was substantially less ORO staining of intracellular lipid droplets when compared with the cells treated with PA alone (Fig. 2a and b). Post-treatment with RSG showed a similar protective role (Additional file 1: Figure S2). In primary mouse Sertoli cells, pre-treatment with RSG also ameliorated PA-induced lipid accumulation (Fig. 2c and d). These results demonstrated that RSG may alleviate PA-induced lipid accumulation.

RSG ameliorates PA-induced cytotoxicity through a PPARγ-dependent pathway

RSG is a PPARγ agonist, so it may exert its protective effects through a PPARγ-dependent pathway. To investigate the involvement of PPARγ-dependent pathway, a set of PPARγ specific siRNAs was transfected into TM4 cells to knock down the expression of PPARγ. Both the MTT assay and ORO staining assay indicated that knocking down PPARγ expression substantially alleviated the protective effects of RSG on PA-induced lipotoxicity (Fig. 3). Therefore, it can be inferred that RSG protects Sertoli cells from PA-induced lipotoxicity through a PPARγ-dependent pathway.

RSG does not suppress PA endocytosis

Decreased lipid accumulation may be due to a decrease in PA endocytosis, a decrease in lipid synthesis, or an increase in lipid catabolism. To evaluate whether RSG affects PA endocytosis, BODIPY FL C16, a PA analogue labeled with a fluorophore, was used to trace the uptake of PA. Notably, RSG pre-treatment did not suppress the endocytosis of PA (Fig. 4). Therefore, the inhibition of PA uptake does not explain the decreased levels of lipid accumulation following RSG treatment.

RSG induces the expression of lipid catabolic genes

To clarify whether the RSG-induced alleviation of lipid accumulation was as a result of increased lipid catabolism or decreased lipid synthesis, the expression levels of

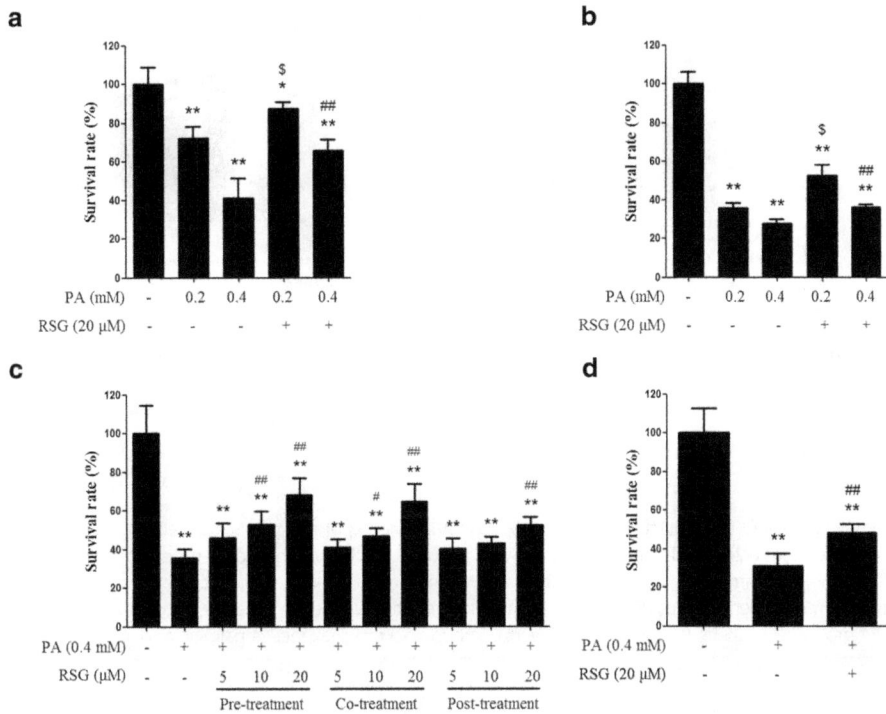

Fig. 1 RSG ameliorates the PA-induced decrease in Sertoli cell viability. (**a** and **b**) An MTT assay was performed with TM4 cells treated with PA for (**a**) 12 h or (**b**) 24 h, with or without RSG pre-treatment. **c** Dose- and time-dependent analysis of the effect of RSG on PA-induced cytotoxicity (MTT assay). **d** An MTT assay was conducted in primary mouse sertoli cells treated with PA for 24 h with or without RSG pre-treatment. Data are presented as the mean ± standard deviation of three independently prepared samples, each with three measurements. $^{*}P < 0.05$ and $^{**}P < 0.01$ vs. control group; $^{$}P < 0.05$ vs. 0.2 mM-PA group; $^{#}P < 0.05$ and $^{##}P < 0.01$ vs. 0.4 mM-PA group. *RSG* rosiglitazone, *PA* palmitic acid, *MTT* 3-(4,5-dimethyl-2-thiazolyl)-2,5-diphenyl-2-H-tetrazolium bromide

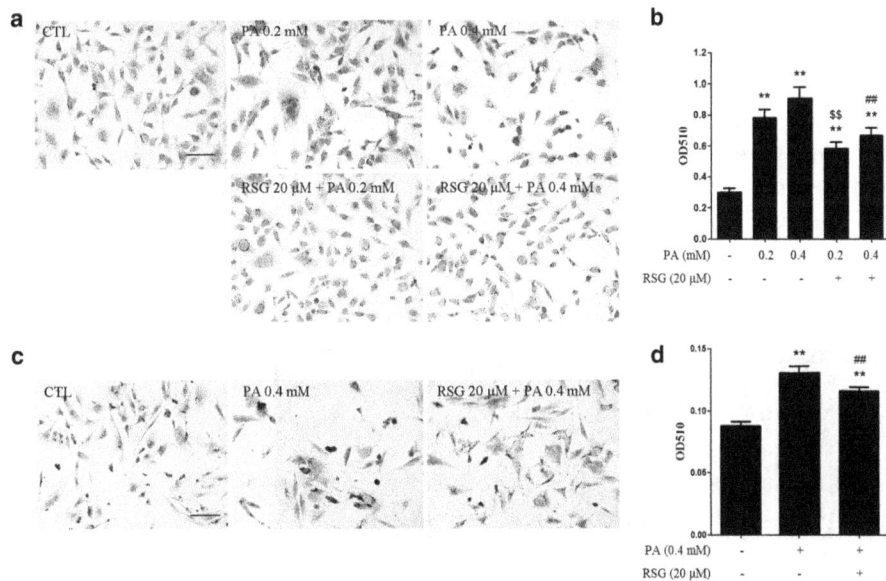

Fig. 2 RSG alleviates PA-induced lipid accumulation in Sertoli cells. TM4 cells (**a** and **b**) and primary mouse Sertoli cells (**c** and **d**) were pre-treated with 20 μM RSG for 2 h, and then treated with 0.2 or 0.4 mM PA for 24 h. **a** and **b** ORO staining of TM4 cells (**a**) and quantification of neutral lipids (**b**). **c** and **d** ORO staining of primary mouse Sertoli cells (**c**) and quantification of neutral lipids (**d**). Data are presented as the mean ± standard deviation of three independently prepared samples, each with three measurements. Scale bar, 100 μm. $^{**}P < 0.01$ vs. control group; $^{$$}P < 0.01$ vs. 0.2-mM PA group; $^{##}P < 0.01$ vs. 0.4 mM-PA group. *RSG* rosiglitazone, *PA* palmitic acid, *ORO* oil red O

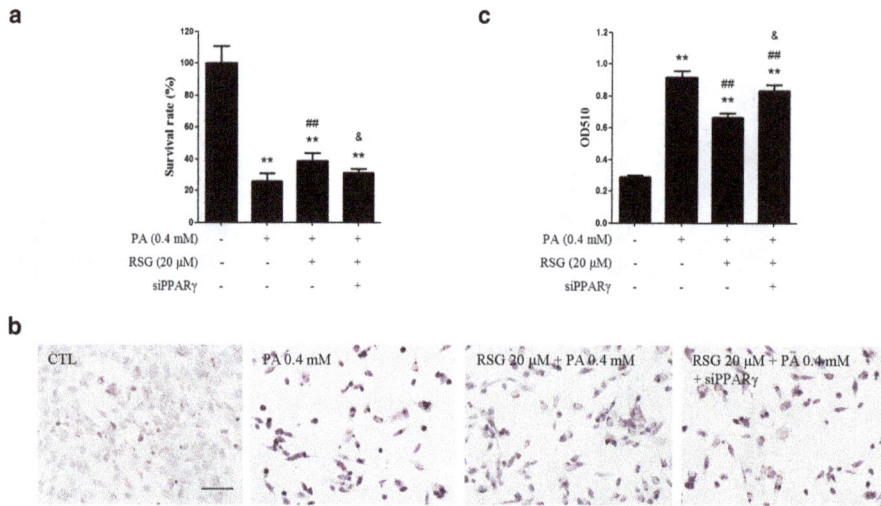

Fig. 3 Knockdown of PPARγ alleviated the protective effects of RSG on PA-induced lipotoxicity in Sertoli cells. TM4 cells were transfected with NC-siRNA or siPPARγ. 6 h after transfection, cells were pretreated with (or without) RSG for 2 h, and then treated with PA for 24 h. **a** MTT assay of TM4 cells. **b** and **c** ORO staining of primary mouse Sertoli cells (**b**) and quantification of neutral lipids (**c**). Data are presented as the mean ± standard deviation of three independently prepared samples, each with three measurements. Scale bar, 100 μm. $^{**}P < 0.01$ vs. control group; $^{##}P < 0.01$ vs. 0.4 mM-PA group; $^{&}P < 0.05$ vs. 0.4 mM-PA + 20 μM-RSG group. *RSG* rosiglitazone, *PA* palmitic acid, *ORO* oil red O

key genes involved in both processes were measured. The results of RT-qPCR indicated that the expression of CPT1A, a gene that mediates fatty acid β-oxidation, was upregulated by PA and was further elevated by RSG (Fig. 5a). Similarly, western blot analysis of CPT1A also reflected these results (Fig. 5b and c). However, the expression of CPT1B, another gene associated with fatty acid oxidation, was also upregulated by PA, but was not affected by RSG (Fig. 5d). In addition, the upregulation of CPT1B (1.41-fold increase) by PA was not as marked as that of CPT1A (2.36-fold increase). DGAT1 and DGAT2, key enzymes that regulate the synthesis of triglyceride from fatty acids, were also detected by qPCR. The results demonstrated that DGAT1 levels were not

significantly altered when compared among the three groups (Fig. 5e); however, DGAT2 mRNA expression was suppressed by PA, which was subsequently restored by RSG treatment (Fig. 5f). These results indicated that only the induction of CPT1A expression by RSG, which in turn led to increased fatty acid oxidation, may be able to explain how RSG decreases lipid accumulation.

RSG ameliorates PA-induced cytotoxicity in HepG2 cells, but not in HUVECs

To validate the specificity of the effect of RSG on different cell types, the present study selected a further two representative cell lines, HepG2 and HUVECs, which were analyzed by MTT assay and ORO staining. As

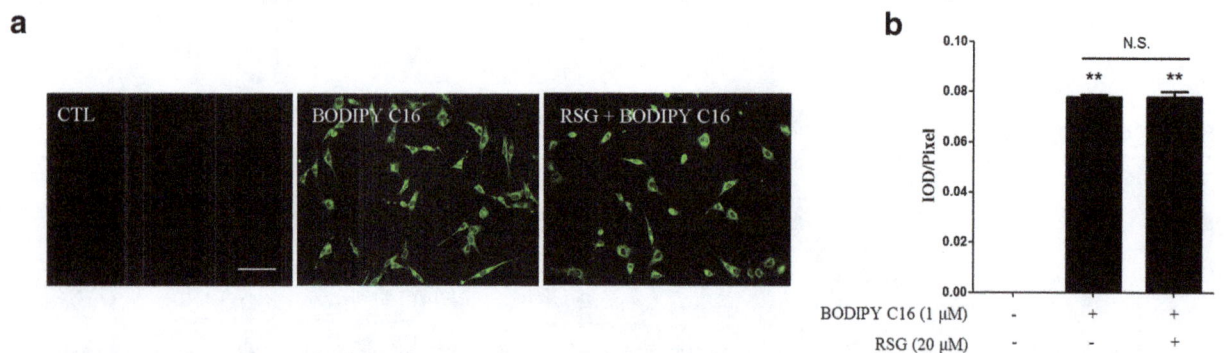

Fig. 4 RSG did not affect PA endocytosis. TM4 cells were pretreated with or without 20 μM RSG for 24 h, and then treated with 1 μM BODIPY FL C16 for 30 min. **a** Fluorescent images were captured with a fluorescence microscope (scale bar, 100 μm), and (**b**) the mean fluorescence intensities were quantified. Data are presented as the mean ± standard deviation of three independent experiments. $^{**}P < 0.01$ vs. control group. N.S., not significant; RSG, rosiglitazone; PA, palmitic acid; BODIPY FL C16, 4,4-difluoro-5,7-dimethyl-4-bora-3a,4a-diaza-s-indacene-3-hexadecanoic acid

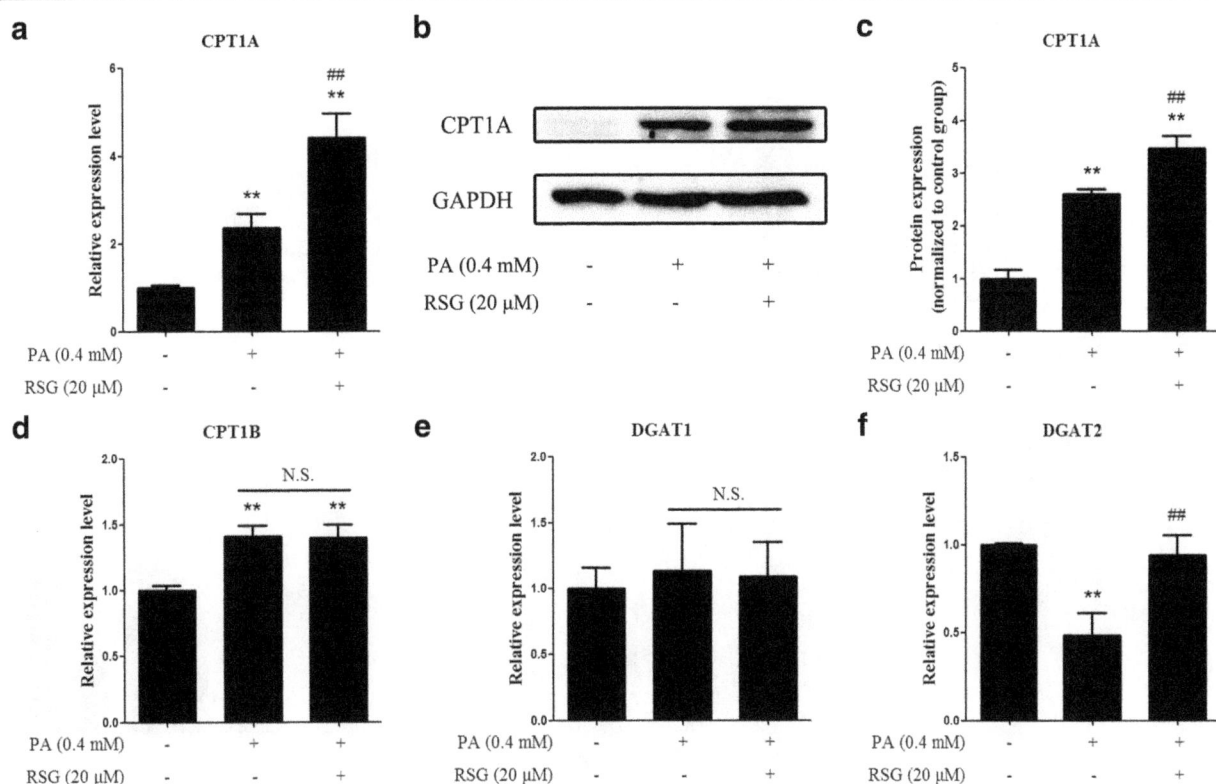

Fig. 5 Effects of RSG on lipid metabolic genes. mRNA expression levels of (**a**) CPT1A, (**d**) CPT1B, (**e**) DGAT1 and (**f**) DGAT2 were assessed using the reverse transcription-quantitative polymerase chain reaction method. **b** Protein expression levels of CPT1A were validated using western blot analysis, and (**c**) quantified by densitometry. Data are presented as the mean ± standard deviation of three independent experiments. $^{**}P < 0.01$ vs. control group; $^{##}P < 0.01$ vs. 0.4 mM-PA group. N.S., not significant; RSG, rosiglitazone; PA, palmitic acid; CPT1A/1B, carnitine palmitoyltransferase 1A/1B; DGAT1/2, diacylglycerol O-acyltransferase 1/2

previously reported, lipid metabolism in Sertoli cells is similar to that observed in hepatocytes [25, 26], thus, HepG2 was selected as a positive control. The results demonstrated that RSG significantly ameliorated the cytotoxicity and lipid accumulation induced by PA in HepG2 cells (Fig. 6a, c and d). In HUVECs, as the negative control, neither PA-induced cytotoxicity nor lipid accumulation was affected by RSG (Fig. 6b, e and f).

Discussion

In non-adipose tissues, lipid accumulation in cells usually leads to cell dysfunction and apoptosis, which is known as lipotoxicity. Saturated fatty acids, such as PA and stearic acid, have been reported to be more toxic than other fatty acids [27]. In the present study, PA, which is the major saturated fatty acid in both plasma and spermatozoa, was selected as the representative saturated fatty acid. In our previous studies, the toxicity of PA on Sertoli cells has been demonstrated (unpublished data). In the present study, the results of the MTT assay also confirmed the toxicity of PA (Fig. 1). Moreover, lipid accumulation in cells caused by PA treatment was observed (Fig. 2), indicating there may be an imbalance of lipid metabolism.

RSG is an anti-diabetic drug and a PPARγ agonist. It has been reported to be beneficial to dyslipidemia, and exert protective effects in cells exposed to fatty acids, including PA [28, 29]. The present study investigated whether RSG protected Sertoli cells from PA-induced toxicity. According to the MTT results, RSG significantly elevated cell survival rates, which were decreased by PA (Fig. 1). In addition, the ORO staining assay indicated that RSG ameliorated the lipid accumulation induced by PA (Fig. 2). Furthermore, knocking down PPARγ by its specific siRNAs significantly abolished the protective effects of RSG (Fig. 3). These results demonstrated that RSG may serve a cytoprotective role in Sertoli cells exposed to PA, and PPARγ play a part in the actions of RSG in Sertoli cells. It is worth mentioning that post-treatment with 20 μM RSG also showed a considerable effect on PA treated Sertoli cells (Fig. 1c and Additional file 1: Figure S2), indicating that RSG has the potential not only in the prevention but also in the therapy of Sertoli cell dysfunction coupled with dyslipidemia.

There are several possible mechanisms by which lipid accumulation may be attenuated in cells induced by fatty acids: i) prevent the endocytosis of fatty acids; ii) inhibit the

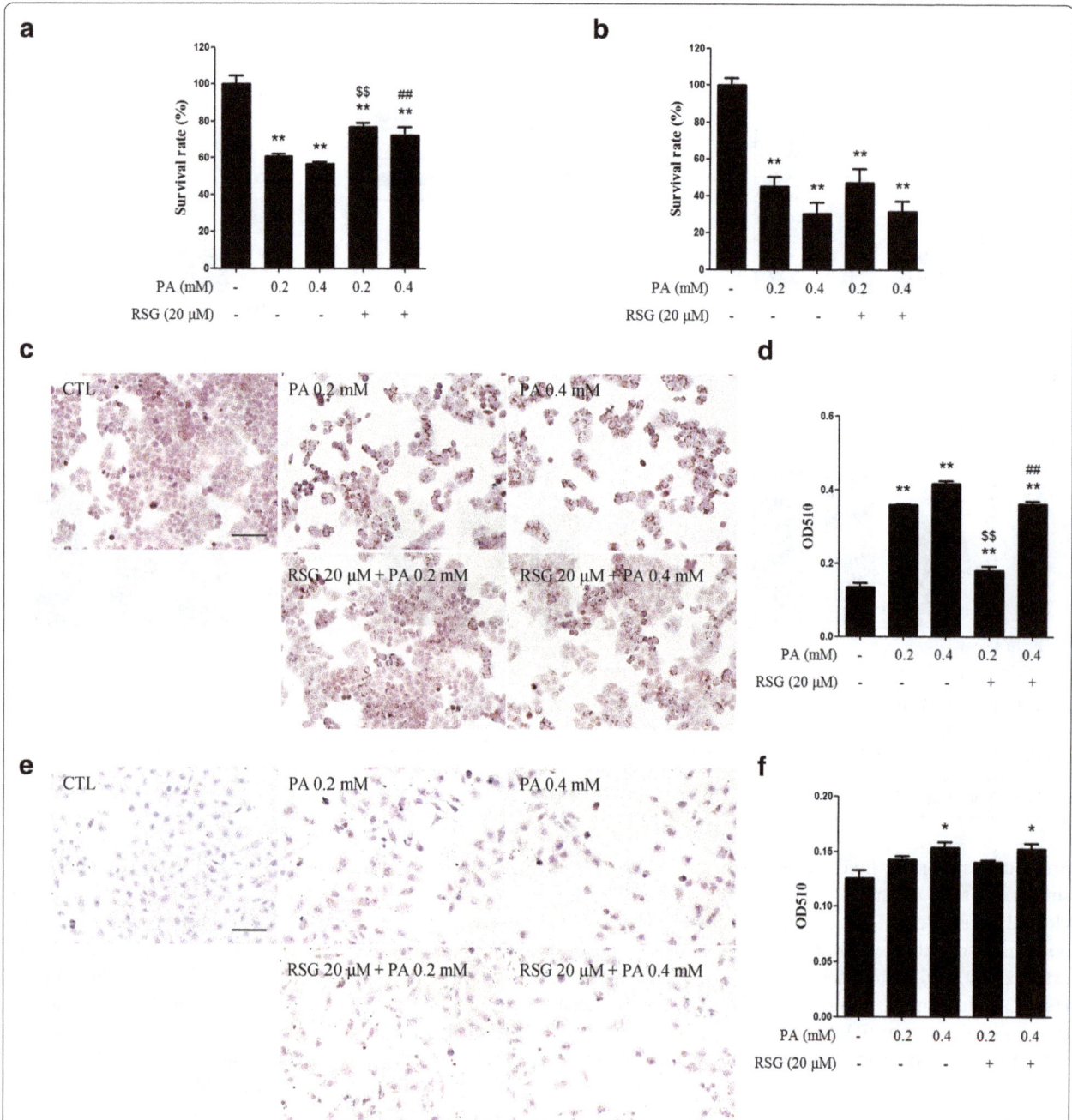

Fig. 6 Effects of RSG on PA-induced cytotoxicity in HepG2 cells and HUVECs. **a** and **b** MTT assay of (**a**) HepG2 cells and (**b**) HUVECs treated with PA for 24 h with or without RSG pre-treatment. **c-f** ORO staining of (**c** and **d**) HepG2 cells and (**e** and **f**) HUVECs. Cells were pre-treated with 20 μM RSG for 2 h, and then treated with 0.2 or 0.4 mM PA for 24 h. **c** and **e** Scale bar, 100 μm. **d** and **f** Quantifications of neutral lipids in cells stained with ORO were also presented. Data are presented as the mean ± standard deviation of three independently prepared samples, each with three measurements. $^*P < 0.05$ and $^{**}P < 0.01$ vs. control group; $^{\$\$}P < 0.01$ vs. 0.2 mM-PA group; $^{\#\#}P < 0.01$ vs. 0.4 mM-PA group. RSG, rosiglitazone; PA, palmitic acid; ORO, oil red O; HUVECs, human umbilical vein endothelial cells

synthesis of triglyceride; and iii) promote the clearance of fatty acids by β-oxidation [30]. To elucidate the mechanism by which RSG alleviates PA-induced lipid accumulation in Sertoli cells, the present study evaluated the uptake of PA after RSG treatment, and detected the expression of genes involved in triglyceride synthesis and β-oxidation.

PA-induced lipid accumulation is accompanied by an increase in fatty acid uptake, as demonstrated by the increased translocation of fatty acid transporters, such as cluster of differentiation-36 (CD36), after PA treatment [31]. Therefore, inhibiting the cellular uptake of fatty acids has an effect on limiting lipotoxicity [32]. To investigate the cellular uptake of PA, a fluorescent PA analogue, BODIPY FL C16, was added to the culture medium of TM4 Sertoli cells. BODIPY FL C16 taken up by cells would exhibit fluorescence inside the cells, which can be observed using a fluorescence microscope [33]. According to the results of the present study, the endocytosis of PA was not significantly different when comparing cells with and without RSG pre-treatment (Fig. 4). Therefore, it could be concluded that RSG does not affect the uptake of PA into Sertoli cells, and thus, the protective effect of RSG on PA-induced lipid accumulation in Sertoli cells may be due to a change in the balance between fatty acid β-oxidation and triglyceride synthesis.

As previously reported, redirection of PA metabolism towards oxidation exerts a protective role in cells against PA-induced toxicity [34]. CPT1s are enzymes that mediate the binding of long-chain fatty acids to carnitine and promote their transport across mitochondrial membranes. Therefore, CPT1s catalyze the rate-limiting step of fatty acid β-oxidation [35]. CPT1A and CPT1B are two isoforms of CPT1s. Upregulation of the expressions of CPT1A and CPT1B leads to a decrease in lipid accumulation [36]. Thus, the expression levels of CPT1A and CPT1B were determined in the present study. The results demonstrated that CPT1A expression increased following PA stimulation, and further upregulation of CPT1A was observed after RSG treatment (Fig. 5a-c). However, although the expression of CPT1B was induced by PA, the extent was not as marked as that observed with CPT1A. Moreover, the expression of CPT1B was not elevated further by RSG treatment (Fig. 5d), which indicated that CPT1B may be not involved in the protective effect of RSG. Taken together, these results suggested that RSG may induce fatty acid oxidation by upregulating CPT1A expression, which in turn may protect Sertoli cells from PA-induced cytotoxicity.

DGATs are enzymes that catalyze the formation of triglycerides from diglycerides, which is the final step in triglyceride synthesis. In mammals, DGAT1 and DGAT2 are the two isoforms of DGATs [37]. Inhibition of either DGAT1 or DGAT2 has been considered to be an attractive target for the treatment of dyslipidemia [38]. However, the effects of DGATs on lipotoxicity remain unclear. For example, in cardiomyocytes, an acute overexpression of DGAT1 serves a protective role; however, prolonged overexpression of DGAT1 causes excessive lipid accumulation and leads to cell dysfunction [39]. Therefore, the effects of DGATs should be considered, depending on the circumstances. In the present study, it was revealed that DGAT1 expression did not change following PA stimulation or RSG pre-treatment (Fig. 5e). On the other hand, DGAT2 expression was markedly decreased by PA treatment, and RSG pretreatment restored its expression (Fig. 5f). As DGAT2 is

an enzyme involved in lipid synthesis, its upregulation by RSG may not explain the induced decrease in lipid accumulation. However, the acute DGAT2 overexpression induced by RSG may be a protective mechanism; nevertheless, it may not compromise the catabolic effect of CPT1A on PA.

Notably, these results regarding the expression of CPT1s and DGATs were quite similar to those of Joung Hoon Ahn et al. [30], who reported the protective effects of oleic acid against PA-induced pancreatic AR42J cell apoptosis. According to their results, DGAT1 expression remained unchanged, while DGAT2 expression was inhibited by PA and upregulated by oleic acid. In addition, CPT1 expression was also induced by PA and further elevated by oleic acid. Both RSG and oleic acid are PPARγ activators [40], thus, it is possible that activation of PPARγ may serve a protective role in PA-induced cell damage. As previously reported, PPARγ is also involved in the regulation of both CPT1s and DGATs [41, 42]. Therefore, it follows that PPARγ may participate in the regulation of fatty acid metabolism, and activation of PPARγ may be an effective treatment for Sertoli cell dysfunction induced by saturated fatty acids.

The effects of RSG on lipid metabolism are dissimilar in different types of tissues [43], possibly due to their different metabolic patterns. As previously reported, lipid metabolism in Sertoli cells is similar to that observed in hepatocytes [25, 26]. Also, the existence of lipid droplets is a feature of Sertoli cells [44], indicating that excessive lipid can be stored as lipid droplets in Sertoli cells. Similarly, hepatocytes also store lipid in large quantities, which is different from other cell types such as epithelial cells [45]. Therefore, the hepatocytic cell line HepG2 and the epithelial cell line HUVEC were selected in the present study as positive and negative controls, respectively. In HepG2 cells, RSG significantly rescued cell viability, which was decreased by PA stimulation (Fig. 6a). In addition, the lipid accumulation induced by PA was also alleviated by RSG (Fig. 6c and d). By contrast, cell viability was not affected by RSG in HUVECs (Fig. 6b). Moreover, the accumulation of lipid droplets in HUVECs after PA treatment was not as marked as that observed in HepG2 and TM4 cells, and RSG did not decrease this lipid accumulation (Fig. 6e and f). Therefore, the effect of RSG in protecting cells from lipotoxicity may be specific to Sertoli cells and hepatocytes, and not to other cell types that do not store excess lipid in large quantities. These results indicated that the pattern of lipid metabolism is similar in Sertoli cells and hepatocytes, and so the treatment strategies used for improving liver steatosis may have potential as a therapy for Sertoli cell dyslipidemia.

Conclusions

The results of the present study demonstrated that RSG ameliorated the toxicity caused by PA in Sertoli cells by inducing CPT1A expression to promote fatty acid oxidation. According to these findings, RSG, and possibly other PPARγ agonists, offer potential in protecting Sertoli cells from saturated fatty acid-induced cytotoxicity. Moreover, TM4 cells appear suitable for analyzing mechanisms involved in Sertoli cell steatosis and its reversal. These results provide novel insights into the development of therapeutic methods for the treatment of Sertoli cell dysfunction coupled with dyslipidemia; however, the curative effect of RSG requires confirmation both in vivo and in clinical trials.

Abbreviations

36B4/RPLP0: Ribosomal protein lateral stalk subunit P0; BODIPY FL C16: 4,4-difluoro-5,7-dimethyl-4-bora-3a,4a-diaza-s-indacene-3-hexadecanoic acid; BSA: Bovine serum albumin; CPT1A/1B: Carnitine palmitoyltransferase 1A/1B; DGAT1/2: Diacylglycerol O-acyltransferase 1/2; DMEM/F12: Dulbecco's modified Eagle's medium/Ham's nutrient mixture F12; DMSO: Dimethyl sulfoxide; FBS: Fetal bovine serum; MTT: 3-(4,5-dimethyl-2-thiazolyl)-2,5-diphenyl-2-H-tetrazolium bromide; ORO: Oil red O; PA: Palmitic acid; PBS: Phosphate buffer saline; PPARγ: Peroxisome proliferator-activated receptor-γ; RSG: Rosiglitazone; RT-qPCR: Reverse transcription-quantitative polymerase chain reaction; SD: Standard deviation

Acknowledgements

The authors would like to sincerely thank Mr. Yong Shao, Mr. Cencen Wang, Ms. Peipei Cheng, Ms. Rong Zeng and Ms. Yanran Zhu for their excellent technical support and assistance during the experiments.

Funding

The present study was supported by the Jiangsu Key Research and Development Program (grant no. BE2016750), Foundation for Key Medical Talents in Jiangsu Province (grant no. ZDRCA2016096), Family Planning Research Project of the Army (grant no. 16JS012), Natural Science Foundation of Jiangsu Province (grant no. BK20170620), China Postdoctoral Science Foundation (grant no. 2017M613434), National Natural Science Foundation of China (grant nos. 81701431, 81701440 and 31701304) and Six Talent Peaks Project in Jiangsu Province (grant no. 2017-WSW-033).

Authors' contributions

XG, PP and BY conceived and designed the experiments. XG, PP, KJ and XH performed the experiments. JJ and XcH performed the statistical analysis. XG, PP, LC, XQ and RM interpreted the results. XG, PP and BY drafted the manuscript. All authors read and approved the final manuscript.

Competing interests

The authors declare that they have no competing interests.

References

1. Nery SF, Vieira MA, Dela Cruz C, Lobach VN, Del Puerto HL, Torres PB, Rocha AL, Reis AB, Reis FM. Seminal plasma concentrations of anti-Mullerian hormone and inhibin B predict motile sperm recovery from cryopreserved semen in asthenozoospermic men: a prospective cohort study. Andrology. 2014;2(6):918–23.

2. Garcia TX, Farmaha JK, Kow S, Hofmann MC. RBPJ in mouse Sertoli cells is required for proper regulation of the testis stem cell niche. Development. 2014;141(23):4468–78.

3. McCabe MJ, Tarulli GA, Laven-Law G, Matthiesson KL, Meachem SJ, McLachlan RI, Dinger ME, Stanton PG. Gonadotropin suppression in men leads to a reduction in claudin-11 at the Sertoli cell tight junction. Hum Reprod. 2016;31(4):875–86.

4. Wang X, Zhao F, Lv ZM, Shi WQ, Zhang LY, Yan M. Triptolide disrupts the actin-based Sertoli-germ cells adherens junctions by inhibiting rho GTPases expression. Toxicol Appl Pharmacol. 2016;310:32–40.

5. Keber R, Rozman D, Horvat S. Sterols in spermatogenesis and sperm maturation. J Lipid Res. 2013;54(1):20–33.

6. Rebourcet D, Darbey A, Monteiro A, Soffientini U, Tsai YT, Handel I, Pitetti JL, Nef S, Smith LB, O'Shaughnessy PJ. Sertoli cell number defines and predicts germ and Leydig cell population sizes in the adult mouse testis. Endocrinology. 2017;158(9):2955–69.

7. Craig JR, Jenkins TG, Carrell DT, Hotaling JM. Obesity, male infertility, and the sperm epigenome. Fertil Steril. 2017;107(4):848–59.

8. Warensjo E, Riserus U, Vessby B. Fatty acid composition of serum lipids predicts the development of the metabolic syndrome in men. Diabetologia. 2005;48(10):1999–2005.

9. Liu C, Fu Y, Li CE, Chen T, Li X. Phycocyanin-functionalized selenium nanoparticles reverse Palmitic acid-induced pancreatic beta cell apoptosis by enhancing cellular uptake and blocking reactive oxygen species (ROS)-mediated mitochondria dysfunction. J Agric Food Chem. 2017;65(22):4405–13.

10. Xiao X, Li H, Qi X, Wang Y, Xu C, Liu G, Wen G, Liu J. Zinc alpha2 glycoprotein alleviates palmitic acid-induced intracellular lipid accumulation in hepatocytes. Mol Cell Endocrinol. 2017;439:155–64.

11. Yan P, Tang S, Zhang H, Guo Y, Zeng Z, Wen Q. Palmitic acid triggers cell apoptosis in RGC-5 retinal ganglion cells through the Akt/FoxO1 signaling pathway. Metab Brain Dis. 2017;32(2):453–60.

12. Tavilani H, Doosti M, Abdi K, Vaisiraygani A, Joshaghani HR. Decreased polyunsaturated and increased saturated fatty acid concentration in spermatozoa from asthenozoospermic males as compared with normozoospermic males. Andrologia. 2006;38(5):173–8.

13. Esmaeili V, Shahverdi AH, Moghadasian MH, Alizadeh AR. Dietary fatty acids affect semen quality: a review. Andrology. 2015;3(3):450–61.

14. Lu ZH, Mu YM, Wang BA, Li XL, Lu JM, Li JY, Pan CY, Yanase T, Nawata H. Saturated free fatty acids, palmitic acid and stearic acid, induce apoptosis by stimulation of ceramide generation in rat testicular Leydig cell. Biochem Biophys Res Commun. 2003;303(4):1002–7.

15. Yang SJ, Choi JM, Chang E, Park SW, Park CY. Sirt1 and Sirt6 mediate beneficial effects of rosiglitazone on hepatic lipid accumulation. PLoS One. 2014;9(8):e105456.

16. Sanchez JC, Converset V, Nolan A, Schmid G, Wang S, Heller M, Sennitt MV, Hochstrasser DF, Cawthorne MA. Effect of rosiglitazone on the differential expression of obesity and insulin resistance associated proteins in lep/lep mice. Proteomics. 2003;3(8):1500–20.

17. Wu J, Wu JJ, Yang LJ, Wei LX, Zou DJ. Rosiglitazone protects against palmitate-induced pancreatic beta-cell death by activation of autophagy via 5'-AMP-activated protein kinase modulation. Endocrine. 2013;44(1):87–98.

18. Meshkani R, Sadeghi A, Taheripak G, Zarghooni M, Gerayesh-Nejad S, Bakhtiyari S. Rosiglitazone, a PPARgamma agonist, ameliorates palmitate-induced insulin resistance and apoptosis in skeletal muscle cells. Cell Biochem Funct. 2014;32(8):683–91.

19. Wang X, Zhao F, Lv ZM, Shi WQ, Zhang LY, Yan M. Triptolide disrupts the actin-based Sertoli-germ cells adherens junctionsby inhibiting rho GTPases expression. Toxicol Appl Pharmacol. 2016;310:32–40.

20. Livak KJ, Schmittgen TD. Analysis of relative gene expression data using real-time quantitative PCR and the 2(−Delta Delta C(T)) method. Methods. 2001;25(4):402–8.

21. Ge X, Chen SY, Liu M, Liang TM, Liu C. Evodiamine inhibits PDGFBBinduced proliferation of rat vascular smooth muscle cells through the suppression of cell cycle progression and oxidative stress. Mol Med Rep. 2016;14(5):4551–8.

22. Karpe F, Dickmann JR, Frayn KN. Fatty acids, obesity, and insulin resistance: time for a reevaluation. Diabetes. 2011;60(10):2441–9.

23. Leamy AK, Egnatchik RA, Shiota M, Ivanova PT, Myers DS, Brown HA, Young JD. Enhanced synthesis of saturated phospholipids is associated with ER stress and lipotoxicity in palmitate treated hepatic cells. J Lipid Res. 2014;55(7):1478–88.

24. Shen Y, Zhao Z, Zhang L, Shi L, Shahriar S, Chan RB, Di Paolo G, Min W. Metabolic activity induces membrane phase separation in endoplasmic

reticulum. Proc Natl Acad Sci U S A. 2017;114(51):13394–9.

25. Oulhaj H, Huynh S, Nouvelot A. The biosynthesis of polyunsaturated fatty acids by rat sertoli cells. Comp Biochem Physiol B. 1992;102(4):897–904.

26. Schleich F, Legros JJ. Effects of androgen substitution on lipid profile in the adult and aging hypogonadal male. Eur J Endocrinol. 2004;151(4):415–24.

27. Pan Z, Wang J, Tang H, Li L, Lv J, Xia L, Han C, Xu F, He H, Xu H, Kang B. Effects of palmitic acid on lipid metabolism homeostasis and apoptosis in goose primary hepatocytes. Mol Cell Biochem. 2011;350(1–2):39–46.

28. Ikeda J, Ichiki T, Takahara Y, Kojima H, Sankoda C, Kitamoto S, Tokunou T, Sunagawa K. PPARγ agonists attenuate palmitate-induced ER stress through up-regulation of SCD-1 in macrophages. PLoS One. 2015;10(6):e0128546.

29. Rogue A, Antherieu S, Vluggens A, Umbdenstock T, Claude N, de la Moureyre-Spire C, Weaver RJ, Guillouzo A. PPAR agonists reduce steatosis in oleic acid-overloaded HepaRG cells. Toxicol Appl Pharmacol. 2014;276(1):73–81.

30. Ahn JH, Kim MH, Kwon HJ, Choi SY, Kwon HY. Protective effects of oleic acid against Palmitic acid-induced apoptosis in pancreatic AR42J cells and its mechanisms. Korean J Physiol Pharmacol. 2013;17(1):43–50.

31. Puthanveetil P, Wang Y, Zhang D, Wang F, Kim MS, Innis S, Pulinilkunnil T, Abrahani A, Rodrigues B. Cardiac triglyceride accumulation following acute lipid excess occurs through activation of a FoxO1-iNOS-CD36 pathway. Free Radic Biol Med. 2011;51(2):352–63.

32. Ahowesso C, Black PN, Saini N, Montefusco D, Chekal J, Malosh C, Lindsley CW, Stauffer SR, DiRusso CC. Chemical inhibition of fatty acid absorption and cellular uptake limits lipotoxic cell death. Biochem Pharmacol. 2015;98(1):167–81.

33. Rambold AS, Cohen S, Lippincott-Schwartz J. Fatty acid trafficking in starved cells: regulation by lipid droplet lipolysis, autophagy, and mitochondrial fusion dynamics. Dev Cell. 2015;32(6):678–92.

34. Henique C, Mansouri A, Fumey G, Lenoir V, Girard J, Bouillaud F, Prip-Buus C, Cohen I. Increased mitochondrial fatty acid oxidation is sufficient to protect skeletal muscle cells from palmitate-induced apoptosis. J Biol Chem. 2010; 285(47):36818–27.

35. Qu Q, Zeng F, Liu X, Wang QJ, Deng F. Fatty acid oxidation and carnitine palmitoyltransferase I: emerging therapeutic targets in cancer. Cell Death Dis. 2016;7:e2226.

36. Zhang YF, Yuan ZQ, Song DG, Zhou XH, Wang YZ. Effects of cannabinoid receptor 1 (brain) on lipid accumulation by transcriptional control of CPT1A and CPT1B. Anim Genet. 2014;45(1):38–47.

37. Liu Q, Siloto RM, Lehner R, Stone SJ, Weselake RJ. Acyl-CoA:diacylglycerol acyltransferase: molecular biology, biochemistry and biotechnology. Prog Lipid Res. 2012;51(4):350–77.

38. Naik R, Obiang-Obounou BW, Kim M, Choi Y, Lee HS, Lee K. Therapeutic strategies for metabolic diseases: small-molecule diacylglycerol acyltransferase (DGAT) inhibitors. ChemMedChem. 2014;9(11):2410–24.

39. Birse RT, Bodmer R. Lipotoxicity and cardiac dysfunction in mammals and drosophila. Crit Rev Biochem Mol Biol. 2011;46(5):376–85.

40. Edvardsson U, Ljungberg A, Oscarsson J. Insulin and oleic acid increase PPARgamma2 expression in cultured mouse hepatocytes. Biochem Biophys Res Commun. 2006;340(1):111–7.

41. Son NH, Park TS, Yamashita H, Yokoyama M, Huggins LA, Okajima K, Homma S, Szabolcs MJ, Huang LS, Goldberg IJ. Cardiomyocyte expression of PPARgamma leads to cardiac dysfunction in mice. J Clin Invest. 2007; 117(10):2791–801.

42. Blanchard PG, Turcotte V, Cote M, Gelinas Y, Nilsson S, Olivecrona G, Deshaies Y, Festuccia WT. Peroxisome proliferator-activated receptor gamma activation favours selective subcutaneous lipid deposition by coordinately regulating lipoprotein lipase modulators, fatty acid transporters and lipogenic enzymes. Acta Physiol (Oxf). 2016;217(3):227–39.

43. Kim JK, Fillmore JJ, Gavrilova O, Chao L, Higashimori T, Choi H, Kim HJ, Yu C, Chen Y, Qu X, Haluzik M, Reitman ML, Shulman GI. Differential effects of rosiglitazone on skeletal muscle and liver insulin resistance in A-ZIP/F-1 fatless mice. Diabetes. 2003;52(6):1311–8.

44. Gautam M, Bhattacharya I, Devi YS, Arya SP, Majumdar SS. Hormone responsiveness of cultured Sertoli cells obtained from adult rats after their rapid isolation under less harsh conditions. Andrology. 2016;4(3):509–19.

45. Liu K, Czaja MJ. Regulation of lipid stores and metabolism by lipophagy. Cell Death Differ. 2013;20(1):3–11.

## 21

Shifting perspectives from "oncogenic" to oncofetal proteins; how these factors drive placental development

Rachel C. West*（iD）, Gerrit J. Bouma and Quinton A. Winger

Abstract

Early human placental development strongly resembles carcinogenesis in otherwise healthy tissues. The progenitor cells of the placenta, the cytotrophoblast, rapidly proliferate to produce a sufficient number of cells to form an organ that will contribute to fetal development as early as the first trimester. The cytotrophoblast cells begin to differentiate, some towards the fused cells of the syncytiotrophoblast and some towards the highly invasive and migratory extravillous trophoblast. Invasion and migration of extravillous trophoblast cells mimics tumor metastasis. One key difference between cancer progression and placental development is the tight regulation of these oncogenes and oncogenic processes. Often, tumor suppressors and oncogenes work synergistically to regulate cell proliferation, differentiation, and invasion in a restrained manner compared to the uncontrollable growth in cancer. This review will compare and contrast the mechanisms that drive both cancer progression and placental development. Specifically, this review will focus on the molecular mechanisms that promote cell proliferation, evasion of apoptosis, cell invasion, and angiogenesis.

Keywords: Cell proliferation, Migration, Invasion, Angiogenesis, Genomic instability, Placenta, Placental insufficiency

Background

During pregnancy, the female body undergoes incredible anatomic, metabolic, and physiological changes in the process of providing for the needs of a developing fetus. One of the most essential developments is the genesis of a placenta, which is critical for hormone production and gas and nutrient exchange between the mother and the fetus [1–3]. Any aberration in these physiological processes can cause devastating placental pathologies like preeclampsia and intrauterine growth restriction (IUGR) [4], leading to severe pregnancy complications [5]. Preeclampsia affects 4–8% of pregnancies in the United States and is attributed as the cause behind 500,000 fetal and 75,000 maternal deaths each year [6, 7]. IUGR also affects 7–9% of newborn infants and is thought to cause up to 50% of unexplained stillbirths [8]. These pregnancy complications can also cause long-term developmental delays and health consequences including;

cerebral palsy, deafness, chronic lung disease, neurodevelopmental delays, and metabolic disorders [9–11], leading to substantial health care costs and emotional burdens on families. Both preeclampsia and IUGR appear to be heritable as they both are associated with an increased likelihood of IUGR and fetal death in subsequent pregnancies of the affected mothers [11]. Additionally, IUGR often occurs frequently in women suffering from placental morbidities such as preeclampsia, and gestational diabetes, putting the mother's life in significant danger as well as the fetus [12].

The conditions affecting fetal growth can either be placental or fetal in origin. Fetal growth is dependent upon the overall health of the fetus, the ability of the mother to metabolize and provide sufficient amounts of substrates necessary for growth, and the competency of the placenta to transport these substrates from the mother to the fetus [13]. However, impaired placental function seems to drive the most severe cases of IUGR [14]. This placental insufficiency is a common phenotype associated with both IUGR and maternal placental co-morbidities including preeclampsia and hypertension

---
* Correspondence: rachcwest2@gmail.com
Department of Biomedical Sciences, Animal Reproduction and Biotechnology Laboratory, Colorado State University, 10290 Ridgegate Circle, Lone Tree, Fort Collins, CO 80124, USA

[15]. Currently, treatments for pathologies caused by placental insufficiency are lacking, with no known treatment for pre-eclampsia other than the immediate delivery of the fetus.

While the understanding of the consequences of IUGR and preeclampsia has increased exponentially over the past few decades, there is still a need to elucidate the underlying cause behind placental insufficiency during development. Understanding what is driving placental insufficiency during early development will be essential in the development of better diagnostic and treatment tools for the prevention and treatment of both pathologies. The delicate interplay between cell proliferation and differentiation could be a key event that malfunctions early on in pregnancy, eventually leading to placental dysfunction.

Typically, when one considers oncogenes it's hard to ignore the profound effects these proteins have during normal homeostasis in adult tissues. These genes promote rampant cell proliferation in otherwise healthy tissues. Proliferative cells eventually begin to migrate towards other organ systems, invading into tissues to form metastatic tumors. However, to only consider oncogenes as "bad" fails to consider the original purposes of these genes. These oncogenic processes are essential during early embryonic, fetal, and placental development and any aberrant signaling by these genes can cause devastating effects on fetal growth. These proteins are responsible for the cancer-like processes that characterize early placental development. However, in direct contrast to carcinogenesis, the placenta uses these factors in a tightly controlled, highly regulated environment. This regulation exploits these factors so that they create a remarkably efficient organ in a short amount of time without the adverse consequences that often come with the expression of oncogenic proteins. Therefore, we propose that oncogenes instead be considered as oncofetal proteins.

This review will focus on the similarities of oncogenic processes like proliferation, escape of apoptosis, cell invasion and migration, angiogenesis, and the signaling pathways that drive these mechanisms in both cancer and placental development. Understanding these parallels between placentation and tumorigenesis will provide insight into not only better ways to treat cancer but also understand how these processes can fail during development leading to placental insufficiency.

Human placental development
Placentation begins with the uterine endometrium changing its structure to prepare for implantation, a process known as decidualization [16]. The fibroblast-like cells of the endometrium transform into secretory decidual cells. These decidual cells comprise an immunoprivileged matrix that protects the implanting embryo from attack by maternal immune cells [17]. It also secretes the histotroph, an endometrial secretion that facilitates implantation and conceptus development during the initial weeks of pregnancy [18]. The histotroph also contains factors that regulate the invasion potential of the early trophoblast cells if an embryo implants [19].

Once fertilization occurs, the zygote travels from the ampulla of the Fallopian tube to enter the endometrial cavity within 3 days [20]. During this journey, the zygote divides and undergoes a series of mitotic divisions to become the morula [21]. Approximately 5 days after fertilization, the morula transforms into a newly expanded blastocyst of 58-cells partitioned into a peripheral layer called the trophectoderm, that will eventually become the placenta and the inner cell mass (ICM), which will become the fetus [22]. Approximately 9 days after fertilization, the blastocyst implants into the uterine wall in a three step process called apposition, adhesion, and invasion [23]. At this timepoint, a multinucleated, primitive syncytium has formed, penetrating the decidua, hollowing out areas of the stromal layer, and forming the lacunae that will eventually be filled with maternal blood [24]. Additionally, by day 9 the progenitor trophoblast cells, cytotrophoblast cells, have begun to form villous structures that will eventually differentiate into the two main cell types of the placenta; the weakly proliferative and fusional syncytiotrophoblast and the terminally differentiated, invasive extravillous trophoblast (EVT) [25]. At day 12 of gestation, cytotrophoblast cells begin to penetrate the primitive syncytium, forming the first primary chorionic villi of the placenta [26]. The cytotrophoblast cells proliferate rapidly and accumulate in floating villi which will differentiate to form the syncytium. This layer of cells will eventually come into contact with the maternal blood [27]. Alternatively, cytotrophoblast cells will also form anchoring villi that will eventually attach to and invade into the mother's decidualized endometrium, myometrium, and eventually her spiral arterioles [28] (Fig. 1). This balance between cytotrophoblast cell proliferation and subsequent differentiation into the invasive and migratory EVT has a marked similarity to how cancer cells form tumors and metastasize.

Cell proliferation
As the placenta begins forming 1 week after fertilization and must begin to facilitate nutrient and gas exchange by the end of the first trimester, rapid and substantial cell proliferation is essential. However, unlike cancer, this cell proliferation is tightly regulated and cells lose their proliferative capacity once they undergo differentiation into the invasive EVT lineage. One group of genes that are responsible for cytotrophoblast cell proliferation are growth factors and their receptors [29]. Epidermal growth factor (EGF), hepatocyte growth factor (HGF), vascular endothelial growth factor (VEGF), and placental

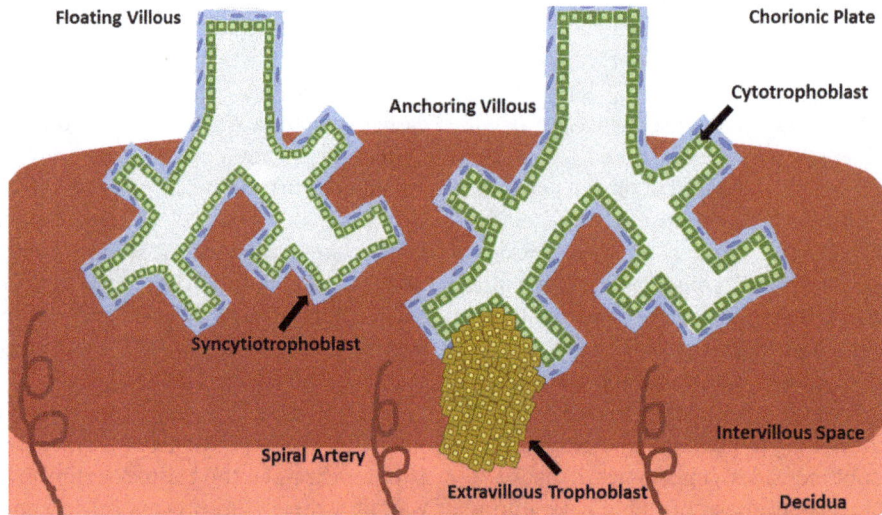

Fig. 1 Early Placental Development. The progenitor cells of the placenta, the cytotrophoblast proliferate rapidly during the first trimester of pregnancy. During this time they also differentiate to become part of the syncytiotrophoblast layer that fuses and becomes the layer of the placenta that comes into contact with the maternal blood. Additionally, cytotrophoblast cells differentiate to become part of the extravillous trophoblast, the cells that invade into the mother's endometrium, seeking out her spiral arteries

growth factor (PLGF), insulin like growth factor (IGF), transforming growth factor (TGF) and their subsequent receptors have all been identified in the cytotrophoblast and are speculated to act in a paracrine and autocrine manner on the differentiated cells of the placenta [30–36]. These growth factors bind to tyrosine kinase receptors on cytotrophoblast cell membranes inducing self-dimerization to activate the MEK/ERK proliferation pathway and the PI3K/Akt anti-apoptosis pathway [37]. These kinase signaling cascades are potent catalysts that influence cell proliferation and survival in many cell types, including the placenta [38]. Gene editing experiments targeting the MAPK pathway in mice was embryonic lethal by E11.5 due to severe placental defects [39]. Additionally, gene disruption of the PI3K/Akt pathway led to depleted cells in the spongiotrophoblast layer (cells of the junctional zone of the mouse placenta, the specific function is still unclear [40]) and decreased vascularization [41]. These data indicate a necessary role for growth factor driven activation of the MAPK/PI3K pathways during early placental development. Interestingly, the phosphorylated forms of ERK1 and ERK2 were only detected in proliferative cytotrophoblast cells until the end of the first trimester. This alludes to their importance in cell proliferation, losing expression once cells begin to terminally differentiate [42].

Additional oncogenic downstream target of the MAPK pathway, JUN has also been implicated in early placental cell proliferation and differentiation. However, different members of the JUN family are expressed at different time points. Messenger RNA for *c-Jun* was found at its highest levels in early gestational placental tissue whereas *jun-B* was at its highest levels between 35 and 40 weeks [43]. The authors of this study concluded that in the placenta *c-jun* is essential

for cytotrophoblast cell proliferation while *jun-B* likely plays a role in terminal differentiation. This conclusion is at least partially supported by another finding using stimulation by epidermal growth factor (EGF) to induce differentiation of human primary cytotrophoblast cells towards the syncytiotrophoblast fate. Cells were treated with EGF for 40 min pulses and, while both c-jun and jun-B mRNA levels rapidly increased 2–4 h after exposure, EGF's effects on jun-B were the most striking. Jun-B was significantly increased in cytotrophoblast cells differentiating towards the syncytiotrophoblast lineage, indicating that EGF and its activation of jun-B is important in the terminal differentiation of cytotrophoblast cells [44]. Interestingly, the hormone adiponectin has also been implicated as an important regulator for the JUN kinase pathway, with a particular emphasis on c-jun regulation. In normal placentas, adiponectin has an antiproliferative effect. However, in gestation diabetes mellitus (GDM) placentas, adiponectin levels are decreased with an increase in cell proliferation, potentially thought to be a contributor to the macrosomia seen in GDM babies. To test whether adiponectin actually inhibits c-Jun in GDM placentas, the choriocarcinoma cell line, BeWo, was treated with high levels of glucose. These high glucose treated cells had significantly lower levels of adiponectin, leading to increased c-Jun protein and increased cell proliferation. Furthermore, addition of adiponectin to high glucose treated cells inhibited c-Jun activation, suppressing cell proliferation [45].

There are also several oncofetal proteins outside of the family of growth factors that promote cell proliferation. For example, our laboratory studies the LIN28-let7-HMGA2 molecular axis. LIN28 is an RNA binding protein considered to be a key molecular factor that regulates the transition from a pluripotent, highly proliferative state to a terminally differentiated cell [46]. One of the main targets of LIN28 is the let-7 family of miRNAs. When cells are highly proliferative, LIN28 negatively regulates the let-7 family. However, as cells begin to differentiate the let-7 family of miRNAs is upregulated and can bind to the 3' UTR of *LIN28* to inhibit its translation into protein [47]. Because of this negative feedback loop, LIN28 and the let-7 s are often inversely expressed in many cancers [48]. In addition to this, increased LIN28 has been correlated with highly aggressive cancers and poor prognosis [49]. The let-7 s also regulate several other oncofetal proteins including HMGA2, c-Myc, RAS, and VEGF [49]. In placental cells, a knockdown of LIN28A led to spontaneous differentiation and syncytialization in human trophoblast cells [50]. Furthermore, knockdown of LIN28B and knockout of both LIN28A and LIN28B leads to trophoblast cells that are driven to differentiate towards only the syncytiotrophoblast lineage, but not extravillous trophoblast cells [51]. Collectively these data suggest that, as with pluripotent cells, LIN28 is an essential gatekeeper in trophoblast cell proliferation and differentiation.

Cell survival

The ability to bypass apoptosis is another hallmark of cancer and is essential during placentation. Again, the growth receptors and receptor tyrosine kinase pathways mentioned above play an important role in cell survival, specifically IGF-1 and IGF-2 binding to IGF-1R [38, 52].The relationship between IGF-1R and the PI3K/Akt and MAPK pathways has been described as a crucial cell protectant in many different cancer cell types [53–56]. In immortalized human placental BeWo cells and in placental tissue explants both IGF1 and IGF2 rescued serum-starved cells from apoptosis [57]. Additionally, mutated IGF1-R in pregnant women leads to both intrauterine and post-natal growth restriction [58] and there is a direct correlation between IGF levels and birth weight [59].

There are two distinct mechanisms the IGF system targets to promote cell survival; the Bcl-2 family and caspase proteins [60]. Increased Bcl-2 expression has been reported in several cancer cell lines and tumors [61–64] and leads to increased cell survival and resistance to chemotherapy treatment [65]. Bcl-2 immunolocalization in the placenta has been described in several papers [66–68]; however its involvement in trophoblast cell apoptosis is still unclear. Soni et al. describe a gradual increase in Bcl-2 expression throughout pregnancy with maximal immunoreactivity occurring at term [69]. Ishihara et al. also suggest that based on their findings that abundant expression of Bcl-2 in term syncytiotrophoblast prevents cell death, allowing for the maintenance of placental mass near the end of pregnancy [66].

Additionally, the IGFs regulate caspase expression. Activation of IGF1-R can prevent cleavage of caspases in both cancer cells and fetal brain cells, preventing apoptosis [70, 71]. In accordance with the findings of Bcl-2 expression, there appears to be no caspase-mediated apoptosis in the syncytiotrophoblast of term villi of the placenta. There was also no response to stimulus-induced apoptosis in syncytiotrophoblast of villous explants from term placental tissue [72]. These data suggest that the syncytiotrophoblast can protect itself against apoptotic signals to continue to function and contribute to fetal growth until the end of pregnancy.

In most cell types, the transcription factor p53 antagonizes IGF signaling to promote apoptosis and cell cycle arrest [73]. Several papers report that p53 closely monitors the IGF-1/Akt pathway and, upon sensing stress, negatively regulates IGF-1/Akt to halt cell proliferation and induce autophagy [74–76]. This negative regulation occurs by p53 transactivating IGF-BP3. The family of IGF-BPs regulates ligand availability to their IGF receptors [77]. It has been shown that a p53-induced accumulation of IGF-BP3 in the extracellular medium of cells can inhibit mitogenic function of IGF-1 in vitro [78]. Increased IGF-BP3 leads to increased complexing to IGF-1, reducing their ability to bind IGF-1R to promote cell survival and proliferation [79]. However, over 50% of human cancers have p53 mutations, preventing it's pro-apoptotic function to promote spontaneous tumorigenesis [80]. In the placenta, increased p53 protein expression in placental villi is correlated with pre-eclampsia [81]. As excessive apoptosis in the villous trophoblast of placental villi is a characteristic of pre-eclampsia, these data suggest that upregulated p53 induces a disproportionate amount of apoptosis, leading to placental insufficiency (Fig. 2).

Finally, another important anti-apoptotic factor often found in cancer is survivin [82]. Belonging to the "inhibitor of apoptosis" family, upregulation of survivin in cancers is directly correlated with apoptotic resistance, increased cell survival, and poor response to chemotherapy [83]. Survivin is yet another anti-apoptotic protein increased by IGF-1. In prostate cancer cells, stimulation with IGF-1 lead to increased survivin expression due to the increased stabilization and translation of survivin mRNA [84]. Alternatively, survivin has also been described as negatively regulated at the transcriptional level by p53 with the surivivin promoter having a p53 binding element although the exact mechanism of regulation by p53 is still poorly understood [82]. In the placenta, survivin is thought to play a crucial role in cell survival and proliferation of trophoblast cells [85, 86]. Messenger RNA levels of survivin were analyzed in first, second, and third trimester placentas of pre-eclamptic women, compared to normal placentas, survivin was significantly decreased. Additionally, survivin levels were directly correlated with severity of pre-eclampsia, with levels

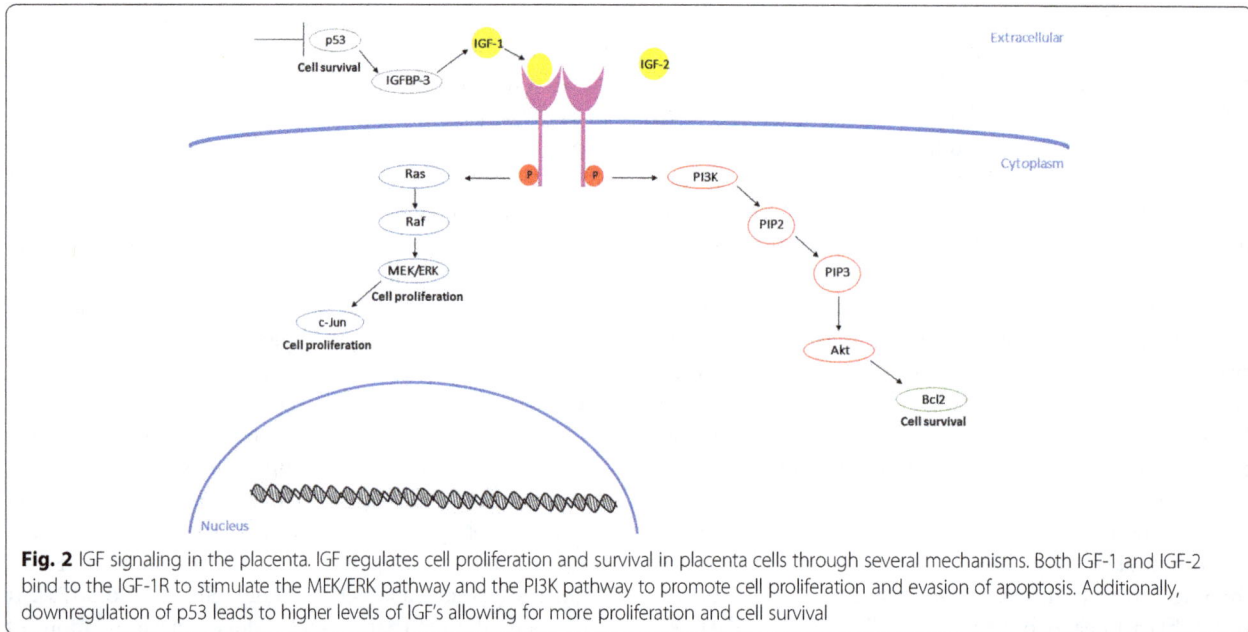

Fig. 2 IGF signaling in the placenta. IGF regulates cell proliferation and survival in placenta cells through several mechanisms. Both IGF-1 and IGF-2 bind to the IGF-1R to stimulate the MEK/ERK pathway and the PI3K pathway to promote cell proliferation and evasion of apoptosis. Additionally, downregulation of p53 leads to higher levels of IGF's allowing for more proliferation and cell survival

decreasing as pre-eclampsia became more severe [87]. Due to the upregulated levels of p53 in pre-eclampsia it has been suggested that the negative regulation of survivin by p53 is a potential cause of the low levels of survivin mRNA found in pre-eclamptic placentas [86].

Cell invasion

Human placentation is unique in that the EVT cells of the placenta invade fully into the maternal decidua to encapsulate and erode the spiral arteries, exposing the placenta to maternal blood [88]. The similarities between cell invasion of EVT cells and cancer cells are striking. However, one key difference is that trophoblast cells adhere to a tightly regulated pattern of proliferation then differentiation and invasion without metastasis into new tissues. Cancer cells proliferate rapidly, eventually seeking out other tissues to metastasize towards. Not surprisingly, many of the same factors are required for both neoplastic cells and trophoblast cells. Some of these requirements for invasion include altered expression of cell adhesion molecules, secretion of proteinases, and epithelial-mesenchymal transition.

In non-invasive cells, there is a network of proteins that harness cells to the extracellular matrix (ECM) and to each other. However, in invasive or metastatic cells, this network is downregulated [89] which allows cells to seek out new tissues. One group of altered proteins is the integrin family. Integrins are a heterodimeric family of cell membrane proteins that are made up of at least 18 α subunits and 8 β subunits [90]. These subunits dimerize to form at least 24 different receptors, allowing them to bind to a variety of different ECM ligands. Because of this diversity, some integrins promote adhesion and some

promote invasion. This review will only focus on the integrins that regulate cell invasion in the placenta.

During placental development, there is a delicate balance between adhesion-promoting integrin expression and invasion-promoting integrins. This balance in early cytotrophoblast cells is regulated in large part by α5β1 and α1β1. In contrast to cancer, cytotrophoblast cells use the invasion-restraining role of α5β1 to balance the invasion-promoting role of α1β1 to tightly regulate the depth of invasion into the mother's decidua [91]. During early gestation, the proliferating cytotrophoblast cells begin to upregulate α1β1 as they differentiate to become more invasive. However, as gestation continues and invasion becomes less of a priority, expression of the α1β1 integrin complex declines [91]. Additionally in pre-eclamptic placental tissue, α1β1 immunostaining is almost nonexistent while the invasion-restraining α5β1 is still detectable at levels similar to normotensive placentas [92]. This suggests that the shallow invasion of uterine vasculature, a hallmark of pre-eclampsia, is at least in part caused by altered integrin expression.

The integrin family is inextricably linked with the TGF- β signaling pathway. TGF- β is both a regulator and regulated by several integrins in many different cell types [93]. Both α1β1 and α5β1 expression is stimulated by TGF- β in fibroblast cells. Additionally, α5β1 has been found to be upregulated by TGF- β in both carcinoma cells and lung cancer cells [93, 94]. As TGF- β is known to have an important role in both the inhibition and promotion of trophoblast cell invasion [95, 96], these data imply that there is a delicate interplay between TGF- β signaling and the regulation of the integrins α5β1 and α1β1 during early placental development.

Another driver of cell invasion shared between cancer and placentation is the loss of expression of the cell adhesion molecule E-cadherin. Found at the adherens junctions of epithelial cells, E-cadherin is a potent promoter of cell-cell adhesion [97]. Known as a suppressor of invasion, decreased function of E-cadherin is directly correlated with invasion and tumor metastasis [98, 99]. E-cadherin also plays a critical role in the maintenance of the epithelial cell phenotype, with a loss of E-cadherin being the final step to trigger the epithelial-mesenchymal transition (EMT) [100], a process that is not only important during early embryonic development but also cancer. E-cadherin is predominantly expressed in anchored placental villi of first and second trimester placentas, gradually becoming down-regulated as cells differentiate to become EVT [101]. The transcription factor Snail, transcriptionally regulates E-cadherin, by binding to the E-box elements found on Snail's promoter region to trigger EMT and has also been suggested to regulate E-cadherin expression in EVT [102]. There is a layer of proliferative, non-invasive EVT cells found in the proximal and distal parts of anchored villi and as these cells undergo EMT to become invasive and migratory, there is a change in E-cadherin expression. However, term placentas from women with HELLP syndrome and pre-eclampsia found a reduction of E-cadherin in EVT cells with an apparent increase in Snail expression [102]. Snail appears to be the main regulator of decreased E-cadherin in most tumor expression and it now appears to be an important regulator of E-cadherin in EVT cells as well. Addtionally, E-cadherin is known to be essential for early embryonic and placental development as E-cadherin $^{-/-}$ mice have severe epithelial trophoblast defects and die at the time of implantation [103].

Finally, the metalloproteinase (MMP) family of proteins is a critical group of enzymes that facilitate invasion. In addition to degrading the ECM, MMPs also can modify cell adhesion molecules like integrins and activate cytokines to stimulate epithelial-mesenchymal transition and drive cell invasion [104]. Several MMPs, including MMP-2, MMP-3, and MMP-9 have been described in different locations in the placenta; however there is evidence to suggest that MMP-9 is the most influential proteinase during placental invasion [105, 106]. MMP-2 and MMP-9 are found at their highest levels in the extravillous cytotrophoblast between 6 and 8 weeks of pregnancy, appearing to facilitate trophoblast invasion into the decidua [107]. Interestingly, MMP expression isn't restricted to the invasive trophoblast cells as MMPs have been described in the endometrial stromal and natural killer cells of the decidua [108]. Furthermore, permissiveness to invasion by the decidua seems to be influenced by the presence of cytotrophoblast cells. This interaction between uterine and trophoblast MMPs could be regulated by the pregnancy hormone, human chorionic gonadotropin (hCG). To stimulate maternal recognition of pregnancy during the first trimester, the developing embryo secretes proteins to decidualized endometrial stromal cells, allowing for upregulation of MMPs [109]. In immortalized JEG-3 cells and in villous tissue explants, addition of hCG to culture medium increased invasion in a dose dependent manner [110, 111]. Interestingly, these data suggest that the uterus has the ability to influence invasion, keeping this process regulated and local. This is in direct contrast to the unregulated and rampant invasion seen in metastatic cancer.

Angiogenesis

Angiogenesis is a mandatory process driving tumor pathogenesis leading to tumor metastasis and poor cancer prognosis. Alternatively, the ability to not only join existing vessels but also to create vessels in avascular tissue is an essential component of placental development. Any aberration in the signaling pathways that drive angiogenesis and vasculogenesis can lead to shallow invasion into the maternal spiral arteries, a known cause of placental insufficiency. The angiopoietin (ANG) and vascular endothelial growth factor (VEGF) families of growth factors are two critical families for vessel development in the placenta [112]. Similar to the balancing and counterbalancing effects of integrins regulating cell invasion, VEGF and placenta growth factor (PlGF) work in a synergistic fashion to promote angiogenesis in a controlled environment [113]. Both growth factors are key components that control two different types of angiogenesis, branching and non-branching. (Fig. 3).

Vasculogenesis begins approximately at 21 days postconception when mesenchymal stem cells inside the mesenchymal villi of the placenta differentiate to become hemangiogenic progenitor cells [114]. These progenitor cells eventually migrate towards the periphery of the villous columns and coalesce to form hemangiogenic cords, the primitive original vessels of the villous [115]. Eventually these cords will mature into a more sophisticated network of vessels, differentiating into intermediate villi with capillary networks of branched vessels [116]. This process is almost totally driven by paracrine signaling of VEGF-A from the cytotrophoblast [114]. VEGF-A works through receptor tyrosine kinase receptors, VEGFR-1 and VEGFR-2, to stimulate branched angiogenesis [117]. Branching angiogenesis requires a series of steps including permeabilization of vascular tissue, degradation of the basement membrane, and increased proliferation and migration of endothelial cells. This leads to the formation of endothelial cell tubes and recruitment of pericytes to the exterior of the capillary, forming a stable vessel [115, 118]. These mechanisms lead to the creation of a network of immature intermediate villi containing superficially located capillaries lying directly beneath the trophoblast layer of the villous

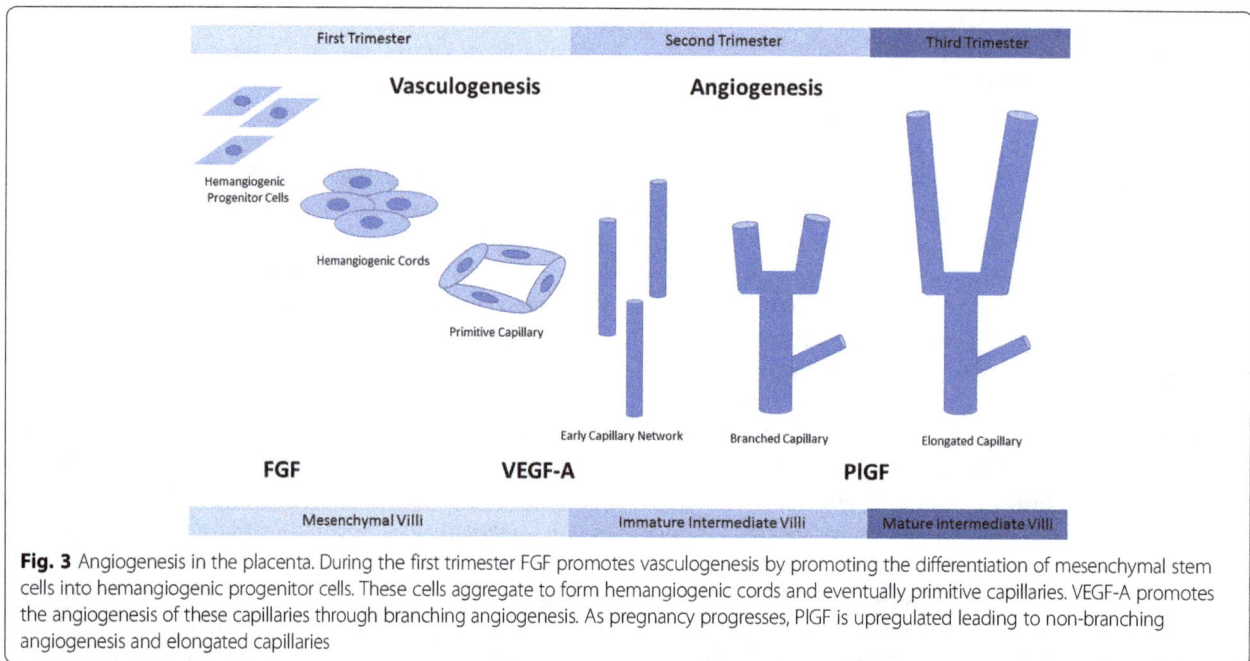

Fig. 3 Angiogenesis in the placenta. During the first trimester FGF promotes vasculogenesis by promoting the differentiation of mesenchymal stem cells into hemangiogenic progenitor cells. These cells aggregate to form hemangiogenic cords and eventually primitive capillaries. VEGF-A promotes the angiogenesis of these capillaries through branching angiogenesis. As pregnancy progresses, PlGF is upregulated leading to non-branching angiogenesis and elongated capillaries

surface [119]. These branched vessels are responsible for the dramatic increase in villous blood vessels facilitating enhanced fetoplacental blood flow to accommodate the rapidly developing fetus [120]. Branching angiogenesis and VEGF-A expression continues to dominate placental vascularization quickly producing a multitude of vessels until approximately the 26th week of gestation [121]. At this point, villous vascularization undergoes a switch from branching to non-branching angiogenesis. At this point, the focus moves from producing more vessels to increasing the length of the existing vessels [122].

Non-branching angiogenesis is driven by another member of the VEGF family of proteins, PlGF. Whereas VEGF-A and VEGFR-2 are expressed at high levels during early pregnancy, waning as pregnancy advances [122]; PlGF is expressed at relatively low levels during the first trimester of pregnancy but increases at 11–12 weeks, reaching peak levels at week 30 of pregnancy [123]. PlGF is thought to have an antagonistic effect on VEGF-A, forming a heterodimer that prevents VEGF-A from activating either VEGF1-R or VEGF2-R [124]. At peak PlGF expression, the immature intermediate villi begin to form the mature intermediate villi. Non-branching angiogenesis leads to the formation of long, thin vessels found at the tips of the villous. These vessels continue to grow in length, eventually surpassing the boundaries of the mature intermediate villi to form terminal villi. Each terminal villous has a thin trophoblast layer covering only one or two capillary coils [125]. These villous structures are critical for diffusional gas exchange from mother to fetus [121] (Fig. 2).

Similarly to cancer, both VEGF and PlGF are regulated by hypoxia. In tumors, hypoxia has been shown to

upregulate both VEGF and VEGFR expression [126–128]. As with tumorigenesis, hypoxia is necessary in early placental development. During the first trimester, placental development occurs in a low-oxygen environment due to the absence of access to maternal circulation [129]. These conditions are considered key to stimulating placental vasculogenesis. In placental fibroblasts, hypoxia upregulates both VEGF mRNA and protein [130]. One mechanism working to regulate VEGF through hypoxia is the glycoprotein Fibronectin. Fibronectin works through its high affinity integrin receptor, $\alpha 5\beta 1$ to stimulate VEGF during angiogenesis of embryos as well as several tumors [131, 132]. Bovine aortic endothelial cells grown in a low pH environment to mimic hypoxia, had increased interactions between fibronectin and VEGF [133]. Additionally, low pH conditions stimulated the secretion of fibronectin into culture medium in human trophoblast cells [134]. Finally, in differentiated placental multipotent mesenchymal stromal cells (PMSCs), $\alpha 5\beta 1$ has been show to interact with fibronectin to promote VEGF-A induced differentiation and migration [135].

Additionally, PlGF is also regulated by low oxygen conditions, albeit in an opposite fashion to VEGF. Human placental cells exposed to low oxygen conditions had decreased PlGF mRNA and protein [121]. Abnormal oxygen levels during early placental development are thought to lead to altered VEGF/PlGF expression leading to pre-eclampsia. For example, in the instances of pre-placental hypoxia where mother, placenta, and fetus are hypoxic (due to high altitude or anemia) there is an increase of VEGF and branched angiogenesis [136]. This phenomenon is also seen in uteroplacental hypoxia, where maternal oxygen levels are normal but there is impaired oxygen circulation throughout the placenta and fetus [137]. However, in instances of post-placental hypoxia where the mother has normal oxygen levels but the fetus is hypoxic, the placenta may become hyperoxic leading to inappropriate levels of oxygen during early development, causing increased levels of PlGF and increased non-branching angiogenesis [138]. This early onset placental hyperoxia often leads to the most severe form of pre-eclampsia, with increased adverse outcomes and fetal mortality [138].

Genomic instability

Genomic instability is widely acknowledged as a hallmark of cancer. Ranging widely from nucleotide mutations to alternations in chromosome number or structure (known as chromosome instability), genomic instability can have major deleterious effects on normal cells [139]. However, some degree of instability appears to be tolerated by cells and has been documented in human embryos. One study analyzed blastomeres from women under 35 years of age that had undergone in vitro fertilization (IVF). Upon analysis, researchers found that 70% of all embryos had some chromosomal genomic abnormality. Additionally, only 9% of the embryos analyzed had a 100% occurrence of diploid blastomeres [140]. This suggests that genomic instability is prevalent in human embryos and potentially explains the low levels of fertility in women compared to other species. Another study analyzed levels of aneuploidy in fertilized oocytes, cleavage stage embryos, and blastocyst stage embryos. There was a large increase in aneuploidy between the fertilized oocyte stage and cleavage stage embryos. As embryos developed to the blastocyst stage, there was a significant decrease in the aneuploidy rate (83% aneuploidy in cleavage stage versus 58% in blastocyst stage). However, while there was a decrease in rates of aneuploidy, there were still high levels of overall chromosomal abnormality [141]. These data suggest that, as with tumors, for rapid placental development to occur a lapse in the cell-cycle checkpoint machinery must occur. Additionally, it has been suggested that this genomic instability actually provides an advantage for embryo implantation [142].

In addition to aneuploidy, extravillous trophoblast cells of the placenta are also polyploid [143]. These cells are analogous to murine trophoblast giant cells that are also invasive. However, rodent trophoblast giant cells have ploidy levels that can reach up to 1024 N compared to the 4–8 N recorded in extravillous trophoblast cells [144]. These cells become polyploid through a process known as endoreduplication, where cells undergo mitosis but fail to divide after DNA replication. Endoreduplication is another phenomenon that occurs in cancer to promote genomic instability [145]. It has been proposed that endoreduplication occurs during times of genomic instability to increase tissue mass while cell proliferation is decreased to prevent propagation of cells with damaged chromosomes [146]. In the placenta, extravillous trophoblast cells invade into the decidua as two different cell types, interstitial cytotrophoblast cells (iCTBs) and endovascular cytotrophoblast cells (eCTBs). The iCTBs are the cells that invade into the decidua, moving as deep as the first third of the myometrium. Once at the myometrium, these cells undergo a final step of differentiation where they undergo endoreduplication to become multinucleated [147]. Similarly to how damaged cells undergo endoreduplication to increase size, it is thought that iCTBs undergo endoreduplication to further penetrate into the myometrium of the uterus.

Finally, even with less priority attributed to cell-cycle checkpoints and DNA repair, there must be some regulation of DNA repair in the placenta for it to develop into a proper functioning organ. Our laboratory is currently focused on the regulation of DNA repair and genome stability in trophoblast cells by the tumor suppressor BRCA1. BRCA1 is a multifunctional protein involved in many different aspects of cell cycle regulation including; regulation of transcription of several proliferation factors, homologous recombination of double-stranded breaks (DSBs), cell-cycle checkpoint regulation, and chromatin remodeling [148]. BRCA1 works to repair DNA damage by acting as a scaffolding protein for other DNA repair proteins and also promotes strand-invasion by interacting with the recombinase protein, Rad51 [149, 150]. Additionally, BRCA1 forms a repressor complex with CtIP and ZNF350. This repressor complex binds to promoter regions of several oncofetal proteins to prevent transcription [151]. One oncofetal proteins target already discussed in the "cell proliferation" section is HMGA2. In addition to promoting cell proliferation, increased levels of HMGA2 causes genomic instability by preventing non-homologous end-joining as well as delaying clearance of γ-H2AX, a marker for DSBs, [152]. BRCA1$^{-/-}$ knockout mice are embryonic lethal before gestational day 7.5 due to dramatic decreases in cell proliferation and poor differentiation of the extraembryonic tissue. These knockout embryos have a complete loss of diploid trophoblast cells with an overabundance of trophoblast giant cells [153]. Interestingly, mouse trophoblast giant cells are polyploid and are potentially accustomed to levels of genomic instability through endoreduplication, which is necessary for trophoblast giant cell function.

Unfortunately, this question will be hard to prove using today's current models of trophoblast cell development. Trophoblast cells derived from first trimester placentas are very difficult to obtain. Additionally these cells are hard to culture, making alternative model systems to study trophoblast development essential. Immortalized cell lines are extensively used as a model for trophoblast development and differentiation. However, these cells present their own shortcomings that make them less than ideal candidates for use. These shortcomings are especially apparent when it comes to studying DNA damage and genomic instability. For example, cytogenetic analysis of the extravillous first trimester Swan71 cell line immortalized with hTert revealed that these cells were near pentaploid in karyotype [136]. This is almost certainly due to chromosomal missegregation during mitosis, leading to a heterogeneous population of aneuploid cells. Additionally, when our lab began using this cell line to investigate BRCA1 in human trophoblast cells we found high levels of markers for DNA damage. We created a BRCA1 knockout trophoblast cell line using CRISPR-Cas9 genome editing to investigate levels of DNA damage by immunostaining for markers of double and single-stranded breaks. Surprisingly, the level of DSBs, as evidenced by immunostaining for γ-H2AX, was indistinguishable between BRCA1 knockout cells (BrKO) and wild-type Swan71 cells (Fig. 4). This high level of double-stranded breakage was confirmed using another marker for DSBs, 53BP1 (data not shown). These data corroborate the idea that immortalized cells suffer from cellular crises when cultured in vitro, resulting in microsatellite and chromosomal instability. Due to this propensity towards genomic instability in culture, immortalized cells are unlikely to provide insight into the role of genomic instability during early placental development. Additionally, this genomic instability of immortalized cells leads to a higher propensity for these cells to behave as cancer cells, no longer regulated in the controlled manner that characterizes trophoblast cells. This creates a need for a better model system to investigate the regulation of oncogenic processes during trophoblast development.

Conclusion

While understanding the consequences of fetal growth restriction has increased exponentially over the past few decades, there is still a need to elucidate the underlying cause behind placental insufficiency during placental organogenesis. Understanding what is driving placental insufficiency during early fetal development will be essential in the development of better diagnostic and treatment tools for the prevention and treatment of IUGR. The ability of placental cells to divide rapidly, differentiate, invade and migrate into tissues, and eventually create their own vascular network makes these cells an ideal system to gain insight into cancer biology and tumor metastasis. Alternatively, as placental pathologies like intrauterine growth restriction (IUGR) and pre-eclampsia are multi-faceted disorders with no known cause, better understanding the molecular mechanisms that drive oncogenic processes will provide better insight into how the early placenta develops. Pre-eclampsia and IUGR are rarely diagnosed until after 20 weeks of gestation, significantly later than pathogenesis begins. Therefore it is critical to start thinking of oncofetal proteins in their original roles, namely as drivers of cell proliferation, differentiation, invasion, and cell survival during early embryogenesis and placental development. Studying how oncofetal proteins drive placentation is essential to facilitate the process of providing better diagnostics for earlier screenings as well as treatment, ensuring the proper care for healthier babies and happier mothers.

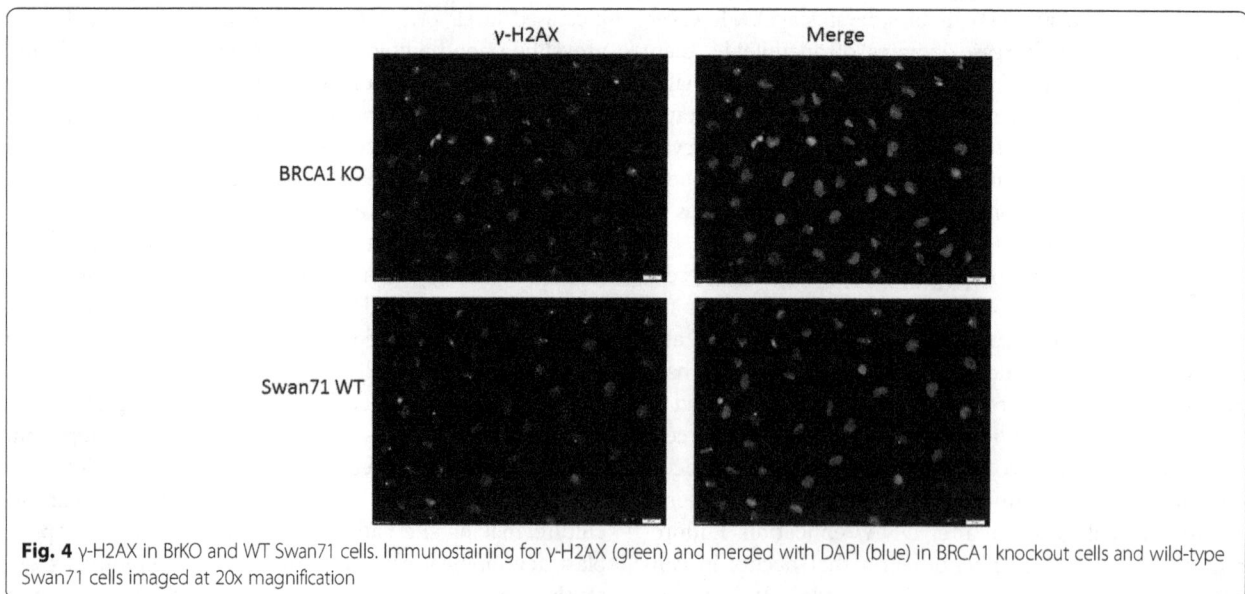

Fig. 4 γ-H2AX in BrKO and WT Swan71 cells. Immunostaining for γ-H2AX (green) and merged with DAPI (blue) in BRCA1 knockout cells and wild-type Swan71 cells imaged at 20x magnification

Acknowledgements

The lab of Claudia Weise for their expertise on genomic instability and help with the immunofluorescence.

Funding

This project was supported by Agriculture and Food Research Initiative Competitive Grant no. 2017-67015-26460 from the USDA National Institute of Food and Agriculture., the Colorado State University College Research Council, and the Colorado State University Vice President for Research Fellowship.

Authors' contributions

RW wrote the article. GB contributed to the outline of the article, contributed to writing by providing sources for the article, edited the manuscript. QW helped formulate the idea of the article, edited the manuscript, served as advisor to Rachel West. All authors read and approved the final manuscript.

Competing interest

Quinton Winger is a member of the Reproductive Biology and Endocrinology editorial board.

References

1. Goplerud JM, Delivoria-Papadopoulos M. Physiology of the placenta--gas exchange. Ann Clin Lab Sci. 1985;15(4):270–8.
2. Hay WW Jr. Placental transport of nutrients to the fetus. Horm Res. 1994;42(4–5):215–22.
3. Freemark M. Placental hormones and the control of fetal growth. J Clin Endocrinol Metab. 2010;95(5):2054–7.
4. Ilekis JV, Reddy UM, Roberts JM. Preeclampsia--a pressing problem: an executive summary of a National Institute of Child Health and Human Development workshop. Reprod Sci. 2007;14(6):508–23.
5. Gude NM, et al. Growth and function of the normal human placenta. Thromb Res. 2004;114(5–6):397–407.
6. Choudhury M, Friedman JE. Epigenetics and microRNAs in preeclampsia. Clin Exp Hypertens. 2012;34(5):334–41.
7. Coolman M, et al. Medical record validation of maternally reported history of preeclampsia. J Clin Epidemiol. 2010;63(8):932–7.
8. Ergaz Z, Avgil M, Ornoy A. Intrauterine growth restriction-etiology and consequences: what do we know about the human situation and experimental animal models? Reprod Toxicol. 2005;20(3):301–22.
9. Ananth CV, Vintzileos AM. Epidemiology of preterm birth and its clinical subtypes. J Matern Fetal Neonatal Med. 2006;19(12):773–82.
10. Hutter D, Kingdom J, Jaeggi E. Causes and mechanisms of intrauterine hypoxia and its impact on the fetal cardiovascular system: a review. Int J Pediatr. 2010;2010:401323.
11. Cosmi E, et al. Consequences in infants that were intrauterine growth restricted. J Pregnancy. 2011;2011:364381.
12. von Beckerath AK, et al. Perinatal complications and long-term neurodevelopmental outcome of infants with intrauterine growth restriction. Am J Obstet Gynecol. 2013;208(2):130 e1–6.
13. Krishna U, Bhalerao S. Placental insufficiency and fetal growth restriction. J Obstet Gynaecol India. 2011;61(5):505–11.
14. Veerbeek JH, et al. Placental pathology in early intrauterine growth restriction associated with maternal hypertension. Placenta. 2014;35(9):696–701.
15. Huppertz B. Placental origins of preeclampsia: challenging the current hypothesis. Hypertension. 2008;51(4):970–5.
16. Dunn CL, Kelly RW, Critchley HO. Decidualization of the human endometrial stromal cell: an enigmatic transformation. Reprod BioMed Online. 2003;7(2):151–61.
17. Mori M, et al. The decidua-the maternal bed embracing the embryo-maintains the pregnancy. Semin Immunopathol. 2016;38(6):635–49.
18. Gellersen B, Brosens JJ. Cyclic decidualization of the human endometrium in reproductive health and failure. Endocr Rev. 2014;35(6):851–905.
19. Brosens JJ, Pijnenborg R, Brosens IA. The myometrial junctional zone spiral arteries in normal and abnormal pregnancies: a review of the literature. Am J Obstet Gynecol. 2002;187(5):1416–23.
20. Cross JC, Werb Z, Fisher SJ. Implantation and the placenta: key pieces of the development puzzle. Science. 1994;266(5190):1508–18.
21. Croxatto HB, et al. Studies on the duration of egg transport in the human oviduct. I. the time interval between ovulation and egg recovery from the uterus in normal women. Fertil Steril. 1972;23(7):447–58.
22. Hardy K, Handyside AH, Winston RM. The human blastocyst: cell number, death and allocation during late preimplantation development in vitro. Development. 1989;107(3):597–604.
23. James JL, Carter AM, Chamley LW. Human placentation from nidation to 5 weeks of gestation. Part II: tools to model the crucial first days. Placenta. 2012;33(5):335–42.
24. Hertig AT, Rock J, Adams EC. A description of 34 human ova within the first 17 days of development. Am J Anat. 1956;98(3):435–93.
25. Staun-Ram E, Shalev E. Human trophoblast function during the implantation process. Reprod Biol Endocrinol. 2005;3:56.
26. Yabe S, et al. Comparison of syncytiotrophoblast generated from human embryonic stem cells and from term placentas. Proc Natl Acad Sci U S A. 2016;113(19):E2598–607.
27. Genbacev O, et al. Hypoxia alters early gestation human cytotrophoblast differentiation/invasion in vitro and models the placental defects that occur in preeclampsia. J Clin Invest. 1996;97(2):540–50.
28. Lyall F, et al. Human trophoblast invasion and spiral artery transformation: the role of PECAM-1 in normal pregnancy, preeclampsia, and fetal growth restriction. Am J Pathol. 2001;158(5):1713–21.
29. Ferretti C, et al. Molecular circuits shared by placental and cancer cells, and their implications in the proliferative, invasive and migratory capacities of trophoblasts. Hum Reprod Update. 2007;13(2):121–41.
30. Ladines-Llave CA, et al. Cytologic localization of epidermal growth factor and its receptor in developing human placenta varies over the course of pregnancy. Am J Obstet Gynecol. 1991;165(5 Pt 1):1377–82.
31. Horowitz GM, et al. Immunohistochemical localization of transforming growth factor-alpha in human endometrium, decidua, and trophoblast. J Clin Endocrinol Metab. 1993;76(3):786–92.
32. Dungy LJ, Siddiqi TA, Khan S. Transforming growth factor-beta 1 expression during placental development. Am J Obstet Gynecol. 1991;165(4 Pt 1):853–7.
33. Maruo T, Mochizuki M. Immunohistochemical localization of epidermal growth factor receptor and myc oncogene product in human placenta: implication for trophoblast proliferation and differentiation. Am J Obstet Gynecol. 1987;156(3):721–7.
34. Clark DE, et al. Localization of VEGF and expression of its receptors flt and KDR in human placenta throughout pregnancy. Hum Reprod. 1996;11(5):1090–8.
35. Maglione D, et al. Isolation of a human placenta cDNA coding for a protein related to the vascular permeability factor. Proc Natl Acad Sci U S A. 1991;88(20):9267–71.
36. Fant M, Munro H, Moses AC. An autocrine/paracrine role for insulin-like growth factors in the regulation of human placental growth. J Clin Endocrinol Metab. 1986;63(2):499–505.
37. Scaltriti M, Baselga J. The epidermal growth factor receptor pathway: a model for targeted therapy. Clin Cancer Res. 2006;12(18):5268–72.
38. Forbes K, et al. Insulin-like growth factor I and II regulate the life cycle of trophoblast in the developing human placenta. Am J Physiol Cell Physiol. 2008;294(6):C1313–22.
39. Hatano N, et al. Essential role for ERK2 mitogen-activated protein kinase in placental development. Genes Cells. 2003;8(11):847–56.
40. Simmons DG, Cross JC. Determinants of trophoblast lineage and cell subtype specification in the mouse placenta. Dev Biol. 2005;284(1):12–24.
41. Yang ZZ, et al. Protein kinase B alpha/Akt1 regulates placental development and fetal growth. J Biol Chem. 2003;278(34):32124–31.
42. Kita N, et al. Expression and activation of MAP kinases, ERK1/2, in the human villous trophoblasts. Placenta. 2003;24(2–3):164–72.
43. Dungy LJ, Siddiqi TA, Khan S. C-jun and jun-B oncogene expression during placental development. Am J Obstet Gynecol. 1991;165(6 Pt 1):1853–6.
44. Dakour J, et al. EGF promotes development of a differentiated trophoblast phenotype having c-myc and junB proto-oncogene activation. Placenta. 1999;20(1):119–26.
45. Chen H, et al. Adiponectin exerts antiproliferative effect on human placenta via modulation of the JNK/c-Jun pathway. Int J Clin Exp Pathol. 2014;7(6):2894–904.

46. Faas L, et al. Lin28 proteins are required for germ layer specification in Xenopus. Development. 2013;140(5):976–86.

47. Guo Y, et al. Identification and characterization of LIN-28 homolog B (LIN28B) in human hepatocellular carcinoma. Gene. 2006;384:51–61.

48. Viswanathan SR, et al. Lin28 promotes transformation and is associated with advanced human malignancies. Nat Genet. 2009;41(7):843–8.

49. Wang T, et al. Aberrant regulation of the LIN28A/LIN28B and let-7 loop in human malignant tumors and its effects on the hallmarks of cancer. Mol Cancer. 2015;14:125.

50. Seabrook JL, et al. Role of LIN28A in mouse and human trophoblast cell differentiation. Biol Reprod. 2013;89(4):95.

51. West RC, McWhorter ES, Ali A, Goetzman LN, Russ JE, Gonzalez-Berrios CL, Anthony RV, Bouma GJ, Winger QA. HMGA2 is regulated by LIN28 and BRCA1 in human placental cells. Biol Reprod. https://doi.org/10.1093/biolre/ioy183.

52. Lotem J, Sachs L. Control of apoptosis in hematopoiesis and leukemia by cytokines, tumor suppressor and oncogenes. Leukemia. 1996;10(6):925–31.

53. Gooch JL, Van Den Berg CL, Yee D. Insulin-like growth factor (IGF)-I rescues breast cancer cells from chemotherapy-induced cell death--proliferative and anti-apoptotic effects. Breast Cancer Res Treat. 1999;56(1):1–10.

54. Peruzzi F, et al. Multiple signaling pathways of the insulin-like growth factor 1 receptor in protection from apoptosis. Mol Cell Biol. 1999;19(10):7203–15.

55. Kennedy SG, et al. The PI 3-kinase/Akt signaling pathway delivers an anti-apoptotic signal. Genes Dev. 1997;11(6):701–13.

56. Scotlandi K, et al. Expression of an IGF-I receptor dominant negative mutant induces apoptosis, inhibits tumorigenesis and enhances chemosensitivity in Ewing's sarcoma cells. Int J Cancer. 2002;101(1):11–6.

57. Harris LK, et al. IGF2 actions on trophoblast in human placenta are regulated by the insulin-like growth factor 2 receptor, which can function as both a signaling and clearance receptor. Biol Reprod. 2011;84(3):440–6.

58. Walenkamp MJ, et al. A variable degree of intrauterine and postnatal growth retardation in a family with a missense mutation in the insulin-like growth factor I receptor. J Clin Endocrinol Metab. 2006;91(8):3062–70.

59. Gibson JM, et al. Regulation of IGF bioavailability in pregnancy. Mol Hum Reprod. 2001;7(1):79–87.

60. Reed JC. Bcl-2 and the regulation of programmed cell death. J Cell Biol. 1994;124(1–2):1–6.

61. Reed JC, et al. Differential expression of bcl2 protooncogene in neuroblastoma and other human tumor cell lines of neural origin. Cancer Res. 1991;51(24):6529–38.

62. Gala JL, et al. High expression of bcl-2 is the rule in acute lymphoblastic leukemia, except in Burkitt subtype at presentation, and is not correlated with the prognosis. Ann Hematol. 1994;69(1):17–24.

63. Chen-Levy Z, Nourse J, Cleary ML. The bcl-2 candidate proto-oncogene product is a 24-kilodalton integral-membrane protein highly expressed in lymphoid cell lines and lymphomas carrying the t(14,18) translocation. Mol Cell Biol. 1989;9(2):701–10.

64. Karnak D, Xu L. Chemosensitization of prostate cancer by modulating Bcl-2 family proteins. Curr Drug Targets. 2010;11(6):699–707.

65. van Golen CM, Castle VP, Feldman EL. IGF-I receptor activation and BCL-2 overexpression prevent early apoptotic events in human neuroblastoma. Cell Death Differ. 2000;7(7):654–65.

66. Ishihara N, et al. Changes in proliferative potential, apoptosis and Bcl-2 protein expression in cytotrophoblasts and syncytiotrophoblast in human placenta over the course of pregnancy. Endocr J. 2000;47(3):317–27.

67. Kim CJ, et al. Patterns of bcl-2 expression in placenta. Pathol Res Pract. 1995; 191(12):1239–44.

68. Ratts VS, et al. Expression of BCL-2, BAX and BAK in the trophoblast layer of the term human placenta: a unique model of apoptosis within a syncytium. Placenta. 2000;21(4):361–6.

69. Soni S, et al. Apoptosis and Bcl-2 protein expression in human placenta over the course of normal pregnancy. Anat Histol Embryol. 2010;39(5): 426–31.

70. Singleton JR, Randolph AE, Feldman EL. Insulin-like growth factor I receptor prevents apoptosis and enhances neuroblastoma tumorigenesis. Cancer Res. 1996;56(19):4522–9.

71. Cao Y, et al. Insulin-like growth factor (IGF)-1 suppresses oligodendrocyte caspase-3 activation and increases glial proliferation after ischemia in near-term fetal sheep. J Cereb Blood Flow Metab. 2003;23(6):739–47.

72. Longtine MS, et al. Caspase-mediated apoptosis of trophoblasts in term human placental villi is restricted to cytotrophoblasts and absent from the multinucleated syncytiotrophoblast. Reproduction. 2012;143(1):107–21.

73. Feng Z, Levine AJ. The regulation of energy metabolism and the IGF-1/ mTOR pathways by the p53 protein. Trends Cell Biol. 2010;20(7):427–34.

74. Feng Z, et al. The coordinate regulation of the p53 and mTOR pathways in cells. Proc Natl Acad Sci U S A. 2005;102(23):8204–9.

75. Budanov AV, Karin M. p53 target genes sestrin1 and sestrin2 connect genotoxic stress and mTOR signaling. Cell. 2008;134(3):451–60.

76. Feng Z. p53 regulation of the IGF-1/AKT/mTOR pathways and the endosomal compartment. Cold Spring Harb Perspect Biol. 2010;2(2):a001057.

77. Forbes K, Westwood M. Maternal growth factor regulation of human placental development and fetal growth. J Endocrinol. 2010;207(1):1–16.

78. Buckbinder L, et al. Induction of the growth inhibitor IGF-binding protein 3 by p53. Nature. 1995;377(6550):646–9.

79. Neuberg M, et al. The p53/IGF-1 receptor axis in the regulation of programmed cell death. Endocrine. 1997;7(1):107–9.

80. Ozaki T, Nakagawara A. Role of p53 in cell death and human cancers. Cancers (Basel). 2011;3(1):994–1013.

81. Sharp AN, et al. Preeclampsia is associated with alterations in the p53-pathway in villous trophoblast. PLoS One. 2014;9(1):e87621.

82. Jaiswal PK, Goel A, Mittal RD. Survivin: a molecular biomarker in cancer. Indian J Med Res. 2015;141(4):389–97.

83. Garg H, et al. Survivin: a unique target for tumor therapy. Cancer Cell Int. 2016;16:49.

84. Vaira V, et al. Regulation of survivin expression by IGF-1/mTOR signaling. Oncogene. 2007;26(19):2678–84.

85. Lehner R, et al. Localization of telomerase hTERT protein and survivin in placenta: relation to placental development and hydatidiform mole. Obstet Gynecol. 2001;97(6):965–70.

86. Muschol-Steinmetz C, et al. Function of survivin in trophoblastic cells of the placenta. PLoS One. 2013;8(9):e73337.

87. Li CF, et al. Reduced expression of survivin, the inhibitor of apoptosis protein correlates with severity of preeclampsia. Placenta. 2012;33(1):47–51.

88. Pollheimer J, Knofler M. Signalling pathways regulating the invasive differentiation of human trophoblasts: a review. Placenta. 2005; 26(Suppl A):S21–30.

89. Farahani E, et al. Cell adhesion molecules and their relation to (cancer) cell stemness. Carcinogenesis. 2014;35(4):747–59.

90. Seguin L, et al. Integrins and cancer: regulators of cancer stemness, metastasis, and drug resistance. Trends Cell Biol. 2015;25(4):234–40.

91. Damsky CH, et al. Integrin switching regulates normal trophoblast invasion. Development. 1994;120(12):3657–66.

92. Zhou Y, et al. Preeclampsia is associated with abnormal expression of adhesion molecules by invasive cytotrophoblasts. J Clin Invest. 1993;91(3): 950–60.

93. Margadant C, Sonnenberg A. Integrin-TGF-beta crosstalk in fibrosis, cancer and wound healing. EMBO Rep. 2010;11(2):97–105.

94. Mise N, et al. Zyxin is a transforming growth factor-beta (TGF-beta)/Smad3 target gene that regulates lung cancer cell motility via integrin alpha5beta1. J Biol Chem. 2012;287(37):31393–405.

95. Huang Z, et al. Transforming growth factor beta1 promotes invasion of human JEG-3 trophoblast cells via TGF-beta/Smad3 signaling pathway. Oncotarget. 2017;8(20):33560–70.

96. Cheng JC, Chang HM, Leung PC. Transforming growth factor-beta1 inhibits trophoblast cell invasion by inducing snail-mediated down-regulation of vascular endothelial-cadherin protein. J Biol Chem. 2013;288(46):33181–92.

97. Pecina-Slaus N. Tumor suppressor gene E-cadherin and its role in normal and malignant cells. Cancer Cell Int. 2003;3(1):17.

98. Vleminckx K, et al. Genetic manipulation of E-cadherin expression by epithelial tumor cells reveals an invasion suppressor role. Cell. 1991;66(1): 107–19.

99. Behrens J, et al. Dissecting tumor cell invasion: epithelial cells acquire invasive properties after the loss of uvomorulin-mediated cell-cell adhesion. J Cell Biol. 1989;108(6):2435–47.

100. Hay ED. An overview of epithelio-mesenchymal transformation. Acta Anat (Basel). 1995;154(1):8–20.

101. Zhou Y, et al. Human cytotrophoblasts adopt a vascular phenotype as they differentiate. A strategy for successful endovascular invasion? J Clin Invest. 1997;99(9):2139–51.

102. Blechschmidt K, et al. Expression of E-cadherin and its repressor snail in placental tissue of normal, preeclamptic and HELLP pregnancies. Virchows Arch. 2007;450(2):195–202.

103. Larue L, et al. E-cadherin null mutant embryos fail to form a trophectoderm epithelium. Proc Natl Acad Sci U S A. 1994;91(17):8263–7.

104. Mehner C, et al. Tumor cell-produced matrix metalloproteinase 9 (MMP-9) drives malignant progression and metastasis of basal-like triple negative breast cancer. Oncotarget. 2014;5(9):2736–49.

105. Cohen M, Meisser A, Bischof P. Metalloproteinases and human placental invasiveness. Placenta. 2006;27(8):783–93.

106. Demir-Weusten AY, et al. Matrix metalloproteinases-2, −3 and −9 in human term placenta. Acta Histochem. 2007;109(5):403–12.

107. Onogi A, et al. Hypoxia inhibits invasion of extravillous trophoblast cells through reduction of matrix metalloproteinase (MMP)-2 activation in the early first trimester of human pregnancy. Placenta. 2011;32(9):665–70.

108. Cohen M, et al. Role of decidua in trophoblastic invasion. Neuro Endocrinol Lett. 2010;31(2):193–7.

109. Tapia-Pizarro A, et al. Human chorionic gonadotropin (hCG) modulation of TIMP1 secretion by human endometrial stromal cells facilitates extravillous trophoblast invasion in vitro. Hum Reprod. 2013;28(8):2215–27.

110. Zygmunt M, et al. Invasion of cytotrophoblastic JEG-3 cells is stimulated by hCG in vitro. Placenta. 1998;19(8):587–93.

111. Prast J, et al. Human chorionic gonadotropin stimulates trophoblast invasion through extracellularly regulated kinase and AKT signaling. Endocrinology. 2008;149(3):979–87.

112. Geva E, et al. Human placental vascular development: vasculogenic and angiogenic (branching and nonbranching) transformation is regulated by vascular endothelial growth factor-a, angiopoietin-1, and angiopoietin-2. J Clin Endocrinol Metab. 2002;87(9):4213–24.

113. Carmeliet P, et al. Synergism between vascular endothelial growth factor and placental growth factor contributes to angiogenesis and plasma extravasation in pathological conditions. Nat Med. 2001;7(5):575–83.

114. Demir R, Seval Y, Huppertz B. Vasculogenesis and angiogenesis in the early human placenta. Acta Histochem. 2007;109(4):257–65.

115. Arroyo JA, Winn VD. Vasculogenesis and angiogenesis in the IUGR placenta. Semin Perinatol. 2008;32(3):172–7.

116. Wang, Y. and S. Zhao, in Vascular Biology of the Placenta. San Rafael (CA). Morgan and Claypool Publishers; 2010.

117. Vuorela P, et al. Expression of vascular endothelial growth factor and placenta growth factor in human placenta. Biol Reprod. 1997;56(2):489–94.

118. Gourvas V, et al. Angiogenic factors in placentas from pregnancies complicated by fetal growth restriction (review). Mol Med Rep. 2012;6(1):23–7.

119. Kingdom J, et al. Development of the placental villous tree and its consequences for fetal growth. Eur J Obstet Gynecol Reprod Biol. 2000; 92(1):35–43.

120. Charnock-Jones DS, Kaufmann P, Mayhew TM. Aspects of human fetoplacental vasculogenesis and angiogenesis. I Molecular regulation. Placenta. 2004;25(2–3):103–13.

121. Ahmed A, et al. Regulation of placental vascular endothelial growth factor (VEGF) and placenta growth factor (PlGF) and soluble Flt-1 by oxygen--a review. Placenta. 2000;21(Suppl A):S16–24.

122. Cerdeira AS, Karumanchi SA. Angiogenic factors in preeclampsia and related disorders. Cold Spring Harb Perspect Med. 2012;2(11). https://doi.org/10.1101/cshperspect.a006585.

123. Saffer C, et al. Determination of placental growth factor (PlGF) levels in healthy pregnant women without signs or symptoms of preeclampsia. Pregnancy Hypertens. 2013;3(2):124–32.

124. Eriksson A, et al. Placenta growth factor-1 antagonizes VEGF-induced angiogenesis and tumor growth by the formation of functionally inactive PlGF-1/VEGF heterodimers. Cancer Cell. 2002;1(1):99–108.

125. Kaufmann P, et al. The fetal vascularisation of term human placental villi. II. Intermediate and terminal villi. Anat Embryol (Berl) 1985;173(2):203–14.

126. Shweiki D, et al. Vascular endothelial growth factor induced by hypoxia may mediate hypoxia-initiated angiogenesis. Nature. 1992;359(6398):843–5.

127. Plate KH, et al. Vascular endothelial growth factor is a potential tumour angiogenesis factor in human gliomas in vivo. Nature. 1992;359(6398):845–8.

128. Tuder RM, Flook BE, Voelkel NF. Increased gene expression for VEGF and the VEGF receptors KDR/Flk and Flt in lungs exposed to acute or to chronic hypoxia. Modulation of gene expression by nitric oxide. J Clin Invest. 1995; 95(4):1798–807.

129. Jauniaux E, et al. Trophoblastic oxidative stress in relation to temporal and regional differences in maternal placental blood flow in normal and abnormal early pregnancies. Am J Pathol. 2003;162(1):115–25.

130. Wheeler T, Elcock CL, Anthony FW. Angiogenesis and the placental environment. Placenta. 1995;16(3):289–96.

131. Kim S, et al. Regulation of angiogenesis in vivo by ligation of integrin alpha5beta1 with the central cell-binding domain of fibronectin. Am J Pathol. 2000;156(4):1345–62.

132. Parsons-Wingerter P, et al. Uniform overexpression and rapid accessibility of alpha5beta1 integrin on blood vessels in tumors. Am J Pathol. 2005;167(1): 193–211.

133. Goerges AL, Nugent MA. pH regulates vascular endothelial growth factor binding to fibronectin: a mechanism for control of extracellular matrix storage and release. J Biol Chem. 2004;279(3):2307–15.

134. Gaus G, et al. Extracellular pH modulates the secretion of fibronectin isoforms by human trophoblast. Acta Histochem. 2002;104(1):51–63.

135. Lee MY, et al. Angiogenesis in differentiated placental multipotent mesenchymal stromal cells is dependent on integrin alpha5beta1. PLoS One. 2009;4(10):e6913.

136. Krebs C, Longo LD, Leiser R. Term ovine placental vasculature: comparison of sea level and high altitude conditions by corrosion cast and histomorphometry. Placenta. 1997;18(1):43–51.

137. Kiserud T, et al. Estimation of the pressure gradient across the fetal ductus venosus based on Doppler velocimetry. Ultrasound Med Biol. 1994;20(3):225–32.

138. Macara L, et al. Structural analysis of placental terminal villi from growth-restricted pregnancies with abnormal umbilical artery Doppler waveforms. Placenta. 1996;17(1):37–48.

139. Yao Y, Dai W. Genomic Instability and Cancer. J Carcinog Mutagen. 2014;5: 1000165. https://doi.org/10.4172/2157-2518.1000165.

140. Vanneste E, et al. Chromosome instability is common in human cleavage-stage embryos. Nat Med. 2009;15(5):577–83.

141. Fragouli E, et al. The origin and impact of embryonic aneuploidy. Hum Genet. 2013;132(9):1001–13.

142. Farquharson RG, Stephenson MD, editors. Early pregnancy. Second edition. Cambridge: Cambridge University Press; 2017. pages cm

143. Cross JC. Genetic insights into trophoblast differentiation and placental morphogenesis. Semin Cell Dev Biol. 2000;11(2):105–13.

144. Zybina EV, Zybina TG. Polytene chromosomes in mammalian cells. Int Rev Cytol. 1996;165:53–119.

145. Hanahan D, Weinberg RA. Hallmarks of cancer: the next generation. Cell. 2011;144(5):646–74.

146. Fox DT, Duronio RJ. Endoreplication and polyploidy: insights into development and disease. Development. 2013;140(1):3–12.

147. Velicky P, Knofler M, Pollheimer J. Function and control of human invasive trophoblast subtypes: intrinsic vs. maternal control. Cell Adhes Migr. 2016; 10(1–2):154–62.

148. Takaoka M, Miki Y. BRCA1 gene: function and deficiency. Int J Clin Oncol. 2018;23(1):36–44.

149. Tibbetts RS, et al. Functional interactions between BRCA1 and the checkpoint kinase ATR during genotoxic stress. Genes Dev. 2000;14(23): 2989–3002.

150. West SC. Molecular views of recombination proteins and their control. Nat Rev Mol Cell Biol. 2003;4(6):435–45.

151. Ahmed KM, Tsai CY, Lee WH. Derepression of HMGA2 via removal of ZBRK1/ BRCA1/CtIP complex enhances mammary tumorigenesis. J Biol Chem. 2010; 285(7):4464–71.

152. Li AY, et al. Suppression of nonhomologous end joining repair by overexpression of HMGA2. Cancer Res. 2009;69(14):5699–706.

153. Hakem R, et al. The tumor suppressor gene Brca1 is required for embryonic cellular proliferation in the mouse. Cell. 1996;85(7):1009–23.

Permissions

All chapters in this book were first published in RBE, by BioMed Central; hereby published with permission under the Creative Commons Attribution License or equivalent. Every chapter published in this book has been scrutinized by our experts. Their significance has been extensively debated. The topics covered herein carry significant findings which will fuel the growth of the discipline. They may even be implemented as practical applications or may be referred to as a beginning point for another development.

The contributors of this book come from diverse backgrounds, making this book a truly international effort. This book will bring forth new frontiers with its revolutionizing research information and detailed analysis of the nascent developments around the world.

We would like to thank all the contributing authors for lending their expertise to make the book truly unique. They have played a crucial role in the development of this book. Without their invaluable contributions this book wouldn't have been possible. They have made vital efforts to compile up to date information on the varied aspects of this subject to make this book a valuable addition to the collection of many professionals and students.

This book was conceptualized with the vision of imparting up-to-date information and advanced data in this field. To ensure the same, a matchless editorial board was set up. Every individual on the board went through rigorous rounds of assessment to prove their worth. After which they invested a large part of their time researching and compiling the most relevant data for our readers.

The editorial board has been involved in producing this book since its inception. They have spent rigorous hours researching and exploring the diverse topics which have resulted in the successful publishing of this book. They have passed on their knowledge of decades through this book. To expedite this challenging task, the publisher supported the team at every step. A small team of assistant editors was also appointed to further simplify the editing procedure and attain best results for the readers.

Apart from the editorial board, the designing team has also invested a significant amount of their time in understanding the subject and creating the most relevant covers. They scrutinized every image to scout for the most suitable representation of the subject and create an appropriate cover for the book.

The publishing team has been an ardent support to the editorial, designing and production team. Their endless efforts to recruit the best for this project, has resulted in the accomplishment of this book. They are a veteran in the field of academics and their pool of knowledge is as vast as their experience in printing. Their expertise and guidance has proved useful at every step. Their uncompromising quality standards have made this book an exceptional effort. Their encouragement from time to time has been an inspiration for everyone.

The publisher and the editorial board hope that this book will prove to be a valuable piece of knowledge for researchers, students, practitioners and scholars across the globe.

List of Contributors

Kailin Yang, Liuting Zeng and Jinwen Ge
Hunan University of Chinese Medicine, Changsha 410208, Hunan Province, China

Tingting Bao
Beijing University of Chinese Medicine, Beijing 100029, Beijing, China

Jiayin Lu, Zixu Wang, Jing Cao, Yaoxing Chen and Yulan Dong
Laboratory of Neurobiology, College of Animal Medicine, China Agricultural University, Haidian, Beijing 100193, People's Republic of China

Jing Ye, Zhiqiu Yao, Wenyu Si, Xiaoxiao Gao, Chen Yang, Ya Liu, Jianping Ding, Weiping Huang, Fugui Fang and Jie Zhou
Anhui Provincial Laboratory of Animal Genetic Resources Protection and Breeding, College of Animal Science and Technology, Anhui Agricultural University, 130 Changjiang West Road, Hefei 230036, Anhui, China

Ya Liu, Jianping Ding, Weiping Huang and Fugui Fang
Anhui Provincial Laboratory for Local Livestock and Poultry Genetic Resource Conservation and Bio-Breeding, 130 Changjiang West Road, Hefei 230036, Anhui, China

Jing Ye, Zhiqiu Yao, Wenyu Si, Ya Liu, Jianping Ding, Weiping Huang, Fugui Fang and Jie Zhou
Department of Animal Veterinary Science, College of Animal Science and Technology, Anhui Agricultural University, 130 Changjiang West Road, Hefei 230036, Anhui, China

Julian K. Christians, Kendra I. Lennie, Maria F. Huicochea Munoz and Nimrat Binning
Department of Biological Sciences, Simon Fraser University, Burnaby, BC, Canada

Kyosuke Kagami, Masanori Ono and Hiroshi Fujiwara
Department of Obstetrics and Gynecology, Graduate School of Medical Sciences, Kanazawa University, Takara-machi 13-1, Kanazawa, Ishikawa 920-8640, Japan

Kyosuke Kagami, Yohei Shinmyo and Hiroshi Kawasaki
Department of Medical Neuroscience, Graduate School of Medical Sciences, Kanazawa University, Takara-machi 13-1, Kanazawa, Ishikawa 920-8640, Japan

Betânia Rodrigues Santos, Sheila Bunecker Lecke and Poli Mara Spritzer
Division of Endocrinology, Gynecological Endocrinology Unit, Hospital de Clínicas de Porto Alegre, Rua Ramiro Barcelos, 2350, Porto Alegre, RS 90035-003, Brazil

Betânia Rodrigues Santos and Poli Mara Spritzer
Department of Physiology, Laboratory of Molecular Endocrinology, Universidade Federal do Rio Grande do Sul (UFRGS), Porto Alegre, Brazil

Sheila Bunecker Lecke
Department of Diagnostic Methods, Universidade Federal de Ciências Médicas de Porto Alegre (UFCSPA), Porto Alegre, Brazil

Dongdong Tang, Xiaojin He and Huan Wu
Reproductive Medicine Center, Department of Obstetrics and Gynecology, The First Affiliated Hospital of Anhui Medical University, Hefei, Anhui, People's Republic of China

Dongdong Tang, Xiaojin He and Huan Wu
Anhui Province Key Laboratory of Reproductive Health and Genetics, Anhui Medical University, Hefei, Anhui, People's Republic of China

Dongdong Tang, Xiaojin He and Huan Wu
Anhui Provincial Engineering Technology Research Center for Biopreservation and Artificial Organs, Hefei, Anhui, People's Republic of China

Zhenyu Huang, Dangwei Peng, Li Zhang and Xiansheng Zhang
Department of Urology, The First Affiliated Hospital of Anhui Medical University, Hefei, Anhui, People's Republic of China

Cheng Li, Hui-Yu Zhang, Yan Liang, Wei Xia, Qian Zhu, Duo Zhang, Zhen Huang, Gui-Lin Liang, Hang Qi, Xiao-Qing He, Jiang-Jing Yuan and Jian Zhang
Department of Gynecology, International Peace Maternity and Child Health Hospital, School of Medicine, Shanghai Jiao Tong University, Shanghai, China

Cheng Li, Zhen Huang, Rui-Hong Xue, Ya-Jing Tan, He-Feng Huang and Jian Zhang
Institute of Embryo-Fetal Original Adult Disease Affiliated to Shanghai Jiao Tong University School of Medicine, Shanghai Jiao Tong University, Shanghai, China

Cheng Li, Rui-Hong Xue, Ya-Jing Tan and He-Feng Huang
Center of Reproductive Medicine, International Peace Maternity and Child Health Hospital, School of Medicine, Shanghai Jiao Tong University, No. 910, Hengshan Rd, Shanghai 200030, China

Yanxin Wu, Wai-Kit Ming, Dongyu Wang, Haitian Chen, Zhuyu Li and Zilian Wang
Department of Obstetrics and Gynecology, The First Affiliated Hospital of Sun Yat-sen University, No. 58 Zhongshan Road 2, Guangzhou 510000, P. R. China

Zhuo Liu, Yanwen Jiang, Yuqiang Qian, Shuxiong Chen, Shan Gao, Lu Chen, Chunjin Li and Xu Zhou
College of Animal Science, Jilin University, 5333 Xian Road, Changchun 130062, Jilin, China

Yongfeng Sun
College of Animal Science and Technology, Jilin Agricultural University, 2888 Xincheng Street, Changchun 130118, Jilin, China

Nirja Chaudhari, Mitali Dawalbhakta and Laxmipriya Nampoothiri
Reproductive-Neuro-Endocrinology Lab, Department of Biochemistry, Faculty of Science, The Maharaja Sayajirao University of Baroda, Vadodara, Gujarat, India

Rodrigo A. Carrasco, Jaswant Singh and Gregg P. Adams
Department of Veterinary Biomedical Sciences, Western College of Veterinary Medicine, University of Saskatchewan, 52 campus drive, Saskatoon, Saskatchewan S7N5B4, Canada

Santosh K. Yadav, Aastha Pandey, Lokesh Kumar, Archana Devi, Bhavana Kushwaha, Rahul Vishvkarma, Jagdamba P. Maikhuri, Singh Rajender and Gopal Gupta
Division of Endocrinology, CSIR-Central Drug Research Institute, BS-10/1, Sector-10, Jankipuram Extension, Sitapur Road, Lucknow 226031, India

Archana Devi, Bhavana Kushwaha, Singh Rajender and Gopal Gupta
Academy of Scientific and Innovative Research (AcSIR), New Delhi 110001, India

Michelle Goldsammler and Erkan Buyuk
Montefiore's Institute for Reproductive Medicine and Health, Department of Obstetrics and Gynecology and Women's Health, Albert Einstein College of Medicine, Montefiore Medical Center, Hartsdale, NY, USA

Zaher Merhi
Department of Obstetrics and Gynecology, Division of Reproductive Biology, NYU School of Medicine, New York, NY, USA

Department of Biochemistry, Albert Einstein College of Medicine, Bronx, NY, USA

F. S. Mennini, A. Marcellusi, R. Viti and C. Bini
Economic Evaluation and HTA (CEIS- EEHTA) - Faculty of Economics, University of Rome "Tor Vergata", Via Columbia, 2, 00133 Rome, Italy

F. S. Mennini and A. Marcellusi
Institute for Leadership and Management in Health - Kingston Hill Campus, Kingston Hill, Kingston upon Thames KT2 7LB, UK

A. Carosso, A. Revelli and C. Benedetto
Gynecology and Obstetrics I, Physiopathology of Reproduction and IVF Unit, Department of Surgical Sciences, University of Torino, S. Anna Hospital, Via Ventimiglia 3, 10126 Torino, Italy

A. Revelli
LIVET Infertility and IVF Clinic, Via Tiziano Vecellio, 3, 10126 Torino, Italy

Xiaotong Wang, Xiaoke Zhang, Lian Hu and Honggang Li
Family Planning Research Institute/Center of Reproductive Medicine, Tongji Medical College, Huazhong University of Science and Technology, Wuhan 430030, China

Xiaoke Zhang
Center for Reproductive Medicine, The Third Affiliated Hospital of Zhengzhou University, Zhengzhou 450052, China

Mahsa Darbandi and Sara Darbandis
Reproductive Biotechnology Research Center, Avicenna Research Institute, Academic Center for Education, Culture and Research, Tehran, Iran

Ashok Agarwal
American Center for Reproductive Medicine, Cleveland Clinic, Cleveland, Ohio 44195, USA

Pallav Sengupta
Department of Physiology, Faculty of Medicine, MAHSA University, Jalan SP2, Bandar Saujana Putra, 42610 Jenjarom, Selangor, Malaysia

Damayanthi Durairajanayagam
Department of Physiology, Faculty of Medicine, Universiti Teknologi MARA, Sungai Buloh Campus, Jalan Hospital, 47000 Sungai Buloh, Selangor, Malaysia

Ralf Henkel
Department of Medical Biosciences, University of the Western Cape, Bellville, Cape Town 7535, South Africa

Mohammad Reza Sadeghi
Reproductive Immunology Research Center, Avicenna Research Institute, Academic Center for Education, Culture and Research, Tehran, Iran

T. Zhao and Z. Y. Shan
Department of Endocrinology and Metabolism, Institute of Endocrinology, First Affiliated Hospital, China Medical University, Shenyang, Liaoning, China

B. M. Chen
The First Affiliated Hospital of Sun Yat-sen University, Guangzhou, China

X. M. Zhao
Chengde Medical University, Chengde, Hebei, China

Xueying Zhang, Ying Xu, Lulu Fu, Dandan Li, Xiaowei Dai, Lianlian Liu, Jingshun Zhang and Lianwen Zheng
Reproductive Medical Center, Department of Obstetrics and Gynecology, The Second Hospital of Jilin University, No. 218 Ziqiang Street, Changchun 130041, Jilin, China

Manhua Cui
Department of Obstetrics and Gynecology, The Second Hospital of Jilin University, No. 218 Ziqiang Street, Changchun 130041, Jilin, China

Xie Ge, Peng Pan, Jun Jing, Xuechun Hu, Li Chen, Xuhua Qiu, Rujun Ma, Kadiliya Jueraitetibaike, Xuan Huang and Bing Yao
Center of Reproductive Medicine, Nanjing Jinling Hospital, Clinical School of Medical College, Nanjing University, Nanjing 210002, Jiangsu, China

Rachel C. West, Gerrit J. Bouma and Quinton A. Winger
Department of Biomedical Sciences, Animal Reproduction and Biotechnology Laboratory, Colorado State University, 10290 Ridgegate Circle, Lone Tree, Fort Collins, CO 80124, USA

Index

www.ingramcontent.com/pod-product-compliance
Lightning Source LLC
Chambersburg PA
CBHW061257190326
41458CB00011B/3698